OXFORD MEDICAL PUBLICATIONS

Prostate Cancer
Biology, Diagnosis, and Management

Prostate Cancer: Biology, Diagnosis, and Management

Edited by

KONSTANTINOS N. SYRIGOS
Consultant Medical Oncologist
Head, Oncology Unit
3rd Department of Medicine
Athens Medical School
Sotiria General Hospital
Athens, Greece

OXFORD
UNIVERSITY PRESS

OXFORD

UNIVERSITY PRESS

Great Clarendon Street, Oxford OX2 6DP

Oxford University Press is a department of the University of Oxford.
It furthers the University's objective of excellence in research, scholarship,
and education by publishing worldwide in

Oxford   New York

Athens Auckland Bangkok Bogotá Buenos Aires Cape Town
Chennai Dar es Salaam Delhi Florence Hong Kong Istanbul Karachi
Kolkata Kuala Lumpur Madrid Melbourne Mexico City Mumbai Nairobi
Paris São Paulo Shanghai Singapore Taipei Tokyo Toronto Warsaw

and associated companies in Berlin   Ibadan

Oxford is a registered trade mark of Oxford University Press
in the UK and in certain other countries

Published in the United States
by Oxford University Press Inc., New York

Oxford University Press 2001

A catalogue record for this title is available from the British Library

Library of Congress Cataloging in Publication Data

Prostate cancer: biology, diagnosis, and management/edited by Konstantinos N. Syrigos.
(Oxford medical publications)
Includes bibliographical references.
1. Prostate – Cancer   I. Syrigos, Konstantinos N.   II. Series.
[DNLM: 1. Prostatic Neoplasms – diagnosis   2. Prostate – physiopathology   3. Prostatic
Neoplasms – therapy. WJ 752 P965527 2001]
RC280.P7 P7584 2001   616.99'463–dc21   2001036248
ISBN 0 19 263185 3 (Hbk: alk. paper)

ISBN 0 19263185 3

10 9 8 7 6 5 4 3 2 1

Typeset by EXPO Holdings, Malaysia
Printed in Great Britain
on acid-free paper by
The Bath Press Ltd, Avon

Preface

This is the second in a series of books on urological malignancies that has been launched by Oxford University Press. In the previous year, Professor Donald G. Skinner and myself, have attempted to review comprehensively bladder cancer, covering in one volume most aspects of this malignancy, from epidemiology and molecular oncology to innovative treatment strategies and palliative medicine. The response to this essay was the stimulus to proceed to a second book addressing another urological malignancy: prostate cancer.

The objective of the preparation of this volume is to provide a single, comprehensive source of information on the discipline of prostate cancer and to furnish a fertile platform for further investigation towards a better understanding of this disease. As the text is particularly directed towards clinicians, efforts have been made to cover important advances in clinical and basic science research, with emphasis on their clinical applications.

Over the last decade, prostate cancer has increasingly become the province of many special interests, including the medical oncologist, urologist, radiotherapist, endocrinologist, palliative care physician, epidemiologist, and biologist. In the age of increasing specialization, where journals, articles, and books addressed to specialists comprise the main source of information for physicians, we feel strongly that there is still a major need for a comprehensive textbook on prostate cancer. Therefore, the purpose of the volume in hand is to present a picture of prostate cancer in its totality and to update the subject in one tome. The present book attempts to cover extensively the area of prostate cancer based on the experience of well-established scientists. The authorship is derived from an international forum and consists primarily of those who have made major contributions in the area they have been asked to discuss. The authors have attempted to combine their clinical experience with the newest advances in the relevant sciences and to highlight the therapeutic aspects of each topic. Emphasis has been given on the multi-disciplinary approach, providing overviews from various expert branches. It is expected that with this methodology specialists associated with prostate cancer will not only get a feeling for the current practice in their own area of interest, but they will also be able to obtain sufficient information about problems presenting in their patients and potential solutions offered by different areas of expertise. The rationale for this policy is the perception that physicians who are acquainted with 'adjacent' specialist branches, who are familiar with basic sciences, and who are able to use this knowledge in the evaluation and treatment of their patients, are in a better position to analyze clinical problems and accordingly help their patients. Finally, management of prostate cancer is surrounded with several controversies regarding the management of localized disease, the role and the pattern of hormonal treatment, and the chemotherapy of hormonal-resistant prostate cancer. In this volume effort has been made to present clearly and evenly all arguments for each approach in sequential chapters.

A comprehensive textbook is inevitably not fully up to date at the time of publication and this applies particularly in the areas where advances have been more rapid. It is therefore a tribute to our distinguished contributors and to the publisher, Oxford University Press, that this edition has appeared within 2 years of its initiation. Gratitude should be extended to our patients, students, and colleagues for providing the contributors with ongoing education, stimulus, and purpose.

Finally, I wish to dedicate this volume to Katerina, Nikolas, and Alexander for their forbearance and support throughout this project.

Konstantinos N. Syrigos, MD, PhD

Contents

Contents

Contributors

Aarnink, G. Rene
Department of Urology, University Hospital Nijmegen, Nijmegen, The Netherlands

Alevyzaki, Fotini, MD
Oncology Unit, 3rd Department of Medicine, Athens Medical School, Sotiria General Hospital, Athens, Greece

Algaba, Fernando, MD
Professor of Pathology, Pathology Section. Fundació Puigvert. Universitat Autónoma de Barcelona, Spain

Athanasiadis, Loukas, MSc, BABCP, UKCP
Consultant Psychiatrist, Psychiatric Hospital, 'AHEPA' Hospital, University of Thessaloniki, Greece

Barista, Ibrahim, MD
Associate Professor of Medical Oncology, Department of Medical Oncology, Hacettepe University, Institute of Oncology, Ankara, Turkey

Beerlage, P. Harrie
Department of Urology, University Hospital Nijmegen, Nijmegen, The Netherlands

Benoit, M. Ronald, MD
Division of Urology, Allegheny General Hospital, Pittsburgh, Pennsylvania, USA

Brendler, B. Charles, MD
Professor and Chief, Section of Urology, Department of Surgery, The University of Chicago, Chicago, IL, USA

Calabró, Fabio
Department of Medical Oncology, San Raffaele Scientific Institute, Rome, Italy

Clements, Richard, MA., BM., BCh., FRCS, FRCR
Consultant Radiologist, Gwent Healthcare NHS Trust, Newport, S. Wales, University of Wales College of Medicine, Cardiff, UK

Closset, Jean
Biochimie et Laboratoire d'Endocrinologie, Tour de Pathologie B23, avenue de l'Hôpital, 3, Université de Liége. Belgique

Dawson, A. Nancy, MD
Professor of Medicine, Director Genito-Urinary Oncology, University of Maryland, Greenbaum Cancer Center, Baltimore, MD, USA

Dearnely, P. David, MA, MD, FRCP, FRCR
Bob Champion Senior Lecturer & Honorary Consultant, Institute of Cancer Research, Royal Marsden NHS Trust, Sutton, Surrey, UK

Denis, J. Louis, FACS
Chairman, Education & Training Division, EORTC, Chief, Oncology Center Antwerp, Department of Urology, Antwerp, Belgium

Farnsworth, E. Wells, PhD
Adjunct Professor of Urology, Northwestern University Medical School, Bloomingdale, IL, USA

Giatromanolaki, Alexandra, MD
Lecturer in Pathology, Democritus University of Thrace, Alexandroupolis, Greece

Gleave, E. Martin, MD, FRCSC, FACS
Head, Department of Surgery, Division of Urology, University of British Columbia, Vancouver General Hospital, Vancouver, B.C., Canada

Goldenberg, S. Larry, MD, FRCSC
Division of Urology, University of British Columbia, Vancouver General Hospital, Vancouver, B.C., Canada

Gravas, A. Stavros, MD, FEBU
Department of Urology, Hygeia General Hospital, Athens, Greece

Griffiths, Keith, FACS
Tenovus Cancer Research Center, University of Wales College of Medicine, Cardiff, UK

Grumet, Campell Sherry, MA, MS
Genetic Cancelor, Prostate Risk Assessment Program, Fox Chase Cancer Center, USA

Harrington, J. Kevin, FRCR, PhD
Associate Professor of Clinical Oncology, NHS Royal Marsden Hospitals, & Molecular Medicine Program, Mayo Clinic, Rochester, USA

Harris, Michael, MD
The Division of Urology, Department of Surgery, The University of Texas Health Sciences Center at San Antonio, and Traverse City, Michigan, USA

Holtgrewe, H. Logan, MD
Associate Professor of Urology, Department of Urology, James Buchanan Brady Urological Institute, Johns Hopkins University School of Medicine, Baltimore, Maryland, USA

Hopkins, L. Jon, MD
Hematology/Oncology Department, National Naval Medical Center, Bethesda, MD, USA

Jager, J. Gerrit
Department of Radiology, University Hospital Nijmegen, Nijmegen, The Netherlands

Kallakury V. S. Bhaskar, MD
Department of Pathology and Laboratory Medicine, Albany Medical College, Albany, NY, USA

Karayiannakis, J. Anastasios, MD, Msc
Assistant Professor of Surgery, 2nd Department of Surgery, University of Thrake, Alexandroupolis, Greece

Kehayas, Platon, MD, FACS
Head, Department of Urology, Hygeia General Hospital, Athens, Greece

Labrie Fernard, MD, PhD
Professor and Director of Research, Prostate Cancer Clinical Research Unit, Quebec, Canada

Leak, A. Jessie, MD
Associate Professor, The University of Texas, MD Anderson Cancer Center, Department of Anesthesiology & Department of Symptom Control and Palliative Care, Houston, Texas, USA

Long, P. John, MD
Assistant Professor of Urology, Tufts University School of Medicine, Boston, Massachusetts, USA

Martiniello-Wilks, Rosetta, PhD
Oncology Research Center, Prince of Wales Hospital, Randwick and Division of Medicine, University of New South Wales, Randwick, Australia

Michalaki, Vicki, MD
Oncology Unit, 3rd Department of Medicine, Athens Medical School, Sotiria General Hospital, Athens, Greece

Messing, M. Edward, MD, FACS
Chairman, Department of Urology, University of Rochester Medical Centre, Rochester, NY, USA

Naslund, J. Michael, MD, MBA
Associate Professor, Division of Urology, Director, Maryland Prostate Center, University of Maryland School of Medicine, Baltimore, Maryland, USA

Nickel, J. Curtis, MD
Professor of Urology, Queen's University Kingston General Hospital, Kingston, ON, Canada

Nutting, M. Christopher, BSc, MBBS, MRCP, FRCP
Clinical Research Fellow, Cancer Research Campaign, Academic Radiotherapy & Oncology, Institute of Cancer Research, Royal Marsden NHS Trust, Sutton, Surrey, UK

Oleyourryk, J. Gregory, MD
Resident, Department of Urology, University of Rochester Medical Center, Rochester, NY, USA
de la Rosette, Jean J. M. C. H.
Head, Department of Urology, University Hospital Nijmegen, Nijmegen, The Netherlands

Ross, S. Jeffrey, MD
Cyrus Strong Merrill Professor of Pathology, Chairman, Department of Pathology and Laboratory Medicine, Albany Medical College, Albany, NY, USA

Russell, J. Pamela, PhD
Director, Oncology Research Center, Prince of Wales Hospital, Randwick and Professor, Division of Medicine, University of New South Wales, Randwick, Australia

Reiter, Eric
Institut National de la Recherche Agronomique (INRA), URA CNRS 1291, Station de Physiologie de la Reproduction des Mammiféres Domestiques, Nouzilly, France

Shepherd, L. David, MD
The Division of Urology, Department of Surgery, The University of Texas Health Sciences Center at San Antonio, Texas, USA
da Silva, Calais Fernando
Chief Service of Urology, Amadora, Portugal

Sivridis, Efthimios, MD, PhD
Associate Professor in Pathology, Director of the Department of Pathology, Democritus University of Thrace, Alexandroupolis, Greece

Sternberg, N. Cora, MD, FACP
Chief, Department of Medical Oncology, San Raffaele Scientific Institute, Rome, Italy

Supkis, Edward D., Jr., MD
Associate Professor, The University of Texas, MD Anderson Cancer Center, Department of Anesthesiology, Houston, Texas, USA

Syrigos, N. Konstantinos, MD, PhD
Consultant Medical Oncologist, Head, Oncology Unit, 3rd Department of Medicine, Athens Medical School, Sotiria General Hospital, Athens, Greece

Thompson, Ian, MD
Professor and Chair, Division of Urology, Department of Surgery, The University of Texas Health Sciences Center at San Antonio, Texas, USA

Yang, J. Ximing, MD, PhD
Assistant Professor, Departments of Pathology and Surgery/Urology, The University of Chicago, Chicago, IL, USA

Vile, G. Richard, PhD
Molecular Medicine Program, Mayo Clinic, Rochester, USA

Voeks, J. Dale, PhD
Oncology Research Center, Prince of Wales Hospital, Randwick and Division of Medicine, University of New South Wales, Randwick, Australia

Zbar, P. Andrew, MD, FRCS, FRACS
Senior Lecturer, Honorary Consultant Surgeon, Professional Surgical Unit, St James' University Hospital, Leeds, UK

Section I

1 | Surgical anatomy of the prostate

Andrew P. Zbar, Fotini Alevyzaki, and Anastasios J. Karayiannakis

Introduction

The role of radical extirpative surgery of the prostate in prostatic carcinoma is controversial. It is clear that in patients with organ-confined disease, low Gleason's histological tumor grade, and low circulating prostate-specific antigen levels, that such a radical approach may be warranted. More recently, there has been a reassessment of prostatic surgical anatomy as it pertains to cancer with the availability of whole-gland specimens and, further, with the introduction of nerve-sparing techniques and urethral sphincter preserving surgery in selected cases. This approach has been advanced over the last decade because of an improved understanding of the neural and peri-prostatic venous anatomy relevant to radical prostatectomy and pelvic lymphadenectomy, which has balanced oncologic clearance with functional outcome.

This chapter briefly outlines the anatomy of the region as it pertains to the management of prostatic cancer, as well as the anatomical factors that influence surgical decision-making.

Prostatic morphology

During the first 3 months of fetal growth, the prostate develops as an epithelial invagination from the prostatic urethra under the influence of the surrounding mesenchyme. Hormonally induced growth is directed on the glandular zone of the prostate, the urogenital sinus, and the external genitalia (1–3). Further outgrowths of the dorsal portion of the mesonephric duct form the inner zone of the prostate gland by invasion of the mesenchyme as branching tubulo-glandular structures. In the female, the urethra develops from the portion that, in the male, is proximal to the opening of the prostatic utricle. The adult prostate undergoes morphologic changes around the time of puberty, increasing to the adult weight of 20 g by about 25 years of age.

There is considerable controversy concerning the gross anatomical interrelationships of the prostate, mostly pertaining to the classical description of the lobes (4). As no true lobar structures exist in the adult prostate, McNeal pointed out the presence of discrete zones of the gland. According to this view, the prostate consists of a peripheral zone representing about 70% of the glandular bulk, a central zone forming 20% gland weight, a transitional zone of 5% of the gland, and a non-glandular anterior fibromuscular zone of stroma (5, 6). This description of morphology has been largely accepted, since the peripheral glandular zone comprises all the apical and most of the posterior sub-capsular area, representing the region of cancer-susceptible tissue. The central zone amalgamates at the confluence of the ejaculatory ducts at the level of the verumontanum, although strict visible separation of the peripheral zone from the central zone is conceptually artificial. It is believed to be of Wolffian ductal origin and less than 1% of all carcinomas of the prostate arise from this zone. The transitional zone is located in a para-urethral position in the mid-prostate and forms the region subject to benign prostatic hyperplasia. Carcinoma in this zone is uncommon (< 20% of all cancers), although histologically it represents isolated tumor formation noted histologically following trans-urethral prostate resection (7, 8). The boundary between this transitional zone and the peripheral zone forms the basis of the 'surgical capsule' morphologically noted between benign and malignant-bearing tissues. The traditional clinical differentiation of the gland into lateral lobes with a central sulcus does not correspond to the histologically separable zones, although it loosely represents lateral and central regional enlargement of the transitional zone.

The prostate is partially invested in a fibrous capsule, mostly coalescing posteriorly and laterally, which is relatively absent towards the glandular apex, providing a minimal barrier at this point for neoplastic infiltration. Although the presence of a true glandular capsule is debated, its invasion, particularly at the point of attachment of the seminal vesicles, represents a specific staging of extra-prostatic spread (9–12). Prostatic carcinoma may spread via lateral extension, lymphatic embolization, or hematogenous dissemination. Local extension occurs through the prostatic capsule directly into the bladder base and seminal vesicles. Rectal and urethral extension is extremely uncommon with Denonvillier's fascia representing a natural fascial barrier to neoplastic invasion. As the prostatic capsule is weaker apically and basally, spread is more commonly observed in these regions, where the prostate meets adjoining organs, and at the entry and exit points of the neurovascular bundles, ejaculatory ducts, and bladder neck.

Topographical anatomy of the prostate

Pelvic fascia

The relations of the prostate are governed by an understanding of the fasciae surrounding the gland. This fascia is dynamic, containing a considerable amount of elastic tissue and smooth muscle. It is continuous with the retroperitoneal fasciae forming broad outer, intermediate, and inner strata. The outer stratum is known as the endopelvic fascia and it lines the inner aspect of the surrounding pelvic musculature, being continuous superiorly with the transversalis fascia. It is fixed to the arcuate line of the pelvis, Cooper's ligament inferiorly, the sacrospinous ligaments, ischial spines, and the tendinous arc of the levator ani plate. The intermediate layer surrounds the pelvic viscera and consists of loose areolar tissue for visceral expansion. It anatomically lines the potential spaces of the pelvic viscera (retropubic, paravesical, rectogenital, and retrorectal (presacral) spaces). The main neurovascular pedicles traverse these spaces and are consequently at risk during their dissection. In specific areas, this stratum condenses in both sexes to form individually recognizable 'ligaments' of the pelvis (cardinal, uterosacral, and lateral rectal). Reflection of the intermediate fascial layer over the pelvic organs forms the visceral layer of pelvic fascia. The inner stratum lies adherent to the undersurface of the peritoneum and covers the rectum as Denonvillier's

fascia, forming the developmental remnant of the rectogenital peritoneal pouch. Under-dissection of this fascia, particularly posterior and lateral to the prostate, may breach invasive tumor, whereas overly aggressive dissection at this point risks inadvertent rectal injury. This fascial barrier to malignancy has also been implicated in the etiology of genital prolapse in the female (13).

Condensation of this fascia anteriorly forms the puboprostatic ligaments, supporting the membranous urethra and the vesico-prostatic sulcus represents the landmark of the dorsal venous complex, early control of which results in relatively bloodless radical prostatectomy. Damage to this fascia in the female has been implicated in stress urinary incontinence and associated urethrocoele, and forms the basis of urethral suspension procedures (14).

Prostatic relations

The prostate is approximately 3 cm × 4 cm × 2 cm and functions as a vehicle for the prostatic urethra (15). It contains anterior, posterior, and lateral surfaces with an inferior apex, which is continuous with the striated urethral sphincter (with histological extension of pericapsular glandular tissue into this region) and a formative base located at the vesico-prostatic junction. Its capsule contains collagen, elastin, and smooth muscle, fusing with Denonvillier's fascia posteriorly and the endopelvic fasciae anterolaterally (16). Anteriorly, the prostate is fixed by the puboprostatic ligaments with the superficial dorsal vein lying lateral to this landmark and draining into the dorsal-venous complex attached to the posterolateral portion of the gland. Laterally, the gland abuts against the pubococcygeal component of the levator ani complex. Both of these landmarks are important for prostatic excision, since lateral prostate dissection and displacement of the fascia off the surface of the levator ani medially is necessary to free the posterolateral prostate, whilst controlling the major venous plexus (17). The cavernosal nerves (as part of the main neurovascular bundle important in erectile function) lay posterolateral to this point of dissection.

Vascular supply

The main arterial supply for the prostate is derived from the inferior vesical artery with a series of small urethral arteries derived from this vessel separately penetrating the prostato-vesical junction posterolaterally in a peri-urethral locale, classically at the 1–5 and the 7–11 o'clock positions. The largest vessels penetrate the posterior portion of the gland and run paraurethrally supplying the transitional zone as principal arteries for nodules of benign prostatic hyperplasia (18). Distinct capsular arteries may occasionally be found coursing with the neurovascular bundles at the lateral margin at the back of the gland.

Newer techniques designed to minimize blood loss during radical prostatectomy take advantage of preliminary control of the main points of venous drainage of the gland. The main dorsal-vein complex ramifies distally over the gland near the urethral sphincter and excessive traction on the prostate without prior venous control may result in torrential hemorrhage from this region. Moreover, blind hemostasis at this point will damage the striated urethral sphincter. The main dorsal vein of the penis passes between the pubic arch and the internal urethral sphincter, trifurcating in to a central superficial branch and two lateral plexi (19). The deep dorsal vein should be triply ligated at this point to free the anterior aspect of the glandular apex. In mobilization of the posterolateral portion of the prostate, the lateral plexi are deliberately sought as they sweep alongside the posterior part of the gland communicating with components of the rectal veins and the vesical plexi. Here they form 3–5 distinct inferior vesical veins, which drain into the internal iliac (hypogastric) vein. These veins are located in the posterior groove of the prostate near the seminal vesicle, often marked by a separate small venous tributary to the tip of the vesicle requiring ligation. Great care should be exercised at this point since the main neurovascular bundle lies immediately subjacent to this area. In the female, this area has extensive and variable communication with the uterine, ovarian, and rectal complexes, although the latter may often be rudimentary. This main venous system forms distinct communications via the pelvic plexi with emissary veins of the pelvic bones (Batson's plexi), representing a well-recognized mechanism for hematogenous spread of prostatic tumor to the axial skeleton (20, 21).

Lymphatic drainage

Most of the prostatic lymphatic drainage is towards the obturator and internal iliac lymph nodes. A small drainage from the gland may pass to the presacral and, rarely, the external iliac lymph node chains with occasional skip sites detected in the pre-aortic lymph node group (22–24). Overall occurrence of lymph node involvement in prostatic carcinoma is variably reported between 20 and 40%, although the incidence of nodal positivity appears to be falling (25, 26). A thorough knowledge of the lymphatic anatomy of the prostate is important for consideration of pelvic lymphadenectomy performed either prior to, or in association with, a radical prostatectomy (either retropubic or perineal).

The exact place of staging pelvic lymphadenectomy as a decision-making procedure for radical prostatectomy is unknown. Improved pre-operative imaging and the development of lymph node decision analysis monograms function as accurate predictors for lymph node metastases, the latter data being based on tumor size, Gleason's grade and pre-operative PSA level (27). Given that a substantial number of node-positive cases will survive long term (28), and with the reduced morbidity of pelvic lymphadenectomy using either limited laparotomy with modified template nodal dissection or laparoscopic pelvic lymphadenectomy (29–32), the exact indications and contra-indications for this procedure remain unclear at the present time (33). It would seem reasonable to contemplate some form of pelvic lymphadenectomy as a preliminary to a radical prostatectomy with strong consideration in early stage T1 and T2 tumors with low grade and low PSA levels in fit patients or in larger local tumors with negative bone scans. The borders of lymph node dissection in the open lymphadenectomy should extend from the external iliac vein laterally, the hypogastric artery posteriorly, and the inguinal ligament distally. Dissection should incorporate the common iliac bifurcation proximally (34), although in those cases undertaken laparoscopically, full clearance of the common iliac vascular confluence is difficult (35), particularly in patients with large bodily habitus, or where there has been prior abdominal surgery (36). The minilaparotomy may be potentially reserved for patients undergoing a radical perineal approach, necessitating a second incision, or in selected cases where the prime modality of treatment is non-surgical (radical radiotherapy or cryoblation). In both, the minilaparotomy and the laparoscopic approach, there is a considerable risk of under-staging.

Neural anatomy

The autonomic nerve supply to the prostate incorporates a sympathetic inflow (pre-ganglionic T 10–12/L 1–2), which promotes smooth muscle and capsular contraction, and an α_1-adrenergic parasympathetic input, which results in acinar secretion, enhancement of pre-prostatic sphincter tone, and reduction in capsular tone (37). These components merge as the hypogas-tric nerves to form the inferior hypogastric (pelvic) plexus. The plexus lies at the level of the seminal vesi-cles as a flattened rectangular neural mass, whose branches embrace the rectum behind the mesorectum and in front of the presacral and Waldeyer's fascia (38, 39). These neural branches course to the rectum, bladder, seminal vesicles, and prostate, traveling with the vessels behind the rectal ampulla. Caudally, the pelvic plexus innervates the prostate, coalescing as the cavernous nerves (or main neurovascular bundle) where they lie at the tip of the seminal vesicle on either side behind the leaf of the endopelvic fascia and more anteriorly subjacent to Denonvillier's fascia (40, 41). The neurovascular bundle travels against the postero-lateral border of the prostate as a discrete trunk lateral to the prostatic venous complex, which serves as a landmark. It is vulnerable during apical glandular dis-section at the 5 and 7 o'clock positions and during dis-section of the rectum. Tumor invasion at these points creates difficulty in prostate dissection since the endopelvic fascia and Denonvillier's fascia are normally excised during the neural skeletonization (42, 43).

Anatomical considerations in prostate oncology

Radical prostatectomy is dependent upon an anatomi-cal definition of the endopelvic fascia as it relates to the prostate gland. Lateral dissection and reflection medi-ally of this fascia off the levator ani exposes Santorini's venous plexus behind the main bulk of the gland at its apex. As already stated, preliminary venous isolation of the deep dorsal-vein complex beneath the puboprosta-tic ligaments and the cavernous plexus posterolaterally, permits mobilization of the prostate in a relatively bloodless field. Excessive traction on the gland, which is not fully mobilized in this way, will lead to serious hemorrhage (44).

The main modifications of radical retropubic prosta-tectomy in the last few years have centered on nerve-sparing and urethral-sparing techniques. These procedures should be used in selected cases where oncologic clearance will not be compromised. Nerve-sparing radical prostatectomy is considered in young patients to preserve erectile function where the primary tumor is organ-confined with lack of invasion at the apex and the back of the gland on trial dissection. During the mobilization, care should be taken to avoid

excessive distraction of the catheter and electrocautery near the main neurovascular bundles (45, 46). Urethral-sparing techniques are desirable for preserva-tion of urinary continence and the striated urethral sphincter musculature, although the true incidence of post-operative stress urinary incontinence following radical retropubic prostatectomy is probably under-reported (47, 48). This approach substantially reduces the incidence of delayed bladder neck contracture and is considered where no tumor is located in the transi-tional zone or at the prostate base, in the absence of a significant median prostatic lobe, and in patients without a history of prior bladder neck surgery. To carry out sphincter sparing, clean transection of the prostato-urethral junction is required in accordance with adequate oncological clearance, whilst at the same time avoiding excessive traction particularly on the posterior urethra (49, 50).

As an alternative to the retropubic approach, radical prostatectomy for cancer may also be achieved via the perineal operator. This approach is uncommonly used and taught in the United Kingdom, although it has been extensively developed in the United States, where it has been shown to be associated with a cancer-related outcome, which is equivalent to that of the abdominal surgeon (51–54). Although this approach is relatively bloodless (when compared with the retropu-bic technique) and provides accurate urethrovesical mucosal apposition, the perineal prostatectomy requires an ancillary approach for pelvic lymph node assessment and is less satisfactory at neural and potency preservation.

A thorough knowledge of deep perineal anatomy is required and much of the dissection uses similar land-marks as employed by the coloproctologist in the per-formance of the perineal component of an abdomen-perineal excision. Here the dissection is carried out to expose the infralevator urogenital diaphragm with due care taken to avoid injury to the levator ani/external anal sphincter complex (55, 56). Exposure and division of the rectourethralis muscle (the most medial component of the levator) is the key to this dissection, permitting the rectum to be swept dorsally and preventing injury (57), outlining the pos-terior prostatic capsule and allowing excision of the prostate *en bloc* with its adherent Denonvillier's fascia. (58, 59) As the posterior prostate is mobilized, an attempt is made to identify the main neurovascular bundle between the apex of the gland and the inner aspect of the levators, although this can often be quite difficult (60–62).

Conclusions

Newer techniques of radical prostatectomy take advantage of a desire to preserve urinary continence and erectile function in organ-confined disease without compromising oncological clearance (63–65). An accurate knowledge of anatomy is required to reduce intraoperative blood loss with the likelihood of neural preservation, whilst maintaining a wide lateral dissection with *en bloc* excision of both the endopelvic and Denonvillier's fasciae. The role and technique of attendant pelvic lymphadenectomy is evolving, given current decision analyses for the expected incidence of involved nodes based on pathological variables of the primary tumor and serum PSA estimations.

References

1. Lowsley OS. The development of the human prostate gland with reference to the development of other structures at the neck of the urinary bladder. *Am J Anat* 1912, **13**, 299.
2. Cunha GR, Chung L WK, Shannon JM *et al.* Hormonal induced morphogenesis and growth rate: role of mesenchymal: epithelial interactions. *Rec Prog Horm Res* 1983, **39**, 559–98.
3. Wilson JD, Griffin JE, Lesken M *et al.* Role of gonadal hormones in development of the sexual phenotypes. *Hum Genet* 1981, **58**, 78–84.
4. Franks LM. Atrophy and hyperplasia in the prostate proper. *J Pathol Bacteriol* 1954, **68**, 617.
5. McNeal JE. Anatomy of the prostate: an historical survey of divergent views. *Prostate* 1980, **1**, 3–13.
6. McNeal JE. Normal and pathologic anatomy of the prostate. *Urology* 1981, **17**(Suppl), 11–16.
7. McNeal JE. Normal histology of the prostate. *Am J Surg Pathol* 1988, **12**, 619–33.
8. McNeal JE, Redwine EA, Freiha FS *et al.* Zonal distribution of prostate adenocarcinoma: crrelation with histological pattern and direction of spread. *Am J Surg Pathol* 1988, **12**, 897–906.
9. Ayala AO, Ro JY, Babarian R *et al.* The prostatic capsule: does it exist? *Am J Surg Pathol* 1989, **13**, 21–27.
10. Wheeler TM. Anatomic considerations in carcinoma of the prostate. *Urol Clin North Am* 1989, **16**, 623–34.
11. American Joint Committee on Cancer. *Manual for staging cancer* (4th edn). JB Lipincott, Philadelphia, 1992, 181.
12. Ohori M, Scardino PT, Lapin SL *et al.* The mechanisms and prognostic significance of seminal vesicle involvement by prostate cancer. *Am J Surg Pathol* 1993, **17**, 1252–61.
13. Zacharin RF. *Pelvic floor anatomy and the surgery of pulsion enterocoele.* Springer-Verlag, New York, 1985.
14. DeLancey JOL. The pubovesical ligament: a separate structure for the urethral supports ('pubo-urethral ligaments'). *Neurourol Urodyn* 1989, **8**, 53.
15. McNeaL JE. The prostate and the prostatic urethra: a morphologic synthesis. *J Urol* 1972, **107**, 1008–16.
16. Walsh PC, Lepor H and Eggleston JC. Radical prostatectomy with preservation of sexual function: anatomical and pathological considerations. *Prostate* 1983, **4**, 473–85.
17. Myers RP. Radical prostatectomy: pertinent surgical anatomy. *Urol Clin North Am* (Atlas) 1994, **2**, 1.
18. Flocks RH. The arterial distribution within the prostate gland: its role in trans-urethral prostatic resection. *J Urol* 1937, **37**, 524.
19. Reiner WG, Walsh PC. Anatomical approach to the surgical management of the dorsal vein and Santorini's plexus during radical retropubic prostatectomy surgery. *J Urol* 1979, **121**, 198–200.
20. Batson OV. The function of the vertebral veins and their role in the spread of metastases. *Ann Surg* 1940, **112**, 138.
21. Dodds PR, Caride VJ, Lytton B. The role of the vertebral veins in the dissemination of prostate cancer. *J Urol* 1981, **126**, 753–5.
22. Golimbu M, Morales P, Al-Askari S, Brown J. Extended pelvic lymphadenectomy for prostate cancer. *J Urol* 1979, **121**, 617–21.
23. Morales P, Golimbu M. The therapeutic role of pelvic lymphadenectomy in prostate cancer. *Urol Clin North Am* 1980, **7**, 623–7.
24. McLaughlin AP, Saltzstein SL, McCullough DL, Gittes RF. Prostate carcinoma: incidence and location of unsuspected lymphatic metastases. *J Urol* 1976, **115**, 89–91.
25. Fowler JE, Whitmore WF. The incidence and extent of pelvic lymph node metastases in apparently localized prostatic carcinoma. *Cancer* 1981, **47**, 2941–7.
26. Petros JA, Catalona WJ. Lower incidence of unsuspected lymph node metastasis in 521 consecutive patients with clinical localized prostate cancer. *J Urol* 1992, **147**, 1574–8.
27. Bluestein D, Bostwick D, Bergstrahl E, Oesterling J. Eliminating the need for bilateral pelvic lymphadenectomy in selected patients with prostate cancer. *J Urol* 1994, **151**, 1315–8.
28. Austenfield MS, Davis BE. New concepts in the treatment of stage D1 adenocarcinoma of the prostate. *Urol Clin North Am* 1990, **17**, 867–8.
29. Steiner MS, Marshall FF. Mini-laparotomy staging pelvic lymphadenectomy (minilap): alternative to standard and laparoscopic pelvic lymphadenectomy. *Urology* 1993, **41**, 201–3.
30. Perrotti M, Gentle DL, Baruda JH *et al.* Mini-laparotomy pelvic lymph node dissection. *J Urol* 1996, **155**, 986–8.
31. Bouillier JA, Hagood PG, Parra RO. Endocavitary (laparoscopic) pelvic lymphadenectomy with specific indications in urologic surgery. *Urology* 1993, **41**(1), 19–25.
32. Kerbl K, Clayman RV, Petros JA *et al.* Staging pelvic lymphadenectomy for prostate cancer: a comparison of

laparoscopic and open techniques. *J Urol* 1993, **150**, 396–8.

33. Patel M, Kateluns PM. Indications for laparoscopic pelvic lymph node dissection in the staging of prostatic carcinoma. *Aust NZ J Surg* 1995, **65**, 233–6.

34. Brendler CB, Cleeve IK, Anderson EE *et al*. Staging pelvic lymphadenectomy for carcinoma of the prostate: risk versus benefit. *J Urol* 1980, **124**, 849–50.

35. Burney TI, Campbell EC, Naslund MJ *et al*. Complications of staging laparoscopic pelvic lymphadenectomy. *Surg Laparosc Endosc* 1993, **3**, 184–90.

36. Loughlin KR, Kavoussi LR. Laparoscopic lymphadenectomy in the staging of prostate cancer. *Contemp Urol* 1992, **4**, 69.

37. Burnett HL. Nitric oxide control of lower genitourinary tract functions-a review. *Urology* 1995, **45**, 1071–83.

38. Schlegel PN, Walsh PC. Neuroanatomical approach to radical prostatectomy with preservation of sexual function. *J Urol* 1987, **138**, 1402–6.

39. Walsh PC, Lepor H, Eggleston JC. Radical prostatectomy with preservation of sexual function: anatomical and pathological considerations. *Prostate* 1983, **4**, 473–85.

40. Lepor H, Gregerman M, Crosby R *et al*. Precise localization of the autonomic nerves from the pelvic plexus to corpora cavernosa: a detailed anatomical study of the adult male pelvis. *J Urol* 1985, **133**, 207–12.

41. Walsh PC, Donker PJ. Impotence following radical prostatectomy: insight into aetiology and prevention. *J Urol* 1982, **128**, 492–7.

42. Lue TF, Zeineh ST, Schmidt RA *et al*. Neuroanatomy of penile erection: its relevance to iatrogenic impotence. *J Urol* 1984, **131**, 273–80.

43. Breza J, Abouserf SR, Orvis BR *et al*. Detailed anatomy ofpenile neurovascular structures: surgical significance. *J Urol* 1989, **141**, 437–43.

44. Hedican SP, Walsh PC. Postoperative bleeding following radical retropubic prostatectomy. *J Urol* 1994, **152**, 1181–3.

45. Catalona WJ, Bigg SW. Nerve-sparing radical prostatectomy: evaluation of results after 250 patients. *J Urol* 1990, **143**, 538–43.

46. Myers RP. Practical pelvis anatomy pertinent to radical retropubic prostatectomy. *AUA Update Series* 1994, **13** (4), 26.

47. Jonler M, Messing EM, Rhodes PR *et al*. Sequelae of radical prostatectomy. *Br J Urol* 1994, **74**, 352–8.

48. Kerr LA, Zincke H. Radical retropubic prostatectomy for prostate cancer in the elderly and the young: complications and prognosis. *Eur Urol* 1994, **25**, 305–11.

49. Andriole GL, Smith DS, Rao G *et al*. Early complications of contemporary anatomical radical retropubic prostatectomy. *J Urol* 1994, **152**, 1858–60.

50. Myers RP. Male urethral sphincteric anatomy and radical prostatectomy. *Urol Clin North Am* 1991, **18**, 211–27.

51. Belt E, Ebert CE, Surber Jr AC. A new anatomic approach in perineal prostatectomy. *J Urol* 1939, **41**, 482.

52. Paulson DF. Radical perineal prostatectomy. *Urol Clin North Am* 1980, **7**, 847–53.

53. Paulson DF. Long term results of radical perineal prostatectomy. *Eur Urol* 1995, **27**, 35.

54. Frazier HA, Robertson JE, Paulson DF. Radical prostatectomy: the pros and cons of the perineal vs. retropubic approach. *J Urol* 1992, **147**, 888–90.

55. Weldon E. Extended radical perineal prostatectomy—an anatomical and surgical study. *J Urol* 1988, **139**, 448(A).

56. Weldon E, Tavel FR. Potency-sparing radical perineal prostatectomy: anatomy, surgical technique and initial results. *J Urol* 1988, **140**, 559–62.

57. McLaren RH, Barrett DM, Zincke H. Rectal injury occuring at radical prostatectomy for prostate cancer: aetiology and treatment. *Urology* 1993, **42**, 401–5.

58. Tobin CE, Benjamin JA. Anatomical and surgical restudy of Denonvillier's fascia. *Surg Gynecol Obstet* 1945, **80**, 373.

59. Villiers A, McNeal JE, Faiha FS *et al*. Invasion of Denonvillier's fascia in radical prostatectomy specimens. *J Urol* 1993, **149**, 793–8.

60. Myers RP, Goellner JR, Cahill DR. Prostate shape, extemal striated urtethral sphincter in radical prostatectomy: the apical dissection. *J Urol* 1987, **138**, 543–50.

61. Van Ophoven A, Roth S. The anatomy and embryological origins of the fascia of Denonvilliers: a medicohistorical debate. *J Urol* 1997, **157** (1), 3–9.

62. Kourambas J, Angus DG, Hosking P, Chou ST. A histological study of Denonvillier's fascia and its relationship to the neurovascular bundle. *Br J Urol* 1998, **82**, 408–13.

63. Walsh PC. Radical retropubic prostatectomy with reduced morbidity: an anatomical approach. *NCI Monogr* 1988, **7**, 133.

64. Roseb MA, Goldstone L, Lapin S, Wheeler T, Scardino PT. Frequency and location of extracapsular extension and positive surgical margins in radical prostatectomy specimens. *J Urol* 1992, **148**, 331–3.

65. Goad JR, Scardino PT. Modification in the technique of radical retropubic prostatectomy to minimize blood loss. *Urol Clin North Am* 1994, **20**, 65–6.

2 | *Physiology of the prostate*

Wells E. Farnsworth

Introduction

The prostate gland is probably one of the least understood and appreciated organs of the body. Its presence is often considered of little benefit to the young and a downright danger to the elderly. It is the source of more clinical problems than is the vermiform appendix with which its presumed uselessness is often equated. Little wonder that many investigators ask what God had in mind in creating this organ.

One of the discouraging realities confronting the prostatologist is that, despite all that has been learned in the past 40 years about both benign prostatic hyperplasia (BPH) and prostatic cancer (PCA), when either of these diseases is detected, the therapeutic battle has already been lost. As Waxman (1) says of PCA, 'primary hormone therapy does not prolong life, its action only postponing or palliating the symptoms'. Bonfiglio and Terry (2) well recognized that 'conceptually, cancer is considered a disease of the cell in which the normal mechanisms of control of growth and proliferation are disturbed. This results in distinctive morphologic alterations of the cell and aberrations of tissue patterns. These cytologic and histologic alterations are the basis of the diagnosis of cancer'. Metastatic potential and predisposition to home to specific organs from cells within a single prostatic tumor, shows the spectrum of growth forces at work that confounds the complete efficacy of any and all cytostatic strategies presently directed toward the arrest of PCA. BPH is less ominous but more ubiquitous, and at least as poorly understood.

This chapter intends to establish the bases—anatomical and physiological—of normal prostatic function, from which succeeding sections of this volume will show the pathological departures of structure and function, which comprise prostatic cancer. While it is recognized that this background information can answer few of the questions posed, it is hoped that, through showing what and where the prostate is, and reviewing the forces at work for actuating its functions, the reader can appreciate the dynamics of prostatic physiology.

Structure

Gross structure

The four major subdivisions of the adult prostate (Fig. 2.1) can best be located in relationship to the prostatic urethra, about which they grow. The prostatic portion of the urethra extends from the bladder neck distally to join, at the urogenital diaphragm, with the membranous urethra. It can be further subdivided at its midpoint into the proximal, or preprostatic segment, which courses backwards to the bladder neck at an angle of 30°, and a distal, or prostatic segment, whose course of direction is nearly vertical. The line of division between segments is the upper end of the verumontanum (V), where the ejaculatory ducts gain access to the urethra. All these features are shown in the midsagittal section (Fig. 2.2) of the prostate of a 22-year-old man. The tissue is stained with the Giemsa solution to show its connective tissue (Fig. 2.1) (3).

Functional anatomy

Figure 2.3 shows schematically the previously unrecognized heterogeneity of the compartments of the prostatic duct system of both the overlying epithelium and the stroma upon which it lies. The presence of the unlike cells within the separate regions offers a credible rationale for a single level of circulating steroid hormones supporting the very different biological activities within these regions. The peculiar competencies of the regions are due, not only to the structural variety and abundance of the stromal cell population, but also to the growth factors (the 'forces at work'), which they

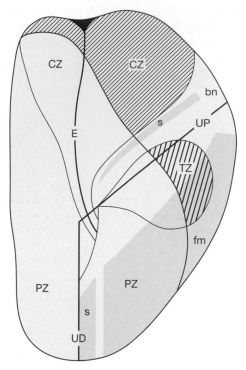

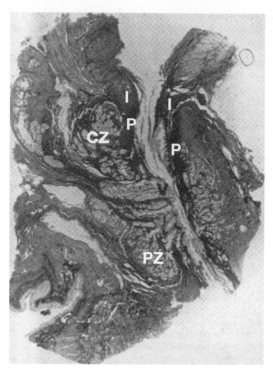

Fig. 2.1 Sagittal diagram of distal prostatic urethral segment (UD), proximal urethral segment (UP), and ejaculatory ducts (E), showing their relationships to a sagittal section of the anteromedial, non-glandular tissues: bladder neck (bn); anterior fibromuscular stroma (fm); preprostatic sphincter (s); distal striated sphincter (s). These structures are shown in relation to a three-dimensional representation of the glandular prostate: central zone (CZ), peripheral zone (PZ), transition zone (TZ). From: McNeal JE, chapter 42, Prostate. In: *Histology for pathologists* (2nd edn) (ed. Steenberg SS). Lippincott-Raven Publishers, Philadelphia, 1997, 997–1017, with permission.

Fig. 2.2 Mid-sagittal section of true prostate from 22-year-old man (van Giesenstain). Internal sphincter (I), preprostatic sphincter (P), central zone/peripheral zone (CZ/PZ), verumontanum and utriculus masculinus (V). From: Blacklock NJ, chapter 16, *Surgical anatomy of the prostate*. In: *Scientific foundations of urology* (1st edn) (Williams DE, Chisholm CD). Butterworth Heinemann, a division of Reed Educational and Professional Publishing, 1976, 113–125, with permission.

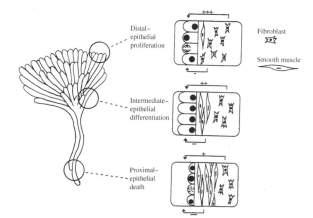

Fig. 2.3 Proposed effects of stromal heterogeneity within the prostatic ductal system. In the distal region, abundant fibroblastic cells may elaborate positive factors, including epithelial proliferation. Increased smooth muscle in the intermediate region may block positive factors or produce factors inhibitory for epithelium, allowing epithelial differentiation. High levels of possible negative factors from the abundant smooth muscle in the proximal region may induce epithelial cell death. From: Nemeth JA, Lee C. Prostatic ductal system in rats: regional variation in stromal organization. *Prostate* 1996, **28**, 124–8; Wiley-Liss, Inc., New York, with permission.

elaborate and impose upon themselves and on the epithelial cells by apocrine and paracrine secretion, respectively (4). It is uncertain whether the epithelial cells of the three regions are actually different or are one cell type, which is adapted in structure and function to the diversity of the stromal environment. Bonkhoff and Remberger (5) suggested that:

(1)   'the abnormal growth of the secretory epithelium in BPH may be related to an increase in total number of androgen-responsive basal cells in the proliferative compartment'; and

(2)   'prostatic cancer derives from the transformed stem cells located in the basal layer that acquire secretory luminal characteristics under androgen stimulus'.

In addition, Aumuller *et al.* (6) show that human prostatic neuroendocrine cells represent a cell lineage of their own, being of neurogenic origin and, therefore, distinct from the urogenital sinus-derived secretory and basal cells. These cells seem to be devoid of androgen receptors from the outset.

Growth factors

In the normal prostate, these peptide cytokines directly, and the sex steroids, androgen and estrogen, indirectly, regulate the gland's growth and homeostasis. Since each may have more than one effect, it is necessary to first introduce them and their sites of origin and action (7, 8).

Basic fibroblast growth factor (bFGF) is an autocrine secretion of the normal prostate. It stimulates proliferation of stromal fibroblasts. The stroma also secretes transforming growth factor-$\beta 1$ (TGF-$\beta 1$) to inhibit stromal proliferation. This antagonizes the mitogenic action of bFGF but extends the half-life of the latter. A third product of the stroma is insulin-like growth factor-1 (IGF-1) that promotes the transformation of prostate epithelial cells from the G1 phase to the S phase of its cell cycle. The mechanism is paracrine secretion of the IGF-1 from the stroma to IGF-1 receptors concentrated in the epithelium.

The epithelial cells elaborate other cytokines. From studies of the androgen-dependent cell lines, LNCaP and ALVA, these appear to secrete epidermal growth factor (EGF) and the closely related transforming growth factor-a (TGF-a). LNCaP cells contain EGF receptors. Epithelial growth is increased by both EGF and, separately, by androgen. Not incidentally, both EGF and androgen additively down-regulate secretion of prostatic acid phosphatase (PAP). In contrast, EGF decreases, but androgen increases, epithelial cell secretion of prostate-specific antigen (PSA).

Hormone action

In this paragraph, only a précis on this topic will be presented, adequate to provide the vocabulary and principal concepts to be encountered, since the subject will be covered in the chapters that follow. Hormones and growth factors are the primary signals of cellular communication. Chemically, the hormones include hydrophilic amino acid derivatives, ranging from the complex polypeptide proteins, e.g. luteinizing hormone (LH), through smaller peptides, e.g. thyrotropin-releasing hormone (TRH), to amino acid derivatives, e.g. catecholamines. In addition, there are the hydrophobic steroid derivatives of cholesterol, including those with an intact steroid nucleus (adrenal and sex steroids) and those in which the B ring of cholesterol has been cleaved (Vitamin D and its derivatives). The response of a tissue to a hormone is determined by the presence of a receptor for the hormone and of a post-receptor machinery to which the receptor is coupled. Each receptor is able to recognize a hormone as an entity distinct from all other substances and, by binding to it, it is able to effect modification of cellular metabolism and/or growth (7, 8).

Hydrophilic hormones

The receptors for the hydrophilic hormones are on the plasma membrane of target cells. Their signaling pathway within the cell typically consists of sequential phosphorylations and dephosphorylations, using protein kinase and phosphatase cascades. These are initiated by the hormone's binding to, and activating of, the receptors on the cell surface, hence enhancing the rate of generation of second messengers such as c-AMP, diacylglycerol (DAG), and calcium ions, which initiate the effect. The effect of these is to activate the cascades and, thereby, mobilize key target proteins, such as transcription factors, that control gene expression or repression.

Hydrophobic hormones

In contrast, the pathways of the hydrophobic hormones are various. The classic genomic action of steroid hormones is through intracellular receptors: After moving passively across the plasma membrane, the steroids bind to specific receptors within the cytoplasm or the nucleus. The resultant hormone–receptor complexes attach to specific target sites within the chromatin.

Non-classical hydrophobic hormone action

While the classic genomic concept of steroid action is the accepted dogma, there are other non-classical modes of behavior of these hormones. These non-classical actions generally occur at the membrane level and are not associated with entry of the hormone into the cell. They take place far more rapidly and use signals that are insensitive to inhibitors of transcription or protein synthesis. Some investigators have suggested that the rapid effects of these steroids are due to a non-specific modification of the fluidity of the plasma membrane. Others, however, question how such an action can explain the rapidity and specificity of the process. Still, as will be discussed below, the rapid effects could be due to a direct interaction of the steroid with a steroid receptor in the plasma membrane. In addition, *in vitro* studies have shown the activation of a second messenger system directly, in the absence of the steroid hormone. This can lead to steroid hormone receptor-mediated cellular responses.

Hormones in and on the prostate

Blood-borne sex steroids

There are two peaks of prostatic growth (9), the first occurring at puberty, when there is a rise in androgen level. The second peak begins at around age 50, when there is an increase in the ratio of estrogen to androgen (10). This second peak is accompanied by the development of BPH (11). A large clinical study (12) also showed a strong trend toward development of BPH associated with increased serum estradiol (E_2) level. In addition, the study revealed that this risk was confined to men with relatively low androgen levels. Thus, the ascent of the estrogen/androgen ratio reflects as much, if not more, the elevation of the serum E_2 as the descent of the serum androgen concentration. As noted above,

BPH is a stromal disease characterized by nodules arising in the peri-urethral transition zone (13), which is the most estrogen-responsive part of the prostate. This proliferation of prostatic stroma, while obviously associated with higher plasma E_2 and urinary estrogen secretion, is not correlated with testosterone levels (14).

Androgens

In the blood of normal men, only about 2% of the testosterone is free (unbound); 60% is bound to the homodimeric β globulin, sex hormone-binding globulin (SHBG), also known as testosterone-binding globulin (TeBG). The remaining 38% are bound to albumin and other proteins, including cortisol-binding globulin (CBG). The formerly-held notion that the 'active' fraction of testosterone is identical to the unbound fraction has been refuted by Pardridge's finding (15) that dissociation of protein-bound hormone can occur in the capillary bed. Therefore, the active fraction delivered to the cells is larger than the free fraction obtained by equilibrium dialysis *in vitro*. The amount of hormone available to enter cells depends on the combination of capillary transit time (see Blood flow, below), the half-time of dissociation, the amount of hormone bound to the various carrier proteins, and the permeability of the cell membrane. Of course, the amount of hormone supplied also depends directly on the capillary density, i.e. the number of capillaries in a unit volume of tissue (16).

Estrogens

Of the circulating estrogen in young men, 75–90% arises from peripheral aromatization, mainly in adipose tissue, of both testosterone to E_2 and androstenedione (DIONE) to estrone (E_1). The testes synthesize the remaining 10–25%. As men grow older, the androgen/estrogen ratio falls, due to the rise in estrogen production and fall in the elaboration of androgen (9). Processes within the prostate also form estrogen. One of these is the aromatase activity present within the stroma. Second, abundant estrone sulfate is taken up from the plasma and hydrolyzed to free E_1 by a stromal sulfatase. The stromal enzyme, 17β-hydroxysteroid dehydrogenase, readily reduces the estrone to the more potent E_2 within the stroma. In a study by Stege and Carlstrom (17), BPH patients had elevated levels of testosterone and non-SHBG-bound testosterone in the presence of normal SHBG and gonadotropin levels. They had elevated levels of DHEA and DHEA sulfate in the presence of normal cortisol levels, presenting as a 'younger' pattern of adrenal response to ACTH as judged by the increments in DHEA and 17a-hydroxprogesterone. Finally, they had elevated ratios of E_1 and DIONE, which suggests that there was an increased peripheral aromatization and subnormal prolactin (Prl) levels.

Prolactin

As detailed in the reviews of Farnsworth (l8) and Costello and Franklin (l9), the non-gonadotrophic hormone prolactin (Prl) greatly enhances the sensitivity of prostatic tissue to androgen. Also, it has effects that are independent of androgens. The Costello group demonstrated that Prl stimulates citric acid production by specific prostatic secretory epithelial cells. This effect is achieved by stimulation of mitochondrial aspartate amino-transferase (mAAT). The net rate of citrate synthesis may be increased, as well, by zinc inhibition of mitochondrial aconitase and, consequently, of citrate oxidation. Recently, it has become known that Prl is produced in many sites besides the pituitary, including the prostate (20, 21). In the prostate, the hormone is produced in highest density within the secretory epithelial cells, as it is shown by the Prl mRNA and it acts as a direct growth and differentiation factor. Prl receptors can be demonstrated mainly in the apical parts of the secretory epithelium and, to a limited extent, in the stroma. Since the epithelial cells are joined by tight junctions, making them inaccessible to circulating Prl, entry to them must be by a secreted ligand, i.e. an autocrine or paracrine substance available to the apically-located Prl receptor. Probably, the Prl-synthesizing cells are of the neuroendocrine– paracrine type. Hypophyseal secretion of Prl is stimulated by the hypothalamic tripeptide TRH and is inhibited by dopamine (22). Prostatic Prl levels are androgen- and Prl-dependent. It is hypothesized that TRH, which is also elaborated by the prostate, may serve as a mediator of Prl in controlling prostatic growth and function. There are several hypothesis as to how Prl functions. Based upon a wide variety of experimental work, it is now believed that the most plausible and readily demonstrable mechanism is the facilitation of irreversible metabolism of testosterone to dihydrotestosterone (DHT) and androsteyediol. However, the mode of action does not appear to be the activation of the enzyme, 5a-reductase. It is more likely that Prl enhances the rate of substrate testosterone entry into the cell, i.e. the increase in the permeability of the prostate plasma membrane to the steroid. It now appears that both androgen and Prl modify biosynthesis of low viscosity prostaglandins within the plasma membrane, perhaps through the mediation of lipoprotein lipase (LPL) (23).

Blood flow

Over a decade ago English *et al.* (24) reported loss of prostatic endothelial cells, associated with castration-induced regression of the rat prostate. Now, Shabsigh *et al.* (25) and Lekas (26) have rediscovered and further investigated this phenomenon. They have found that the rapid and significant reduction in blood flow to the mature rat ventral prostate, but not to the urinary bladder, precedes the appearance of apoptosis in the prostate epithelial cells. Its time of appearance coincides with the time of apoptotic changes in the prostatic vascular endothelial and stromal cells, indicating that androgen supports survival of the vascular and stromal cells, as well as those of the epithelial compartment. Not surprisingly, androgen receptors, but not their blood vessels, are observed in both compartments of the ventral and dorsal prostate. The Shabsigh group, on noting that the prostate endothelial cells are not known to express androgen receptor, suggest that there may be some paracrine action whereby 'the expression of the prostate endothelial cell survival protein (growth factor) is being produced by the androgen receptor-positive prostate epithelial and stromal cells in response to androgen stimulation'. Lekas *et al.*, similarly, suggest that the decrease in blood flow could be the result of a general effect of decreased metabolism or be caused by stimulation or inhibition of a specific vasoregulatory factor, e.g. the potent vasoconstrictor, endothelin-1, or the vasodilator nitric oxide, both of which are produced in the prostate and are possibly regulated by androgen. Farnsworth (27) has shown that androgen ablation inhibits the ability of androgen-responsive prostate cancer cells to produce the specific endothelial mitogen, vascular endothelial growth factor (VEGF), a potent angiogenic agent. The menstrual ebb and flow of estrogen levels in the female, and the significant fall in this hormone's blood concentration at menopause through its direct effect on the uterine vascular cells, is familiar to everyone. The majority of the vasoprotective effects of estrogens appear to be directly on vascular cells—even in men. The estrogen receptor (ER) mediates many of the known cardiovascular effects of estrogen, and is expressed in the vascular cells of both males and females (28, 29). Unfortunately, no special attention has been given to regulation of prostatic blood flow.

Secretory products of the prostate

Williams-Ashman (30), like Mann (31) before him, noted that 'the secretions of the accessory glands and semen are a veritable cornucopia of chemical oddities'. Probably the most extraordinary of these is the great quantity of citric acid produced, which contributes to the ejaculated semen. But, prostatic intermediary metabolism, its androgen sensitivity, and especially this bounteous level of citricogenesis, have been grievously overlooked for many years (32). The obvious anomaly would be a defect in the operation of the Krebs cycle: an inability to oxidize the citric acid. However, the enzyme aconitase, which converts citric acid to isocitric acid, was found to be abundant in the human prostate (33). It has also been demonstrated that the full tricarboxylic acid cycle functions in the rat ventral prostate (34, 35). In addition, Barron and Huggins (36) showed that human prostate tissue does respire, although at the modest rate of tumor tissue. The predominant pathway of energy production is glycolytic, not anaerobic, but hypoxic. The limited ability of the prostate to oxidize citrate posed another question: If citrate is not metabolized, where does the cell obtain the 4-carbon dicarboxylic keto acid, oxaloacetate, which must be condensed with acetyl CoA, obtained from glycolysis, to make citrate? It has been shown the presence of abundant transaminase activity (37). These aminotransferase enzymes can handily convert amino acids, principally aspartic acid, in this case, to the needed oxaloacetate. Costello and Franklin (38) have developed an elaborate hypothesis (Fig. 2.4), whereby, upon androgen stimulation, the transaminase is evolved in prostatic mitochondria. Farnsworth (39, 40) has shown an amino acid transport function, which is stimulated by androgen in *vitro* to deliver the needed amino acid to the mitochondrial enzyme, while Costello and Franklin (38) have confirmed Farnsworth 's hypothesis that citrate secretion from the prostate is driven by a Na^+-citrate transporter, coupled to $(Na^+ + K^+)$-ATPase activity (Fig. 2.5). More recently, Swinnen and Verhoeven (4l) have confirmed the findings of Nyden and Williams-Ashman (42) and Farnsworth and Brown (35) that androgen also drive lipid biosynthesis and the elaboration of the enzyme, fatty acid synthase, employing citrate as substrate. The amount of citrate deployed into fatty acids, for incorporation into plasma mem-

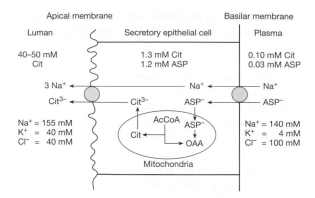

Fig. 2.4 Proposed distribution and transport of citrate and aspartate in prostate secretory epithelial cells. A high affinity, Na^+-coupled aspartate transporter at the basilar membrane is responsible for the import of aspartate against a concentration gradient. Intracellular aspartate is converted to citrate, the apical membrane contains an Na^+-coupled citrate transporter, which is necessary for the secretion of citrate against a large concentration gradient. This Na^+-coupled citrate transporter results in Cit^{3-}, rather than Cl^-, being the major anion in prostatic fluid. Although not represented in the illustration, the luminal Na^+ concentration will likely vary in proportion to the Cit^{3-} concentration. From: Costello LC, Franklin RB. Concepts of citrate production and secretion by prostate. 1. Metabolic relationships. *Prostate* 1991, **18**, 25–46; Wiley-Liss, Inc., New York, with permission.

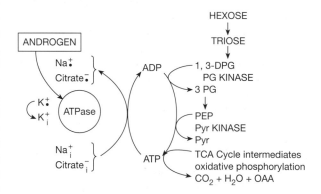

Fig. 2.5 Proposed model for regulation of prostatic metabolism and secretion by androgen. Increased Na^+ efflux facilitates uptake of glycolyzable substrates. Concurrent loss of citrate reduces product inhibition of citric acid synthesis, permitting a more rapid flow of carbon through the glycolytic pathway to form more citrate. Rate of glycolysis is accelerated by provision of more ADP from ATP, thus hastening activities of phosphoglycerate kinase and probably pyruvate kinase. The extra ADP permits an accelerated rate of oxidative phosphorylation to provide, along with glycolysis, the additional ATP needed to meet the requirements of the microtubules and adenylate cyclase From: Farnsworth WE. Prostate plasma membrane receptor: a hypothesis. *Prostate* 1991, **19**, 329–352: Wiley-Liss, Inc., New York, with permission.

branes, is better appreciated when it is remembered that synthesis of 1 mol of palmitate requires 8 mol of citrate.

While not investigated in prostate tissue, it is important to note that hypoxic conditions enhance glucose uptake by cells and tissues (43), a response than can be mimicked by exposure of cells to pharmacologic inhibitors of oxidative phosphorylation. Glucose transport is acutely stimulated through enhanced Glut-l and Glut-4 glucose transporter function. Moreover, hypoxia, *per se*, acts through hypoxia-inducible factor 1 (HIF-l)-enhanced Glut-l transcription. In cancer cells more details of this process will be found below.

As noted above, a number of other materials are characteristic, by nature or abundance, of the prostate (44) .Of the proteins, PAP, PSA, and the plasminogen activators (Pas) are most familiar. Both PAP and PSA can leak into the serum. Elevation of the concentration of these in the blood, including the free fraction of PSA (45), has long been a diagnostic index of likely PCa metastasis. In their review of plasminogen activators, Kircheimer and Binder (46) make clear that it is the tissue-type PA (t-PA) that is responsible for practically all vascular fibrinolysis, through activation of the conversion of plasminogen to plasmin.

Zinc is present in high concentration in seminal plasma. Zinc ions inhibit 5α-reductase, the enzyme that reduces testosterone to DHT. Costello and Franklin (19) find that zinc ions inhibit both mitochondrial aconitase and consequently citrate oxidation. Although in some species a part of the prostatic Zn is associated with the enzyme, carbonic anhydrase, this is not true in human prostate.

Seminal emission is a sequential process. The first fraction is richest in spermatozoa, indicating that epididymal efflux precedes products of the reproductive accessory glands. Fructose, pepsinogens, some proteases, and enzymes are found in the last fraction, and the plasminogen activators and the citric acid occupy the intermediate portion.

Hypoxia and metabolic control

Evidently, the relative hypoxia of the prostate is not due to defective blood flow, nor to inadequate vascularization of the gland. Rather, it seems to reflect a limited demand for oxygen, notably due to the marked diversion of citric acid from the tricarboxylic cycle, as discussed above, and to competing mechanisms, which

establish this ischemia. Thus, the low QO_2 appears to be the normal homeostatic setting for the normal prostate. Reichlin (47) notes that, in engineering formulations of feedback, three controlled variables can be identified: a sensing element that detects the concentration of the controlled variable; a reference input that defines the proper control levels; and an error signal that determines the output of the system. The reference input is the set point of the system.

As will be discussed below, several quite separate factors participate in sustaining this intrinsic set point of prostatic oxygenation. These include the extent of proliferation, the extent of vascularization, and the rate of blood flow. Hormone levels, growth factors, and the nervous system affect all of these, in turn. As mentioned above, one can say that prostatic-relative hypoxia reflects an extraordinarily modest demand for oxygen; not a deficiency of supply .The organism has a normal cardiac output and blood pressure. What is limiting is the size (density) of the prostatic capillary bed plus a vascular tone prohibiting a blood flow rate comparable to that in organs like the heart, liver, kidney, etc.. Just as in tumor cells, hypoxia promotes a compensatory glycolytic rate, enhances the lactate concentration, and causes macrophages to release several growth factors, bFGF, tumor necrosis factor α (TNF-α), vascular endothelial growth factor (VEGF), also known as vascular permeability factor (VPF), and hypoxia-inducible factor-l (heme oxygenase-l). In addition, another endogenous angiogenesis inhibitor, angiostatin, has been identified (48). This internal fragment of plasminogen, specifically blocks angiogenesis and the growth (proliferation) of endothelial cells (49). It is probable liberated from the plasminogen by proteases such as uPA.

Vascular endothelial growth factor (VEGF)

This is a specific endothelial cell mitogen, produced both in tumors and normal cultured cells in response to hypoxia, including the prostate (7). The VEGF gene appears to respond to ischemia in the same way as does the erythropoietin gene. Its oxygen-sensing capability is thought to be due to a direct effect of the oxygen tension on a heme-containing protein. A 28-base-pair element, within the 5′ promoter of VEGF, mediates hypoxia-inducible transcription, much as does the hypoxia-inducible factor-l binding site within the erythropoietin 3′ enhancer.

VEGF can induce the hormone, endothelin-l (see below), to produce bFGF. The latter may then act upon angiogenesis as a secondary autocrine or intracrine cytokine. The action of bFGF can be modulated by TGF-β through its inhibition of bFGF-induced cell migration and protease production. bFGF stimulates urokinase plasminogen activator (uPA) expression, which, in turn, activates latent TGF-β. The activated TGF-β stimulates plasminogen activator inhibitor (PAI-1) synthesis that inhibits uPA to shut down subsequent TGF-β activation and bFGF activity. Obviously, these several interactions create a loop to closely regulate both TGF-β and bFGF effects. TGF-β also functions as a biphasic regulator of bFGF-induced angiogenesis: at low concentrations, TGF-β stimulation the bFGF effect, whereas, at high concentration, it inhibits bFGF action, *in vitro*.

The rate and extent of angiogenesis is also influenced by the extracellular matrix, whose components modulate vascular endothelial cell adhesion, migration, proliferation, morphogenesis, and responsiveness to angiogenic cytokines (50). Thus, metalloproteinases, which Stearns *et al.* (5l) have demonstrated to be secreted by human prostate cancer cells, facilitate formation of new microvessels by their proteolytic attack on the extracellular macromolecules. However, just as with the dynamic equilibrium of VEGF vs. PAI-l, there is elaboration by prostatic epithelial cells of Interleukin-10, which inhibits angiogenesis.

Hypoxia affects not only neovascularization, but also the level of blood supplied to the capillary bed. Endothelial cells produce vasodilators such as prostaglandin and nitric oxide (NO) and vasoconstrictors, such as thromboxane and endothelin-l (ET-l). ET-1 is probably the most potent vasoconstrictive peptide known (7). It is markedly prominent in prostatic glandular epithelium but of minimum concentration in the stroma. ET-1 mediates a powerful contraction of human prostatic smooth muscle, without the mediation of α_1 adrenergic or dihydropyridine-sensitive calcium channels or the synthesis of prostaglandins. The release of ET-1 from cultured endothelial cells is stimulated both by hypoxia and ischemia and also by a wide variety of other agents, including insulin, catecholamines, thrombin, arginase vasopressin, and various ions. Atrial natriuretic peptide and prostaglandin inhibit its secretion. Accumulation of ET-l also inhibits its own secretion, substantially more to the abluminal than to the luminal side of endothelial cells. This indicates that it probably functions more as a paracrine than an endocrine hormone. While Langenstroer (52) postulated that ET-1 has this effect on the prostate, the growth of epithelial cells from BPH

is not affected by ET-1 (53). From experiments with cultured rat smooth muscle cells, Rajegepala *et al.* (54) concluded that some of the vascular effects of angiotensin-II, thought to be unique to this hormone, are mediated by ET-1. Other data, derived from non-prostatic activities, may help explain the functions and interactions of these two different hormones. For example, Gomez-Garre *et al.* (55) find that both these hormones evoke similar responses in mesangial cells of the rat kidney: mitogenesis and production of matrix protein, acting through Angio-II and ET-1, respectively (56). Similarly, Bell *et al.* (57) show, in blood flow studies of two rat tumors, a direct, although not identical, response to both hormones. More provocative, and perhaps illuminating, is the study of Jahan *et al.* (58) of the direct effects of ET-l and Angio-II on cell-cycle progression in rat aorta smooth muscle cells in primary culture: these agents have no effect on the cell cycle of GO cells, whereas platelet-derived growth factor (PDGF) stimulates the entry of GO cells into the G1 phase without further progression to the S and M phases. However, when these cells are brought to the G1 phase by PDGF treatment, they are stimulated by ET-l and by Angio-II to undergo progression to the S and M phases. Thus, both hormones, though not initiators, are promoters of cell cycle progression by smooth muscle cells.

Nitric oxide

Counterbalancing the depressor effects of ET-l is the dilator NO, which is also produced by endothelial cells. Their antagonistic actions, coupled with those of the autonomic nervous system, determine vascular tone. NO is produced in the endothelial cells from L-arginine by nitric oxide synthase (NOS) (59), an enzyme stimulated not only by ET-1, but also by IGF-1 and VEGF. Evidently, NO mediates aspects of VEGF-signaling required for endothelial cell proliferation and organization *in vitro*. There is biochemical and immunohistochemical evidence (60) of catalytically active NOS in both the transition zone (site of BPH) and peripheral zone (site of PCa).

Heme oxygenase

Yet another agent contributing to homeostasis of blood flow rate, through effects on the vascular endothelium, is the heme oxygenase enzyme, HO-l. Whereas the expression of endothelial NOS gene is suppressed by hypoxia, the expression of heme oxygenase, the enzyme catalyzing production of carbon monoxide (CO), is up-regulated by hypoxia (61). When mammalian cells are subjected to hypoxia, transcription of genes encoding erythropïietin, VEGF, and, as one might expect, the glycolytic enzymes aldolase A, enolase 1, and lactic dehydrogenase (62). Heme oxygenase is responsible for the breakdown of heme to CO and biliverdin. CO is a vasodilator, which suppresses the production of ET-1 and PDGF-B by endothelial cells (63). In the prostate, Hedlund *et al.* (64) found that the arginine–NO pathway may have a role in the control of smooth muscle activity and/or in secretory neurotransmission. The expression of HO-l is increased in both BPH and malignant prostate tissue (65). Now, through use of *in vivo* electrode measurements, Movsas *et al.* (66) show that hypoxic regions exist in human prostate carcinoma. In fact, Zhong *et al.* (67) have found that hypoxia-inducible factor 1 can be detected even in normoxic PC-3 cells. In contemplating the wide assortment of agents and processes so tightly regulating the oxygenation of prostatic tissue, it is crucial to remember that all these are subject to quantitative and probably qualitative adaptive changes accompanying depletion or repletion of the circulating androgen level: the set point (68, 69).

Contractile activity

It is generally accepted that, in symptomatic BPH, besides the increase in tissue mass described above, there is a dynamic contractile component related to smooth muscle tone (70). Elbadawi and Goodman (7l) provide an exhaustive review of the autonomic innervation of male genital glands. Farrell (72) showed that ejaculation could be induced by pilocarpine in dogs that had been cannulated so as to permit collection of just prostatic fluid. Refinements of the cannulation procedure by Huggins and Sommers (73) made possible quantitation of efflux and assessment of the effect of hornones. A similar study of the cannulated rat ventral prostate (74) showed that there is a steady tonically stimulated retrograde secretion, which is blocked by atropine and by antiadrenergic drugs. In addition, there is an antegrade flow, which is increased by both pilocarpine and catecholamines. The finding that the action of pilocarpine can be blocked by Dibenzyline or reserpine suggested that this action is mediated by catecholamincs. This action was considered to reflect a shift in the rate of cellular efflux and not as variations in the extent of muscular contraction since there was

not any visible evidence of the latter. Bruschini *et al.* (75), repeating these same experiments in the dog, showed that secretion is evoked by cholinergic stimulation, whereas urethral contractions, which effectively express the secretion into the lumen, are due to sympathetic stimulation. More recent work by Jacobs and Story (76) and by Wang *et al.* (77) suggest that, in the rat prostate, emission of seminal fluid from the prostatic urethra occurs in response to smooth muscle contraction, caused by adrenergic action on α_1 receptors. Extensive neuroanatomical and neurophysiological investigations (78) in the rat now make clear that the predominant adrenergic input to the prostate is from the short adrenergic neurons, while the close relationship of cholinergic nerves to glandular epithelium is suggestive of a secretory function.

There are different interpretations of the likely mechanism of action of cholinergic agonists. For example, Jacobs and Story (76) demonstrated release of the growth factor EGF by pilocarpine and surmised that EGF secretion represents a true cholinergic response and not a reflex α-adrenergic activity. A more recent study of the potentiation and inhibition of neuronal nicotinic receptors by atropine (79) invites reinterpretation of these relationships. However, it has been clearly shown that EGF secretion into rat prostatic fluid is under both α_1-adrenergic and cholinergic control (76). Apparently, receptor agonists can cause contraction of the smooth muscle to expel fluid from the rat prostate. On the other hand, carbachol induces direct epithelial cell secretion through a mechanism other than contraction of the smooth muscle of the gland.

Hormonal control

Both prostatic weight and the volume of the gland's secretion vary directly with testosterone level. However, since the concentration of protein and PAP does not vary with androgen level, it appears that the composition of prostatic fluid is under neural, not hormonal, control (80, 81).

Pharmacology

Our knowledge of how smooth muscle tone and contraction of the human bladder neck, surgical capsule, and prostatic stroma are driven began with the demonstration by Caine *et al.* (82) that treatment of BPH tissue with the mixed α_1/α_2-adrenal receptor antagonist phenoxybenzamine will reduce urethral resistance and thereby increase uroflow, accompanied by symptomatic

relief. As reviewed by Andersson *et al.* (83), while phenoxybenzamine is clinically effective and has a high
affinity for both α_1- and α_2-adrenal receptors, the contractile properties are mediated principally by α_1-
adrenal receptors. In addition, there is a significant
incidence and severity of adverse effects of phenoxybenzamine arising from interactions independent of the
α_1-adrenal receptors. Clinically, therefore, a preferred
agent is prazosin, which is active only on the α_1-recep-
tor. Autoradiography (70) indicates that 85% of prazosin is localized in the fibromuscular stroma, with a
much lower density (15%) on the glandular epithelium.
Based on other findings, which show that stroma and
epithelium exist in a similar ratio, it is estimated that >
95% of the α_1-receptor in human prostate is associated
with the stroma.

The innovative experiments of Guh *et al.* (84)
provide a plausible explanation of the effects of noradrenaline on the tone of the hyperplastic prostate. They
found that ouabain, at a concentration insufficient by
itself to cause contraction, elicits an increase in tone,
following repeated stimulation by noradrenaline or an
electric field. This is interpreted as showing that the
increased tone is due to increased Ca^{2+} entry and
decreased Ca^{2+} extrusion through the Na^+/Ca^{2+}
exchange system as a consequence of Na^+ pump inhibition by this cardiac glycoside.

Standley *et al.* (85) showed that IGF-I enhances (Na^+
+ K^+)-ATPase activity in vascular smooth muscle cells
(VSMC). It has been rapid and long-lasting effects. The
early (rapid), but not the long-lasting, effect is diminished, in part, by an inhibition of Na^+/H^+ exchange. As
mentioned above, the (Na^+ + K^+)-ATPase is an important mediator of vascular tone, $[Ca^{2+}]$, intracellular pH
and growth. The fact that IGF-I is secreted locally by
VSMC and endothelial cells suggests that this growth
factor (hormone) may regulate local blood flow and
short-term vascular growth. Since long-term activity of
the pump is diminished by use of a specific inhibitor of
the Na^+/H^+ exchange, perhaps part of the activity of
the pump is due to increased intracellular Na^+ and/or
intracellular pH.

Muscarinic activity

Unlike the abundant and clear-cut information about
adrenal receptors, knowledge of cholinergic participation in contractile and secretory activity is limited. As
noted earlier, the presence of muscarinic cholinergic
receptors has been well-documented in human and rat

prostates. But, while cholinergic agonists are known to
cause contraction of a number of smooth muscles,
including the urinary bladder, urethra, and prostatic
capsule, Caine *et al.* (82) did not observe any cholinergic contraction of prostate adenoma. However, by use
of both radioligand-binding and subtype-specific antibodies, the M1 subtype of the muscarinic receptor was
found to be present in BPH and was, in fact, the predominant (75%) subtype there (8l, 86). Two possible
functions of these receptors in the human prostate are
stimulation of prostatic secretion and growth. As
Famsworth and Lawrence (74) and Wang *et al.* (77)
showed in the rat prostate, cholinergic stimulation produces a steady, low level of secretion without histologic
evidence of muscle contraction. In the human prostate,
the anatomic location of muscarinic receptors
(specifically the M1 type) on the glandular epithelium
makes the possibility of a secretory role for muscarinic
receptors an attractive hypothesis. Since the M1 receptor from BPH immunoprecipitates with α subunits of
the G proteins, it is postulated that G12, perhaps the
M1 receptor, affects cell growth of the adenoma,
through phospholipase C. This enzyme hydrolyzes
phosphatidylinositol—bis—phosphate to inositol
trisphosphate (IP3) and diacylglycerol, stimulates
arachidonic acid release, and opens calcium channels.
Gutkind (87) showed that, when cell cultures, transfected with genes coding for M1, M3, and M5, are
treated with the muscarinic agonist carbachol, they
undergo transformation. Ruggieri *et al.* (86) proposed
that these muscarinic receptors, linked to the PI system,
stimulate the proliferation of LNCaP cells but not their
production of PSA.

Contractile activity

In 1993, Langenstroer *et al.* (52) presented the first
detailed characterization of endothelin in the human
prostate and showed that ET-1 is markedly prominent
in the glandular epithelium, but of minimum concentration in the stroma. Isometric tension studies revealed
that the contractile response to ET-1 is not affected by
indomethacin, terazosin, or nifedipine, but that extracellular calcium is a common requirement for both ET-
l and phenylephrine to elicit this contraction. Thus,
ET-1, an epithelial secretion product, mediates a potent
contraction of human prostatic smooth muscle cells
that is not mediated via á$_1$ adrenergic, or dihydropyridine-sensitive calcium channels or prostaglandin synthesis.

Androgen effects

The effects of androgen deprivation have been studied in the rabbit prostatic urethra and the dog prostate. The sensitivity of the adrenergic contractile response in the dog prostate (88) is not affected by androgen deprivation; nor is α-adrenergic contractile activity in the dog prostate regulated by androgen. The rabbit prostatic urethra (89) does respond to androgen deprivation by a decrease in electrically evoked relaxation, probably due to an impairment of the relaxing ability of the smooth muscle in response to NO.

Acknowledgements

I thank the following for gracious help and moral support: Drs Leslie Costello, Renty Franklin, Chung Lee, John McNeal, and Mr. Robert Kelley and Ms Katherine Sugg.

References

1. Waxman J. Hormonal aspects of prostatic cancer; a review. *Roy Soc Med* 1985, **78**, 125–35.
2. Bonfiglio TA, Terry R. The pathology of cancer. In: *Clinical oncology. A multidisciplinary approach* (6th edn) (ed. Rubin P). Am Cancer Soc, Rochester 1983, 20–9.
3. Blacklock NJ. Surgical anatomy. In: *Scientific foundations of urology* (2nd edn) (ed. Chisholm GD, Williams DS). William Heinemann Med Books, London 1982, 473–85.
4. Nemeth JA, Lee C. Prostatic duct system in rats: regional variation in stromal organization. *Prostate* 1996, **28**, 124–8.
5. Bonkhoff H, Remberger K. Differentiation pathways and histogenetic aspects of normal, hyperplastic and neoplastic prostate: a stem cell model. *Prostate* 1996, **28**, 98–106.
6. Aumilller G, Leonhardt M, Janssen M *et al.* Neurogenic origin of human prostate endocrine cells. *Urology* 1999, **53**, 1041–8.
7. Farnsworth WE. Prostate stroma: physiology. *Prostate* 1999, **38**, 60–72.
8. Farnsworth WE. Roles of estrogen and SHBG in prostate physiology. *Prostate* 1996, **28**, 17–23.
9. Levine AC, Kirschenbaum A, Gabrilove JL. The role of sex steroids in the pathogenesis and maintenance of benign prostatic hyperplasia. *Mt Sinai J Med* 1997, **64**, 20–5.
10. Krieg M, Weisser H, Tunn S. Potential activities of androgen metabolizing enzymes in human prostate. *Steroid Biochem Molec Biol* 1995, **53**, 395–400.
11. Krieg M, Nass R, Tunn S. Effect of aging on the endogenous levels of 5α-dihydro-testosterone, testosterone, estradiol, and estrone in epithelium and stroma of normal and hyperplastic human prostate. *J Clin Endocrinol Metab* 1993, **77**, 375–81.
12. Gann PH, Hennekens CH, Longcope C *et al.* A prospective study of plasma hormone levels, nonhormonal factors, and development of benign prostatic hyperplasia. *Prostate* 1995, **26**, 40–9.
13. McNeal JE. Anatomy of the prostate: an historical survey of divergent views. *Prostate* 1980, **1**, 3–13.
14. Seppelt U. Correlation among prostate stroma, plasma estrogen levels and urinary estrogen excretion in patients with benign prostatic hypertrophy. *J Clin Endocrinol Metab* 1978, **47**, 1230–5.
15. Pardridge WM. Transport of protein-bound hormones into tissue *in vivo. Endocrine Revs* 1981, **2**, 103–23.
16. Deering RE, Bigler SA, Brown M *et al.* Microvascularity in benign prostatic hyperplasia. *Prostate* 1985, **26**, 111–15.
17. Stege R, Carlstrom K. Testicular and adrenocortical function in healthy men and in men with benign prostatic hyperplasia. *J Steroid Biochem Molec Biol* 1992, **42**, 357–62.
18. Farnsworth WE. Estrogen in the etiopathogenesis of BPH. *Prostate* 1999, **41**, 263–74.
19. Costello LC, Franklin RB. Concepts of citrate production and secretion by prostate, 2. Hormonal relationships in normal and neoplastic prostate. *Prostate* 1991, **19**, 181–205.
20. Ben-Jonathan N, Mershon JL, Allen DL *et al.* Extrapituitary prolactin: distribution, regulation, functions, and clinical aspects. *End Revs* 1996, **17**, 639–69.
21. Nevalainen MT, Valve EM, Ingleton PM *et al.* Prolactin and prolactin receptors are expressed and functioning in human prostate. *J Clin Invest* 1997, **99**, 618–27.
22. Farnsworth WE. TRH: mediator of prolactin in the prostate? *Med Hypotheses* 1993, **41**, 450–4.
23. Hang J, Rillema JA. Prolactin effects on lipoprotein lipase (LPL) activity and on LPL mRNA levels in cultured mouse mammary gland explants. *Proc Soc Exptl Biol Med* 1997, **216**, 98–203.
24. English HE, Drago JR, Santen RJ. Cellular response to androgen depletion and repletion in the rat ventral prostate: autoradioraphy and morphometric analysis. *Prostate* 1985, **7**, 41–51.
25. Shabsigh A, Chang DT, Heitjan DF *et al.* Rapid reduction in blood flow in the rat ventral prostate gland after castration: preliminary evidence that androgens influence prostate size by regulating blood flow to the prostate gland and prostate epithelial cell survival. *Prostate* 1998, **36**, 201–6.
26. Lekas E, Johansson M, Widmark A *et al.* Decrement of blood flow precedes the involution of the ventral prostate in the rat after castration. *Urol Res* 1997, **25**, 309–14.
27. Farnsworth WE. Prostate stroma: physiology. *Prostate* 1999, **38**, 60–72.
28. Karas RH, Gauer EA, Bieber HE *et al.* Growth factor activation of the estrogen receptor in vascular cells

occurs via a mitogen-activated protein kinase-independent pathway. *Clin Invest* 1998, **101**, 2851–61.

29. Farhat MY, Lavigne MC, Remwell PW. The vascular protective effects of estrogen. *FASEB* 1996, **10**, 615–24.

30. Williams-Ashman HG. Discussion. In: *National Cancer Institute Monograph 12: Biology of Prostate and Related Tissues*, 1963, 250.

31. Mann T. Biochemistry of the prostate gland and its secretion. In: *National Cancer Institute Monograph 12: Biology of Prostate and Related Tissues*, 1963, 235–249.

32. Costello L. Commentary: Intermediary metabolism of normal and malignant prostate: a neglected area of prostate research. *Prostate* 1998, **34**, 303–4.

33. Barron ESG, Huggins C. The citric acid and aconitase content of the prostate. *Proc Soc Exptl Biol Med* 1946, **62**, 195–6.

34. Williams-Ashman HG. Changes in the enzymatic constitution of the ventral prostate induced by androgenic horD1ones. *Endocrinology* 1954, **54**, 121–9.

35. Farnsworth WE, Brown JR. Androgen on prostatic biosynthetic reactions. *Endocrinology* 1961, **68**, 978–86.

36. Barron ESG, Huggins C. The metabolism of the prostate: transamination and citric acid. *J Urol* 1946, **55**, 385–90.

37. Barron ESG, Huggins C. The metabolism of the prostate: transamination and citric acid. *J Urol* 1946, **55**, 385–90.

38. Costello LC, Franklin RB. The intermediary metabolism of the prostate: a key to understanding the pathogenesis and progression of prostate malignancy. *Oncology* 2000, **59**, 269–82.

39. Farnsworth WE. Activities of the androgen-responsive receptor of the prostatic plasma membrane. *Invest Urol* 1977, **15**, 75–7.

40. Farnsworth WE. Prostate plasma membrane receptor: a hypothesis. *Prostate* 1991, **19**, 329–52.

41. Swinnen JV, Verhoeven G. Androgens and the control of lipid metabolism in human prostate cells. *J Steroid Biochem Molec Biol* 1998, **65**, 191–8.

42. Nyden SJ, Williams-Ashman HG. Influence of androgens on synthetic reactions in ventral prostate tissue. *Am J Physiol* 1953, **172**, 588–600.

43. Behrooz A, Ismai1-Beigi F. Stimulation of glucose transport by hypoxia: signals and mechanisms. *News Physiol Sci* 1999, **14**, 105–10.

44. Farnsworth WE. Physiology and biochemistry of prostatic secretion. In: *Scientific foundations of urology* (2nd edn) (ed. Chisholm GD, Williams DI). Wil1iam Heinemann Medical Books, London 1982, 485–90.

45. Lechevalier E, Eghazarian C, Ortega J-C *et al*. Kinetics of post biopsy levels of serum free prostate-specific antigen and percent free prostate-specific antigen. *Urology* 1999, **53**, 731–5.

46. Kirchheimer JC, Binder BR. Plasminogen activators. In: *The prostate as an endocrine gland* (ed. Farnsworth WE, Ablin RJ). CRC Press, Boca Raton 1990, 37–45.

47. Reichlin S. Neuroendocrinology. In: *William's textbook of endocrinology* (9th edn) (ed. Wilson JD, Foster DW, Kronenberg HM *et al*.). WB Saunders, Philadelphia 1998, 165–248.

48. Cao Y, Ti RW, Davidson O *et al*. Kringle domains of human angiostatin. Characterization of the antiproliferative activity on endothelial cells. *J Biol Chem* 1996, **271**, 29461–7.

49. Gately S, Twardowski P, Stack MS *et al*. The mechanism of cancer-mediated conversion of plasminogen to the angiogenesis inhibitor angiostatin. *Proc Natl Acad Sci USA* 1997, **94**, 10868–72.

50. Quian X, Wang TN, Rothman VL *et al*. Thrombospondin-l modulates angiogenesis in vitro by up-regu1ation of matrix metalloproteinase-9 in endothelial cells. *Exptl Cell Res* 1997, **235**, 403–12.

51. Stearns ME, Rhim J and Wang M. Interleukin 10 (IL-I0) inhibition of primary human prostate cell-induced angiogenesis: IL-10 stimulation of tissue inhibitor of metalloproteinase-l and inhibition of matrix metalloproteinase MMP-2/MMP-9 secretion. *Clin Cancer Res* l999, **5**, 189–96.

52. Langenstroer P, Tang R, Shapiro E *et al*. Endothelin-l in human prostate: tissue levels, source of production and isometric tension studies. *J Urol* 1993, **149**, 495–9.

53. Grant ES, Brown T, Roach A *et al*. In vitro expression of endothelin-l (ET-1) and the ET_A and ET_B ET receptors by prostatic epitheliun and stroma. *J Clin Endocrinol Metab* 1997, **82**, 508–513.

54. Rajagolalan S, Laursen, JB, Borthayre A *et al*. Role for endothelin-l in angiotensin II-mediated hypertension. *Hypertension* 1997, **30**, 29–34

55. Gomez-Garre D, Ruiz-Ortega M, Ortego M *et al*. Effects and interactions of endothelin-l and angiotensin II on matrix protein expression and synthesis and mesangial growth. *Hypertension* 1996, **27**, 885–92.

56. Stojilkovic SS, Catt KJ. Expression and signal transduction pathways of endothelin receptors in neuroendocrine cells. *Frontiers in Neuroendocrinology* 1996, **17**, 327–69.

57. Bell KM, Prise VE, Shaffi KM *et al*. A comparative study of tumour blood flow modification in two rat tumour systems using endothelin-l and angiotensin II: influence of tumour size on angiotensin II response. *Int J Cancer* 1996, **67**, 730–8.

58. Jahan H, Kobayashi S, Nishimura J *et al*. Endothelin-l and angiotensin II act as progression but not competence growth factors in vascular smooth muscle cells. *Eur J Pharmacol* 1996, **295**, 261–9.

59. Harrison DG. Nitric oxide and nitric oxide synthase. *J Clin Invest* 1997, **100**, 2153–7.

60. Burnett AL, Macquire MP, Chamness SL *et al*. Characterization and localisation of nitric oxide synthase in the hunan prostate. *Urology* 1995, **45**, 435–9.

61. Liu Y, Christou H, Morita T *et al*. Carbon monoxide and nitric oxide suppress the hypoxic induction of vascular endothelial growth factor gene via the 5′ enhancer. *J Biol Chem* 1998, **273**, 15257–62.

62. Semenza GL, Jiang B-H, Lemg SW *et al*. Hypoxia response elements in the enolase A, enolase 1, and lactate dehydrogenase A gene promoters contain essential binding sites for hypoxia-inducible factor 1. *J Biol Chem* 1996, **271**, 32529–37.

63. Kourembanas S, Morita T, Liu Y *et al*. Mechanisms by which oxygen regulates gene-expression and cell-cell

interaction in the vasculature. *Kidney International* 1997, **51**, 438–43.

64. Hedlund P, Ekstrom P, Larsson B *et al*. Heme oxygenase and NO-synthase in the human prostate-relation to adrenergic, cholinergic and peptide-containing nerves. *J Autonom Nervous System* 1997, **63**, 115–26.

65. Maines MD, Abrahamsson PA. Expression of heme oxygenase-l (HSP32) in human prostate: normal, hyperplastic, and tumor tissue distribution. *Urology* 1996, **47**, 727–33.

66. Movsas B, Chapman JD, Horwitz EM *et al*. Hypoxic region exists in human prostate carcinoma. *Urology* 1999, **53**, 11–8.

67. Zhong H, Agani F, Baccala AA *et al*. Increased expression of hypoxia inducible factor-1α in rat and human prostate cancer. *Cancer Res* 1998, **58**, 5280–4.

68. Franck-Lissbrant I, Haggstrom S, Damber JE *et al*. Testosterone stimulates angiogenesis and vascular regrowth in the ventral prostate in castrated adult rats. *Endocrinology* 1998, **139**, 451–6.

69. Sordello S, Bertrand N, Plouet J. Vascular endothelial growth factor is up-regulated *in vitro* and *in vivo* by androgens. *Biochem Biophys Res Commun* 1998, **251**, 287–90.

70. Kenny B, Ballard S, Blagg J *et al*. Pharmacological options in the treatment of benign prostatic hyperplasia. *J Medicinal Chem* 1997, **40**, 1293–315.

71. Elbadawi A Goodman DC. Autonomic innervation of accessory male genital glands. In: *Male accessory sex glands* (ed. Spring-Mills E, Hafez ESS). Elsevier/North-Holland, Amsterdam, 1980, 101–28.

72. Farrell JI. Studies of the secretion of the prostate gland. I. A method of collecting the pure secretion of the dog. II. Factors influencing the secretion of prostatic fluid III. Some properties of the prostatic secretion of the dog. *Tr Am A Genito Urin Surgeons* 1931, **24**, 221–30.

73. Huggins C, Sommer JL. Quantitative studies of prostatic secretion. III. Simultaneous measurement of size and secretion of the canine prostate and the interaction of androgenic and estrogenic substances thereon. *J Exper Med* 1953, **97**, 663–80.

74. Farnsworth WE, LawrenceMH. Regulation of prostatic secretion in the rat. *Proc Soc Exptl Biol Med* 1965, **119**, 373–6.

75. Bruschini H, Schmidt RA, Tanagho EA. Neurologic control of prostatic secretion in the dog. *Invest Urol* 1978, **15**, 288–90.

76. Jacobs SC, Story MT. Exocrine secretion of epidermal growth factor by the rat prostate: effect of adrenergic agents, cholinergic agents, and vasoactive intestinal peptide. *Prostate* 1988, **13**, 79–87

77. Wang JM, McKenna KE, Lee C. Determination of prostate secretion in rats: effect of neurotransmitters and testosterone. *Prostate* 1991, **18**, 289–301.

78. McVary KT, McKenna KE, Lee C. Prostate innervation. *Prostate* 1998, **8** (Suppl), 2–13.

79. Zwart R, Vijverberg HPM. Potentiation and inhibition of neuronal nicotinic receptors by atropine: competitive and noncompetitive effects. *Molec Pharmacol* 1997, **52**, 886–95.

80. Huggins C. The prostate secretion. *Harvey Lect* 1947, **42**, 148–93.

81. Luthin GR, Wang P, Zhou H *et al*. Role of M1 receptor-G protein in cell proliferation in the prostate. *Life Sci* 1997, **60**, 963–8.

82. Caine M, Raz S and Zeigler M. Adrenergic and cholinergic receptors in the human prostate, prostate capsule and bladder. *Brit J Urol* 1975, **47**, 197–202.

83. Andersson KE, Lepor H and Wyllie MG. Prostatic a-adrenoceptors and uroselectivity. *Prostate* 1997, **30**, 202–15.

84. Guh JH, Ko FN, Chueh S-C *et al*. Ouabain-induced increases in the resting tone of human hyperplastic prostate following repeated noradrenaline and electric field stimulation. *Brit J Pharmacol* 1996, **117**, 1716–20

85. Standley PR, Zhang F, Zayas RM *et al*. IGF-I regulation of Na^+-K^+-ATPase in rat arterial smooth muscle. *Am J Physiol* 1997, **273**, 113–121.

86. Ruggieri MR, Colton MD, Wang P *et al*. Human prostate muscarinic receptor subtypes. *J Pharmacol Exper Ther* 1995, **274**, 976–82.

87. Gutkind JS, Novotny EA, Brann MR *et al*. Muscarinic acetylcholine receptor subtypes as agonist-dependent oncogenes. *Proc Biol Acad Sci USA* 1991, **88**, 4703–7

88. Lin AT-L, Chen M-T, Chiang H *et al*. Effect of orchiectomy on the alpha-adrenergic contractile response of dog prostate. *J Urol* 1995, **154**, 1930–3

89. Holmquist F, Persson K, Bodker A *et al*. Some pre- and postjunctional effects of castration. Rabbit isolated corpus cavernosa and urethra. *J Urol* 1994, **152**, 1011–6.

3 | Pituitary hormone receptors of the prostate

Eric Reiter and Jean Closset

Introduction

The organogenesis and secretory activity of the prostate gland are under hormonal control. Androgens play a major role in this regulation during both development and adult life (1). Moreover, androgen depletion very rapidly induces apoptosis in the prostate (2). Yet although essential, androgens alone are not sufficient to induce normal growth of the prostate or to ensure its normal functioning. Furthermore, non-androgenic hormones must be involved in the proliferation of prostate cancer cells that do not respond to anti-androgen therapy and thus become androgen independent (3, 4). It is paradoxical, furthermore, that testosterone levels decrease with age in men, whilst the incidence of prostatic diseases increases dramatically (5, 6).

Non-androgenic steroids and some peptide hormones and growth factors can exert synergistic or antagonistic effects on the prostate (1, 4). Furthermore, prostatic cells secrete numerous growth factors: nerve growth factor, insulin-like growth factors, epidermis-derived growth factor, transforming growth factors, fibroblast growth factors, platelet-derived growth factor (7–9). These growth factors play an important role in regulating prostatic growth through autocrine or paracrine control mechanisms. Relationships between the stromal and epithelial compartments of the gland are also involved in prostate physiology and physiopathy (1, 10, 11). In this context, identifying the endocrine and intraprostatic factors that control prostate function, and understanding their mechanisms of action, are important objectives, given the very high incidence of prostate diseases in men.

Pituitary hormones act on the prostate

It has long been established that regression of the prostate is more pronounced after hypophysectomy combined with castration than after castration alone (12–14). Recent work by Varani *et al.* shows that pituitary extracts are required for successful maintenance of human prostate tissue, non-malignant or malignant, for several days in organ culture (15). Prolactin (PRL) was initially believed to be the only pituitary hormone acting on the prostate, but it has recently been shown that growth hormone (GH), luteinizing hormone (LH), and follicle-stimulating hormone (FSH) are also important in normal and pathological development of the prostate (16, 17). Specific receptors for these three hormones have been detected by various approaches in human and/or rodent prostates, and co-expression of some of these receptors with their specific hormonal ligands has been evidenced in various normal and pathological situations (Fig. 3.1). The aim of the present chapter is to detail the available data concerning expression of pituitary hormone receptors in the prostate and the related functional consequences.

Prolactin receptors

High-affinity receptors for prolactin (PRL-R) are expressed in the prostate (18–20). PRL stimulates the proliferation (21, 22) and differentiation (23) of prostate cells. In intact and hypophysectomized rats, PRL injections increase the weight of the gland (24) and enhance RNA/DNA synthesis in all the lobes (25). Hyperprolactinemia, induced by combined androgen/estrogen treatment, is responsible for the development of inflammation (26), dysplasia, and adenocarcinoma (27) in the dorsolateral lobes of the gland. These effects are completely reversed in the presence of bromocriptin (26–28). Wennbo *et al.* generated several lines of transgenic mice overexpressing PRL and observed that prostate weight was 20 times higher in these mice than in wild-type (*wt*) animals (29). Symmetrically, male mice with targeted disruption of the PRL gene display a significantly lower prostate weight than their *wt* counterparts (30, 31). PRL-R gene knock-out mice have also been generated, but prostate

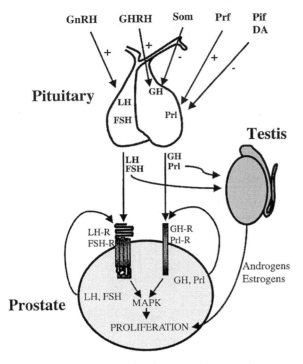

Fig. 3.1 Hypothetical mode of action of pituitary hormones on the prostate: GnRH, gonadotropin-releasing hormone; GHRH, growth hormone releasing hormone; Som, somatostatin; Prf, prolactin-releasing factor; Pif, prolactin-inhibitory factor; DA, dopamine; MAPK, mitogen-activated protein kinase.

function has not yet been evaluated in these animals (32). All these effects may be due in part to the stimulating action of PRL on testicular steroidogenesis (33), but PRL can also act directly through its receptors and subsequently enhance 5-reductase activity and receptivity to androgens (34–38).

More recently it has been demonstrated that PRL can also exert androgen-independent effects on the prostate (39, 40). In the rat, PRL increases the zinc and citrate concentrations in the lateral prostate (23, 41) and the activity of mitochondrial aspartate aminotransferase (40). These effects are completely independent of androgens. We have also shown that in all the lobes of the rat prostate, and independently of androgens, PRL can stimulate synthesis of certain major proteins: the C3 subunit of prostatein in the ventral lobes, probasin and RWB in the dorsolateral lobes (42). These same effects of PRL were observed in the presence of Finasteride and in explant cultures (42).

The exact role of PRL in human prostate pathology is not yet clear. Circulating PRL levels increase with age, so the PRL concentration is high when prostate diseases develop (43, 44). Yet conflicting results have been reported, showing either increased (45, 46) or unchanged PRL levels in the case of benign prostatic hyperplasia (BPH), but increased levels in patients with prostatic carcinoma (47). The recent observation that PRL is produced in the prostate itself (48, 49) may partially explain these differences. It also suggests that PRL-R could be involved in both systemic and autocrine/paracrine regulations. In addition, it is now well established that PRL-R can activate the MAPK (mitogen-activated protein kinase) signaling cascade and hence promote cell proliferation in response to PRL (50).

Growth hormone receptors

Expression of the GH receptor (GH-R) throughout the male reproductive system, including the prostate gland, was demonstrated in 1990 (51). Since then, we have shown that short-term GH treatment stimulates prostatic expression of androgen receptor, IGF-I, and IGF-I receptor in hypophysectomized immature rats (38). We were unable to determine in this model, however, whether these effects were mediated by GH-R, by the IGF-I receptor, or whether they resulted from stimulation of testicular steroidogenesis following hormone treatment. We later demonstrated effects of GH treatment on adult GH-deficient dwarf rats and on hypophysectomized and castrated normal adult rats (52). In both models, hormone treatment induced an increase in the levels of prostatein C3 subunit, probasin, and RWB RNAs, thus affecting the different lobes of the prostate. This series of experiments showed, moreover, that the role of GH is at least partly distinct from that of androgens and modulated by GH or IGF-I receptors, expressed in large quantities in the rat prostate (38, 52). In run-on assays it was shown that GH stimulates C3 and probasin gene transcription, while IGF-I stimulates the latter (52). The presence of sequences resembling the consensus for STAT 5 in the promoters of the C3 and probasin genes (the 5′ regulating end region of the RWB gene is still unknown) may explain these results. Moreover, the prostates of transgenic mice over-expressing bovine GH weigh considerably more than those of wild-type mice, as observed in two laboratories using different lines (29, 53). Nguyen *et al.*, furthermore, have recently demonstrated the important role played by GH, during fetal life, in the differentiation of the male reproductive tract including the prostate (54). The observation that prostate weight is significantly reduced in IGF-I gene knock-out mice confirms that IGF-I may mediate the effects of GH on the gland (55).

Regarding the potential role of GH in prostate diseases, we have shown that cell lines derived from human tumors (lines LNCaP and PC3) and rat tumors (lines MAT-Lu, MAT-LiLu, and PIF-I) express more transcripts corresponding to GH-R and binding protein than normal tissue (52). Like the PRL-R, the GH-R can induce the MAPK signaling pathway and thus mediate proliferation (56). These data suggest that GH may be directly involved in prostate cancer, an hypothesis supported by a recent study by Jungwirth *et al.* (57). These authors showed a highly significant inhibitory effect of MZ-4–71, a novel antagonist of growth hormone releasing hormone, on *in vivo* proliferation of different prostate tumor cell lines. When the tumorigenous and androgen-independent cell lines DU-145 and PC-3 were xenografted into nude mice, and when Dunning R-3327 AT-1 cells were transplanted into rats, animals treated with MZ-4–71 showed a considerably diminished tumor volume as compared to control animals. Systematic studies in humans are now necessary to establish whether the promising results obtained with these experimental models can be achieved in man. If so, molecules like MZ-4–71 could be candidates for treating androgen-independent prostate tumors. Other investigators have obtained improved clinical performances of patients with hormone-refractory prostate cancer by using a combination of dexamethasone, triptorelin, and a somatostatin analog (lanreotide) at doses capable of decreasing GH production in the pituitary gland (58). In studies on acromegalic, GH-deficient, and healthy subjects, furthermore, chronic excesses of GH and IGF-I were shown to cause prostate overgrowth and further rearrangement phenomena, but not prostate cancer (59, 60). Some of these effects were reversed by treatment with octreotide, which normalizes the circulating levels of both GH and IGF-I (59). Finally, an epidemiological study has demonstrated a strong positive association between IGF-I plasma levels and prostate cancer risk (61). Together, these spectacular results should lead to viewing the GH/IGF-I axis as important in prostate pathologies.

Gonadotropin receptors

It is well known that LH, by stimulating testicular steroidogenesis, plays a major role in prostate physiology. The idea that LH might also act directly on the prostate gland is very recent, the first results having been published in 1995. By cloning the gene encoding the LH/CG receptor (LH/CG-R), investigators were able to show that the receptor belongs to the seven-transmembrane-domain receptor family (62, 63) and that it is also present in non-gonadal tissues (64). These

data prompted us to look for LH/CG-R in the rat prostate.

Specific LH/CG-R transcripts were detected in the prostates of normal adult rats and a binding site was evidenced, with characteristics similar to those described for the gonadal LH/CG-R (K_a: 6.0×10^9 M^{-1}) (65, 66). LH/CG-R was found to be mainly expressed in the epithelium of the ventral lobe. In explant cultures of normal adult-rat prostates, LH induced a significant dose-dependent stimulation of cAMP (65). A subsequent publication by others has confirmed these results (67).

The heterogeneous distribution of LH/CG-R within the gland and the observed stimulation of cAMP by LH in prostate explant cultures suggest that LH plays a physiological role in the rat prostate. Yet expression of traditional markers of prostate function (C3, probasin, RWB) appears unaffected by this hormone. The differential display technique was used to search for LH-regulated genes in prostates from hypophysectomized and castrated rats, where indirect effects of androgens are impossible (68). The study revealed eight different genes whose expression is significantly stimulated by LH, including the gene encoding ribosomal protein S 23. Interestingly, none of these clones were regulated by androgens, suggesting that LH and androgens use independent signaling pathways to regulate gene transcription in the prostate.

It is now worth addressing the question: is LH involved in human prostate diseases? Recently, Tao *et al.* (69) showed that the LH/CG receptor gene is expressed in the prostates of patients with BPH and cancer. Dirnhofer *et al.* have also evidenced its expression in the prostates of certain BPH and cancer patients (17). In addition, these authors detected transcripts for the gonadotropin alpha subunit, for LH beta, and in some cases, for FSH beta and the FSH receptor, thus opening new avenues for future research. Here again, the possibility of pituitary-independent actions of these hormones should be considered. That gonadotropins might stimulate mitogenic activity in prostatic cells, possibly via an autocrine/paracrine mechanism, is a realistic hypothesis, given the role played by many G-protein-coupled receptors in normal growth control and tumorigenesis (70).

Conclusions and prospects

Growth hormone, LH, and to a lesser extent FSH, must now be viewed as hormones which, along with steroids and prolactin, act directly on the prostate. Further work must be carried out to fully characterize the action of GH, LH, and FSH, and extend our knowledge of the action of prolactin. Human pathologies involving selective hypersecretion of these hormones (acromegaly, hyperprolactinemia, and gonadotropinoma) represent very interesting models for studying the effects of these hormones on the prostate and the mechanisms involved. Activating and inactivating mutations in LH/CG-R, as well as inactivating mutations in FSH-R, also represent potentially interesting models for assessing the roles of the corresponding hormones in the function and pathogenesis of the human prostate (71–72). It is now possible to produce transgenic mice over-expressing, specifically in the prostate, a hormone or receptor gene (thanks to transgenes whose expression is controlled by the probasin and C3 gene 5′ regulating end regions (73–75). These should be most useful in attempts to understand the physiological roles of all four hormones so as to evaluate their possible involvement in disease. Various lines of gene knock-out mice are now available and constitute models for studying how pituitary hormones affect the prostate (e.g. 30, 32, 55, 76–78). Organ culture methods are also particularly adapted to evaluating a single hormone's effects on the gland (15). Finally, experiments carried out in nude mice or *in vitro* on tumor cell lines should also contribute to evaluating the importance of PRL, GH, LH, and FSH receptors in human prostate diseases.

References

1. Cunha GR, Donjacour AA, Cooke PS *et al.* The endocrinology and developmental biology of the prostate. *Endocr Rev* 1987, **8**, 338–62.

2. Isaacs JT. Antagonistic effect of androgens on prostatic cell death. *Prostate* 1984, **5**, 545–57.

3. Schröder FH. Endocrine therapy for prostate cancer: Recent developments and current status. *Br J Urol* 1993, **71**, 633–40.

4. Wilding G. Endocrine control of prostate cancer. *Canc Surv* 1995, **23**, 43–62.

5. Davidson JM, Chen JJ, Crapo L *et al.* Hormonal changes and sexual function in aging men. *J Clin Endocrinol Metab* 1983, **57**, 71–7.

6. Nankin HR, Calkins JH. Decreased bioavailable testosterone in aging normal and impotent men. *J Clin Endocrinol Metab* 1986, **63**, 1418–20.

7. Story MT. Polypeptide modulators of prostatic growth and development. *Cancer Surv* 1991, **11**, 123–46.

8. Steiner MS. Role of peptide growth factors in the prostate: a review. *Urology* 1993, **42**, 99–110.

9. Sinowatz F, Amselgruber W, Pendl J *et al.* Effects of hormones on the prostate in adult and aging men and animals. *Microsc Res Techn* 1995, **30**, 282–92.

10. Cunha GR, Sekkingstad M, Meloy BA. Heterospecific induction of prostatic development in tissue recombinants prepared with mouse, rat, rabbit and human tissues. *Differentiation* 1983, **24**, 174–80.

11. Cunha GR, Chung LWK, Shannon JM *et al.* Hormone induced morphogenesis and growth: role of mesenchymal epithelial interactions. *Recent Prog Horm Res* 1983, **39**, 559–98.

12. Hunggins C, Russell PS. Quantitative effects of hypophysectomy on testis and prostate of dogs. *Endocrinol* 1946, **39**, 1–7.

13. Grayhack JT, Bunce PL, Kearns JW *et al.* Influence of the pituitary on prostatic response to androgen in the rat. *Bull Johns Hopkins Hosp* 1955, **96**, 154–321.

14. Brendler H. Adrenalectomy and hypophysectomy for prostate cancer. *Urology* 1973, **2**, 99–102.

15. Varani J, Dame MK, Wojno K *et al.* Characteristics of nonmalignant and malignant human prostate in organ culture. *Lab Invest* 1999, **79**, 723–31.

16. Reiter E, Hennuy B, Bruyninx M *et al.* Effects of pituitary hormones on the prostate. *Prostate* 1999, **38**, 159–65.

17. Dirnhofer S, Berger C, Hermann M *et al.* Coexpression of gonadotropic hormones and their corresponding FSH- and LH/CG-receptors in the human prostate. *Prostate* 1998, **35**, 212–20.

18. Aragona C, Friesen HG. Specific prolactin binding site in the prostate and testis of rats. *Endocrinol* 1975, **97**, 677–84.

19. Barkey RJ, Shani J, Amit T *et al.* Specific binding of prolactin to seminal vesicle, prostate, and testicular homogenates of immature, mature and aged rats. *J Endocrinol* 1977, **74**, 163–73.

20. Thompson SA, Johnson MP, Brooks CL. Biochemical and immunohistochemical characterization of prolactin binding in rat ventral, lateral and dorsal prostate lobes. *Prostate* 1982, **3**, 45–58.

21. Grayhack JT. Pituitary factors influencing growth of the prostate. *NCI Monog* 1963, **12**, 189–99.

22. Negro-Vilar A, Saad WA, McCann SM. Evidence for a role of prolactin in prostate and seminal vesicle growth in immature animals. *Endocrinol* 1977, **100**, 729–37.

23. Costello LC, Franklin RB. Effect of Prolactin on the prostate. *Prostate* 1994, **24**, 162–66.

24. Smith C, Assimos D, Lee C *et al.* Metabolic action of prolactin in regressing prostate: independent of androgen action. *Prostate* 1985, **6**, 49–59.

25. Prins GS, Lee C. Biphasic response of the rat lateral prostate to increasing levels of serum prolactin. *Biol Reprod* 1983, **29**, 938–45.

26. Tangbanluekal L, Robinette CL. Prolactin mediates estradiol-induced inflammation in the lateral prostate of Wistar rats. *Endocrinol* 1993, **132**, 2407–16.

27. Lane KE, Leav I, Ziar J *et al.* Suppression of testosterone and estradiol-17?-induced dysplasia in the dorsolateral prostate of Noble rats by bromocriptin. *Carcinogenesis* 1997, **18**, 1505–10.

28. Bosland MC, Ford H, Horton L. Induction of high incidence of ductal prostate adenocarcinomas in NBL/Cr

and Sprague–Dawley Hsd:SD rats treated with a combination of testosterone and estadiol-17? or DES. *Carcinogenesis* 1995, **16**, 1311–7.

29. Wennbo H, Kindblom J, Isaksson OGP *et al.* Transgenic mice overexpressing the prolactin gene develop dramatic enlargement of the prostate gland. *Endocrinol* 1997, **138**, 4410–5.

30. Horseman ND, Zhao W, Montecino-Rodriguez E *et al.* Defective mammopoiesis, but normal hematopoiesis, in mice with a targeted disruption of the prolactin gene. *EMBO J* 1997, **16**, 6926–35.

31. Steger RW, Chandrashekar V, Zhao W *et al.* Neuroendocrine and reproductive functions in male mice with targeted disruption of the prolactin gene. *Endocrinol* 1998, **139**, 3691–5.

32. Ormandy CJ, Camus A, Barra J *et al.* Null mutation of the prolactin receptor gene produces multiple reproductive defects in the mouse. *Genes Dev* 1997, **11**, 167–78.

33. Dombrowicz D, Sente B, Closset J *et al.* Dose-dependent effects of human prolactin on the immature hypophysectomized rat testis. *Endocrinol* 1992, **130**, 695–700.

34. Yamanaka H, Kirdani RY, Saroff J *et al.* Effects of testosterone and prolactin on rat prostatic weight, 5α-reductase and arginase. *Am J Physiol* 1975, **229**, 1102–10.

35. Baraneo JLS, Legnani B, Chiauzzi VA *et al.* Effects of prolactin on androgen metabolism in androgen target tissues of immature rats. *Endocrinol* 1982, **109**, 2188–95.

36. Jones R, Riding PR, Parker MG. Effect of prolactin or testosterone induced growth and protein synthesis in rat accessory sex glands. *J Endocr* 1983, **96**, 407–16.

37. Prins GS. Prolactin influence on cytosol and nuclear androgen receptors in the ventral, dorsal and lateral lobes of the rat prostate. *Endocrinol* 1987, **120**, 1457–64.

38. Reiter E, Bonnet P, Sente B *et al.* Growth hormone prolactin stimulate androgen receptor, insulin-like growth factor-I and IGF-I receptor levels in the prostate of immature rats. *Mol Cell Endocrinol* 1992, **88**, 77–87.

39. Nevalainen MT, Valve EM, Mäkelä SI *et al.* Estrogen and prolactin regulation of rat dorsal and lateral prostate in organ culture. *Endocrinol* 1991, **129**, 612–22.

40. Franklin RB, Costello LC. Prolactin stimulates transcription of mitochondrial aspartate a m i n o -transferase of prostate epithelial cells. *Mol Cell Endorinol* 1992, **90**, 27–32.

41. Rui H, Purvis K. Hormonal control of prostate function. *Scand J Urol Nephrol* 1988, **107** (Suppl), 32–8.

42. Reiter E, Lardinois S, Klug M *et al.* Androgen-independent effects of prolactin on the different lobes of the rat prostate. *Mol Cell Endocrinol* 1995, **112**, 113–22.

43. Vekemans M, Robyn C. Influence of age on serum prolactin levels in women and men. *Br Med J* 1975, **4**, 738–9.

44. Hammond GL, Kontturi M, Maattala P *et al.* Serum FSH, LH and prolactin in normal males and patients with prostatic diseases. *Clin Endocrinol* 1977, **7**, 129–35.

45. Saroff J, Kirdani RY, Chu M *et al.* Measurments of prolactin and androgens in patients with prostatic diseases. *Oncology* 1980, **37**, 46–52.

46. Odoma S, Chisholm GD, Nicol K *et al.* Evidence for the association between blood prolactin and androgen receptor in BPH. *J Urol* 1985, **133**, 717–20.

47. Harper ME, Peeling WB, Cowley T *et al.* Plasma steroid and protein hormone concentration in patients with prostatic carcinoma, before and during estrogen therapy. *Acta Endocrinol* 1976, **81**, 409–26.

48. Nevalainen MT, Valve EM, Ingelton PM *et al.* Prolactin and Prolactin receptors are expressed and functioning in the human prostate. *J Clin Invest* 1997, **99**, 618–27.

49. Nevalainen MT, Valve EM, Ahonen T *et al.* Androgen-dependent expression of prolactin in rat prostate epithelium *in vivo* and in organ culture. *FASEB J* 1997, **11**, 1297–307.

50. Bole-Feysot C, Goffin V, Edery M *et al.* Prolactin (PRL) and its receptor: actions, signal transduction pathways and phenotypes observed in PRL receptor knockout mice. *Endocr Rev* 1998, **19**, 225–68.

51. Lobie PE, Breipohl W, Garcia-Aragon J *et al.* Cellular localization of the growth hormone receptor/binding protein in the male and female reproductive systems. *Endocrinol* 1990, **126**, 2214–21.

52. Reiter E, Kecha O, Hennuy B *et al.* Growth Hormone directly affects the function of thc different lobes of the rat prostate. *Endocrinol* 1995, **136**, 3338–45.

53. Ghosh PK, Bartke A. Effects of the expression of bovine growth hormone on the testes and male accessory reproductive glands in transgenic mice. *Transgenic Res* 1993, **2**, 79–83.

54. Nguyen AP, Chandorkak A, Gupta C. The role of growth hormone in fetal mouse reproductive tract differentiation. *Endocrinol* 1996, **137**, 3659–66.

55. Baker J, Hardy MP, Zhou J *et al.* Effects of an IGF-I gene null mutation on mouse reproduction. *Mol Endocrinol* 1996, **10**, 903–18.

56. Vanderkuur JA, Butch ER, Waters SB *et al.* Signaling molecules involved in coupling growth hormone receptor to mitogen-activated protein kinase activation. *Endocrinol* 1997, **138**, 4301–7.

57. Jungwirth A, Schally AV, Pinski J *et al.* Inhibition of *in vivo* proliferation of androgen-independent prostate cancers by an antagonist of growth hormone-releasing hormone. *Br J Cancer* 1997, **75**, 1585–92.

58. Koustilieris M, Tzanela M, Dimopoulos T. Novel concept of antisurvival factor (ASF) therapy produces an objective clinical response in four patients with hormone-refractory prostate cancer: case report. *Prostate* 1999, **38**, 313–6.

59. Colao A, Marzullo P, Ferone D *et al.* Prostatic hyperplasia: an unknown feature of acromegaly. *J Clin Endocrinol Metab* 1998, **83**, 775–9.

60. Colao A, Marzullo P, Spiezia S *et al.* Effect of growth hormone (GH) and insulin-like growth factor I on prostate diseases: an ultrasonographic and endocrine study in acromegaly, GH deficiency, and healthy subjects. J Clin Endocrinol Metab 1999, 84, 1986–1991.

61. Chan JM, Stampfer MJ, Giovannucci E *et al.* Plasma insulin like growth factor-I and prostate cancer risk: a prospective study. *Science* 1998, **279**, 563–6.

62. McFarland KC, Sprengel R, Phillips HS *et al.* Lutropin-choriogonadotropin receptor: an unusual member of G protein-coupled receptor family. *Science* 1989, **245**, 494–9.

63. Loosfelt H, Misrahi M, Atger M *et al.* Cloning and sequencing of porcine LH-hCG receptor cDNA; variants lacking transmembrane domain. *Science* 1989, **245**, 525–8.

64. Rao CV. The beginning of a new era in reproductive biology and medicine : Expression of low levels of functional luteinizing hormone/human chorionic gonadotropin receptors in non gonadal tissues. *J Physiol Pharmacol* 1996, **47**, 41–53.

65. Reiter E, McNamara M, Closset J *et al.* Expression and functionality of luteinizing hormone/chorionic gonadotropin receptor in the rat prostate. *Endocrinol* 1995, **136**, 917–23.

66. Roche PC, Ryan RJ. The LH/hCG receptor. In: *Luteinizing hormone action and receptors* (ed. Ascoli M). CRC Press, Florida 1985, 17–56.

67. Tao YX, Lei ZM, Woodworth SH *et al.* Novel expression of luteinizing hormone/chorionic gonadotropin receptor gene in rat prostates. *Mol Cell Endocrinol* 1995, **111**, 9–12.

68. Reiter E, Poncin J, Hennuy B *et al.* Luteinizing hormone increases the abundance of various transcripts, independently of the androgens, in the rat prostate. *Biochem Bioph Res Co* 1997, **233**, 108–12.

69. Tao YX, Bao S, Ackermann DM *et al.* Expression of luteinizing hormone/human chorionic gonadotropin receptor gene in benign prostatic hyperplasia and in prostate carcinomas in humans. *Biol Reprod* 1997, **56**, 67–72.

70. Gutkind JS. The pathways connecting G protein-coupled receptors to the nucleus through divergent mitogen-activated protein kinase cascades. *J Biol Chem* 1998, **273**, 1839–42.

71. Themmen APN, Martens JWM, Brunner HG. Activating and inactivating mutations in LH receptors. *Mol Cell Endocrinol* 1998, **145**, 137–42.

72. Tapanainen JS, Aittomäki K, Min J *et al.* Men homozygous for an inactivating mutation of the follicle-stimulating hormone (FSH) receptor gene present variable suppression of spermatogenesis and fertility. *Nat Genet* 1997, **15**, 205–6.

73. Maroulakou IG, Anver M, Garrett L *et al.* Prostate and mammary adenocarcinoma in transgenic mice carrying a rat C3(1) simian virus 40 large tumor antigen fusion gene. *Proc Natl Acad Sci USA* 1994, **91**, 11236–40.

74. Greenberg NM, De Mayo FJ, Sheppard PC *et al.* The rat probasin gene promoter directs hormonally and developmentally regulated expression of a heterologous gene specifically to the prostate in transgenic mice. *Mol Endocrinol* 1994, **8**, 230–9.

75. Greenberg NM, De Mayo FJ, Finegold MJ *et al.* Prostate cancer in a transgenic mouse. *Proc Natl Acad Sci USA* 1995, **92**, 3439–43.

76. Liu JP, Baker J, Perkins AS *et al.* Mice carrying null mutations of the genes encoding insulin like growth factor I (IGF-I) and type 1 IGF-I receptor (IGF-I-R). *Cell* 1993, **75**, 59–72.

77. Acampora D, Mazan S, Tuorto F *et al.* Transient dwarfism and hypogonadism in mice lacking Otx1 reveal prepubescent stage-specific control of pituitary levels of GH, FSH and LH. *Development* 1998, **125**, 1229–39.

78. Lee SL, Sadovsky Y, Swirnoff AH *et al.* Luteinizing hormone deficiency and female infertility in mice lacking the transcription factor NGFI-A (Egr-1). *Science* 1996, **273**, 1219–21.

4 | Microbiology of the prostate in health and disease

J. Curtis Nickel

Introduction

The prostate holds a privileged position. Situated just below the bladder, it is separated from the outside microbial-dense world by a long protective urethra. Traditional dogma believes the prostate to be a sterile organ unless the patient suffers from clinically evident prostatitis or lower urinary tract infection. But is this the case? This chapter will explore the microbiology of prostatitis, benign prostatic hyperplasia, prostate cancer, as well as the normal asymptomatic prostate gland without any evidence of disease. This chapter will have clinical implications for physicians and urologists dealing with men with prostate problems, whether they are infectious, benign, or malignant.

Acute bacterial prostatitis

Acute bacterial prostatitis presents with clinical signs and symptoms of fever, dysuria, obstructive voiding, and exquisitely tender and perhaps boggy prostate on digital rectal examination. It is very rare, tends to occur spontaneously, and is associated with a generalized infection of the glandular and stromal components of the prostate gland. It is almost always associated with bacterial cystitis and many times associated with generalized bacteremia or even septicemia.

The majority of acute prostatitis patients present with an Enterobacteriaceae infection (1). These gram-negative bacilli are considered to be normal gastro-intestinal flora in humans. Typically, *Escherichia coli* represents 80% of the infections in acute prostatitis. The remaining 10–15% of additional bacterial prostatitis infections are caused by *Serratia*, *Klebsiella*, *Proteus*, and *Pseudomonas aeruginosa*. The gram-positive enterococci account for 5–10% of infections.

True bacterial prostatitis is easily diagnosed and the bacteria are almost always eradicated with wide-spectrum antibiotic therapy. Occasionally a prostatic abscess will occur that needs to be surgically drained. Acute bacterial prostatitis does not appear to be related to the chronic prostatitis syndromes listed below.

Chronic bacterial prostatitis

Chronic bacterial prostatitis is characterized by recurrent episodes of lower urinary tract infections (cystitis) and uropathogens detected in prostate-specific specimens (expressed prostatic secretion, post-prostatic massage urine or semen). Patients may complain of genito-urinary and perineal pain or discomfort between these acute episodes but, in many cases, the patients are asymptomatic. In most series, chronic bacterial prostatitis typically accounts for only about 5–10% of prostatitis patients (2). *Escherichia coli* is the most prevalent organism, but other Enterobacteriaceae and *Pseudomonas* are also typically found (Table 4.1). It is believed that enterococcus may have an etiologic role but the role of other gram-positive organisms, which typically colonize the distal urethra (*Staphylococcus epidermidis*, *Corynebacterium* spp., *Staphylococcus saprophyticus*, and *Bacteroides* spp.), as a cause of prostatitis remains controversial.

Table 4.1 Microbiology of bacterial prostatitis

80%	*Escherichia coli*
10–15%	*Serratia*
	Klebsiella
	Proteus
	Pseudomonas
5–10%	Enterococci

Table 4.2 National Institutes of Health (NIH) classification and definition of the categories of the prostatitis syndromes

Category I
Acute bacterial prostatitis—acute infection of the prostate gland.
Category II
Chronic bacterial prostatitis—recurrent urinary tract infection
Chronic infection of the prostate
Category III
Chronic pelvic pain syndrome (CPPS)—discomfort or pain in the pelvic region
No demonstrable infection using standard culture techniques
Category IIIA
Inflammatory CPPS
Significant number white cells in semen/expressed prostatic secretion/urine specimen after prostate massage (VB3)
Category IIIB
Non-inflammatory CPPS
Insignificant number white cells in semen/expressed prostatic secretion/urine specimen after prostate massage (VB3)
Category IV
Asymptomatic inflammatory prostatitis (AIP)
Evidence of inflammation and/or infection in biopsy, semen, expressed prostatic secretion, urine specimen after prostate massage
No symptoms

Chronic abacterial prostatitis/chronic pelvic pain syndrome

The vast majority of patients who present with prostatitis-like symptoms will not grow uropathogens on prostate-specific cultures. These patients have previously been referred to as chronic non-bacterial prostatitis or prostatodynia. Because it has become recognized that many of the symptoms referred to as chronic prostatitis may not be related to the prostate gland at all (and subsequently promote inappropriate therapy), the Consensus Meeting of the National Institutes of Health Workshop on Chronic Prostatitis (3) reclassified this category as chronic pelvic pain syndrome (Table 4.2). This large category of patients was further subdivided into the inflammatory type (Category IIIA) and non-inflammatory type (Category IIIB) based on the presence or absence of white blood cells detected on prostate specific specimens.

Controversy persists both in the literature and at prostatitis meetings on the etiology of this syndrome. Popular theories (4) include intraprostatic ductal reflux (perhaps associated with dysfunction obstructive voiding), immunologic causes, chemical etiology, neuromuscular/neurogenic or microbiological causes for the symptoms present in this syndrome. A very popular theory presented by many researchers is that this particular syndrome is caused by organisms thought to be presumed non-pathogens, rarely cultured organisms, cryptic non-culturable organisms, or even viruses (Table 4.3).

The author has presented the various arguments in the debate as to whether or not chronic pelvic pain syndrome is a microbial infectious disease or not in a recent review (5). Since this topic is so controversial, a summary of that extensive review is warranted.

There is empiric support for the concept that many patients with prostatitis may have a microbiological etiology for their syndrome. Most patients presenting with chronic prostatitis are treated with antibiotics (6, 7, 8), despite the fact that most cultures remain negative. This therapeutic paradox can be explained by the fact that many patients with no demonstrable infection respond to antibiotic therapy (9). Other studies have shown that serial repetitive prostatic massage specimens of expressed prostatic fluid identify more organisms than an initial single localization study (10).

While the consensus that most gram-positive organisms were seldom causative for the symptoms of prostatitis, it is now generally agreed that *Streptococcus faecalis* may cause chronic bacterial prostatitis and

Table 4.3 Possible microbiological agents in 'abacterial prostatitis/chronic pelvic pain syndrome'

Possible prostate pathogens:
coagulase-negative staphylococcus
Chlamydia sp.
Ureaplasma sp.
anaerobic bacteria
yeast (*Candida*)
Trichomonas sp.
Corynebacterium sp.
Acknowledged (?) prostate non-pathogens:
diphtheroids
Lactobacilli sp.
Cryptic non-culturable organisms:
'biofilm bacteria'
viruses
cell-wall deficient bacteria
micro-organisms yet to be discovered

related recurrent enterococcal bacteruria (11, 12). Our group has isolated coagulase-negative bacteria in a culture of expressed prostatic secretion, as well as similar organisms in prostate biopsies (13). Others have also implicated coagulase-negative *Staphylococcus* in this disease (14, 15). Most investigators believe that coagulase-negative staphylococci localized to prostate specific specimens, including prostate biopsies, represent only colonization.

The evidence in respect to *Chlamydia trachomatis* is extremely conflicting and confusing. *Chlamydia trachomatis* has been identified in 20–56% of patients presenting with chronic prostatitis employing culture, immunologic, molecular biological, and even biopsy techniques (16, 17, 18, 19, 20, 21, 22, 23, 24, 25, 26). However studies done by the same and other investigations employing cultures and serology could not confirm *Chlamydia trachomatis* as an etiologic agent in idiopathic prostatitis (27, 28, 29, 30). Anti-chlamydial antibody titers prostatic fluid was noted in 12% of control patients (31). A large molecular biological study of prostate tissue biopsies only detected chlamydia in 1% of men with chronic prostatitis (32).

Other investigators have suggested that *Ureoplasma urealyticum* may be an important cause of chronic prostatitis. Investigators have found high *Ureoplasma urealyticum* concentrations in 8–13% of patients with prostatitis (33, 34, 35). However other investigators were unable to implicate *Ureoplasma urealyticum* in patients with non bacterial prostatitis (36, 37).

Some investigators believe that observations on the high prevalence of *Trichomonas* in patients with prostatitis support an association between this organism and the syndrome (38, 39, 40, 41, 42). However others (43) seldom isolated *T. vaginalis* from the urethras in men with chronic prostatitis syndrome.

Anaerobic bacteria (44), yeast such as *Candida* (45, 46, 47), viruses (48, 49), and cell-wall deficient microorganisms (50) have been implicated in prostatic inflammation. Similarly, diphtheroids and *Corynebacterium* species (51, 52), usually acknowledged as prostate non-pathogens, have also been suggested as potential etiologic agents of disease.

Our group has shown that bacteria may not show up in expressed prostatic secretion and other prostate-specific specimens because of their protected 'biofilm' mode of growth within prostatic ducts or within obstructed ducts and glans of the prostate (53, 54). A recent study (55) demonstrated that men with inflamed expressed prostatic secretion (EPS) were more likely to have bacterial isolation, positive cultures for anaerobic

bacteria, higher total bacterial counts, and more bacterial species isolated in prostate biopsy cultures than men without EPS inflammation (even if the cultures were negative). Employing molecular biological methods (preliminary chain reaction) to evaluate a well-defined population of men with chronic idiopathic prostatitis, one group (32) determined that 8% of biopsies showed positive PCR assays for one or more specific micro-organisms. Broad spectrum PCRs demonstrated tetracycline-resistant and coating sequences in 25% of subjects and 16SrRNAs in 77% of the patients. Investigators also found a strong correlation between inflammation in expressed prostatic secretion and detection of 16SrRNA in prostate tissue. All these findings suggest that fastidious and non-cultureable micro-organisms may be important in the etiology of chronic inflammatory prostatitis.

Benign prostatic hyperplasia

Kohnen and Drock (56) discovered that up to 98% of surgically rejected prostates removed for benign prostatic hyperplasia (BPH) contained at least some foci of significant prostatic inflammation. This finding has been confirmed by other researchers (57). Gorelick *et al.* (58) discovered that 21% of patients undergoing prostatectomy yielded a positive, single-organism bacterial growth in prostate tissue. In a study recently completed in our institution (59), we noted that 100% of specimens demonstrated some degree of prostatic inflammation while 44% of the prostate specimens demonstrated bacterial growth. Of the organisms cultured from the deep prostatic chips, 87% were potentially uropathogenic. These findings suggest that inflammation and bacteria (uropathogenic and non-uropathogenic) are routinely associated in prostate glands in men with benign prostatic hyperplasia.

Prostate cancer

Inflammation is frequently observed in association with prostate cancer. It sometimes also confounds the detection of prostate cancer through its potential effect on PSA levels. Prostatitis, and more specifically bacterial prostatitis, was first shown to influence PSA shortly after it was released for general use (60). Adequate treatment with appropriate antibiotics for acute prostatitis usually results in subsequent normalization of serum PSA levels. Chronic inflammation of the prostate in a patient who developed biopsy proven granulomatous prostatitis secondary to bacillus calmette-guerin (BCG) for carcinoma of the urinary bladder was likewise demonstrated to be associated with elevated serum PSA (61). A recent investigation revealed an elevated serum PSA level in 71% of patients with acute prostatitis, 15% of patients with chronic prostatitis, and 6% with non-bacterial prostatitis, but none with prostatodynia (62). In patients with bacterial prostatitis, the serum PSA level decreased to normal after antimicrobial therapy in most cases in this series.

In 700 men who underwent prostate needle biopsy for elevated PSA or abnormal digital rectal examination, 27% have histological evidence of prostatitis (63). The majority (94%) had chronic inflammation, 6% had acute inflammation, and 0.2% had granulomatous changes. In another study, serum PSA values significantly correlated with the extent of histologically proven acute and chronic active prostatitis, whereas no correlation was noted between PSA and chronic inactive prostatitis (64). In this study, acute and chronic prostatitis was defined as acute (or chronic, respectively) infiltrate with neutrophils in the glands, whereas chronic inactive prostatitis indicated only chronic inflammatory infiltrate in the glands and stroma.

Molecular biological studies performed on sterile biopsies of patients with prostate cancer prior to radical prostatectomy, suggests the presence of asymptomatic organisms within the prostate (Alexander, University of Maryland, personal communication). The implications of these findings, if duplicated, will be important as we study the microbiology of the prostate in benign and malignant prostate disease.

The normal prostate

There is some evidence, albeit controversial, that the normal prostate gland has a commensal flora. In acute bacterial prostatitis (which is a very, very rare condition) there is a generalized overwhelming of the entire prostate gland by a particularly uropathogenic organism. In chronic bacterial prostatitis, on the other hand, most patients are asymptomatic between episodes of recurrent lower urinary tract infections or cystitis. It may be that these patients have colonization of their prostate by potentially uropathogenic bacteria that only cause clinical problems when they are released into the rest of the lower urinary tract. The evidence presented in the preceding sections demonstrates that many innocuous, and perhaps non-pathogenic, bacteria are present in studies of patients with chronic prostatitis/chronic pelvic pain syndrome. These organisms include gram-positive bacteria such as *Staphylococcus epidermidis*, *Staphylococcus saprophyticus*, diphtheroids, *Corynebacterium*, *Chlamydia*, *Ureoplasma*, and perhaps other micro-organisms as well. The studies however failed to prove that these organisms were implicated in the symptoms. They might just be innocent bystander colonizers of the prostate gland. Evidence was also presented in the preceding section as to the very common occurrence of inflammation and bacteria in patients being investigated and treated for BPH and prostate cancer. Likewise, there has been no proven association between inflammation and bacteria in these benign and malignant diseases of the prostate gland. Unfortunately, no well-designed study has ever been attempted in a control population to determine the presence of these various micro-organisms in the healthy prostate. As such, this question of whether or not the prostate is a sterile organ (particularly in health) remains unanswered.

Clinical implications

While our knowledge of the microbiology of the prostate gland is interesting, confusing, and conflicting, it does appear to have some practical implications for clinical practice (Table 4.4). The clinical syndrome of acute bacterial prostatitis is well-defined, the most common organisms are both known and accepted, and this knowledge is already being used to direct effective antibiotic therapy for this syndrome. Similarly in chronic bacterial prostatitis, which by definition includes only uropathogenic bacteria, the best antibiotic therapy (fluoroquinolines and trimethroprim penetrate the prostate gland and ducts better than other antibiotics) is recognized. Although the optimal

Table 4.4 Microbiology of the prostate: clinical lessons

1. The prostate may not be a sterile organ.
2. Prostatic micro-organisms may or may not be involved in the symptoms suffered by patients with chronic prostatitis.
3. Inflammation and/or infection may be involved in the pathogenesis of BPH and prostate cancer.
4. Inflammation and/or infection may be associated with elevated PSA.
5. Antibiotic prophylaxis is warranted in prostate surgery.

duration of therapy is unknown, 4–6 weeks of antibiotic treatment results in amelioration and cure in the majority of this rare group. Because of the distinct possibility that chronic abacterial prostatitis/chronic pelvic pain syndrome is secondary to some presumed non-pathogenic, *Chlamydia trachomatis*, *Ureaplasma urealyticum*, or a non-cultureable micro-organism, it would seem prudent that all patients who present with this syndrome (particularly with those with the inflammatory category) be treated at least once with a wide-spectrum antibiotic. Based on the evidence, fluoroquinolones such as ofloxacin or alternatively a combination of trimethoprim and a tetracycline (either sequentially or concurrently) would be recommended to cover the vast majority of these organisms. Because bacteria, particularly potentially uropathogenic bacteria, have been identified in prostate glands of many patients with benign prostatic hyperplasia, all patients undergoing transurethral surgery for BPH should be considered for antibiotic prophylaxis. Similarly, prostate cancer patients who undergo prostate manipulation (biopsy, radical prostatectomy, radioactive seed implantation) should also be considered for prophylactic therapy. Patients with genito-urinary pain symptoms (symptoms of acute/chronic prostatitis/chronic pelvic pain syndrome) and an elevated PSA should be considered for a full course of antibiotics and a repeat PSA before proceeding to a prostate biopsy (Fig. 4.1).

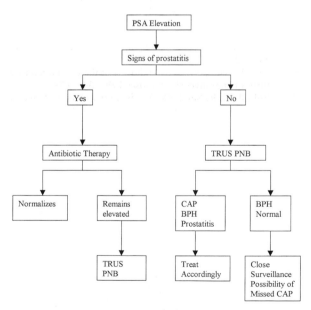

Fig. 4.1 Management approach for serum PSA elevation: BPH, benign prostatic hyperplasia. (Adapted with permission from Letran JL, Brawer MK. Prostate specific antigens and prostatitis. In: *Textbook of prostatitis* (ed. Nickel JC. ISIS, Oxford UK, 1999.)

Conclusions

The prostate is not always a sterile organ, particularly when associated with prostate disease (prostatitis, BPH, prostate cancer). There is some evidence that it may not be a sterile organ in patients with a normal healthy prostate as well. There may or may not be a population of bacteria that would include a normal non-pathogenic flora with occasional asymptomatic colonization by potentially uropathogenic bacteria. These uropathogenic bacteria in the prostate do pose a risk to the patient, particularly if they suffer from recurrent urinary tract infections, symptomatic prostatic inflammation, or require prostate manipulation for BPH and/or prostate cancer. The entire story of the microbiology of the prostate gland remains to be told.

References

1. Nadler R, Schaeffer A. Lower urinary tract cultures. In: *Textbook of prostitis* (ed. Nickel JC). ISIS, Oxford UK 1999.
2. Weidner W, Schiefer HG, Krauss H *et al.* Chronic prostatitis: a thorough search for etiologically involved micro-organisms in 1,461 patients. *Infection* 1991, **19** (Suppl 3), 119–25.
3. National Institutes of Health/National Institute of Diabetes and Digestive and Kidney Disease. *Summary Statement: Workshop on Chronic Prostatitis*. Bethesda, December, 1995.
4. Nickel JC. Prostatitis: myths and realities. *Urology* 1998, **51**, 362–66.
5. Nickel JC, Downey J, Hunter D, Clark J. Prevalence of prostatitis-like symptoms in a population based study using the National Institutes of Health chronic prostatits symptom index. *J Urol* 2001, **165**, 842–5.
6. Collins MM, Stafford RS, O'Leary MP *et al.* How common is prostatitis? A national survey of physician visits. *J Urol* 1998, **159**, 1224–8.
7. Moon TD. Questionnaire survey of urologists and primary care physicians' diagnostic and treatment practices for prostatitis. *Urology* 1997, **50**, 543–7.
8. Nickel JC, Nigro M, Valiquette L *et al.* Diagnosis and treatment of prostatitis in Canada. *Urology* 1998, **52**, 797–802.
9. Nickel JC, Corcos J, Afridi S *et al.* Antibiotic therapy for chronic inflammatory (NIH Category II/IIIA) prostatitis. *J Urol* 1998, **159**, 272A.
10. Hennenfent BR, Feliciano AE Jr. Changes in white blood cell counts in men undergoing thrice-weekly prostatic massage, microbial diagnosis and antimicrobial therapy for genitourinary complaints. *Br J Urol* 1998, **81**, 370–6.
11. Bergman B. On the relevance of gram-positive bacteria in prostatitis. *Infection* 1994, **22**, S221.
12. Drach GW. Problems in diagnosis of bacterial prostatitis: Gram-negative, gram-positive and mixed infections. *J Urol* 1974, **111**, 630–6.

13. Nickel JC, Costerton JW. Coagulase-negative staphylococcus in chronic prostatitis. *J Urol* 1992, **147**, 398–400.

14. Bergman B, Wedren H, Holm SE. *Staphylococcus saprophyticus* in males with symptoms of chronic prostatitis. *Urology* 1989, **34**, 241–5.

15. Drach GW. Prostatitis: Man's hidden infection. *Urol Clin North Am* 1975, **2**, 499–520.

16. Mardh PA, Colleen S. Chlamydia in chronic prostatitis. *Scand J Urol Nephrol* 1972, **9**, 8–16.

17. Shortliffe LM, Sellers RG, Schachter J. The characterization of nonbacterial prostatitis: search for an etiology. *J Urol* 1992, **148**, 1461–6.

18. Bruce AW, Chadwick P, Willet WS *et al.* The role of chlamydia in genitourinary disease. *J Urol* 1981, **126**, 625–9.

19. Bruce AW, Reid G. Prostatitis associated with *Chlamydia trachomatis* in 6 patients. *J Urol* 1989, **142**, 1006–7.

20. Kuroda K, Sawamura Y, Tajima M *et al.* Detection of *Chlamydia trachomatis* in urethra of patients with urogenital infection. *Hinyokika Kiyo* 1989, **35**, 453–6.

21. Nilsson S, Johanisson G, Lycke E. Isolation of *C. trachomatis* from the urethra and prostatic fluid in men with signs and symptoms of acute urethritis. *Acta Dermatol Venereol* 1981, **61**, 456–9.

22. Weidner W, Arens M, Krauss H *et al. Chlamydia trachomatis* in 'abacterial' prostatitis: microbiological, cytological and serological studies. *Urol Int* 1983, **38**, 146–9.

23. Poletti F, Medici MC, Alinovi A *et al.* Isolation of *Chlamydia trachomatis* from the prostatic cells in patients affected by nonacute abacterial prostatitis. *J Urol* 1985, 134, 691–693.

24. Abdelatif OM, Chandler FW, McGuire BSJ. Chlamydia trachomatis in chronic abacterial prostatitis: demonstration by colorimetric in situ hybridization. *Hum Pathol* 1991, **22**, 41–4.

25. Shurbaji MS, Gupta PK, Myers J. Immunohistochemical demonstration of chlamydial antigens in association with prostatitis. *Mod Pathol* 1998, **1**, 348–51.

26. Koroku M, Kumamoto Y, Hirose T. A study on the role of chlamydia trachomatis in chronic prostatitis—analysis of anti-Chlamydia trachomatis specific IgA in expressed prostate secretion by western-blotting method. *Kansenshogaku Zasshi* 1995, **69**, 426–37.

27. Mardh PA, Ripa KT, Colleen S *et al.* Role of *Chlamydia trachomatis* in non-acute prostatitis. *Br J Vener Dis* 1978, **54**, 330–14.

28. Colleen S, Mardh PA. Effect of metacycline treatment on non-acute prostatitis. *Scand J Urol Nephrol* 1975, **9**, 198–204.

29. Mardh PA, Ripa KT, Colleen S. Role of *Chlamydia trachomatis* in non-acute prostatitis. *Br J Vener Dis* 1978, **54**, 330–44.

30. Berger RE, Krieger JN, Kessler D *et al.* Case-control study of men with suspected chronic idiopathic prostatitis. *J Urol* 1989, **141**, 328–31.

31. Shortliffe LM, Wehner N. The characterization of bacterial and nonbacterial prostatitis by prostatic immunoglobulins. *Medicine* 1986, **65**, 399–414.

32. Krieger JN, Riley DE, Roberts MC *et al.* Prokaryotic DNA sequences in patients with chronic idiopathic prostatitis. *J Clin Microbiol* 1996, **34**, 3120–8.

33. Weidner W, Brunner H, Krause W. Quantitative culture of ureaplasma urealyticum in patients with chronic prostatitis or prostatosis. *J Urol* 1980, **124**, 622–5.

34. Fish DN, Danziger LH. Antimicrobial treatment for chronic prostatitis as a means of defining the role of *Ureaplasma urealyticum. Urol Int* 1993, **51**, 129–32.

35. Isaacs JT. *Ureaplasma urealyticum* in the urogenital tract of patients with chronic prostatitis or related symptomatology. *Br J Urol* 1993, **72**, 918–21.

36. Mardh PA, Colleen S. Search for uro-genital tract infections in patients with symptoms of prostatitis. Studies on aerobic and strictly anaerobic bacteria, mycoplasmas, fungi, trichomonads and viruses. *Scand J Urol Nephrol* 1975, **9**, 8–16.

37. Meares EM. Prostatitis vs. 'prostatosis': a clinical and bacteriological study. *JAMA* 1973, **224**, 1372–5.

38. Gardner WJr, Culberson D, Bennett B. *Trichomonas vaginalis* in the prostate gland. *Arch Weidner Pathol Lab Med* 1996, **110**, 430–2.

39. Drummand AC. Trichomonas infestation of the prostate gland. *Am J Surg* 1936, **31**, 98.

40. Kawamura N. Trichomoniasis of the prostate. *Jpn J Clin Urol* 1973, **27**, 335.

41. Kurnatowska A, Kurnatowski A, Mazurek L *et al.* Rare cases of prostatitis caused by invasion of *Trichomonas vaginalis. Wiad Parazytol* 1990, **36**, 229–36.

42. Kuberski T. *Trichomonas vaginalis* associated with nongonoccal urethritis and prostatitis. *Sex Transm Dis* 1980, **7**, 135–6.

43. Krieger JN, Egan KJ. Comprehensive evaluation and treatment of 75 men referred to chronic prostatitis clinic. *Urology* 1991, **38**, 11–9.

44. Nielsen ML, Justesen J. Studies on the pathology of prostatitis. A search for prostatic infections with obligate anaerobes in patients with chronic prostatitis and chronic urethritis. *Scand J Urol* Nephrol 1974, **8**, 1–6.

45. Campbell TB, Kaufman L, Cook JL. Asperigillosis of the prostate associated with an indwelling bladder catheter: case report and review. *Clin Infect Dis* 1992, **14**, 942–4.

46. Golz R, Mendling W. Candidosis of the prostate: a rate form of endomycosis. *Mycoses* 1991, **34**, 381–4.

47. Indudhara R, Singh SK, Vaidynanthan S *et al.* Isolated invasive *Candidal prostatitis. Urol Int* 1992, **48**, 362–4.

48. Benson PJ, Smith CS. Cytomegalovirus prostatitis *Urology* 1992, **40**, 165–7.

49. Doble A, Harris JR, Taylor-Robinson D. Prostatodynia and herpes simplex virus infection. *Urology* 1991, **38**, 247–8.

50. Domingue GJ. Cryptic bacterial infection in chronic prostatitis: diagnostic and therapeutic implications. *Curr Opin Urol* 1998, **8**, 45–9.

51. Domingue GJ, Human LG, Hellstrom WJ. Hidden microorganisms in 'abacterial' prostatitis/prostatodynia. *J Urol* 1997, **157**, 243.

52. Riegel P, Ruimy R, De Briel D *et al. Corynebacterium seminale* sp., a new species associated with genital infections in male patients. *J Clin Microbiol* 1995, **33**, 2244–9.

53. Nickel JC, Costerton JW. Bacterial localization in antibiotic-refractory chronic bacterial prostatitis. *Prostate* 1993, **23**, 107–14.

54. Nickel JC. Bacterial biofilms in urology. *Infect Urol* 1998, **11** (6), 169–75.

55. Berger RE, Krieger JN, Rothman I *et al.* Bacteria in the prostate tissue of men with idiopathic prostatic inflammation. *J Urology* 1997, **157**, 863–5.

56. Kohnen PW, Drach GW. Patterns of inflammation and prostatic hyperplasia: a histologic and bacteriologic study. *J Urol* 1979, **121**, 755–60.

57. Odunjo EO, Elebute EA. Chronic prostatitis and benign prostatic hyperplasia. *Br J Urol* 1971, **43**, 333–7.

58. Gorelick JI, Senterfit LB, Vaughan EDJ. Quantitative bacterial tissue cultures from 209 prostatectomy specimens: findings and implications. *J Urol* 1988, **139**, 57–60

59. Nickel JC *et al.* Asymptotic inflammation and/or infection in benign prostatic hyperplasia. *Br J Urol* 1999, **84**, 976–81.

60. Dalton DL. Elevated serum PSA due to acute bacterial prostatitis. *Urology* 1989, **33**, 465.

61. Bahnson RR. Elevation of prostate specific antigen from bacillus calmette-guerin induced granulomatous prostatitis. *J Urol* 1991, **146**, 1368–9.

62. Pansadoro V, Emiliozzi P, Defidio L *et al.* Prostate specific antigen and prostatitis in men under fifty. *Europ Urology* 1996, **30**, 24–7.

63. Socher S, O'Leary MP, Richie JP *et al.* Prevalence of prostatitis in men undergoing biopsy for elevated PSA or abnormal digital rectal exam. *J Urol* 1996, **155** (suppl), 425A.

64. Hasui Y, Marutsuka K, Asada Y *et al.* Relationship between serum prostate specific antigen and histological prostatitis in patients with benigh prostatic hyperplasia. *Prostate* 1994, **25**, 91–6.

5 | *Lower urinary tract symptoms and benign prostatic hyperplasia*

H. Logan Holtgrewe

Introduction

Within a text devoted to prostate cancer, it is, indeed, appropriate to include a chapter dealing with benign prostatic hyperplasia (BPH): another disorder arising in the same organ; a disorder that is more common than is prostate cancer. Both these diseases can cause comparable symptoms. Unfortunately, as is described by other authors within these proceedings, when prostate cancer produces symptoms, the malignancy is often beyond cure.

Yet it remains the responsibility of the physician managing a patient with lower urinary tract symptoms (LUTS) and suspected BPH to remember that his or her first responsibility is to exclude two life-threatening conditions; the symptoms of which can replicate benign prostatic and urinary disorders.

The first is prostate cancer—the subject of this text. Ornstein and co-workers (1) recently published sobering data. Despite prior screening and serum prostate specific antigen (PSA), digital rectal examination (DRE), and the performance of systematic prostatic-needle biopsies, when indicated, based on abnormalities of either of these tests, more than 15% of men in their series who underwent transurethral resection of the prostate (TURP) with a diagnosis of BPH were found to have unsuspected clinical-relevent cancers within pathological specimens (T1B or greater). A high suspicion must be constantly maintained and continued surveillance must be an ongoing part of the therapy of men with LUTS and BPH. The second is carcinoma *in situ* of the bladder, which is usually associated with microscopic hematuria and is a less difficult diagnostic problem, especially given the high probability of positive urine cytologies associated with this disorder (2).

When the physician is satisfied, through the employment of those existing diagnostic tools currently available, that the patient has a benign urological condition, attention can then be directed toward resolution of the patient's symptoms; the complaint that has prompted his desire for medical assistance. The United States Agency for Health Care Policy and Research (AHCPR), an agency of the Federal Government of the United States of America has published guidelines for the evaluation and management of LUTS and BPH (3). Based upon the world's available urological literature at the time of its publication in 1994, this document contains valuable information and guidance toward the evaluation of the symptomatic male. The Consensus Committee of the World Health Organization (WHO), in its International Consultation on BPH held in Paris, created recommendations for the evaluation of men with lower urinary-tract symptoms and benign prostatic hyperplasia very similar to those published by AHCPR (4).

Essential in the evaluation of a man with LUTS is a careful medical history and physical examination, including a DRE. A urinalysis and serum creatinine is also mandatory as is, in the view of this author, a PSA—especially in the light of the work of Ornstein cited above. In a 1997 poll of American urologists conducted by the American Urological Association and the Gallup Organization of Princeton, New Jersey, it was determined that 92% of American urologists obtain a PSA in the evaluation of men presenting with lower urinary tract symptoms (5).

Quantification of the patient's symptoms is then established using the self-administered AUA Symptom Index (6) or the International Prostate Symptom Score (IPSS) (7). These are identical symptom indices with the exception that the IPSS Index contains an eighth quality of life question not present in the AUA Symptom Index. Extremely important in determining the decision, as regards therapy, is the impact that the patient's symptoms have upon his quality of life. In an effort to determine more about the impact of the patient's symptoms, Barry and co-workers published a

BPH Impact Index (8). This four-question patient-conducted self-assessment helps to decide whether or not the patient's symptoms are severe enough to justify any type of therapeutic intervention, either medical or surgical.

The AHCPR guidelines discuss other optional investigative studies, which can be helpful in assessing the patient's status. One of these studies is the uroflow rate. However, the value of uroflow studies has been challenged by the work of Feneley and co-workers (9), who reported substantial variations in voiding of a single individual on various urinations. Further, Reynard and co-workers (10) reported a significant increase in Q-max with each successive voiding when multiple flow studies were performed on a single individual over a period of time. While extremely popular among urologists, the true value of a urinary flow rate remains questionable. In point of fact, patients care little about their flow rate, only about their symptoms.

More complex urodynamic and pressure flow studies are the only methods available to definitively prove the presence or absence of outlet obstruction. Abrams and co-workers (7) believe that such procedures are mandatory prior to any surgical intervention. It is highly questionable in this author's view, however, whether these invasive and costly procedures can be justified in the evaluation of a man who is not going to undergo surgical treatment but is going to be treated medically or with watchful waiting. Such investigative studies are not advocated by Gerber and co-workers (11), who state that complex urodynamics do not predict the response to medical management. Citing the lack of predictive value, their invasiveness, and cost, McConnell (12) regards urodynamic studies as optional even before surgical intervention.

The routine evaluation of the upper urinary tract by either intravenous pyelography or renal sonogram is not recommended by either the AHCPR or the WHO guidelines. In a man with no flank symptoms, no history of previous urological abnormalities (aside from his lower urinary tract symptoms), and in the absence of hematuria, either gross or microscopic, these guidelines state there is no merit in performing upper-tract visualization. Such procedures are costly and contribute nothing to the final decision in the selection of management. Should there be co-existing abnormalities in the urinary tract, such as hematuria, then obviously upper-tract studies would be indicated based upon the existence of co-morbidity.

Neither is there any evidence that a diagnostic cystoscopy to determine the 'need to treat' is of any value in the view of the AHCPR and WHO Guidelines. Invasive, costly, and uncomfortable to the patient, a diagnostic cystoscopy is not of value. Once surgery has been determined to be the therapy of choice, knowledge concerning anatomy of the prostate (prostate configuration and presence or absence of the median lobe) is of some importance. Cystoscopy is often indicated to clarify these anatomical details.

Pathophysiology of lower urinary tract symptoms

Physicians and urologists worldwide have for decades traditionally referred to a man of 50 years of age or older presenting with slowing urinary stream, hesitancy, urgency, frequency, nocturia, and the feeling of incomplete bladder-emptying as having 'prostatism'. Tradition has attributed the onset of these symptoms to the man's prostate gland having enlarged. Recent epidemiological work has clarified this issue substantially. Today we know that many men presenting with these symptoms do, indeed, have prostate enlargement due to benign prostatic hyperplasia. Many others, however, do not. There currently exists inadequate data to confirm what percentage of symptomatic men have true BPH versus those who are simply symptomatic without any significant prostate gland enlargement. Abrams (7) advocates the use of the term lower urinary tract symptoms (LUTS), a descriptive not a pathological term. Other diagnostic tests and undertakings should then be employed to determine the precise pathophysiological problem causing the patient's symptoms.

Recent epidemiological work has also clarified another misconception long held within the urological community—that prostate volume was unrelated to progression of disease, degree of symptoms, uroflow rates, or patient age. Jacobsen and co-workers (13) report that men with prostates of 30 ml or larger experience a three-fold greater incidence of acute retention. Men between ages 40 and 49 years with moderate or severe symptoms had a risk rate of urinary retention of 3–1000 as compared to a rate of 35–1000 for men aged 70–79 years. These investigators also reported that men with peak flow rates of less than 12 ml/s had a four times greater risk of acute retention than did men with better flow rates. Girman (14) reported that the odds of having moderate or severe symptoms increase with age. Adjusting for age, this investigator found that men with prostate volumes of 50 ml or larger were 3.5 times more likely to have moderate or severe symptoms and 2.4 times more likely to have a peak flow rate of less than 10 ml/s as compared to men with smaller prostates. It, thus, appears that prostate volume is related to age, symptom levels, flow rates, and the probability of development of future adverse events.

Sanda and co-workers (15) have reported a familial incidence of BPH. They reported mean prostate volumes of men with three or more family members with BPH as being 82.7 ml whereas men with sporadic BPH had volumes of only 55.5 ml. Since both groups had comparable androgen levels, Sanda and co-workers concluded that genetic and not androgenic factors were responsible for the differences. Further, symptoms levels appear to have a relationship to the development of future adverse events. Barry and co-workers (16) reported that men with baseline mild, moderate, and severe symptoms experienced a 10%, 24%, and 39% rate of prostate surgery, respectively, during the four years of their study.

Lower urinary tract symptoms are not a surrogate for benign prostatic hyperplasia. It is essential that the physician managing men with LUTS understand this. Even current medical literature continues to confuse this issue. Many recent papers published on the management of 'BPH' are in fact studies of men presenting with lower urinary tract symptoms. It is essential that the physician evaluating men with lower urinary tract symptoms understand clearly that all men with LUTS do not have BPH. This is a very important point as can be seen in subsequent discussion in this chapter since this determination makes a great deal of difference in the strategies of management employed in symptom relief.

Therapeutic options

As recently as the mid-1980s, the only strategies of management available to the symptomatic male were surgery or watchful waiting. In 1962, American urologists performed a mean of 101 transurethral resections of the prostate (TURP) per year (17). In 1986, TURP constituted 38% of all major surgeries performed by American urologists, and activities centered on this single operation comprised 25% of their total professional workload (17). The number of TURPs performed in the United States Medicare program (health care for patients over 65 years of age) reached a peak of 258 000 procedures in 1987. The number of TURPs has steadily fallen to 94 000 in 1998 (Health Care Financing Administration BESS Data 1998) (Fig. 5.1) (18). Comparable declines in the incidence of TURP in the surgical treatment of LUTS and BPH have occurred worldwide (19).

The reasons for the decline in number of TURPs is multifactorial. There has become an increasing awareness of the fact that many men with lower urinary tract symptoms do not experience a high incidence of subsequent complications. Wasson and co-workers (20), in their trial of symptomatic men randomized to either TURP or watchful waiting, reported a very low incidence of major complications among the men randomized to watchful waiting during their 3-year study,

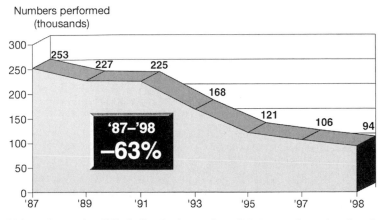

Fig. 5.1 The decade of 1987–98 has witnessed a 63% decline in the number of TURPs performed within the USA Medicare program (men 65 years of age and over).

despite the fact that many of these men had significant symptoms levels.

Clearly the greatest reduction has been related to the advent of medical management. The extent of penetration of medical management in the treatment of men with LUTS was documented by the American Urological Association (AUA) Gallup Poll conducted in 1997 (5). American urologists reported that their first treatment recommendation for men with moderate symptoms (AUA score 8–19) was medical management 25% of the time. Their first recommendation for men with severe symptoms (AUA score of 20 or more) was medical management 55% of the time. Also leading to the decline in the number of TURPs has been the advent of multiple-device therapies for lower urinary tract symptoms and benign prostatic hyperplasia. Thus, the armamentarium of the urologist has become greatly expanded. The patient now has multiple options. It is important that both the physician and patient alike understand these options, their respective harms and benefits, and their probabilities of achieving symptom relief. The remainder of this chapter will undertake to provide basic data concerning the currently available means of managing LUTS and BPH.

The patient who, after evaluation, is found to have refractory urinary retention, upper tract damage, renal insufficiency, bladder damage, bladder calculi, or recurrent urinary tract infections secondary to obstruction, must have surgical correction of their obstructive uropathy. Medical therapy has no role in the management of such patients. Currently, it remains unclear as to whether or not newer device therapies would have a role in this scenario.

Medical therapy

Three forms of medical therapy for LUTS and BPH currently exist:

(1) the pharmacological family of alpha-blocking agents;

(2) hormonal agents—5α-reductase inhibitors; and

(3) phytotherapy using plant extracts.

Alpha-blocking agents

Caine and co-workers first described the use of the non-selective alpha-blocking agent, phenoxybenzamine (21–23) in the management of men with lower urinary tract symptoms. The work of these authors was then supplemented and expanded by Lepor (24–26) and Shapiro (27–30). These investigators reported that there appeared to be relaxation of smooth muscle tone in the prostatic stroma, prostatic capsule, bladder neck, and peri-urethral tissues bringing about a potential relief of LUTS in many men (31). Popular alpha-blocking agents in worldwide use today are the selective long-acting alpha-adrenoreceptor antagonists, terazosin, doxazosin, and tamsulosin. Their popularity has been related to their simplicity in use at once-a-day dosage, and to their apparent specificity to smooth muscle of the lower urinary tract. Lepor has reported that the improvement in symptoms associated with terazosin therapy is dose-dependent. Men receiving placebo, 2 mg, 5 mg, or 10 mg of terazosin experienced a 30% improvement of symptoms of 40%, 51%, 57%, and 69%, respectively (32). Lepor recommends upward titration of dosage until symptoms are relieved or to a maximum dose of 20 mg. Roehrborn and co-workers (33) found a 37.8% improvement in the AUA Symptom Score in doxazosin-treated men versus an 18.4% improvement in their placebo group. Yet, this group of investigators found that the improvement in peak flow rates of the treated versus the placebo group was a minimal 2.2 ml/s. It would seem rather questionable that a patient could determine such a minimal improvement in flow rate.

Lepor postulates that the beneficial affect of terazosin on symptoms is not exclusively mediated by reduction in outlet obstruction (34). He bases this in part on a study of two managed groups of symptomatic men, one with peak urinary flow rates greater than 15 ml/s and the other with peak flow rates of less than 15 ml/s in which both groups were found to have identical symptom improvement. The work of Witjes and co-workers (35) adds additional data. In two studies, investigators found significant symptom improvement in both urodynamically documented obstructed and urodynamically documented unobstructed men.

A deficiency in existing clinical studies using alpha-blocking agents is the lack of long-term evaluations. Despite the millions of doses of alpha-blockers that have been prescribed worldwide, the urological literature is still deficient in data concerning long-term outcomes. In a 42-month terazosin open-label, multicenter study (31), Lepor has reported a mean sustained 40% improvement in the Boyarsky score and a sustained 3 ml/s improvement in Q-max rates at 42 months. However, data are available on only 47 men (9.5% of the initial 494 men entered into the study). A second study was a 4-year long-term efficacy and safety trial of doxazosin (36). This study enrolled men who had previously been part of a double-blinded, placebo-controlled study. Of those patients with 48-month data, all had sustained symptomatic improvement, yet 4-year data were available on only 28 men. Despite their popularity and worldwide use, long-term information remains lacking.

Tamsulosin, a selective alpha-1A adrenoreceptor antagonist, is being advocated due to its exclusive specificity to the smooth muscle of the prostatic stroma, thus eliminating the cardiovascular and other side-effects associated with the less selective alpha-1 agents. This lack of cardiovascular effect has been heralded by its advocates as allowing the drug to be given initially at therapeutic levels without the titration required for terazosin and doxazosin. Abrams and co-workers (37) reported the findings of a randomized, placebo-controlled 7-week trial. Boyarsky symptom improvement was 28% in the tamsulosin group versus 17% improvement in the placebo group. Of interest in this study was a 28% reduction in bladder pressure at peak flow in the tamsulosin group versus an increase of 7.5% in bladder pressure in the placebo group. There appeared to be no significant differences in blood pressure between the tamsulosin and placebo groups. Comparable outcomes were reported in another randomized trial of 12-week duration by Abrams and co-workers (38). Chappel and co-workers (39) in their concluded that tamsulosin was associated with a 35% improvement in the Boyarsky symptom score versus 25% for placebo. These authors reported adverse events were comparable in both the tamsulosin and the placebo groups. In an 8-week trial comparing tamsulosin versus terazosin, Lee and associates (40) concluded that both these agents were equally effective in achieving symptom relief but the tamsulosin had a superior safety profile.

Lowe (41), in an evaluation of the effect of tamsulosin in men already on monotherapy for hypertension, found no clinically significant changes in blood pressure, pulse rates, electrocardiographic findings, or halter monitor findings associated with the addition of tamsulosin to the already existing hypertensive regiment. This prompted Lowe to suggest that no adjustment in programs of monotherapy are required when tamsulosin is added to treat LUTS. It would seem from the available literature that tamsulosin produces, at least in the short term, symptom relief comparable with other alpha-1 blocking agents but exerts less or no effect on the cardiovascular system, thus isplaying a lesser toxicity profile. However, only short-term findings exist in the current medical literature. More long-term data is needed. If the existing short-term studies are substantiated by evaluations of longer duration, it might seem that tamsulosin could emerge as the alpha-blocking agent of choice for normotensive men with LUTS, reserving the alpha-1 blocking agents for treatment of LUTS in men with co-xisting hypertension and in whom the concurrent cardiovascular affects of these alpha-blocking agents yields an additional benefit.

Phytotherapeutic agents

Described by their manufacturers as plant extracts and food supplements, these agents are exempt from the control of the Food and Drug Administration (FDA) of the United States. These agents have been popular in Europe and other parts of the world for many years. In recent months there has been an increasing entry of these agents in the use of treatment of LUTS in the United States. Studies have been undertaken to identify their natural ingredients and the pathophysiology of their alleged symptoms improvement. Most phytotherapeutic agents seem to contain fatty acids, free fatty alcohols, tiriterpenes, and sterols (42). Which, if any of these ingredients, are effective on the prostate seems unclear. It is also unclear as to the absorption rates of these agents (42). Rhodes and co-workers (43) evaluated these agents for 5α-reductase activity and found none. Double-blinded, randomized, placebo-controlled studies evaluating phytotherapies are clearly indicated. Further, their use should be compared to those of the alpha-blocking agents and the hormonal altering agents. Until such time as more information becomes available regarding their efficacy, durability and mode of action, the role of phytotherapeutic agents in management of men with lower urinary tract symptoms will remain unclear.

5α-Reductase inhibitors

Walsh and co-workers (44) describe patients who had a congenital form of psuedohermaphroditism secondary to deficient dihydrotestosterone (DHT) levels, which was related to 5α-reductase activity. Such men have unpalpable prostates. This and other work (45, 46) led to the concept that an inhibitor of 5α-reductase could block DHT production and, thus, impact on the prostate gland. Finasteride is a type II 5α-reductase inhibitor. As such, it blocks the conversion from testosterone to DHT (45, 47). Clinical studies in North America revealed a sustained DHT reduction and a concomitant reduction in prostate volumes at 24 and 36 months (48, 49). This prostate volume reduction was associated with reduction in symptoms and some improvement in uroflow rates. Moore and co-workers (50) found DHT reductions of 72% in peripheral blood and prostate reduction of 30% along with uroflow rate increases of 1.5 ml and PSA reductions in 50% in their cohort of investigated men taking finasteride. These changes were sustained in their cohort of 70 men over an interval of 5 ears.

The histological effects of finasteride on the prostate have been evaluated by several investigators. Marks and co-workers (51) documented PSA reductions from baseline of 48% and DHT reductions of 74% in peripheral blood. Prostate volume reductions are reported at 21%. These authors conducted prostate biopsies finding a linear correlation between pretreatment inner glandular epithelial components and finasteride-induced prostate volume decreases, leading the authors to conclude that finasteride causes a major suppression of prostate epithelium most pronounced in the inner gland and that of the transition zone. Montironi and co-workers (52) report an increase in stroma/epithelial ratios and acini cellular atrophy within the transition zone in men receiving finasteride. Rittmaster and co-workers (53) confirmed these findings by using immunostaining for tissue transglutaminase, a marker for apoptosis and program cell death. The authors suggest that finasteride causes prostate involution through epithelial cell atrophy. These microscopic cellular findings would seem to correlate with clinical symptoms. Tewari and co-workers (54) found that symptomatic responders to finasteride therapy experienced a 44.8% reduction in transition zone volumes in comparison with only a 16% reduction in non-responders. The urodynamic impact of finasteride has been studied by Tammela and co-workers (55) who reported that finasteride achieved moderate decreases in bladder outlet obstruction but only occasionally relieved obstruction completely.

PSA alteration of men receiving finasteride has been well documented in the literature. Guess and co-workers (56) report that finasteride reduces PSA by approximately 50% over pre-therapy levels after an interval of 6 months or longer. Theses authors recommend that men receiving finasteride should have their PSA doubled and then compared with either age-independent or age-adjusted norms for untreated men.

These authors suggest that when PSA is used in this method its sensitivity and specificity is similar to that achieved in untreated men. Matzkin and co-workers (57) reported that, although finasteride reduces both total and free PSA levels, mean to total free assay ratios remain unchanged. Thus, the free to total PSA ratios currently used to help differentiate benign from malignant processes remained valid during finasteride treatment. Narayan and co-workers (58) report that finasteride has no effect on serum levels of prostatic acid phosphatase.

Periodic gross hematuria can occasionally be a problem associated with men with enlarged prostates. Puchner and co-workers (59) have reported the beneficial effect of finasteride in controlling this clinical syndrome. While there exists no contemporary literature confirming its efficacy, this author has found that finasteride is of benefit in men with recurring hematospermia when other more serious conditions of the prostate have been excluded.

Adverse events experienced with finasteride are almost entirely confined to sexual dysfunction. Nickel and co-workers (60) reported adverse events in their finasteride and placebo group to be identical with the exception of sexual events. Their finasteride group experienced a 15.8% incidence in impotence versus a 6.3% incidence in their placebo group. Ejaculatory disorders occurred in 7.7% of finasteride group versus 1.7% in the placebo group. Tollin and co-workers (61) reported that finasteride has no effect on the bone turnover or bone density. In the largest study of the side-effects of finasteride, including 14 772 men, Wilton and co-workers (62) reported the following adverse events: impotency or ejaculatory failure, 2.1%; loss of libido, 1%; gynecomasty, 1.4%. No drug-related deaths were reported in this large study.

Choosing between alpha-blockers and finasteride

Recent clinical studies have contributed greatly to the proper selection of medical therapy. The co-operative, multi-centered Veterans Administration (VA) study of Lepor and co-workers (63) reported that finasteride was only little more effective than placebo in a 1-year, double-blinded, placebo-controlled study made up of four arms (placebo, terazosin, finasteride, and combination terazosin/finasteride). Mean changes in these respective groups were as follows: AUA Symptom Indices reductions, −2.6, −3.2, −6.1, and −6.2; uroflow increases (minimal in all arms), +1.4, +1.6, +2.7, and

+3.2 ml/s; and prostate volume changes (obtained by ultrasound) from baseline of +1.3%, –16.8%, +1.3%, and –18.8%. The mean baseline prostate volumes of the men in all four arms were approximately equal but uniformly small (38.4 ml, 37.5 ml, 36.2 ml, 37.2 ml). If a symptomatic man does not have significant transitional zone enlargement due to BPH, he will fail to respond to finasteride. If the patient's prostate is not enlarged at baseline, reduction in its size could hardly be expected to be beneficial. Because of the small mean prostate volumes of the men in the VA study, it can be inferred that the large majority of the enrolled patients did not have significant BPH-induced transitional zone hypertrophy and were, thus, doomed to finasteride failure from the very inception of the VA study.

Confirming the importance of prostate volume as a predictor to finasteride response is the work of Boyle and co-workers (64). These investigators conducted a meta-analysis of the finasteride arms of six large international trials. All men given finasteride or placebo were divided into groups based upon their baseline prostate volumes. If the baseline volume of the prostate was below 40 ml, finasteride was no more effective than placebo in symptom relief. However, if the prostate volume was 40 ml or greater, there was improvement in symptom scores over placebo; the larger the prostate, the greater the improvement. These findings lead Boyle to conclude that finasteride therapy should be reserved for men with prostate volumes of 40 ml or greater.

Prostate volume, as determined by digital rectal exam (DRE), is recognized as being somewhat inaccurate. Roehrborn and co-workers (65) have documented that when the finger of the experienced urologist deems the prostate to be 40 g or larger, this determination invariably underestimates the gland's true volume as measured by transrectal ultrasound, thus questioning the validity of the use of this easy, cost-effective examination to establish the approximate prostate volume. However, the clinical assessment of prostate size now appears to be further assisted by the recent work of Roehrborn (66) showing that PSA levels are a reliable surrogate for prostate volumes. This work reveals that the higher the PSA the larger is the prostate gland. This assumes that prostate cancer has been excluded, based upon currently available diagnostic methods. This work further reveals that men with a PSA below 1.4 ng/dl do not have enlarged prostates. Above 1.4 ng/dl, the prostate size escalates in volume as the PSA level increases.

The largest and longest, randomized, double-blinded, clinical trial to date on the medical management of

LUTS and BPH is the Proscar Long-Term Efficacy and Safety Study (PLESS). Finasteride, when compared to placebo during the 4-year interval of the PLESS trial, reduced the risk rate of acute urinary retention by 57% and the need for surgical intervention by 55%. These data may have a significant impact on the long-term management of men with enlarged prostates. It appears it is now possible to arrest the progression of BPH with the resultant reduced risk of acute urinary retention and the future need of operative intervention. In men with truly enlarged glands due to BPH, this is an attribute not currently proven for any other form of medical management. During the 4 years of the PLESS study, those men on placebo experienced a 14% mean increase in prostate volume, while those on finasteride experienced a sustained 18.0% reduction (66, 67). Roehrborn and co-workers (66), through analysis of the PLESS data, report that PSA at 1.4 ng/ml distinguishes between two different clinical entities: men with true BPH and enlarged prostates; and men with bothersome symptoms but whose prostates are normal in size. Moreover, these authors reported that higher PSA levels predict future worsening symptom-severity, as well as future prostatic growth, identifying those men with potentially more progressive BPH attended with worsening symptoms, worsening uroflow rates, and increased risks of acute urinary retention and the need for prostatic surgery. These authors state that patients with PSA levels of less than 1.4 ng/ml are likely to have smaller prostates and little chance of progressive symptoms and much lower risks of acute retention and the need for BPH related surgery.

Finasteride offers a new dimension to the armamentarium of the urologist in the management of BPH—prevention—the ability to block the progression of what is now known to be a progressive disease attended with its significant future adverse events. This ability to alter the natural history of BPH is finasteride's greatest attribute.

Which family of medical therapies is best? Alpha-blockers can provide rapid symptom-relief in most men and are effective in men irrespective of prostate volume. Yet, the long-term effectiveness and durability of these agents has been documented in but a scant number of patients. There exists no data to demonstrate that alpha-blockers prevent progression of BPH. Finasteride, on the other hand, is suitable only in those men with prostate glands of 40 ml or greater, and men with PSA levels of 1.4 ng/ml or greater, where the drug has been shown to reduce transition zone volume, block future BPH growth, and reduce the risk rate of acute urinary retention and the need for surgery. Combination therapy using both alpha-blocker and finasteride provides the advantages of rapid onset of symptom relief associated with the prevention of future prostatic growth. However, this adds to the cost of therapy.

Device therapies

An array of 'less invasive' device therapies have evolved. All have the same common denominator—destroying and reducing the volume of prostate adenoma through the delivery of heat. They differ in the means of that delivery. Prostate treatment temperatures below 45°C (hyperthermia) are unassociated with tissue destruction and, according to Abbou and co-workers, are of no clinical benefit (68).

Lasers

Coagulation (free beam) laser prostatectomy (VLAP)

This technique has been described by Kabalin (69). It brings about coagulation of prostate tissue and its overlying urothelium through the creation of multiple coagulated 'lesions'. The necrosed tissue must then slough causing variable degrees of post-operative difficulties, including urinary retention, dysuria, and urinary infection. Nevertheless, in a multi-centered trial of the YAG laser prostatectomy by Kabalin and co-workers (70), 1-year post-treatment outcomes revealed mean reductions of 60% in AUA symptom indices, 105% increase in uroflow rates, and a 38% reduction in residual urine volumes with no mortalities, a serious complication rate of only 3.8%, and a 1-year re-operation rate of 2.7%—results challenging those achieved with TURP and with a much lower morbidity rate and equal re-operation rate.

Jung and co-workers (71) in a perspective, randomized trial of VLAP versus TURP, reported that symptomatic improvement occurred in all men. However, while urodynamically documented pre-operative obstruction was relieved in all TUR patients, it was relieved by VLAP only in those men with prostate volumes less than 50 ml, prompting these authors to limit VLAP to glands less than that size. Long-term outcome reports are rare. Kabalin (72) reported a 3-year follow-up on a series of 227 men but only 10 of these had complete 3-year data.

Contact laser vaporization of the prostate

A technique described by Gomella (73) creates, through its vaporization of prostate tissue and its overlying urethral epithelium cavitation defects similar to those created by TURP, thus, theoretically avoiding the morbidity associated with the tissue sloughing of VLAP. The operative time to cavitate the prostate tissue becomes a factor in larger glands, again limiting this technique to glands below 30 to 50 g (73). Yet, Gomella reports that serum fluid shifts and blood loss with laser vaporization technique are less than those of TURP (74). In a perspective, randomized trial of vaporization versus TURP, Ekrengren (75) reported significantly less intra-operative blood loss, fluid reabsorption, and greater cardiovascular stability with laser vaporization than with TURP. Outcomes studies for the vaporization technique are scant. None report outcomes beyond several months. Results appear to be similar to VLAP with lesser immediate post-operative dysuria and retention (76). Both VLAP and the evaporation techniques require general or regional anesthesia.

Interstitial laser coagulation (ILC)

This technique has been described by Muschter (77). By insertion of the laser bundle through the prostatic urothelium into the adenoma, prostatic urothelium is spared. The concept is that post-operatively the coagulated adenoma is reabsorbed rather than sloughed, therefore, reducing morbidity. Twelve-months outcomes data reported by Muschter (77) using the Nd:YAG laser revealed a mean AUA symptom index reduction from pre- to post-operative of 25.4–6.2 and an increase in Q-max of 7.7–17.6 cc/s. Schettini and co-workers (78) reported 12-months outcomes using the Indigo-diode laser with mean AUA indices reductions of 22.6–9.2 and mean increases in Q-max from 7.9 to 15 cc/s. Similar 12-months outcomes are reported by Arai and co-workers (79): mean AUA symptoms indices reductions from 20.4 to 7.4 and mean Q-max indices from 7.4 to 11.1 cc/s. Its advocates report the procedure can be performed under topical and local anesthesia with analgesia supplement.

Laser prostatectomy is being performed far less frequently in the interval between American Urological Association Gallup Poll surveys of American urologists in 1994 (80) and 1995 (75). Overall, the laser techniques (VLAP, vaporization and ILC) yield outcomes, at least in the short term, approach but do not equal

Table 5.1   Transurethral microwave thermotherapy outcomes

Study	Patients (no)	Symptom score Baseline	Symptom score 12 months	Q-max (cc/s) Baseline	Q-max (cc/s) 12 months
Prostatron 2.0					
Blute	150	13.7	5.4	8.5	11.3
Devone	818	13.3	3.5	8.8	12.6
Prostatron 2.5					
de la Rosette	116	17.5	7.1	9.6	14.5
de Wildt	85	17.6	8.0	9.4	14.9
Targis T3					
Ramsey	154	20.1	8.8	9.3	13.4
Mayer	110	20.8	10.0	7.8	11.6

those achieved with TURP. Complications aside from prolonged catheter drainage are less with the laser therapies than associated with TURP. Longer term outcomes and data concerning the need for repeat surgical intervention or repeat medical therapy following laser therapy are currently lacking. Until such data, especially those dealing with durability, are available, the ultimate role of laser is unclear.

Thermal therapy (TUMT)

At writing, two devices are currently approved for use in the United States by the Food and Drug Administration (FDA): the Prostatron (EDAP Technomed) using the 2.0 software and the Targis System (T3-Urologix). The Prostatron uses monopole antennae and, because of the wavelengths employed, requires shielding of the room in which therapy is given. The Targis antennae is dipolar and requires no room-shielding. Both techniques employ concurrent urethral cooling during therapy (81). Larson (82) compared the Prostatron and Targis antennae in an *in vitro* study using tissue-equivalent phantoms. He felt the Targis antennae provided a more targeted heating

pattern and had a more efficient thermal-energy delivery. The study raised the possibility that these properties could translate into clinical advantage *in vivo*.

Twelve-months outcomes for Prostatron 2.0, Prostatron 2.5, and Targis (T3) are compared in Table 5.1. Comparison of Prostatron 2.0, Targis (T3), and Donier Urowave versus Sham is depicted in Table 5.2. Trials comparing TUMT and TURP have been reported by Dahlstrand (83) and d'Ancona (84) (Table 5.3). Although TUMT achieves significant symptom improvement, at 12 months it is less than that achieved with TURP. Uroflow rates after TUMT are significantly inferior to TURP. In a perspective, randomized trial of Prostatron 2.5 versus TURP utilizing urodynamics pre- and post-operatively, Ahmed (85) found that all urodynamic parameters improved significantly in their TURP patients. TUMT patients experienced a mean reduction in AUA symptom indices from 18.4 to 5.2, but none of their objective urodynamic variables improved.

Long-term outcome studies are rare but two deserve attention. Hallin and Berlin (86) reported on Prostatron 2.0 and found only 23% of men were satisfied at 4 years after therapy and that two-thirds

Table 5.2   Transurethral microwave thermotherapy versus SHAM

Study	Patients (no)	Follow-up Month	TUMT PRE	TUMT POST	SHAM PRE	SHAM POST	TUMT PRE	TUMT POST	SHAM PRE	SHAM POST
			Symptom score				Q-max (cc/s)			
Nawrocki (Prostatron 2.0)	120	6	19.0	9.5	17.5	9.5	8.8	9.4	9.9	9.5
Blute (Targis T3)	111	6	20.3	10.8	23.0	17.3	7.9	11.9	7.5	9.4

Table 5.3 Transurethral microwave thermotherapy vs TURP

Study	Patients (no)	Follow-up Month	Symptom score TUMT		Symptom score TURP		Q-max (cc/s) TUMT		Q-max (cc/s) TURP	
			PRE	POST	PRE	POST	PRE	POST	PRE	POST
Dahlstrand (Prostatron 2.0)	69	12	12.1	2.2	13.6	0.6	8.6	12.6	8.6	18.9
D'Ancona	52	12	18.3	5.7	16.7	3.5	10.0	16.9	9.3	18.6

required supplemental BPH treatment. Keijzers and co-workers (87), also reporting on Prostatron 2.0, found that 41% of their cohort of 231 patients required post-TUMT invasive pretreatment and that 17% were retreated with medication during the 5-year follow-up after TUMT. Baseline prostate volume did not modify these outcomes. These two studies do not in themselves establish a lack of durability of TUMT, but they do establish the need for more long-term data before judgement can be made regarding the role of TUMT in the armamentarium of BPH therapies.

Transurethral needle ablation of the prostate (TUNA)

TUNA technique has been described elsewhere (88). Low-level radiofrequency energy is delivered into prostate adenoma by shielded needles inserted through the prostatic urothelium into the adenoma. Deployment of the needles is determined by prostate volume guided by transrectal ultrasound. The number of 'lesions' of coagulation is again dependent upon prostate volume. Zlotta and co-workers (89) studied the pathology specimens removed by open prostatectomy on 10 men who 1–46 days before had received TUNA therapy. Examination revealed severe thermal damage and de-intervation of alpha receptors and sensory nerves in the TUNA-treated areas, prompting these authors to suggest that this could be an explanation for the clinical effects of TUNA. In a randomized trial of urodynamically proven obstructed men to TURP versus TUNA, Mostafid and co-workers (90) found that both treatments significantly reduced symptoms. While the TURP group at 6 months had statistically significant reductions in detrusor pressure at Q-max, the TUNA group had clinically irrelevant improvement in obstruction. Long-term outcome data for TUNA are scant. Schulman (91) reported 3-year data on 48 men. AUA symptoms indices were reduced from a mean of 21.6 to 8.5 at 3 years, Q-max increased from 9.9 to 16.9 ml/s. All authors reporting on TUNA describe complication rates well below those experienced with TURP.

Surgical therapy

Long-term outcome studies of TURP report overwhelming symptom relief. AHCPR guidelines (3) report a global subjective median probability of symptom improvement after TURP of 88%. Further, TURP achieves an 80% decline in pre-operative to post-operative symptom score. Malone (92) in a 5–8-year follow-up study in the United Kingdom, found that of those men presenting pre-operatively with urinary retention, 93% were asymptomatic post-operatively, whereas only 76% of elective symptomatic patients were asymptomatic post-operatively. Fowler (93), in a study of patients' perception of post-operative TURP results, reported that of those men presenting pre-operatively with urinary retention or severe symptoms, 93% experienced improvement, whereas those with only moderate symptoms pre-operatively experienced a 72% improvement, leaving 15% unchanged and 6% worse. Fowler found the same pattern of improvement in quality-of-life indices. These data contain a valuable lesson in patient selection. TURP works best in those patients who need it most. Moreover, Barry and co-workers (94) found that TURP does not lengthen life. In their outcomes study comparing the course of men undergoing immediate TURP versus those managed with watchful waiting, the TURP group experienced a 1-month loss of life expectancy. These data call into question the concept that early prostatectomy lengthens life by avoiding subsequent urinary complications and the risks associated with deferring surgery to a time when the patient is older and a poorer operative candidate.

The selection of the type of surgical intervention should be based upon prostate-gland configuration, patient desires, and the surgeon's experience and preference. Of all prostatectomies performed for BPH under the Medicare program in the United States, 93% are done transurethrally (95). Mebust (96) found that of 3885 TURPs, 37% produced 10 g or less of tissues and 65% produced 20 g or less. Citing comparable outcomes, fewer complications, fewer bladder neck contractures, shorter hospitalization, and lower costs, Orandi (97), Soonwalla (98), and Sirle (99), favor transurethral incision of the prostate (TUIP) for glands of less than 30 g in size. Given its higher morbidity, greater length of hospital stay, and lack of patient acceptance, open prostatectomy currently is reserved for those cases where a co-existing bladder disorder is corrected at the same time of prostate surgery, for those glands exceeding the volume with which the resectionist feels comfortable, and for those few men with orthopedic disorders preventing their placement in a dorsal lithotomy position. The reported series of open prostatectomy for BPH are very dated, with few recent studies. Mortality and morbidity comparisons to current TURP and TUIP data are, thus, unreliable and unfair.

There are obvious limits to the volume of prostate adenoma that can be resected by TURP in a safe interval of time. There is no established maximum duration of time but intervals beyond 1 h should probably be avoided. This constraint will then affect how much tissue the urologist can resect, which will vary greatly depending upon the surgeon's training, experience, and expertise. Safety and prudence should compel urologists to honestly recognize their resection limitations and confine TURP to these. Current concepts in the technique of open prostatectomy for BPH (100), TURP (101), and TUIP (102) are described elsewhere.

Transurethral electrovaporization of the prostate

Transurethral electrovaporization of the prostate is a modified form of TURP and is described elsewhere (103). The standard resectoscope loop used in TURP is replaced with a variety of commercially available roller balls or a thick wedged-shaped loop through which cutting current, much greater than that used for routine TURP, is delivered. Vaporization and desiccation removes tissue with reduced bleeding. The technique's similarity to that of TURP, so familiar to all urologists, provides an easy learning curve. Kaplan and co-workers (104) reported mean AUA symptom indices reductions from 17.8 to 5.9 at 12 months and mean

Q-max increases from 7.8 to 17.5 in 33 patients. Of these, 96% had their catheters removed at 24 h and were discharged home in one day. The authors reported no adverse affect on erectile dysfunction but 92% of patients had retrograde ejaculation. However, long-term outcomes remain unavailable.

Conclusions—which therapy should be chosen?

Which of the array of available therapies is best? A review of the literature based upon documented urodynamic outcomes of therapies prompted Bosch (105) to establish the following rank order of urodynamic efficacy in relieving obstruction—from the most efficient to the least: open prostatectomy, TURP, TUIP, laser, alpha-blockers, TUMT, androgen deprivation and, finally, placebo. The rank order of the respective risks, harms, and complications of these therapies are exactly the same. While open prostatectomy is most effective, so are its mortality and morbidity the highest—and so down the list. Patients are interested in symptom relief. They cannot appreciate, nor are they concerned about, urodynamic results. Many men are willing to accept a lesser outcome of symptom relief while assuming less risk and avoiding surgery. The final decision must rest with the patient who has been informed by his urologist of the currently available therapies, their probability of symptom relief, and their various harms and risks.

References

1. Ornstein DK, Garresh SR, Smith DS *et al.* The impact of systemic prostate biopsy on prostate cancer incidence symptomatic benign prostatic hyperplasia undergoing transurethral resection of the prostate. *J Urol* 1997, **157**, 880–4.
2. Catalona WJ. Urothelial tumors of the urinary tract. In: *Campbell's Urology* (6th edn) (ed. Walsh P, Retik A, Stamey T *et al.*). WB Saunders, Philadelphia, 1992, 1102–25.
3. McConnell J, Barry M, Bruskewitz R *et al.* Benign prostatic hyperplasia. *Diagnosis and Treatment Clinical Guidelines*, Number 8. AHCPR Publications, February 1994, No. 94–0582. Rockville MD, Agency for Health Care Policy and Research, Public Health Service, US Department of Health and Human Services.
4. Mebust W, Roizo R, O'Leary M *et al.* Correlations between pathology, clinical symptoms and the course of the disease. In: *The Proceedings of the International*

Consultation on benign prostatic hyperplasia (BPH) (ed. Cockett A, Khoury S, Aso Y *et al.*). Scientific Communications International Ltd, Channel Island 1991, 433–51.

5. American Urological Association. *American Urological Association/Gallup Survey of 1997.* Baltimore, Maryland.

6. Barry MJ, Fowler FJ, O'Leary MP *et al.* The American Urological Association symptom index for benign prostatic hyperplasia. *J Urol* 1992, **148**, 1549–57.

7. Abrams P, Blaivas J, Griffiths D *et al.* The objective evaluation of bladder outlet obstruction (urodynamics). In: *The 2nd International Consultation on benign prostatic hyperplasia (BPH).* (ed. Cockett A, Khoury S, Aso Y *et al.*). Scientific Communications International Ltd, Channel Islands, 1993, 115–32.

8. Barry MJ, Fowler FJ, O'Leary MP *et al.* Measuring disease specific health status in men with benign prostatic hyperplasia. *Medical Care* 1995, **33** (Suppl 4), AS145-AS155.

9. Feneley MR, Dunsmeier WD, Pearce J *et al.* Reproducibility of uroflow measurement: experience during a double-blind, placebo-controlled study of doxazosin in benign prostatic hyperplasia. *Urology* 1996, **47**, 658–63.

10. Reynard JM, Peters TJ, Linn C *et al.* The value of multiple free flow studies in men with lower urinary tract symptoms. *Br J Urology* 1996, **77**, 813–8.

11. Gerber GS, Kim JH, Contreras BA *et al.* An observational urodynamic evaluation of men with lower urinary tract symptoms treated with doxazosin. *Urology* 1996, **47**, 840–4.

12. McConnell JD. Why pressure flow studies should be optional and not mandatory for evaluating men with benign prostatic hyperplasia. *Urology* 1994, **44**, 156–8.

13. Jacobsen SJ, Girman CJ, Guess JA *et al.* Natural history of prostatism: longitudinal changes in voiding symptoms in community dwelling men. *J Urol* 1996, **155**, 595–610.

14. Girman CJ, Jacobsen SJ, Guess HA *et al.* Natural history of prostatism: Relationship among symptoms, prostate volume and peak urinary flow rate. *J Urol* 1995, **153**, 1510–5.

15. Sanda MG, Doehring BC, Binkowitz B *et al.* Clinical and biological characteristics of familial benign prostatic hyperplasia. *J Urol* 1997, **157**, 876–902.

16. Barry MJ, Fowler FJ, Lin B *et al.* The natural history of patients with benign prostatic hyperplasia as diagnosed by North American urologists. *J Urol* 1997, **157**, 10–5.

17. Holtgrewe HL, Mebust W, Dowd J *et al.* Transurethral prostatectomy: practice aspects of the dominant operation in American urology. *J Urol* 1989, **141**, 248–53.

18. Health Care Financing Administration BESS Data, 1998.

19. Holtgrewe HL, Bay-Nielsen H, Carlsson P *et al.* The economics of the management of lower urinary tract symptoms and benign prostatic hyperplasia. In: *Proceedings of the 4th Interntional Consultation on BPH.* July 2–5, 1997, Paris, France. (ed. Khoury S, Chatelain C and Griffiths K). Scientific Communications International Ltd, Channel Islands 1998, 535–58.

20. Wasson J, Reda DJ, Bruskewitz RC *et al.* A comparison of transurethral surgery with watchful waiting for moderate symptoms of benign prostatic hyperplasia: the Veterans Affairs Cooperative Study Group on transurethral resection of the prostate. *New Engl J Med* 1995, **332**, 75–9.

21. Caine M, Perlberg S, Maretyk S. A placebo-controlled double blind study of the effect of phenoxybenzamine in benign prostatic obstruction. *Br J Urol* 1978, **50**, 551–4.

22. Caine M, Pfau A, Perlberg S. The use of alpha adrenergic blockers in benign prostatic obstruction. *Br J Urology* 1976, **48**, 258–63.

23. Caine M, Raz S, Ziegler M. Adrenergic and cholinergic receptors in the human prostate, prostatic capsule and bladder neck. *Br J Urol* 1975, **27**, 193–7.

24. Lepor H, Dixon C, Slawin K *et al.* BPH—A glimpse into the future. *AUA News* 1997, **2** (6), 12–4.

25. Lepor H, Kaplan SA, Klinberg I *et al.* Doxazosin for benign prostatic hyperplasia: Long term efficacy and safety in hypertensive and normotensive patients. *J Urol* 1997, **157**, 525–50.

26. Lepor H, Williford WO, Barry MJ *et al.* The efficacy of terazosin, finasteride or both in benign prostatic hyperplasia. Veterans Affairs Cooperative Studies. *New Engl J Med* 1996, **335**, 533–9.

27. Shapiro E, Hartonto V, Lepor H. Quantifying the smooth muscle content of the prostate using double immunoenzymatic staining and color assisted image analysis. *J Urol* 1992, **147**, 1167–70.

28. Shapiro E, Hartonto V, Lepor H. The response to alpha-blockade in benign prostatic hyperplasia is related to the percent area density of prostate smooth muscle. *Prostate* 1992, **21**, 297–307.

29. Shapiro E, Lepor H. Alpha 1 adrenergic receptors in canine lower genitourinary tissues: insight into development and function. *J Urol* 1987, **138**, 979–83.

30. Shapiro E, Lepor H. Pathophysiology of clinical benign prostatic hyperplasia. In: *Urologic clinics of North America* (ed. Lepor H). WB Saunders, Philadelphia, 1995, **22** (2), 285–99.

31. Lepor H. Long term efficacy and safety of terazosin in patietns with benign prostatic hyperplasia. Terazosin Research Group. *Urology* 1995, **45**, 406–13.

32. Lepor H, Baumann M, Shapiro E. The alpha adrenergic binding properties of terazosin in the human prostate adenoma and canine brain. *J Urol* 1998, **140**, 644–67.

33. Roehrborn CG, Siegel RL. Safety and efficacy of doxazosin in benign prostatic hyperplasia: a pooled analysis of three double blind, placebo-controlled studies. *Urology* 1996, **48**, 406–15.

34. Lepor H, Shapiro E. Characterization of the alpha 1 adrenergic receptors in human benign prostatic hyperplasia. *J Urol* 1994, **132**, 1226–9.

35. Witjes WP, Rosier FW, deWilt MJ *et al.* Urodynamic and clinical effects of terazosin therapy in patients with symptomatic benign prostatic hyperplasia. *J Urol* 1996, **155**, 1117–23.

36. Lepor H, Nieder A, Feser J *et al.* Effect of terazosin on prostatism in men with normal and abnormal peak urinary flow rates. *Urology* 1997, **49**, 476–80.

37. Abrams P, Speakman M, Stott M *et al.* A dose-ranging study of the efficacy and safety of tamulosin, the first prostate-selective alpha 1A-adrenoceptor antagonist, in patients with benign prostatic obstruction (symptomatic benign prostatic hyperplasia). *Br J Urol* 1997, **80**, 587–96.

38. Abrams P, Schulman CC, Voage S. Tamulosin, a selective alpha 1c-adrenoceptor antagonist: a randomized, controlled trial in patients with benign prostatic obstruction (symptomatic BPH). The European Tamulosin Study Group. *Br J Urology* 1995, **76**, 325–6.

39. Chapple CR, Wyndaele JJ, Nordling J *et al.* Tamulosin, the first prostate-selective alpha 1A adrenoceptor antagonist. A meta-analysis of two randomized placebo-controlled, multi-center studies in patients with benign prostatic obstruction (symptomatic BPH). European Tamulosin Study Group. *Europ Urology* 1996, **29**, 155–67.

40. Lee E, Lee C. Clinical comparison of selective and non-selective alpha 1A adrenoceptors antagonists in benign prostatic hyperplasia: Studies on tamulosin in a fixed dose and terazosin in increasing doses. *Br J Urology* 1997, **80**, 606–11.

41. Lowe FC. Coadministration of tamulosin and three antihypertensive agents in patients with benign prostatic hyperplasia: pharmacodynamic effect. *Clinical Therapy* 1997, **19**, 730–42.

42. Fitzpatrick JM, Braeckman J, Denis L *et al.* The medical management of BPH with agents other than hormones or alpha-blocker. In: *Proceedings of the 3rd International Consultation on Benign Prostatic Hyperplasia (BPH)* (ed. Cockett AT, Aso Y, Khoury S *et al.*). Scientific Communications International Ltd, Channel Islands 1995, 489–501.

43. Rhodes L, Primica RL, Berman C *et al.* Comparison of finasteride (Proscar), a 5 alpha-reductase inhibitor and various commercial plant extracts in *in vitro* and *in vivo* 5 alpha-reductase inhibition. *Prostate* 1993, **22**, 43–51

44. Walsh PC, Madden JD, Harrod MJ *et al.* Familial incomplete male pseudohermaphroditism, type 2: decreased dihydrotestosterone formation in pseudovaginal perineoscrotal hypospadias. *New Engl J Med* 1974, **291**, 944–9.

45. Brooks TR, Berman C, Garnes D *et al.* Prostatic effects induced in dogs by chronic or acute oral administration of 5 alpha-reductase inhibitors. *Prostate* 1986, **9**, 65–73.

46. McConnell J, Wilson J, Geroge F *et al.* Finasteride, an inhibitor of 5 alpha-reductase suppresses prostatic dihydrotestosterone in men with benign prostatic hyperplasia. *J Clin Endocrin* 1992, **73**, 505–8.

47. Rittmaster RS, Stoner E, Thompson DL *et al.* Effect of MK-906, a specific 5 alpha-reductase inhibitor on serum androgens and androgen conjugates in normal men. *J Andrology* 1989, **10**, 259–62.

48. Stoner E. Maintenance of clinical efficacy with finasteride therapy for 24 months in patients with benign prostatic hyperplasia: the Finasteride Study Group. *Arch Intern Med* 1994, **154**, 83–8.

49. Stoner E. Three year safety and efficacy data on the use of finasteride in the treatment of benign prostatic hyperplasia. *Urology*, **43**, 284–92.

50. Moore E, Bracken B, Bremmer W *et al.* Proscar: five year experience. *Europ Urology* 1995, **28**, 304–9.

51. Marks LS, Partin AW, Gormley CJ *et al. Prostate* tissue composition and response to finasteride in men with symptomatic benign prostatic hyperplasia. *J Urol* 1997, **157**, 2171–80.

52. Montironi R, Valli M, Fabris G. Treatment of benign prostatic hyperplasia with 5 alpha-reductase inhibitor: morphological changes in patients who fail to respond. *J Clin Pathol*, 1997, **49**, 324–8.

53. Rittmaster RS, Norman RW, Thomas LN *et al.* Evidence of atrophy and apoptosis in the prostate of men given finasteride. *J Clinic Endocrin & Metabolism* 1996, **81**, 814–9.

54. Tewari A, Sinohara K, Narayan P. Transition zone volume and transition zone ratio: predictor of uroflow response to finasteride therapy in benign prostatic hyperplasia patients. *Urology* 1995, **45**, 258–64.

55. Tammela TL, Dontturi MJ. Long term effects of finasteride on invasive urodynamics and symptoms in the treatment of patients with bladder outflow obstruction due to benign prostatic hyperplasia. *J Urol* 1995, **154**, 1466–9.

56. Guess HA, Gormley GJ, Stoner E *et al.* The effect of finasteride on prostate specific antigen: Review of available data. *J Urol* 1996, **155**, 3–9.

57. Matzkin H, Barak M, Braf Z. Effect of finasteride on free and total serum prostatic specific antigen in men with benign prostatic hyperplasia. *Br J Urol* 1996, **78**, 405–8.

58. Narayan P, Tewari A, Jacob G *et al.* Differential suppressions of serum prostatic acid phosphatase and prostate specific antigen by 5 alpha-reductase inhibitor. *Br J Urol*, **75**, 642–6.

59. Puchner PS, Miller MI. The effects of finasteride on hematuria associated with benign prostatic hyperplasia: a preliminary report. *J Urol* 1995, **154**, 1779–82.

60. Nickel JC, Fradet Y, Boake RC *et al.* Efficacy and safety of finasteride therapy for benign prostatic hyperplasia: results of a 2 year randomized controlled trial (The PROSPECT Study). PROscar safety plns efficacy Canadian two-year study. *Canad Medic Assoc J* 1996, **155**, 1251–9.

61. Tollin SR, Rosen HN, Zurowski K *et al.* Finasteride therapy does not alter bone turnover in men with benign prostatic hyperplasia—a clinical research center study. *J Clinic Endocrin* 1996, **81**, 1031–40.

62. Wilton L, Pearce G, Edet L *et al.* The safety of finasteride used in benign prostatic hypertrophy: a non-interventional observational cohort study in 14,772 patients. *Br J Urol* 1996, **78**, 379–84.

63. Lepor H, Williford WO, Barry MJ *et al.* The efficacy of terazosin, finasteride or both in benign prostatic hyperplasia. Veterans Affairs Cooperative Studies. *New Engl J Med* 1996, **335**, 533–9.

64. Boyle P, Gould AL, Roehrborn CG. *Prostate* volume predicts outcome of treatment of benign prostatic hyperplasia with finasteride: meta-analysis of randomized clinical trials. *Urology* 1996, **48**, 398–405.

65. Roehrborn CG, Chinon HK, Fulghorn PF *et al.* The role of transabdominal ultrasound in the pre-operative

evaluation of patients with benign prostatic hypertrophy. *J Urol* 1986, **135**, 1190–3.

66. Roehrborn C, Boyle P, Gould A *et al*. Serum prostate specific antigen (PSA) is a predictor of prostate volume in men with benign prostatic hyperplasia. *Urology* 1999, **53**, 581–9.

67. McConnell JD, Bruskewitz R, Walsh P *et al*. The effect of finasteride on the risk of acute urinary retention and the need for prostate treatment among men with benign prostatic hyperplasia. *New Engl J Med* 1998, **338**, 557–62.

68. Abbou CC, Payan C, Viens-Bitker E *et al*. Transrectal and transurethral hyperthermia versus shaw treatment in benign prostatic hyperplasia: a double-blind, randomized multi-center trial. *Br J Urol* 1995, **76**, 619–25.

69. Kabalin J. Laser prostatectomy. In: *Surgery of the prostate* (ed. Resnick M, Thompson I). Churchill Livingston, New York, 1998, 267–75.

70. Kabalin J, Gill H, Leach G *et al*. Prospective multicenter Pro Lose II clinical trial of neodymium: yttrium-aluminum-garnet laser prostatectomy. *Urology* 1997, **50**, 63–7.

71. Jung P, Mattelaer P, Wolff J *et al*. Visual laser ablation of the prostate: Efficacy evaluated by urodynamics and compared toTURP. *Europ Urology* 1996, **30**, 418–25.

72. Kabalin J, Bite G, Doll S. Neodymium: YAG laser coagulation prostatectomy: 3 years of experience with 227 patients. *J Urol* 1996, **155**, 181–95.

73. Gomella L. Contact laser prostatectomy. In: *Surgery of the prostate* (ed. Resnick M, Thompson I). Churchill Livingston, New York, 1998, 283–7.

74. Gomella L, Lotfi M, Reagan G. Laboratory parameters following contact laser ablation of the prostate for benign prostatic hypertrophy. *Techniques in Urology* 1995, **2**, 168–75.

75. Ekengren J, Hahn R. Complications during transurethral vaporization of the prostate. *Urology* 1996, **48**, 424–9.

76. Narayan P, Tewari A, Aboseif S *et al*. A randominzed study comparing visual laser ablation and transurethral evaporation of the prostate in the management of benign prostatic hyperplasia. *J Urol* 1995, **154**, 2083–90.

77. Muschter R, Hofstetterr A. Interstitial laser therapy outcomes in benign prostatic hyperplasia. *J Endourology* 1995, **9**, 129–33.

78. Schettini M, Diana M, Fortunator P *et al*. Interstitial laser coagulation of the prostate: 12 month follow-up. *Br J Urol* 1997, **80**, 217A.

79. Arai Y, Okubo K, Okada T *et al*. Interstitial laser coagulation for management of benign prostatic hyperplasia: a Japanese experience. *J Urol* 1998, **159**, 1961–9.

80. American Urological Association. *Gallup Survey of 1994*. Baltimore, MD, American Urological Association, 1994.

81. Ramsey E. Office treatment of benign prostatic hyperplasia. In: *Urologic clinics of North America* (ed. Holtgrewe HL), **25** (4), 571–80.

82. Larson T, Blute M, Tri J *et al*. Contrast heating patterns and efficiency of the Prostatron and Targis microwave antennae for treatment of benign prostatic hyperplasia. *Urology* 1998, **51**, 908–13.

83. Dahlstrand C, Walden M, Geirson G *et al*. Transurethral microwave thermotherapy versus transurethral resection for symptomatic benign prostatic obstruction: A Prospective randomized study with a 2-year follow-up. *Br J Urol* 1995, **76**, 614–20.

84. D'Ancona FCH, Francisca EAE, Witjes WPJ *et al*. Thermotherapy versus transurethral resection for benign prostatic hyperplasia. *J Urol* 1997, **158**, 120–3.

85. Ahmed M, Bell T, Lawrence W *et al*. Transurethral microwave thermotherapy (Prostatron version 2.5) compared with transurethral resection of the prostate for the treatment of benign prostatic hyperplasia: a randomized, controlled, parallel study. *Br J Urology* 1997, **79**, 181–5.

86. Hallin A, Berlin T. Transurethral microwave thermotherapy for benign prostatic hyperplasia: Clinical outcomes after 4 years. *J Urol* 1998, **159**, 459–64.

87. Keijzers G, Francisca E, d'Ancona F *et al*. Long-term results of lower energy transurethral microwave thermotherapy. *J Urol* 1990, **159**, 1966–72.

88. Naslund MJ. Transurethral needle ablation of the prostate. *Urology* 1997, **50**, 167–71.

89. Zlotta A, Raviv G, Perry M *et al*. Possible mechanisms of transurethral needle ablation of the prostate on benign prostatic hyperplasia symptoms: a neurohistochemical study. *J Urol* 1997, **157**, 894–9.

90. Mostafid A, Harrison N, Thomas P *et al*. A prospective randomized trial of interstitial radiofrequency therapy versus transurethral resection for the treatment of benign prostatic hyperplasia. *Br J Urol* 1997, **80**, 116–21.

91. Schulman C, Zlotta AR. Transurethral needle ablation (TUNA) of the prostate: clinical experience with three years follow-up in patients with benign prostatic hyperplasia (BPH). *Br J Urol* 1997, **80**, 201A-217A.

92. Malone P, Cook A, Edmonson R. Prostatectomy: Patients perception and long term follow-up. *Br J Urol* 1988, **61**, 234–9.

93. Fowler F, Wennberg J, Timothy R *et al*. Symptom status and quality of life following prostatectomy. *JAMA* 1988, **259**, 3018–25.

94. Barry M, Mulley A, Fowler F *et al*. Watchful waiting versus immediate transurethral resection for symptomatic prostatism. *JAMA* 1988, **259**, 3010–6.

95. Health Care Financing Administration (HCFA), Washington DC 1998.

96. Mebust W, Holtgrewe HL, Cockett A *et al*. Transurethral prostatectomy: Evaluating 3,885 patients. *J Urol* 1989, **141**, 243–7.

97. Orandi A. Transurethral incision of the prostate compared with transurethral resection of the prostate in 132 matching cases. *J Urol* 1987, **138**, 810–15.

98. Soonawalla P, Pardonani D. Transurethral incision versus transurethral resection of the prostate: a subjective and objective analysis. *Br J Urol* 1992, **70**, 174–9.

99. Sirle L, Ganabathi K, Zimmern P *et al*. Transurethral incision of the prostate: An objective and subjective evaluation of long-term efficacy. *J Urol* 1992, **147**, 1303–9.

100. Isacksen R, Waters W. Suprapubic prostatectomy. In: *Surgery of the prostate* (ed. Resnick M, Thompson I). Churchill Livingston, New York 1998, 309–15.

101. Holtgrewe HL. Transurethral prostatectomy. In: *Surgery of the prostate* (ed. Resnick M, Thompson I). Churchill Livingston, New York 1998, 241–7.

102. Sall M, Bruskewitz R. Transurethral incision of the Prostate. In: *Surgery of the prostate* (ed. Resnick M, Thompson I). Churchill Livingston, New York 1998, 257–62.

103. Te A, Sontarosa R, Kaplan S. Transurethral electrovaporazation of the prostate. In: *Surgery of the prostate* (ed. Resnick M, Thompson I). Churchill Livingston, New York 1998, 295–301.

104. Kaplan S, Sontarosa R and Te A. Electrovaporazation of the prostate for symptomatic benign prostatic hyperlasia: the 1-year experience. *J Urol* 1996, **155**, 405A.

105. Bosch J. Urodynamic effects of various treatment modalities for benign prostatic hyperplasia. *J Urol* 1997, **158**, 2034–9.

Section II

6 | *Epidemiology and etiology of prostate cancer*

Ibrahim Barista

Epidemiology

Prostate cancer (PC) is the most common malignancy and second cause of cancer death in American men. It is estimated that there would be 179 300 new cases and 37 000 deaths from PC in the United States (US) in 1999, and that a man has a 1/6 chance of developing PC during his lifetime (1). PC predominantly affects elderly men whose life expectation is short and who are likely to be afflicted by other potential fatal conditions. Many with asymptomatic disease may die from other causes before they need symptomatic treatment.

There has been a striking rise in PC incidence over the past two decades. This can be attributed to several factors, including an increase in the use of prostate-specific antigen (PSA) screening, a heightened awareness of PC, and possibly an increased life expectancy (2). The data suggest that rather than a true increase in the prevalence of PC, we may be diagnosing more cases from the pool of men with latent, previously unsuspected disease, and that these diagnoses occur at an earlier, more localized stage of the disease process (3). In contrast to the prevalence of the disease, the age-adjusted mortality has increased at a much slower pace.

The incidence and mortality rates for PC vary widely between different populations, with very low rates in the Far East, moderate rates in southern and Western Europe, and very high rates in northern Europe and the United States of America (USA). PC is much more common in developed than developing countries. There is a 70- to 80-fold range of incidence in the world, from about 3 per 100 000 among Asians in the Far East to over 200 among African-American men in USA.

The clonal growth of partially transformed cells results in morphologically identifiable premalignant lesions, termed prostatic intra-epithelial neoplasia (PIN). Autopsy studies reveal that PIN precedes the development of carcinoma by 10 years or more (4). These lesions are usually detected following prostate surgery, which is most frequently performed for the treatment of benign prostatic hyperplasia (BPH), a common condition among elderly men. In a worldwide comparative autopsy series, Breslow *et al.* reported on latent carcinoma in seven areas namely, Hong Kong, Singapore, Sweden, Germany, Jamaica, Israel, and Uganda (5). The lowest relative frequencies were observed for Chinese in Hong Kong and Singapore. Intermediate prevalences were observed for Israelis and black Ugandans. The prevalence was highest for Caucasians in Sweden and Germany, and for black Jamaicans. The frequency of small latent carcinomas was 12.3% in all areas investigated and did not vary with age. Rates with larger carcinomas increased sharply with age and showed an area-to-area variation resembling that of clinical carcinoma. In a similar autopsy series, there was no consistent trend in latent non-infiltrative type tumors, related to race or age (6). It is likely, therefore, that genetic predisposition facilitates the role of environmental factors acting in the second (or promotion) phase of carcinogenesis, according to the multi-step theory of cancer development (7, 8).

Etiology and risk factors

Risk factors for PC include age, race, positive family history, dietary fat intake, and vasectomy (9). Indeed, there are many others being investigated. It should be remembered, however, that PC most likely results from interplay between these factors, rather than being caused by a single factor alone.

Age

Age is the most important risk factor. PC rarely occurs in men under age 40, and it reaches a peak in the

eighth decade. It is well established that a large proportion of older men harbor indolent prostate cancers
of no threat to their health. Autopsy studies show that
60–70% of men over 80 years old have some histologic evidence of cancer in their prostates (9).
Different lines of evidence suggest that the initiating
events in PC appear very early during life. Men in
their 30s and 40s have a high incidence of small foci
of cancer or PIN, whereas older men have larger
lesions, implying a stepwise progression (10). It is
speculated that the initiating event in PC occurs at
puberty during the abrupt and massive increase of
steroid hormone production (11).

Race

A number of epidemiologic studies have demonstrated
striking racial differences in PC incidence and mortality. Despite marked improvements in the diagnosis and
treatment of PC, racial differences in incidence and
mortality have shown little change (12). A study from
the National Cancer Institute based on the data
extracted from the Surveillance, Epidemiology, and
End Results Program (SEER), as well as census data,
reveal that African-American men living in the US have
a higher incidence rate of clinical PC than do white
men of similar education and socio-economic classes
(13). Critical analysis does not support the hypothesis
that socio-economic status can account for the racial
differences observed in PC.

The most recent cancer statistics from the American
Cancer Society suggest a stage for stage survival advan-
tage for white men over African-American men (1).
These statistics show an overall 5-year relative survival
of 95% for white men versus 81% for African-
American men. There is no evidence that African-
American men are treated differently than white men.
Therefore, racial differences in PC survival, at least in
part, may reflect differences in tumor biology (12).

It is well established that the incidence rate of PC
among Japanese in the US is higher than that among
Japanese in Japan, although the rate observed among
the migrants is still low compared with that among
whites in the US. This implies that lifestyle characteristics may play a major role in prostatic carcinogenesis.
However, Shimizu and associates demonstrated that a
major part of this difference is again due to different
detection strategies for PC between populations, and
the true difference in the incidence is much smaller (on
the order of only 2–3-fold) (14).

Family

Several studies have reported that male first-degree relatives of an affected man are two to three times more
likely to develop PC, compared with men in the general
population (15–17). Gronberg *et al.* demonstrated a 4-
fold increased positive concordance rate in monozy-
gotic twins when one of them had PC (18). This finding
provides further support for a genetic predisposition in
the pathogenesis of PC.

True hereditary PC is a rare disorder (about 9% of
PCs) and was first described by Carter *et al.* in 1992
(19). The diagnostic criteria included the presence of
more than three affected family members in three successive generations, or two family members who developed the disease before age 55 years. Based on data
from a recent large population-based cohort study,
Gronberg and co-workers recommend that men with at
least two close relatives with PC should undergo testing
for PSA and a digital rectal examination annually
between the ages 50 years and 70 years, ages at which
patients are usually offered curative treatment for
localized tumors (20).

Three independent segregation analyses from the
USA and Sweden have shown an autosomal dominant
inheritance mode of hereditary PC (19–22). According
to these studies, the frequency of susceptibility gene in
the population is 0.3–1.67%, and the risk of PC by age
85 years is 63–89% among carriers of the gene, and
3–5% among non-carriers. Because hereditary PC is an
autosomal trait, women may transmit the deleterious
allele to their sons. Thus, simple questioning for a
family history of PC in the father and paternal uncles
of a patient is not sufficient. One must recognize the
possibility of maternal transmission and extend the
pedigree to maternal uncles, cousins, and grandparents.
An early age at onset of PC within the pedigree should
increase one's awareness of the possibility of hereditary
PC. Moreover, clustering of PC has also been reported
in more distant relative pairs, such as
grandfather–grandson, uncle–nephew, first cousins and
second cousins (23).

Chromosomal alterations

As with other malignancies, much work has been done
to identify the operative molecular events in PC.
Classical cytogenetic analysis is limited by the low
mitotic rate and poor growth of PC cells, the

overgrowth of fibroblasts, and the poor morphology of metaphase spreads (24). Despite these difficulties, various marker chromosomes have been detected.

Loss of heterozygosity

Loss of heterozygosity (LOH) involving specific chromosomes has been demonstrated in PCs. These studies imply the existence of multiple potential tumor-suppressor genes that may contribute to the pathogenesis of PC (25, 26). Carter *et al.* studied allelic loss in PC using polymorphic DNA probes for chromosomes that contain documented and putative tumor-suppressor genes (3p, 7q, 9q, 10q, 11p, 13q, 17p, 18q) (27). The majority (61%) of the tumors exhibited allelic loss on at least one of the chromosomes examined. The regions most frequently deleted were found on the long arms of chromosomes 10 and 16. High rates of loss of alleles on chromosome 8p were also reported in these tumors (28, 29).

Tumor-suppressor genes

The retinoblastoma (*Rb*) gene product, which functions to suppress cell division by preventing cells in the G1 phase of cell division from entering the S phase, has been implicated in PC (30–32). It is estimated that 20% of PCs possess *Rb* mutations, and this number could increase due to the LOH on chromosome 13 involving the *Rb* locus.

The reported incidence of *p53* in localized PC varies considerably, ranging from zero to 80%. Although most early studies suggested infrequent *p53* gene alterations in early-stage PC, increasing evidence is mounting to suggest that loss of *p53* tumor-suppressor function may be an important step in disease progression (33).

The loss of the long arm of chromosome 10 is detected in 30–60% of PCs (27, 34, 35). A new tumor-suppressor gene *PTEN/MMAC1*, was isolated recently at 10q23 and mutations were detected in PC cell lines (36). Cairns and associates screened 80 prostate tumors by microsatellite analysis and found chromosome 10q23 to be deleted in 23 cases (35). *PTEN/MMAC1* may be an important tumor-suppressor in PC, and the inactivation of *PTEN/MMAC1* may be an important secondary genetic event that contributes to PC progression.

Previous studies demonstrated that *CD44*, which is located on human chromosome 11 at p13, is a metastasis suppressor gene for PC. The expression of *CD44*

both at mRNA and protein levels is down-regulated during PC progression, and this correlates with higher tumor grade, aneuploidy, and distant metastasis (37). In a recent study, hypermethylation of the *CD44* gene was observed in 31 of 40 primary PC specimens, 3 of 4 distant organ site metastases, and 4 of the 40 matched normal tissues (38).

Proto-oncogenes

The up-regulation of *bcl-2* protein is one of the key alterations observed in androgen-independent PC. The expression of *bcl-2* may confer growth advantage to PC cells, as well as resistance to therapeutic cell death induction (26).

PCs have been shown to express higher amounts of *c-myc* compared with normal prostate tissue of benign prostatic hyperplasia (39).

It is generally accepted that structural or numerical alterations of *ras* genes at DNA level are rare in PC. A study in the US showed that the frequency of *ras* mutations were low (4%) but, when they did occur, they were associated with advanced metastatic disease (40). In contrast, Anwar and associates suggested that *ras* gene mutations occur at significant frequencies (24%) in clinically diagnosed PC (41). The latter study examined prostatic tissue from Japanese men, raising the possibility that significant differences may exist in genetic events associated with PC in American men versus Japanese men.

No amplification has been found for *c-sis* and *c-fos* genes in PC, suggesting altered regulation at the transcript level in cells overexpressing the protein (42). Likewise, the data on *Her2/neu* expression in PC are controversial (42). *RET* appeared to be overexpressed in high-grade PIN and PC when compared with its expression level in benign prostatic secretory epithelium (43).

E-cadherin and alpha-catenin

E-cadherin, the product of the gene on chromosome 16q22, is a cell-adhesion molecule that has a role in the growth and development via mediation of cell-to-cell interaction. Using immunohistochemistry, a correlation between decreased E-cadherin expression and metastatic progression was demonstrated (44). Preliminary results suggest that LOH in this region occur in approximately 25% of PCs analyzed (25).

Other cell-adhesion molecules

Based on the finding of E-cadherin gene losses and reduced expression, an interest has focused on other cell-adhesion molecules that could play a role in prostate tumorigenesis. Hsieh and co-workers demonstrated that expression of C-CAM1, an immunoglobulin-like cell-adhesion molecule (CAM), was diminished in both PIN and cancer lesions (45). A subsequent study of the same group indicated that the intracellular domain of the C-CAM1 molecule is critical for inhibiting the growth of PC, suggesting that C-CAM1 interactive protein(s) may dictate prostate carcinogenesis (46).

HPC1 (hereditary prostate cancer 1) gene

A familial PC gene, responsible for about 5–10% of all PCs, has been mapped to chromosome 1(1q24–25) (47, 48). The *HPC1* locus appears to increase the risk of early-onset PC (48).

BRCA (breast cancer-associated) genes

An increased risk of PC has also been observed in the relatives of breast cancer patients in several population-based studies (15, 49). Genetic epidemiologic data have suggested that some cases of PC could be linked to breast cancer-associated genes *BRCA1* (50–53) and *BRCA2* (53, 54). According to the available information, it appears that contribution of germline *BRCA1* or *BRCA2* mutations to overall incidence of PC is very small (55).

Androgens

Males who have diminished androgen production due to castration, hypogonadism, or enzyme defects of androgen metabolism (e.g. 5α-reductase) have minimal risk for PC (3, 9, 56). A prospective cohort study revealed that high plasma levels of testosterone before diagnosis were associated with increased risk of PC, and an inverse trend was seen with levels of sex hormone-binding globulin (SHBG) (57).

Ross and co-workers demonstrated that young African-American men have higher circulating testosterone level than their white counterparts and suggested that these higher androgen levels could promote cancer growth, leading to the observed higher rates of cancer in African-American men (58). The same investigators compared serum testosterone concentrations in young adult Japanese men with those of young adult whites and African-Americans in the US, but found no significant differences. However, these white and African-American men had significantly higher values of 3α, 17β androstanediol glucuronide (31% and 25% higher, respectively) and androsterone glucuronide (50% and 41% higher, respectively) than Japanese subjects. These two androgens are indices of 5α-reductase activity. Their results raise the possibility that reduced 5α-reductase activity has a role in producing the low PC incidence rates among Japanese (59).

Hill and colleagues measured urinary steroid levels of African-American and North American white men compared with those of black South African men and discovered lower levels of urinary androsterone and testosterone in the latter group (60). African-American and white men in North America, however, had similar urinary androgen levels. These urinary hormone levels were found to be diet-dependent. When South African black men were fed a Western diet, isocaloric with African diet but supplying 40% of calories from fat and 70% of protein from animal resources, their urinary estrogen and androgen levels increased significantly. Conversely, African-American and North American white men, when fed a vegetarian diet, showed a decrease in urinary estrogen and androgen levels (60). This study suggests that dietary factors may modify the testicular hormone activity.

Androgen receptor

The androgen receptor (AR) gene resides on the long arm of the X chromosome and belongs to the superfamily of ligand-dependent transactivation factors. It appears that AR gene alterations in PCs are much more frequent than originally suggested. These genetic defects include point mutations, variations in the length of trinucleotide repeats, or gene amplification (61–63). Schoenberg *et al.* described a patient with metastatic disease with 24 CAG repeats (that encode polyglutamine region of AR) in this region of the AR gene from normal tissue, but a mixture of 24 CAG and 18 CAG in the AR gene from the tumor tissue (61). A series of epidemiologic studies have suggested that the increased risk of developing PC in African-Americans is related to a reduced frequency of CAG repeat numbers in this population (64–68). A shorter glutamine-repeat length predicts for a higher risk, higher grade, and more advanced stage of PC at diagnosis, and for earlier onset of disease (66, 67, 69, 70).

SRD5A2 (steroid 5α-reductase type II) gene

The human *SRD5A2* gene, located on the short arm of chromosome 2, encodes the type II steroid 5α-reductase, which converts testosterone to a more bioactive compound, dihydrotestosterone. Reichardt and co-workers examined the distribution of a dinucleotide repeat in low-risk Asian Americans, high-risk African-Americans, and intermediate-risk non-Hispanic whites (71). They found this marker to be more polymorphic than previously reported, with some alleles being specific to African-Americans. In a subsequent study, the same group analyzed *SRD5A2* gene for mutations (72). They reported one amino acid substitution, V89L, which replaced valine at codon 89 with leucine. This common and panethnic substitution was a 'germline' DNA polymorphism, and it reduced *in vitro* steroid 5α-reductase activity. This substitution was particularly common among Asians and may explain the low risk for PC in this population.

Growth factors

Many PC cells express growth factors and their receptors that are not produced by normal prostate epithelium. These factors include insulin-like growth factor (IGF) -I and -II, epidermal growth factor (EGF), transforming growth factor (TGF)-α, keratinocyte growth factor (KGF), fibroblast growth factor (FGF), and others. These factors are important in the stromal epithelial cross-talk. Some of these factors stimulate (e.g. bFGF) (73) whereas others repress (e.g. TGF-β) (74) epithelial cells with respect to growth, differentiation, and apoptosis.

A strong positive association was observed between IGF-I levels and PC risk (75). This association was independent of baseline PSA levels. KGF, also known as FGF-7, seems to have a dual role as a growth factor and a differentiating agent. A series of reports suggested aberrant expression of KGF or its receptor in the development and progression of human malignancies, including PC (76). Interestingly, it has been shown that in early stages, PC cells start to produce their own KGF, which could be a growth advantage. However, in later stages, the KGF receptor is not expressed anymore on these cancer cells (77).

Prostate-specific antigen (PSA)

Studies have suggested that PSA may serve to modulate IGF function in prostate cancer by blocking the interaction between IGF and its binding protein, insulin-like growth factor-binding protein (IGFBP) (78, 79). In addition to its role as an indicator of PC, PSA may also inhibit the growth of blood vessels associated with cancer progression; however, when PC progression occurs in spite of elevations of PSA, the local angiogenic stimulators overcome the effects of PSA and dominate (80).

Dietary factors

Fat

The ecologic studies have shown strong positive correlations between PC incidence and per capita fat consumption (81, 82). Armstrong and Doll found that the PC mortality in 32 countries was highly associated with total fat consumption, a finding similar to that for breast cancer (83). Subsequent studies showed a positive association between some component of animal fat and risk for PC (84, 85). The relatively higher rates observed among Japanese who have migrated to US suggest that dietary factors play an etiologic role in the occurrence of PC. African-Americans may also have a higher intake of dietary fats and this may contribute to PC promotion (86).

Most case-control studies (86–96) of dietary fat and PC have found positive associations (86–94) (Table 6.1). However, two case-control studies have failed to confirm this finding (95, 96). Cohort studies (97–104) of dietary fat and PC have been less consistent. Observations on Seventh-day Adventists (97, 98), in Japanese who live in Hawaii (99), and Lutheran men (100), have also revealed weak associations or no associations with animal products. A study of US male health professionals (101) observed an association between high-grade/advanced PC and intake of saturated fat, particularly from red meat, and a study of US male physicians (93) observed an association with consumption of red meat. There are many problems associated with the conduct and interpretation of retrospective dietary studies. For example, the accuracy of recall may be debatable in elderly patients, and the current or recent diet may be less relevant to a disease process which may have been initiated many years ago (105).

Regarding the mechanisms of carcinogenesis, it has been postulated that dietary fat may lead to the increased production and bioavailability of sexual hormones. The promoting effect of a high-fat diet on carcinogenesis may also be the result of an accelerated

Table 6.1 Dietary fat and prostate cancer

Author, year (reference no.)	Study type	No. of cases/ controls	Source of fat (intake)	Results, RR or OR (95% CI)
Graham 1983 (87)	Case-control	260/260	Total fat Animal fat	2.04, CI not given, $P < 0.05$ 2.99, CI not given, $P < 0.01$
Talamini 1986 (88)	Case-control	166/202	Meat Milk/dairy products	1.7 (1.0–2.8), $P = 0.05$ 2.5 (1.3–4.7), $P < 0.05$
Ross 1987 (89)	Case-control	284/284	Total fat	1.9, CI not given, $P < 0.05$, for blacks 1.6, CI not given, $P < 0.05$, for whites
Ohno 1988 (95)	Case-control	100/100	Total fat	1.32 (0.76–2.32)
Kolonel 1988 (90)	Case-control	452/899	Saturated fat	1.70 (1.0–2.8) only for age $\geq$ 70
Mettlin 1989 (91)	Case-control	371/371	Animal fat Milk Milk	1.26 (0.76–2.07) 1.92 (1.05–3.50) 2.49 (1.27–4.87) for frequent consumption
West 1991 (92)	Case-control	358/679	Total fat	2.9 (1.0–8.4), for aggressive tumors, only for age $\geq$ 68
Gann 1994 (93)	Case-control	120/120	Red meat	2.5 (0.9–6.7), $P = 0.07$
Whittemore 1995 (86)	Case-control	1655/1645	Saturated fat	2.8 (1.5–5.2) for aggressive tumors
Andersson 1995 (96)	Case-control	256/252	Total fat	0.7 (0.4–1.1)
Vlajinac 1997 (94)	Case-control	101/202	Total fat	1.95 (0.68–5.57)
Snowdon 1984 (97)	Cohort	99/–	Meat Eggs Cheese Milk	1.3 1.3 1.4 1.5 3.6 (when all four animal products were combined)
Mills 1989 (98)	Cohort	180/–	Beef	1.21 (0.83–1.75)
Severson 1989 (99)	Cohort	174/–	Saturated fat Total fat	1.00 (0.68–1.46) 0.87 (0.58–1.31)
Hsing 1990 (100)	Cohort	149/–	Meat	0.8 (0.5–1.3)
Giovannucci 1993 (101)	Cohort	300/–	Total fat Red meat	1.79 (1.04–3.07), $P = 0.06$, 2.64 (1.21–5.77), $P = 0.02$, both for advanced cases
Harvei 1997 (102)	Cohort	141/–	Alpha-linolenic acid Palmitic acid Palmitoleic acid	2.0 (1.1–3.6) 2.3 (1.1–4.7) 2.8 (1.5–5.1) for the highest quartiles of intake
Veierod 1997 (103)	Cohort	72/–	Total fat Skim milk	1.3 (0.6–2.8) for the highest quintile of intake 2.1 (1.2–3.6)
Schuurman 1999 (104)	Cohort	642/–	Total fat Saturated fat	1.02 (0.95–1.09) 1.09 (0.92–1.28)

RR: relative risk; OR: odds ratio; CI: confidence interval.

formation of arachidonic acid and subsequently of prostaglandins (106, 107).

Retinoids

Vitamin A is a generic term for all substances that possess the biologic properties of retinol. It may be ingested either as a preformed vitamin or as provitamin. These compounds are potent antioxidants and may exert a protective effect against epithelial tumors. Many studies have reported on the putative relation between vitamin A or β-carotene intake and PC.

Unfortunately, there is no consistent evidence of protection from PC. In a large population-based study, Whittemore *et al.* (86) failed to find any clear and consistent association between PC and intake of vitamin A or carotenes or consumption of foods high in carotenoid content. Most other case-control studies have also yielded controversial results (87, 89–92, 94, 95, 108) (Table 6.2). The data from cohort studies (100, 109, 110) are equally inconsistent, showing either no association (109, 110) or a positive association (100). In two of these studies (90, 100) the effect was restricted to a certain age range.

Table 6.2   Dietary vitamin A or B-carotene and prostate cancer

Author, year (reference no.)	Study type	No. of cases controls	Source	Results, RR or OR (95% CI)
Graham 1983 (87)	Case-control	260/260	Vitamin A	1.64 (CI not given), for age < 70 1.97 (CI not given), for age ≥ 70
Ross 1987 (89)	Case-control	284/284	Vitamin A	0.8, P > 0.05, for blacks 0.9, P > 0.05, for whites
			Carotene	0.6, P > 0.05, for blacks 1.0, P > 0.05, for whites
Kolonel 1988 (90)	Case-control	452/899	Vitamin A	0.8 (0.5–1.3) for age < 70 2.0 (1.3–3.1) for age ≥ 70
			Carotene	1.0 (0.6–1.6) for age < 70 1.5 (0.9–2.3) for age ≥ 70, for higher quartiles of intake
Ohno 1988 (95)	Case-control	100/100	Beta-carotene	2.86 (1.36–6.04), for age ≥ 70, for low intake
Mettlin 1989 (91)	Case-control	371/371	Beta-carotene	0.60 (0.37–0.99) 0.30 (0.13–0.66), for age < 69, for high intake
West 1991 (92)	Case-control	358/679	Vitamin A	1.0 (0.6–1.7) for ages 45–67 1.6 (0.9–2.7) for ages 68–74
			Carotene	0.8 (0.5–1.2) for ages 45–67 1.4 (0.9–2.4) for ages 68–74
Whittemore 1995 (86)	Case-control	1655/1645	Vitamin A	RR not given, no association
Vlajinac 1997 (94)	Case-control	101/202	Retinol Retinol equivalent	0.69 (0.50–1.24) 1.64 (1.01–2.67)
Cook 1999 (108)	Case-control	631/2204	β-Carotene	0.68 (0.46–0.99)
Paganini-Hill 1987 (109)	Cohort	93/–	Total vitamin A Carotene	1.2* no association 1.0* no association
Hsing 1990 (100)	Cohort	149/–	Vitamin A	2.8 (1.4–5.8) for age < 75 0.4 (0.2–0.9) for age ? 75
			Carotene	1.9 (1.0–3.7) for age < 75 0.2 (0.1–0.6), for age ? 75
Giovannucci 1995 (110)	Cohort	773/–	Total retinol equivalent Retinol without supplements	1.13 (0.88–1.44) 1.30 (1.03–1.66)

RR: relative risk; OR: odds ratio; CI: confidence interval.
*Calculated from data provided in paper.

Observational epidemiological studies have indicated that individuals with diets high in fruits and vegetables, particularly those rich in β-carotene, are at lower risk of cancer, suggesting a role for β-carotene in the primary prevention of cancer. A recent nested case-control study indicated that β-carotene supplementation may reduce risk of PC among those with low baseline levels (108).

Vegetables

Evidence of a protective effect of fruit and vegetables is weak and inconsistent (111). Increasing consumption of beans, lentils and peas, tomatoes, raisin, dates, and other dried fruit were all associated with significantly decreased PC risk (98). This may be explained by the fact that men on vegetarian or high-fiber diets have lower testosterone and plasma estradiol levels. Fibers excreted in feces may bind sex steroids, thereby lowering plasma levels by increased fecal excretion (3).

Vitamin E

There are insignificant data on vitamin E to draw meaningful conclusions about its possible association with PC. Two studies suggest an inverse association. In the first study, the participants of the Alpha-Tocopherol, Beta Carotene Cancer Prevention Study Group (male smokers after 5–8 years of dietary supplementation) who received alpha-tocopherol had fewer cancers of the prostate and colorectum than those who did not receive alpha-tocopherol (112). In the second study, 50 mg of alpha-tocopherol per day—a moderate dose of the antioxidant vitamin E—reduced PC incidence by 32% and PC deaths by 41% in a group of male smokers in Finland (113).

Micronutrients

Micronutrient intake and PC risk have been the subject of several studies, but no consistent relationship has emerged (114, 115).

Isoflavonoids/soy products

Decreased PC risk has been found in Adventist men (98) who eat a lot of beans, lentils, peas, and some dried fruits (all sources of isoflavonoids), and in men of Japanese ancestry in Hawaii (99) who eat rice and tofu, a soybean product that contain isoflavonoids in large quantities. These observations had led Adlercreutz and associates to hypothesize that high phyto-estrogen levels may inhibit the growth of PC in Japanese men, which may explain the low mortality from prostatic cancer in that country (116).

The Asian diet, and to a lesser extent, vegetarian and Mediterranean diets, are not only low in fat, but also a rich source of plant estrogens. These phyto-estrogens, lignans, flavonoids, and isoflavonoids may be protective against PC as they are inhibitors of 5α-reductase and 17β-hydroxysteroid dehydrogenase (117).

Lycopene/tomato products

Dietary consumption of the carotenoid lycopene (mostly from tomato products) has been associated with a lower risk of PC in several studies (98, 110, 118). In a large prospective cohort study, Giovannucci and colleagues found that consumption of lycopene, a non-provitamin A carotenoid, was inversely related to PC risk, especially for aggressive disease (110).

Selenium

Glutathione peroxidase, an enzyme that protects cells from oxidative damage, is selenium-dependent. Recently, the efficacy of 200 μg/day of selenomethionine was evaluated in a placebo-controlled intervention study of 1312 patients with non-melanoma skin cancer (119). There was a 3- to 4-fold lower incidence of PC among those who received the selenium (relative risk [RR] = 0.29, $P < 0.001$).

Vitamin D and sunlight

In 1990, Schwartz and Hulka first hypothesized that vitamin D deficiency is a potential risk factor for PC (120). The hypothesis was based on a series of related observations. First, the incidence of PC increases with age and the elderly are known to be vitamin D deficient. Second, there is a high incidence of PC in blacks who have a reduced capacity to produce vitamin D_3. Third, is the increased incidence of PC in migrant Asians as they adopt a Western diet that contain less vitamin D_3 than they are accustomed to.

There is evidence that ultraviolet (UV) radiation may protect against PC. An inverse correlation was shown between UV radiation exposure and PC (121). The countries with the highest death rates, namely, Denmark, Sweden, and Iceland, have low exposure to

UV light, as do patients living in northeastern parts of the USA where death from PC is the highest. The protective effect of UV light may be mediated through vitamin D. Using a nested case-control design, Corder *et al.* (122) found that lower prediagnostic serum levels of 1,25-dihydroxyvitamin D (1,25-D), a vitamin D metabolite, were significantly associated with an increased risk of clinically detected PC, particularly in men with low levels of 25-dihydroxyvitamin D (odds ratio [OR] = 0.41). A subsequent nested case-control study (123), however, failed to support these findings.

Miller and associates showed that the human PC cells express biologically active vitamin D_3 receptors (124). Additional preliminary evidence of a role of 1,25(OH)$_2$D is that genetic polymorphisms of the vitamin D receptor gene, which may correlate with activity of the receptor, predict the risk of PC (68, 125).

In a study providing indirect support to these findings, higher consumption of calcium was found to be related to advanced PC, as it suppressed the formation of 1,25(OH)$_2$D, and higher intake of fructose was found to be related to a lower risk of advanced prostate cancer, as it stimulated 1,25(OH)$_2$D production (126).

Vasectomy

Occlusion of vas deferens by surgical means is an important family planning method and is referred to as 'vasectomy'. There has been concern over a positive association between vasectomy and PC since the late 1980s when Honda *et al.* first reported findings from their population-based case-control study (127). Regarding the pathogenetic mechanism, it has been sug-

Table 6.3 Summary of findings on vasectomy and prostate cancer

Author, year (reference no.)	Study type	No. of cases/controls	Results OR/RR (95% CI)
Ross 1983 (132)	Case-control	110/110	0.5 (0.2–1.6)*
Honda 1988 (127)	Case-control	216/216	1.4 (0.9–2.3) 2.2 (1.0–4.8) for 20–29 years since vasectomy 4.4 (0.9–21.0) for ≥ 30 years since vasecotmy
Rosenberg 1990 (129)	Case-control	220/1531	3.5 (2.1–6.0) (cancer controls) 5.3 (2.7–10.0) (non-cancer controls). no association with years since vasectomy
Mettlin 1990 (130)	Case-control	614/2588	1.7 (1.1–2.6) association with years since vasectomy
Spitz 1991 (133)	Case-control	343/360	1.6 (1.1–2.3) 2.2 (1.1–4.3) for ≥ 27 years since vasectomy
Hayes 1993 (134)	Case-control	965/1292	1.1 (0.8–1.7) for whites 1.6 (0.5–4.8) for blacks 1.5 (0.8–2.7) for ≥ 20 years since vasectomy 2.0 (1.0–4.0) for age < 35
Hsing 1994 (131)	Case-control	138/638	2.0 (0.7–6.1) (hospital cancer controls) 6.7 (2.1–21.6) (neighborhood controls)
John 1995 (135)	Case-control	1642/1636	1.1 (0.83–1.3)
Zhu 1996 (136)	Case-control	175/258	0.86 (0.57–1.32)
Platz 1997 (137)	Case-control	175/978	1.48 (0.80–2.72)
Sidney 1991 (138)	Cohort	135/–	1.0 (0.7–1.6) no association with years since vasectomy
Nienhuis 1992 (139)	Cohort	1/–	0.44 (0.1–4.0)
Giovannucci 1993 (140)	Cohort Retrospective	96/–	1.56 (1.03–2.37) 1.89 (1.14–3.14) for ≥ 20 years since vasectomy
Giovannucci 1993 (141)	Cohort Prospective	300/–	1.66 (1.25–2.21) 1.85 (1.26–2.72) for ≥ 22 years since vasectomy

RR: relative risk; OR: odds ratio; CI: confidence interval.

* CI not provided, and calculated from the tabular data in the article.

gested that vasectomy may increase the risk for PC because vasectomized men have higher levels of circulating testosterone. Alternatively, vasectomy may induce anti-sperm antibodies, and an immunologic reaction may be responsible for elevation of PC rates (128).

A number of case-control (127, 129–137) and cohort (138–141) studies have examined the association between vasectomy and PC (Table 6.3). The results of the case-control studies have been inconsistent: some studies have reported a positive association (127, 129–131), one a negative association (132), others little or no association (133–137). Conflicting results have also been reported from cohort studies: Sidney *et al.* (138), and Nienhuis *et al.* (139) found no association between vasectomy and PC risk, while Giovannucci *et al.* (140, 141) found modestly increased relative risks.

The risk of PC in relation to time since vasectomy and age at vasectomy have also been inconsistent (Table 6.3). Sidney *et al.* (138) found no difference in PC risk according to age at vasectomy. However, Hayes *et al.* (134), found that men who had been vasectomized at age 34 years or younger experienced a higher risk for PC, while men who had undergone a vasectomy at age 35 years or older did not have an increased risk. In contrast, Giovannucci *et al.* (140) reported an increase in risk for men who had a vasectomy at age 40 years or older. A major concern in the study of vasectomy and PC has been detection bias (135). Vasectomized men may be more likely to subsequently visit a urologist, resulting in an increased chance of being diagnosed with PC (142). In summary, the association—if there exists any—between increased risk for PC and vasectomy, is weak (143, 144). On the basis of currently available data, no changes in family planning policies with regard to vasectomy are warranted (145).

Smoking

Only a few (127, 146, 147) case-control studies have found some association between smoking and incident PC, whereas others (89, 148, 149) have contradicted these results (Table 6.4). Cohort studies (98–100, 150–153) of smoking and death from PC, however, have been more consistent. The largest three (100, 150, 151) prospective studies found a modest (risk ratios < 2) association between current smoking and early death from PC. Men who were cigarette smokers at the time of enrollment in the study had a 34% higher death rate from PC than never-smokers during the 9

years of follow-up (152). It appears that cigarette smoking adds little, if anything, to the risk of developing PC (9).

Alcohol

Alcoholic beverage consumption has been reported to be causally related to malignant tumors of the oral cavity, pharynx, larynx, esophagus, and liver, and there is growing, but as yet inconclusive, evidence that it is related to a rather moderate increase in risk for malignancies at other major organ sites, including the prostate (154, 155). Significantly increased risks of PC have been shown in a large cohort of alcoholics from Denmark (155) and among alcoholics from Sweden who were less than 65 years of age, but not among those who were age 65 or older (154). Likewise, Hayes and co-workers reported the first dose–response relation between alcoholic beverage consumption and risk of PC: significantly elevated risks were seen between those who had 22–56 drinks per week (OR = 1.4, 95% confidence interval [CI] 1.0–1.8) and 57 or more drinks per week (OR = 1.9, 95% CI 1.3–2.7) in comparison to never-users (156). However, with respect to potentially modifiable risk factors, most sizeable case-control (89, 91, 127, 146, 147, 157) and cohort studies (98–100) on PC and alcohol failed to show an association (Table 6.4). Overall, alcohol has not generally been considered a risk factor for PC. Interestingly, alcoholics might have a lower risk of PC than non-drinkers because of the alterations in liver metabolism of testosterone (158).

Obesity/body mass index

Some case-control (88, 159) and cohort studies (97, 103, 153, 160) have suggested that men with high body mass and those who are obese as adults have an increased risk of PC; however, others (86, 92, 98, 161) have failed to confirm this association.

Physical activity/life-style

Level of physical activity has been found to be inversely associated with risk (96, 162), but the data are inconsistent with other studies that showed an association or positive relation (86, 92, 153, 163).

Table 6.4 The association between smoking or alcohol and prostate cancer

Author, year (reference no.)	Study type	Association with smoking	Association with alcohol
Ross 1987 (89)	Case-control	Negative	Negative
Honda 1988 (127)	Case-control	Positive	Negative
Mettlin 1989 (91)	Case-control	–	Negative
Slattery 1993 (146)	Case-control	Positive (little support)	Negative
van der Gulden 1994 (147)	Case-control	Positive	Negative
Hayes 1996 (156)	Case-control	–	Positive
Lumey 1997 (148)	Case-control	Negative	–
Rohan 1997 (149)	Case-control	Negative	–
Lumey 1998 (157)	Case-control	–	Negative
Mills 1989 (98)	Cohort	Negative	Negative
Severson 1989 (99)	Cohort	Negative	Negative
Hsing 1990 (100)	Cohort	Positive	Negative
Hsing 1991 (150)	Cohort	Positive	–
Adami 1992 (154)	Cohort	–	Positive (in alcoholic patients)
Tonnesen 1994 (155)	Cohort	–	Positive (in alcoholic patients)
Coughlin 1996 (151)	Cohort	Positive	–
Rodriguez 1997 (152)	Cohort	Positive	–
Cerhan 1997 (153)	Cohort	Positive	–

Socio-economic status

In general, socio-economic status is not an important risk factor for the development of PC (13, 99, 164, 165).

Farming

Of 24 studies of farming and PC reviewed by Blair and Zahm (166), 17 showed an increased risk, although only in 10 were results significant. Farmers are likely to spend more time outdoors exposed to the sun. However, presently farmers are also exposed to several other risk factors in their work, e.g. pesticides and fer-

tilizers. The increased risk may be multifactorial, including exposure to some agricultural chemicals and to a lesser extent also associated with cadmium, a common although minor ingredient in fertilizers (158). Hence, one study has shown that farmers experience increased PC risk associated with the acres sprayed with pesticides, while other farm exposures examined were not related to PC risk (167).

Other occupational risk factors

No occupational risk factors for PC have been identified and confirmed. Only cadmium compounds and pesticides have been linked with any consistency to an increased PC risk. Cohort studies published in the 1960s and 1970s suggested slightly increased risk among rubber and tire-manufacturing workers (168, 169). Using sound data on exposure, Aronson and co-workers found elevated risks among those employed in the water-transport and aircraft-manufacturing industries (170). Other groups at elevated risk included metal-product fabricators, structural-metal erectors, and railway-transport workers.

In a case-referent study from the Netherlands, significantly elevated risks were found for food manufacturers and book-keepers, as well as those employed in administration, storage, or farm labors. An elevated risk was found in the study for farm laborers, but not for farm owners or for agriculture in general. In addition, a statistically significant excess risk was found for subjects who reported frequent occupational exposure to cadmium (171). In a small study from England, 136 nuclear power plant employees were investigated (172); these men had a 2.36-fold higher risk of developing PC than that expected from control populations. The main risk factors were supposedly tritiated chromium, iron, cobalt, and, perhaps more importantly, zinc.

Cadmium

The prostate gland contains the highest level of zinc of all the organs in body (173). Zinc is required in several enzymes involved in replication and repair of DNA and RNA. Cadmium is an inhibitor of zinc metabolism. Cadmium has recently been accepted by the International Agency for Research on Cancer as a Category 1 (human) carcinogen (174). High levels of cadmium may result from industrial exposure in those who work with batteries, paint, and cigarette manufacturing, and in other occupations. Cadmium has been associated with human PC in some (82, 92, 175), but not all (89, 169), epidemiologic studies. These data do not, however, establish a definitive connection between cadmium and PC.

Benign prostatic hyperplasia

An issue of major clinical importance is whether men with BPH are at elevated risk of cancer of the prostate. Armenian *et al.* reported two studies in which men with BPH were found to be at relatively high risk of cancer (176). In their case-control study, the authors found that hospitalization for a non-cancerous prosta-

tic disease was associated with a relative risk of 5.1 of developing PC. Greenwald and co-workers, however, found no association between BPH and PC (177).

Viruses

Several types of viruses have been isolated from cancer cells, such as human papillomavirus, cytomegalovirus, and herpesvirus, but no definitive links between PC and viruses have been established (9).

Sexual behavior

Considerable attention has been paid to patterns of sexual behavior and the development of PC. Bacterial prostatitis, particularly a history of gonorrhea, has been suggested as an increased risk factor for PC (3). Although extensively studied, there is very little evidence supporting the association.

Diabetes mellitus

In a case-control study, Steenland *et al.* reported that for diabetic men, the relative risk for all cancers was 1.38 (95% CI 1.00–1.91); the elevated risk was particularly evident for colorectal and PC (178). Currently, there is only scant information on diabetes as a risk factor.

Conclusions

Given the similar prevalence rates for histologic cancers at autopsy, it appears that although genetics may play a role in PC etiology, environmental factors appear to have a major role in PC biology, perhaps acting as promoters. If we look more analytically at the etiological factors, including those emerging from epidemiological surveys, there is a mixture of genetic and environmental factors, which interact with the age and the hormonal status of male subjects at risk. Genetic factors, such as race and familial predisposition, cannot be modified. There is, however, a possibility that environmental factors may be brought under control.

From a public health perspective, dietary factors appear to hold the most promise for prevention.

Although no specific prevention can be proposed at the present time, the results from dietary intake studies support the concept that a high-fiber, low-fat, and possibly β-carotene-rich diet may protect men against the development of PC. Furthermore, the potential preventive properties of soya products and lycopenes are being investigated. Another approach to lower PC mortality is early diagnosis through screening. In principle, cancer screening should be targeted at individuals who are likely to have the particular disease in preclinical, detectable, and curable form, and who are at high risk of ultimately suffering and/or dying from this disease. Men in high-risk groups, including African-Americans and those with a family history of PC may be screened at an earlier age. Finally and hopefully, a genetic test to diagnose an inherited predisposition to PC may become available in the near future. This would make it possible to diagnose cancer-prone individuals in advance and diagnose their tumors at an early stage while there is still a possibility of cure.

Acknowledgments

The author gratefully acknowledges the critical review of the manuscript and constructive comments by Associate Professor Omrüm Uzun, MD, and Professor Dincer Firat, MD.

References

1. Landis SH, Murray T, Bolden S *et al.* Cancer statistics, 1999. *CA Cancer J Clin* 1999, **49**, 8–31.
2. Karp JE, Chiarodo A, Brawlet O *et al.* Prostate cancer prevention: Investigational approaches and opportunities. *Cancer Res* 1996, **56**, 5547–56.
3. Haas GP, Sakr WA. Epidemiology of prostate cancer. *CA Cancer J Clin* 1997, **47**, 273–87.
4. Sakr WA, Haas GP, Cassin BF *et al.* The frequency of carcinoma and intraepithelial neoplasia of the prostate in young male patients. *J Urol* 1993, **150**, 379–85.
5. Breslow N, Chan CW, Dhom G *et al.* Latent carcinoma of the prostate at autopsy in seven areas. *Int J Cancer* 1977, **20**, 680–8.
6. Yatani R, Chigusa I, Akazaki K *et al.* Geographic pathology of latent prostatic carcinoma. *Int J Cancer* 1982, **29**, 611–6.
7. Carter HB, Piantadosi S, Isaacs JT. Clinical evidence for and implications of the multistep development of prostate cancer. *J Urol* 1990, **143**, 742–6.
8. Pavone-Macaluso M. Epidemiology, prevention and screening for prostate cancer. *Eur Urol* 1996, **29** (Suppl 2), 49–53.
9. Pienta KJ, Esper PS. Risk factors for prostate cancer. *Ann Intern Med* 1993, **118**, 793–803.
10. Sakr WA, Grignon DJ, Crissman JD *et al.* High grade prostatic intraepithelial neoplasia (HGPIN) and prostatic adenocarcinoma between the ages of 20–69: an autopsy study of 249 cases. *In Vivo* 1994, **8**, 439–43.
11. Diamandis EP, Yu H. Does prostate cancer start at puberty? *J Clin Lab Anal* 1996, **10**, 468–9 (letter).
12. Morton RA Jr. Racial differences in adenocarcinoma of the prostate in North American men. *Urology* 1994, **44**, 637–45.
13. Baquet CR, Horm JW, Gibbs T *et al.* Socioeconomic factors and cancer incidence among blacks and whites. *J Natl Cancer Inst* 1991, **83**, 551–7.
14. Shimizu H, Ross RK, Bernstein L. Possible underestimation of the incidence rate of prostate cancer in Japan. *Jpn J Cancer Res* 1991, **82**, 483–5.
15. Cannon L, Bishop DT, Skolnick M *et al.* Genetic epidemiology of prostate cancer in the Utah Mormon genealogy. *Cancer Surv* 1982, **1**, 47–69.
16. Steinberg GS, Carter BS, Beaty TH *et al.* Family history and the risk of prostate cancer. *Prostate* 1990, **17**, 337–47.
17. Spitz MR, Currier RD, Fueger JJ *et al.* Familial patterns of prostate cancer: a case-control analysis. *J Urol* 1991, **146**, 1305–7.
18. Gronberg H, Damber L, Damber JE. Studies of genetic factors in prostate cancer in a twin population. *J Urol* 1994, **152**, 1484–7.
19. Carter BS, Beaty TH, Steinberg GD *et al.* Mendelian inheritance of familial prostate cancer. *Proc Natl Acad Sci USA* 1992, **89**, 3367–71.
20. Gronberg H, Wiklund F, Damber JE. Age specific risks of familial prostate carcinoma. A basis for screening recommendations in high risk populations. *Cancer* 1999, **86**, 477–83.
21. Gronberg H, Damber JE, Damber L *et al.* Segregation analysis of prostate cancer in Sweden: support for a dominant heritage. *Am J Epidemiol* 1997, **146**, 552–7.
22. Schaid DJ, McDonell SK, Blute ML *et al.* Evidence for autosomal dominant inheritance of prostate cancer. *Am J Hum Genet* 1998, **62**, 1425–38.
23. Cannon-Albright L, Thomas A, Goldgar GE *et al.* Familiality of prostate cancer in Utah. *Cancer Res* 1994, **54**, 2378–85.
24. Kallioniemi OP, Visakorpi T. Genetic basis and clonal evolution of human prostate cancer. *Adv Cancer Res* 1996, **68**, 225–55.
25. Isaacs WB, Bova GS, Morton RA *et al.* Molecular genetics and chromosomal alterations in prostate cancer. *Cancer* 1995, **75**, 2004–12.
26. Bruckeheimer EM, Gjertsen BT, McDonnell TJ. Implications of cell death regulation in the pathogenesis and treatment of prostate cancer. *Semin Oncol* 1999, **26**, 382–98.
27. Carter BS, Ewing CM, Ward WS *et al.* Allelic loss of chromosomes 16q and 10q in human prostate cancer. *Proc Natl Acad Sci USA* 1990, **87**, 8751–5.
28. Bergerheim USR, Kunimi K, Collins VP *et al.* Deletion mapping of chromosomes 8, 10, and 16 in human prostatic carcinoma. *Genes Chromosom Cancer* 1991, **3**, 215–20.

29. Bova GS, Carter BS, Bussemakers JG *et al.* Homozygous deletion and frequent allelic loss of chromosome 8p22 loci in human prostate cancer. *Cancer Res* 1993, **53**, 3869–73.

30. Bookstein R, Shew J, Chen P *et al.* Suppression of tumorigenicity of human carcinoma cells by replacing mutated a mutated Rb gene. *Science* 1990, **247**, 712–5.

31. Bookstein R, Rio P, Madreperla SA *et al.* Promoter deletion and loss of retinoblastoma gene expression in human prostate carcinoma. *Proc Natl Acad Sci USA* 1990, **87**, 7762–6.

32. Phillips SM, Barton CM, Lee SJ *et al.* Loss of the retinoblastoma susceptibility gene (RB1) is a frequent and early event in prostatic tumorigenesis. *Br J Cancer* 1999, **70**, 1252–7.

33. Heidenberg HB, Bauber JJ, Mc Leod DG *et al.* The role of the p53 tumor-suppressor gene in prostate cancer: a possible biomarker? *Urology* 1996, **48**, 971–9.

34. Isaacs WB, Carter BS. Genetic changes associated with prostate cancer in humans. *Cancer Surv* 1991, **11**, 15–24.

35. Cairns P, Okami K, Halachmi S *et al.* Frequent inactivation of PTEN/MMAC1 in primary prostate cancer. *Cancer Res* 1997, **57**, 4497–5000.

36. Li J, Yen C, Liaw D *et al.* PTEN, a putative protein tyrosine phosphatase gene mutated in human brain, breast, and prostate cancer. *Science* 1997, **275**, 1943–7.

37. Gao AC, Lou W, Dong JT *et al.* CD44 is a metastasis suppressor gene for prostatic cancer located on human chromosome 11p13. *Cancer Res* 1997, **57**, 846–9.

38. Lou W, Krill D, Dhir R *et al.* Methylation of the CD44 metastasis suppresser gene in human prostatic cancer. *Cancer Res* 1999, **59**, 2329–31.

39. Fleming WH, Hamel A, MacDonald R *et al.* Expression of the c-myc protooncogene in human prostatic carcinoma and benign prostatic hyperplasia. *Cancer Res* 1986, **46**, 1535–8.

40. Carter BS, Epstein JI, Isaacs WB. Ras gene mutations in human prostate cancer. *Cancer Res* 1990, **50**, 6830–2.

41. Anwar K, Nakakuki K, Shiraishi T *et al.* Presence of *ras* oncogene mutations and human papilloma virus DNA in human prostate carcinomas. *Cancer Res* 1992, **52**, 5991–6.

42. Strohmeyer TG, Slamon DJ. Proto-oncogenes and tumor-suppressor genes in human urological malignancies. *J Urol* 1994, **151**, 1479–97.

43. Dawson DM, Lawrence EG, MacLennan GT *et al.* Altered expression of RET proto-oncogene product in prostatic intraepithelial neoplasia and prostate cancer. *J Natl Cancer Inst* 1998, **90**, 519–23.

44. Umbas R, Schalken JA, Aalders TW *et al.* Expression of the cellular adhesion molecular E-cadherin is reduced or absent in high-grade prostate cancer. *Cancer Res* 1992, **52**, 5104–9.

45. Hsieh JT, Luo W, Song W *et al.* Tumor-suppressive role of an androgen-regulated epithelial cell-adhesion molecule (C-CAM) in prostate carcinoma cells revealed by sense and antisense approaches. *Cancer Res* 1995, **55**, 190–7.

46. Hsieh JT, Earley K, Pong RC *et al.* Structural analysis of the C-CAM1 Molecule for its tumor-suppression function in human prostate cancer. *Prostate* 1999, **41**, 31–8.

47. Smith JR, Freije D, Carpten JD *et al.* Major susceptibility locus for prostate cancer on chromosome 1 suggested by a genome-wide search. Science 1996, **74**, 1371–4.

48. Grönberg H, Xu J, Smith JR *et al.* Early age at diagnosis in families providing evidence of linkage to the hereditary prostate cancer locus (*HPC1*) on chromosome 1. *Cancer Res* 1997, **57**, 4707–9.

49. Tulinius H, Egilsson V, Olafsdottir GH *et al.* Risk of prostate, ovarian, and endometrial cancer among relatives of women with breast cancer. *BMJ* 1992, **305**, 855–7.

50. Arason A, Barkardottir RB, Egilsson V. Linkage analysis of chromosome 17q markers and breast-ovarian cancer in Icelandic families, and possible relationship to prostate cancer. *Am J Hum Genet* 1993, **52**, 711–7.

51. Ford DF, Easton DF, Bishop DT *et al.* Risk of cancer in BRCA1-mutation carriers. *Lancet* 1994, **343**, 692–5.

52. Langston AA, Stanford JL, Wicklund KG *et al.* Germline *BRCA1* mutations in selected men with prostate cancer. *Am J Hum Genet* 1996, **58**, 881–5 (letter).

53. Struewing JP, Hartge P, Wacholder S *et al.* The risk of cancer associated with specific mutations of BRCA1 and BRCA2 among Ashkenazi Jews. *N Engl J Med* 1997, **336**, 1401–8.

54. Wooster R, Bignell G, Lancaster J *et al.* Identification of the breast cancer susceptibility gene BRCA2. *Nature* 1995, **378**, 789–92.

55. Lopez-Otin C, Diamandis EP. Breast and prostate cancer: An analysis of common epidemiological, genetic, and biochemical features. *Endocr Rev* 1998, **19**, 365–96.

56. Imperato-McGinley J, Gautier T, Zirinsky K *et al.* *Prostate* visulization studies in males homozygous and heterozygous for 5?-reductase deficiency. *J Clin Endocrinol Metab* 1992, **75**, 1022–6.

57. Gann PH, Hennekens CH, Ma J *et al.* Prospective study of sex hormone levels and prostate cancer. *J Natl Cancer Inst* 1996, **88**, 1186–26.

58. Ross RK, Bernstein L, Judd H *et al.* Serum testosterone levels in young black and white men. *J Natl Cancer Inst* 1986, **76**, 45–8.

59. Ross RK, Bernstein L, Lobo RA *et al.* 5-alpha-reductase activity and risk of prostate cancer among Japanese and US white and black males. *Lancet* 1992, **339**, 887–9.

60. Hill PW, Wynder EL, Garbaczewski H *et al.* Diet and urinary steroids in black and white North American men and black South African men. *Cancer Res* 1979, **39**, 5101–5.

61. Schoenberg MP, Hakimi JM, Wang S *et al.* Microsatellite mutation (CAG $_{24?? 18}$) in the androgen receptor gene in human prostate cancer. *Biochem Biophys Res Commun* 1994, **198**, 74–80.

62. Takahashi H, Furusato M, Allsbrook WC *et al.* Prevalence of androgen receptor gene mutations in latent prostatic carcinomas from Japanese men. *Cancer Res* 1995, **55**, 1621–4.

63. Taplin ME, Bubley GJ, Shuster TD *et al.* Mutation of the androgen-receptor gene in metastatic androgen-independent prostate cancer. *N Engl J Med* 1995, **332**, 1393–8.

64. Coetzee GA, Ross RK. Re: Prostate cancer and the androgen receptor. *J Natl Cancer Inst* 1994, **86**, 872–3.

65. Irvine RA, Yu MC, Ross RK *et al*. The CAG and GGC microsatellites of the androgen receptor gene are in linkage disequilibrium in men with prostate cancer. *Cancer Res* 1995, **55**, 1937–40.

66. Hardy DO, Scher HI, Bogenreider T *et al*. Androgen receptor CAG repeat lengths in prostate cancer: Correlation with age of onset. *J Clin Endocrinol Metab* 1996, **81**, 4400–5.

67. Stanford JL, Just JJ, Gibbs M *et al*. Polymorphic repeats in the androgen receptor gene: Molecular markers of prostate cancer risk. *Cancer Res* 1997, **57**, 1194–8.

68. Ingles SA, Ross RK, Yu MC *et al*. Association of prostate cancer risk with genetic polymorphisms of in vitamin D receptor and androgen receptor. *J Natl Cancer Inst* 1997, **89**, 166–70.

69. Hakimi JM, Schoenberg MP, Rondinelli RH *et al*. Androgen receptor variants with short glutamine or glycine repeats may identify unique subpopulations of men with prostate cancer. *Clin Cancer Res* 1997, **3**, 1599–608.

70. Kantoff P, Giovannucci E, Brown M. The androgen receptor CAG repeat polymorphism and its relationship to prostate cancer. *Biochim Biophys Acta* 1998, **1378**, C1–C5.

71. Reichardt JKV, Makridakis N, Henderson BE *et al*. Genetic variability of the human *SRD5A2* gene: Implications for prostate cancer risk. *Cancer Res* 1995, **55**, 3973–5.

72. Makridakis N, Ross RK, Pike MC *et al*. A prevalent missense substitution that modulates activity of prostatic steroid 5α-reductase. *Cancer Res* 1997, **57**, 1020–2.

73. Story MT. Polypeptide modulators of prostatic growth and development. *Cancer Surv* 1991, **11**, 123–46.

74. Wilding G. Response of prostate cancer cells to peptide growth factors: Transforming growth factor-?. *Cancer Surv* 1991, **11**, 147–63.

75. Chan JM, Stampfer MJ, Giovannucci E *et al*. Plasma insulin-like growth factor-I and prostate cancer risk: a prospective study. *Science* 1998, **279**, 563–6.

76. Culig Z, Hobisch A, Cronauer MV *et al*. Androgen receptor activation in prostatic tumor cell lines by insulin-like growth factor-I, keratinocyte growth factor, and epidermal growth factor. *Cancer Res* 1994, **54**, 5474–8.

77. Jenster G. The role of androgen receptor in the development and progression of prostate cancer. *Semin Oncol* 1999, **26**, 407–21.

78. Cohen P, Graves HC, Peehl DM *et al*. Prostate-specific antigen (PSA) is an insulin-like growth factor binding protein-3 protease found in seminal plasma. *J Clin Endocrinol Metab* 1992, **75**, 1046–53.

79. Cohen P, Peehl DM, Graves HC *et al*. Biological effects of prostate-specific antigen as an insulin-like growth factor binding protein-3 protease. *J Endocrinol* 1994, **142**, 407–15.

80. Fortier AH, Nelson BJ, Grella DK *et al*. Antiangiogenic activity of prostate specific antigen. *J Natl Cancer Inst* 1999, **91**, 1635–40.

81. Howell MA. Factor analysis of international cancer mortality data and per capita food consumption. *Br J Cancer* 1974, **29**, 328–36.

82. Blair A, Fraumeni JF. Geographic patterns of prostate cancer in the United States. *J Natl Cancer Inst* 1978, **61**, 1379–84.

83. Armstrong B, Doll R. Environmental factors and cancer incidence and mortality in different countries, with special reference to dietary practices. *Int J Cancer* 1975, **15**, 617–31.

84. Rose DP, Boyar AP and Wynder EL. International comparisons of mortality rates for cancer of the breast, ovary, prostate, and colon, and per capita food consumption. *Cancer* 1986, **58**, 2363–71.

85. Giovannucci E. Epidemiologic characteristics of prostate cancer. *Cancer* 1995, **75**, 1766–77.

86. Whittemore AS, Kolonel LN, Wu AH *et al*. Prostate cancer in relation to diet, physical activity, and body size in blacks, whites, and Asians in the United States and Canada. J *Natl Cancer Inst* 1995, **87**, 652–61.

87. Graham S, Haughey B, Marshall J *et al*. Diet in the epidemiology of the carcinoma of the prostate gland. *J Natl Cancer Inst* 1983, **70**, 687–92.

88. Talamini R, La Vecchia C, Decarli A *et al*. Nutrition, social factors and prostatic cancer in a Northern Italian population. *Br J Cancer* 1986, **53**, 817–21.

89. Ross RK, Shimizu H, Paganini-Hill A *et al*. Case-control studies of prostate cancer in blacks and whites in southern California. *J Natl Cancer Inst* 1987, **78**, 869–74.

90. Kolonel LN, Yoshizawa CN and Hankin JH. Diet and prostatic cancer: a case-control study im Hawaii. *Am J Epidemiol* 1988, **127**, 999–1012.

91. Mettlin C, Selenkas S, Natarajan N *et al*. Beta-carotene and animal fats and their relationship to prostate cancer risk. A case-control study. *Cancer* 1989, **64**, 605–12.

92. West DW, Slattery ML, Robison LM *et al*. Adult dietary and prostate cancer risk in Utah: a case-control study with special emphasis on aggressive tumors. *Cancer Causes Control* 1991, **2**, 85–94.

93. Gann PH, Hennekens CH, Sacks FM *et al*. A prospective study of plasma fatty acids and risk of prostate cancer. *J Natl Cancer Inst* 1994, **86**, 281–6.

94. Vlajinac HD, Marinkovic JM, Ilic MD *et al*. Diet and prostate cancer: a case-control study. *Eur J Cancer* 1997, **33**, 101–7.

95. Ohno Y, Yoshida O, Oishi K *et al*. Dietary beta-carotene and cancer of the prostate: a case-control study in Kyoto, Japan. *Cancer Res* 1988, **48**, 1331–6.

96. Andersson SO, Baron J, Wolk A *et al*. Early life risk factors for prostate cancer: a population-based case-control study in Sweden. *Cancer Epidemiol Biomarkers Prev* 1995, **4**, 187–92.

97. Snowdon DA, Phillips RL, Choi W. Diet, obesity and risk of fatal prostate cancer. *Am J Epidemiol* 1984, **120**, 244–50.

98. Mills PK, Beeson WL, Phillips RL *et al*. Cohort study of diet, life style, and prostate cancer in Adventist men. *Cancer* 1989, **64**, 598–604.

99. Severson RK, Nomura AM, Grove JS *et al*. A prospective study of demographics, diet, and prostate cancer among men of Japanese ancestry in Hawaii. *Cancer Res* 1989, **49**, 1857–60.

100. Hsing AW, McLaughlin JK, Schuman LM *et al*. Diet, tobacco use, and fatal prostate cancer: results from the

Lutheran Brotherhood Cohort Study. *Cancer Res* 1990, **50**, 6836–40.

101. Giovannucci E, Rimm EB, Colditz GA *et al.* A prospective study of dietary fat and risk of prostate cancer. *J Natl Cancer Inst* 1993, **85**, 1571–9.

102. Harvei S, Bjerve KS, Tretli S *et al.* Prediagnostic level of fatty acids in serum phospholipids: w-3 and w-6 fatty acids and the risk of prostate cancer. *Int J Cancer* 1997, **71**, 545–51.

103. Veierod MB, Laake P, Thelle DS. Dietary fat intake and risk of prostate cancer: a prospective study of 25,708 Norwegian men. *Int J Cancer* 1997, **73**, 634–8.

104. Schuurman AG, van den Brandt PA, Dorant E *et al.* Association of energy and fat intake with prostate carcinoma risk. Results from the Netherlands cohort study. *Cancer* 1999, **86**, 1019–27.

105. Rowley KH, Mason MD. The aetiology and pathogenesis of prostate cancer. Clin Oncol R Coll Radiol 1997, 9, 213–218.

106. Karmali RA. Prostaglandins and cancer. CA Cancer J Clin 1983, 33, 322–332.

107. Woutersen RA, Appel MJ, van Garderen-Hoetmer A *et al.* Dietary fat and carcinogenesis. *Mutat Res* 1999, **443**, 111–27.

108. Cook NR, Stampfer MJ, Ma J *et al.* Beta-Carotene supplementation for patients with low baseline levels and decreased risks of total and prostate carcinoma. *Cancer* 1999, **86**, 1783–92.

109. Paganini-Hill A, Chao A, Ross RK *et al.* Vitamin A, Beta-carotene, and the risk of cancer: a prospective study. *J Natl Cancer Inst* 1987, **79**, 443–8.

110. Giovannucci E, Ascherio A, Rimm EB *et al.* Intake of carotenoids and retinol in relation to risk of prostate cancer. *J Natl Cancer Inst* 1995, **87**, 1767–76.

111. Giles G, Ireland P. Diet, nutrition and prostate cancer. *Int J Cancer* 1997, **10**, 13–7.

112. The Alpha-Tocopherol, Beta Carotene Cancer Prevention Study Group. The effects of vitamin E and beta carotene on the incidence of lung cancer and other cancer in male smokers. *N Engl J Med* 1994, **330**, 1029–35.

113. Heinonen OP, Albenes D, Virtamo J *et al.* Prostate cancer and supplementation with α-tocopherol and β-carotene: incidence and mortality in a controlled trial. *J Natl Cancer Inst* 1998, **90**, 440–6.

114. Nomura AM, Stemmermann GN, Lee J *et al.* Serum micronutrients and prostate cancer in Japanese Americans in Hawaii. *Cancer Epidemiol Biomarkers Prev* 1997, **6**, 487–91.

115. Key T. Micronutrients and cancer aetiology: the epidemiological evidence. *Proc Nutr Soc* 1994, **53**, 605–14.

116. Adlercreutz H, Markkanen H, Watanabe S. Plasma concentrations of phyto-oestrogens in Japanese men. *Lancet* 1993, **342**, 1209–10.

117. Morton MS, Turkes A, Denis L *et al.* Can dietary factors influence prostatic disease? *BJU International* 1999, **84**, 549–54.

118. Gann PH, Ma J, Giovannucci *et al.* Lower prostate cancer risk in men with elevated plasma lycopene levels: results of a prospective analysis. *Cancer Res* 1999, **59**, 1225–30.

119. Clark LC, Combs GR Jr, Turnbull BW *et al.* Effects of selenium supplementation for cancer prevention in patients with carcinoma of the skin: a randomized controlled trial. Nutritional Prevention of Cancer Study Group. *JAMA* 1996, **276**, 1957–63.

120. Schwartz GG, Hulka BS. Is vitamin D deficiency a risk factor for prostate cancer? (Hypothesis). *Anticancer Res* 1990, **10**, 1307–12.

121. Hanchette CL, Schwartz GG. Geographical patterns of prostate cancer mortality: evidence for a protective effect of ultraviolet radiation. *Cancer* 1992, **70**, 2861–9.

122. Corder EH, Guess HA, Hulka BS *et al.* Vitamin D and prostate cancer: a prediagnostic study with stored sera. *Cancer Epidemiol Biomarkers Prev* 1993, **2**, 467–72.

123. Gann PH, Ma J, Hennekens CH *et al.* Circulating vitamin D metabolites in relation to subsequent development of prostate cancer. *Cancer Epidemiol Biomarkers Prev* 1996, **5**, 121–6.

124. Miller GJ, Stapleton GE, Ferrara JA *et al.* The human prostatic carcinoma cell line LNCaP expresses biologically active, specific receptors for $1\alpha,25$-dihydroxyvitamin D_3. *Cancer Res* 1992, **52**, 515–20.

125. Taylor JA, Hirvonen A, Watson M *et al.* Association of prostate cancer with vitamin D receptor gene polymorphism. *Cancer Res* 1996, **56**, 4108–10.

126. Giovannucci E, Rimm EB, Wolk A *et al.* Calcium and fructose intake in relation to risk of prostate cancer. *Cancer Res* 1998, **58**, 442–7.

127. Honda GD, Bernstein L, Ross RK *et al.* Vasectomy, cigarette smoking, and age at first sexual intercourse as risk factors for prostate cancer in middle-aged men. *Br J Cancer* 1988, **57**, 326–31.

128. Anderson DJ, Alexander NJ, Fulgham DL *et al.* Immunity to tumor-associated antigens in vasectomized men. *J Natl Cancer Inst* 1982, **69**, 551–5.

129. Rosenberg L, Palmer JR, Zauber AG *et al.* Vasectomy and the risk of prostate cancer. *Am J Epidemiol* 1990, **132**, 1051–5.

130. Mettlin C, Natarajan N, Huben R. Vasectomy and prostate cancer risk. *Am J Epidemiol* 1990, **132**, 1056–61.

131. Hsing AW, Wang RT, Gu FL *et al.* Vasectomy and prostate cancer risk in China. *Cancer Epidemiol Biomarkers Prev* 1994, **3**, 285–8.

132. Ross RK, Paganini-Hill A, Henderson BE. The etiology of prostate cancer: what does the epidemiology suggest? *Prostate* 1983, **4**, 333–44.

133. Spitz MR, Fueger JJ, Babaian RJ *et al.* Vasectomy and the risk of prostate cancer. *Am J Epidemiol* 1991, **134**, 108–9.

134. Hayes RB, Pottern LM, Greenberg R *et al.* Vasectomy and prostate cancer in US blacks and whites. *Am J Epidemiol* 1993, **137**, 263–9.

135. John EM, Whittemore AS, Wu AH. Vasectomy and prostate cancer: results from a multiethnic case-control study. *J Natl Cancer Inst* 1995, **87**, 662–9.

136. Zhu K, Stanford JL, Daling JR *et al.* Vasectomy and prostate cancer: a case-control study in a health maintenance organization. *Am J Epidemiol* 1996, **144**, 717–22.

137. Platz EA, Yeole BB, Cho E *et al.* Vasectomy and prostate cancer: a case-control study in India. *Int J Epidemiol* 1997, **26**, 933–8.

138. Sidney S, Quesenberry CP Jr, Sadler MC *et al.* Vasectomy and the risk of prostate cancer in a cohort of multiphasic health-checkup examinees: second report. *Cancer Causes Control* 1991, **2**, 113–6.

139. Nienhuis H, Goldacre M, Seagroatt V *et al.* Incidence of disease after vasectomy: a record linkage retrospective cohort study. *BMJ* 1992, **304**, 743–6.

140. Giovannucci E, Tosteson TD, Speizer FE *et al.* A retrospective cohort study of vasectomy and prostate cancer in US men. *JAMA* 1993, **269**, 878–82.

141. Giovannucci E, Ascherio A, Rimm EB *et al.* A prospective cohort study of vasectomy and prostate cancer in US men. *JAMA* 1993, **269**, 873–7.

142. Howards SS, Peterson HB. Vasectomy and prostate cancer: chance, bias, or a causal relationship? *JAMA* 1993, **269**, 913–4 (editorial).

143. Guess HA. Is vasectomy a risk factor for prostate cancer? *Eur J Cancer* 1993, **29A**, 1055–60.

144. Pienta KJ, Goodson JA, Esper PS. Epidemiology of prostate cancer: Molecular and environmental clues. *Urology* 1996, **48**, 676–83.

145. Farley TM, Meirik O, Mehta S *et al.* The safety of vasectomy: Recent concerns. *Bull World Health Organ* 1993, **71**, 413–9.

146. Slattery ML, West DW. Smoking, alcohol, coffee, tea, caffeine, and theobromine: risk of prostate cancer in Utah (United States). *Cancer Causes Control* 1993, **4**, 559–63.

147. van der Gulden JWJ, Verbeek ALM, Kolk JJ *et al.* Smoking and drinking habits in relation to prostate cancer. *Br J Urol* 1994, **73**, 382–9.

148. Lumey LH, Pittman B, Zang EA *et al.* Cigarette smoking and prostate cancer: no relation with six measures of lifetime smoking habits in a large case-control study among U.S. whites. *Prostate* 1997, **33**, 195–200.

149. Rohan TE, Hislop TG, Howe GR *et al.* Cigarette smoking and risk of prostate cancer: a population-based case-control study in Ontario and British Columbia, Canada. *Eur J Cancer Prev* 1997, **6**, 382–8.

150. Hsing AW, McLaughlin JK, Hrubec Z. Tobacco use and prostate cancer: 26-year follow-up of US veterans. *Am J Epidemiol* 1991, **133**, 437–41.

151. Coughlin SS, Neaton JD, Sengupta A. Cigarette smoking as a predictor of death from prostate cancer in 348,874 men screened for the Multiple Risk Factor Intervention Trial. *Am J Epidemiol* 1996, **143**, 1002–6.

152. Rodriguez C, Tatham LM, Thun MJ *et al.* Smoking and fatal prostate cancer in a large cohort of adult men. *Am J Epidemiol* 1997, **145**, 466–75.

153. Cerhan JR, Torner JC, Lynch CF *et al.* Association of smoking, body mass, and physical activity with risk of prostate cancer in the Iowa 65+ Rural Health Study (United States). *Cancer Causes Control* 1997, **8**, 229–38.

154. Adami HO, McLaughlin JK, Hsing AW *et al.* Alcoholism and cancer risk: a population-based cohort study. *Cancer Causes Control* 1992, **3**, 419–25.

155. Tonnesen H, Moller H, Andersen JR *et al.* Cancer morbidity in alcohol abusers. *Br J Cancer* 1994, **69**, 327–32.

156. Hayes RB, Brown LM, Schoenberg JB *et al.* Alcohol use and prostate cancer risk in US blacks and whites. *Am J Epidemiol* 1996, **143**, 692–7.

157. Lumey LH, Pittman B, Wynder EL. Alcohol use and prostate cancer in U.S. whites: no association in a confirmatory study. *Prostate* 1998, **36**, 250–5.

158. Ekman P, Pan Y, Li C *et al.* Environmental and genetic factors: a possible link with prostate cancer. *Br J Urol* 1997, **79** (Suppl 2), 35–41.

159. Grönberg H, Damber L, Damber JE. Total food consumption and body mass index in relation to prostate cancer risk: a case-control study in Sweden with prospectively collected exposure data. *J Urol* 1996, **155**, 969–74.

160. Andersson SO, Wolk A, Bergstrom R *et al.* Body size and prostate cancer: a 20-year follow-up study among 135 006 Swedish construction workers. *J Natl Cancer Inst* 1997, **89**, 385–9.

161. Nomura A, Heilbrun LK, Stemmerman GN. Body mass index as a predictor of cancer in men. *J Natl Cancer Inst* 1985, **74**, 319–323.

162. Hartman TJ, Albanes D, Rautalahti M *et al.* Physical activity and prostate cancer in the Alpha-Tocopherol, Beta-Carotene (ATBC) Cancer Prevention Study (Finland). *Cancer Causes Control* 1998, **9**, 11–8.

163. Giovannucci E, Leitzmann M, Spiegelman D *et al.* A prospective study of physical activity and prostate cancer in male health professionals. *Cancer Res* 1998, **58**, 5117–22.

164. Ernster VL, Winkelstein W Jr, Selvin S *et al.* Race, socioeconomic status, and prostatic cancer. *Cancer Treat Rep* 1977, **61**, 181–7.

165. van der Gulden JWJ, Kolk JJ, Verbeek ALM. Socioeconomic status, urbanization grade, and prostate cancer. *Prostate* 1994, **25**, 59–65.

166. Blair A, Zahm SM. Cancer among farmers. *Occup Med* 1991, **6**, 335–54.

167. Morrison H, Savitz D, Semenciw R *et al.* Farming and prostate cancer mortality. *Am J Epidemiol* 1993, **137**, 270–80.

168. Kipling M, Waterhouse J. Cadmium and prostatic carcinoma. *Lancet* 1967, **1**, 730–1.

169. Kolonel L, Winkelstein W Jr. Cadmium and prostatic carcinoma. *Lancet* 1977, **2**, 566–7.

170. Aronson KJ, Siemiatycki J, Dewar R *et al.* Occupational risk factors for prostate cancer: results from a case-control study in Montréal, Québec, Canada. *Am J Epidemiol* 1996, **143**, 363–73.

171. van der Gulden JWJ, Kolk JJ, Verbeek ALM. Work environment and prostate cancer risk. *Prostate* 1995, **27**, 250–7.

172. Rooney C, Beral V, Maconochie N *et al.* Case-control study of prostatic cancer in employees of the United Kingdom Atomic Energy Authority. *BMJ* 1993, **307**, 1391–7.

173. Kerr WK, Keresteci AG, Mayoh H. The distribution of zinc within the human prostate. *Cancer* 1960, **13**, 550–4.

174. International Agency for Research on Cancer. *Cancer. Cadmium, mercury, beryllium and the glass industry.* IARC Monogr 58 Lyon: IARC, 1994.

175. Sorahan T, Waterhouse JAH. Cancer of the prostate among nickel-cadmium battery workers. *Lancet* 1985, **1**, 459 (letter).

176. Armenian HK, Lilienfeld AM, Diamond EL *et al.* Relation between benign prostatic hyperplasia and

cancer of the prostate. A prospective and retrospective study. *Lancet* 1974, **2**, 115–7.

177. Greenwald P, Kirmss V, Polan AK *et al*. Cancer of the prostate among men with benign prostatic hyperplasia. *J Natl Cancer Inst* 1974, **53**, 335–40.

178. Steenland K, Nowlin S, Palu S. Cancer incidence in the National Health and Nutrition Survey I. Follow-up data: diabetes, cholesterol, pulse and physical activity. *Cancer Epidemiol Biomarkers Prev* 1995, **4**, 807–11.

7 | *Screening of prostate cancer*

Gregory J. Oleyourryk and Edward M. Messing

Introduction

Screening for a chronic disease is defined as the use of testing in an asymptomatic general or defined population to determine if members are likely to have that particular disease. Diagnostic testing of symptomatic patients that present with signs and/or symptoms must be distinguished from screening, although both may permit the early detection of a specific disease. Those who are deemed likely to have the disease by the screening test are then further evaluated, and individuals in whom the disease is eventually diagnosed are usually recommended to receive treatment for the screened disease. The ultimate goal of screening is to detect and treat the disease earlier than it would have been diagnosed through standard medical care in which testing in the absence of signs and/or symptoms had not occurred. The screening process is considered successful not only if screened individuals are diagnosed earlier but, most importantly, experience reduced mortality and/or morbidity from the disease (1). If screening proves to decrease cancer-specific mortality in a defined population, we must determine the optimal testing procedures, intervals, and sequences to effect detection of that disease sufficiently early to permit institution of successful, and ideally, low morbidity treatment.

For a screening program to be practical, the disease must meet certain criteria. It must be detectable with minimal harm and expense at a stage in which effective treatment can be administered. It must be a serious, relatively common health concern, and occur in a population defined by easily ascertainable demographics and risk factors. There must be some apparent benefit for treatment at early stages, compared to treatment at later stages when the disease would normally have been diagnosed had symptoms and/or signs led to its detection, particularly for disease outcome, but also for disease and treatment-related morbidity. Finally, the disease must have a pre-clinical phase of many months to years, during which the disease is detectable but undiagnosed because it is still asymptomatic. Prostate cancer is a disease that fits many of these criteria, although the benefits of screening, and certainly the details of its practical application, remain subjects of considerable debate.

The sensitivity, specificity, and predictive values of a screening test are used to assess its value in detecting a disease. Sensitivity, the proportion of subjects with the disease who have a positive screening test, is defined as the number of subjects with a positive test who actually have the disease, divided by the total number of subjects with the disease regardless of whether the screening test is positive or negative. This value represents the ability of the test to identify every possible diseased subject. The ideal is 100%, not missing one subject with the disease.

Specificity, the proportion of subjects without the disease who have a negative test, is defined as the number of subjects with a negative test who do not have the disease, divided by the total number of subjects without the disease regardless of whether the screening test is positive or negative. In contrast to sensitivity, specificity represents how accurate the test is in discerning diseased from non-diseased individuals. The ideal situation of 100% specificity would imply that the test was positive only for diseased subjects, and there were no subjects without the disease who have positive results (false-positives). A very difficult part of developing a screening tool is having one with both high sensitivity *and* high specificity, as one is often decreased while trying to improve the other. Goals should be directed at finding a test that safely catches all diseased subject (high sensitivity), while at the same time is cost-effective by including as few disease-free individuals as possible (high specificity).

Unfortunately, sensitivity and specificity cannot easily be determined for prostate cancer because the actual prevalence of the disease remains unknown. Thus, for prostate cancer, positive predictive value (PPV) is often used to determine the accuracy of available tests. Mathematically, PPV is defined as the number of positive tests in subjects with the disease (true-positives), divided by the total number of people with positive tests (true-positives plus false-positives). The PPV is particularly important because the higher it is, the lower the number of unnecessary biopsies. If the specificity or PPV are too low, the number of false-positive tests, and thus the number of needlessly performed biopsies may be unacceptably high.

Also critical to understanding the application of screening programs, and the interpretation of its benefits, is the concept of lead- and length-time biases. If screening only detects cancers at an earlier time but does not alter the progression of the disease or the eventual outcome, screened individuals will appear to have an increased survival time (from disease detection to demise) but their longevity (their age at death) will not be changed. This is 'lead-time bias' and can confound the authenticity of early survival data. Length-bias sampling occurs because the biological variability in the population of cancers predisposes screening tests to detect slower-growing cancers, which have longer pre-symptomatic phases, when they are detectable if screened for, while rapidly growing ones are missed because they proliferate to a symptomatic and incurable stage between screens. Another type of length-bias, termed 'over-diagnosis' occurs when slow-growing tumors that would never cause death, and thus never need treatment, are found. This skews survival results in favor of screening. Either way, length-time bias can give the impression that screening increases survival. Before any conclusions can be made about the true benefits of any screening practice, these phenomena must be considered when interpreting survival results.

Prostate cancer screening

Prostate cancer is the fourth most important cancer for men worldwide, in regard to prevalence, mortality, and morbidity, with a significantly higher incidence in developed countries (2). This year's estimates once again predict its incidence to be the highest of any non-cutaneous cancer in Americans of either gender, 179 300 new cases, and almost twice the number of the next most commonly diagnosed cancer in men (3). The mortality from prostate cancer in the United States in 1999 is estimated to be 37 000, second only to lung cancer (3). Although it is not generally considered to be as aggressive as other malignancies, a man in North America diagnosed with prostate cancer in his mid-60s is more likely to die of this cancer than of any other cause (4). When prostate cancer screening programs are used routinely, the stages of the disease at diagnosis are lower (earlier) than those found in historical control cases (5, 6). Finding the cancer at an earlier stage should theoretically avoid future prostate cancer related morbidities and mortality, as the disease is not generally curable once it has escaped the confines of the prostate gland and immediately adjacent tissues. Although there is an apparent stage shift at diagnosis, there has not yet been a proven decrease in morbidity and mortality. However, recent evidence suggests that a decline in prostate cancer morality is beginning to occur (7).

The biology of prostate cancer is appropriate for screening with a technically simple assay that has relatively high PPV, and a long pre-clinical phase leading to the ability to detect cancers over five years before they would have been clinically evident (8). Critics of prostate cancer screening maintain that the expenses, anxiety, and morbidities of the screening tests, subsequent work-up, and treatments may outweigh its benefits. Despite the high incidence and mortality rates they still appropriately cite that prostate cancer is primarily a disease of older men (with other competing causes of demise), is a relatively slow-growing malignancy, and is often found as a microscopic, latent variant that may never need treatment (9). The debate over whether prostate cancer screening is beneficial continues and will be discussed at the end of this chapter.

Methods of prostate cancer screening

Physical examination: digital rectal exam

The digital rectal exam (DRE) by itself is a relatively poor screening modality. While it may be the simplest, it is not necessarily the most cost-effective screening method, as it actually requires a physician's visit instead of a blood test, and many men have such an aversion to undergoing it that they decline any screening intervention. Moreover, there is considerable subjectivity in the interpretation of this examination.

Up to 90% of patients now being diagnosed with organ-confined disease (or even disease extending just beyond the prostatic capsule), underwent biopsy because of abnormalities on prostate-specific antigen (PSA) testing, having had DREs that would not have prompted biopsy (10). In fact, it has been reported that DRE alone fails to increase the proportion of organ-confined cancers detected (11). Catalona *et al.* reported that DRE alone would have missed approximately 40% of cancers and PSA alone would have missed about 25% of patients with histologically organ-confined prostate cancer of sufficient volume (e.g. over 0.5 cc) or grade (Gleason score > 5) to merit treatment. However, the two combined, increased the prostate cancer detection rate to 78% in a mixed screening and referred population (5). At the current time, it appears most appropriate to use DRE in conjunction with PSA, as complimentary tests.

Transrectal ultrasound

Transrectal ultrasound (TRUS) with 5 and 7 MHz probes, is not much more unpleasant than rectal exam and clearly can evaluate areas of the prostate containing potential lesions that are not easily reachable by an examiner's finger. Additionally, it is an accurate means of assessing prostate volume (using the formula: $0.52 \times$ width $\times$ length $\times$ height), which can then be divided into the serum PSA concentration to give the 'PSA density' (PSA/prostate volume). Also, measurement of the transitional zone's volume can be done during ultrasound, which further helps in the screening process (see below).

Some investigators argued that TRUS was more sensitive than DRE, as well as enhancing the accuracy and safety of biopsy (12). However, studies like that of Reissigl *et al.* found that up to 65% of prostates with biopsy proven cancer had a previous TRUS reported as 'normal' (10), and it has been very common to find ultrasonically normal areas of the gland that contain considerable amounts of cancer. Furthermore, hypoechoic areas on TRUS are not very specific for prostate cancer. Bangma *et al.* reported minimal (3%) loss of cancer detection, with a 17% reduction in the number of biopsies when TRUS was omitted from a screening protocol that included DRE, PSA, and TRUS (13). They found that it was not cost-effective, and only minimally added to the prediction of a positive biopsy. While it can occasionally pick up cancers that may not be detected by DRE or PSA, the high false-positive rate makes the technique undesirable for general screening use. The modality's other drawback as a screening tool is the considerable inherent subjectivity in the performance and interpretation of the test. Despite earlier contentions supporting its use as a screening tool, its inability to distinguish normal from malignant tissue is disappointing, and currently now is used primarily to guide biopsy needles into specific regions of the prostate and adjacent structures.

Prostate-specific antigen

Prostate-specific antigen (PSA) is a serine protease produced by prostate epithelial cells and secreted into seminal fluid. Both malignant and normal prostate cells secrete this enzyme, but when a cancer disrupts the gland's architecture, the levels in the systemic circulation often rise. PSA was originally discovered by Hara *et al.*, and further characterized to be an immunologically unique compound whose production is relatively specific for the prostate gland by Wang *et al.* (14, 15). Over the past 10 years, its use in screening efforts and early detection has drastically changed the diagnosis and management of prostate cancer. The sheer number of patients has changed considerably, as well as the clinical and pathological stages of detected prostate cancers. It has even prompted the creation of a new clinical stage category, T1c. Unlike DRE and TRUS, measurements of PSA are objective and quantitative. However, a physician's interpretation of the significance of a specific level, and the variability of that level in normal and disease states, are not as precisely defined. Today, serum PSA is considered the best method detect early stage prostate cancer, yet of course, it has its limitations as well (5, 16).

The traditional cut-off indicating suspicion for cancer, and for biopsy, has been greater than 4 ng/ml. Greater than 70% of patients with what is believed to be biologically significant prostate cancer that is organ-confined, have serum PSA levels greater than 4 ng/ml (17). In comparison, only 25% of patients with pathologically proven benign prostatic hyperplasia (BPH) fall into this PSA range. Also, in studies of volunteers, PSA values greater than 4 ng/ml are seen in only 8–15% of men 50 years of age and older (18). The PPV (the proportion of individuals with a positive who actually have the disease) of an initial elevated PSA in a man greater than 50 is dependent on the degree of elevation of PSA. The PPV is 64% if the PSA is greater than 10 ng/ml. For levels between 4 ng/ml and 10 ng/ml the PPV is approximately 25% (18). Those patients with a PSA value in this range occupy a diagnostic 'gray zone', in which the PSA concentration identifies the patients as high risk (25% cancer rate versus a 4% rate for the general population over 50), but specificity is poor because 75% of biopsy findings are negative (19).

Concerns about prostate cancer screening with serial PSAs have been raised, the first of which is that the test is not ideally sensitive. In several large screening series roughly 20–30% of men with seemingly biologically significant prostate cancer, based on histologic grade and cancer volume, still confined to the prostate (i.e. exactly the men screening is supposed to help), have PSAs under 4 ng/ml (16). Thus, the test isn't sensitive (true-positives/true-positives and false-negatives) enough, and should be combined with DRE if prostate cancer screening is to be performed. Indeed, 80% of men with PSAs under 4 ng/ml, who have biologically important prostate cancer, have cancer confined to the prostate gland, once again emphasizing the importance of not relying exclusively on PSA (16).

The detection of prostate cancer in its curable stages requires the use of a relatively low PSA cut-off point for screening. However, the specificity of PSA for cancer detection is limited because of its high-false positive rate when a low cut-off is used, causing unnecessary biopsies (20). Because the disease occurs almost exclusively in middle-aged and elderly men, in whom BPH is ubiquitous, this lack of specificity (true-negatives/true-negatives and false-positives) leads many men who do not have prostate cancer, but who do have elevated PSAs, to go through the expense, morbidity, unpleasantness, and obvious anxiety that an elevated PSA and its evaluation provoke.

The widespread use of PSA as a screening device has led to an increase in the number of prostatic ultrasounds performed and biopsies taken. The number of cancers detected has increased and the stages of the cancers detected are earlier than for cancer detected prior to the widespread use of PSA as a screening tool (21). Indeed, those in whom cancer is detected under circumstances of repeated screening have organ-confined disease nearly 80% of the time (6). Whether this is a sufficiently early lead-time to detect cancer before micro-metastasis occur is not yet known, however, Catalona *et al.* reported that in men who in initial screening had PSA values that were less than 4 ng/ml, with follow-up of up to 5 years, 2.6% had prostate cancer found on subsequent screening (16). As would be expected, the proportion of men with clinically advanced cancer was significantly lower in those detected through serial PSA screenings (2%) than in those detected by the initial screen (6%), since preva-

lence cases were picked up by the initial screen (22). This shows the value of serial screening with PSA even with an initial 'normal' value. In addition, since 80% of men with prostate cancer detected, who have PSA below 4 ng/ml (mostly because of abnormalities on DRE), have organ-confined disease, the advantage for including DRE with PSA in regular screening becomes apparent.

At the other end of the spectrum, an additional concern about screening for prostate cancer is that the test may be *too* sensitive. Screening may be detecting the tiny focuses of well-differentiated cancer that many middle-aged and elderly men have in their prostates, and are found incidentally at autopsy (6, 16). There have been estimates that *ad lib* screening still detects only 20% of all men with any cancer at all within their prostates—but that this may still be detecting the disease in, and giving treatment to, men who never were likely to experience any ill-effects from prostate cancer. Advocates for PSA screening have argued that such 'autopsy cancers' are so small that they would not be expected to elevate serum PSA or to be detected by random needle biopsies. However, it is possible that if PSA were elevated from BPH, a biopsy may find an 'autopsy' cancer incidentally, which may be indistinguishable from more significant large-volume cancer. If even a small proportion of the enormous pool of men with 'autopsy cancers' were being diagnosed (and treated) by PSA, this would be a strong argument against wide-scale screening. Currently, the evidence indicates that this is not happening. The distribution of histologic grades (well, moderately, or poorly differentiated tumors) appears very similar in PSA screening populations to what it was in the pre-PSA era (15–20% well-differentiated, 50–60% moderately differentiated, and 20–35% poorly differentiated) (23). One would expect a significant shift to well-differentiated tumors if PSA screening was enabling the detection of a significant percentage of the 'autopsy cancers' (which are almost always well-differentiated.)

Despite these considerations, assuming a man is medically stable and willing to undergo treatment for prostate cancer, it is very difficult not to proceed to TRUS-guided biopsy for PSA levels over 4 ng/ml (that are unexplained by recent infections, instrumentation, or other episodes that are known to elevate the PSA transiently) or for a suspicious DRE. Yet with serum PSA, the high false-positive rate of up to 75% has been a major criticism. To improve the specificity of serum-PSA levels, by reducing the number of false-positives, alternative methods of analyzing the PSA value to enhance its clinical significance have been suggested.

PSA density

One possible way to enhance the specificity of PSA, and diminish the high false-positive rate associated with BPH, is to use the PSA density (PSAD), the ratio of serum PSA to the prostate volume, as measured by TRUS (24). Using the formula $0.52 \times$ width $\times$ length $\times$ height, the volume of the prostate can be best estimated and then divided into the PSA to better estimate the cancer risk in relation to volume adjusted PSA values. This may help one decide if a mildly elevated PSA really warrants a biopsy in someone with a large prostatic volume.

Benson *et al.* believed using PSAD could reduce the number of negative biopsies by about 50%; however, nearly half of the organ-confined prostate cancers, the ones most desirous to find, would be missed as well (24). Moreover, it has been reported that prostate size is not a good predictor of PSA because of the tremendous amount of variability in the relative amount of epithelium in a prostate gland. Bangma *et al.* Reported that using PSAD cut-off of 0.12 ng/ml/cc, in combination with DRE, reduced the number of biopsies by 28%, at the expense of missing 11% of the cancers (13). In reality, of course, the biopsy is often done regardless of the PSAD, since the patient is already undergoing the ultrasound procedure. For these reasons, PSAD is rarely used to determine who should undergo biopsy, but can be useful in deciding if a biopsy should be repeated in a patient with a negative biopsy and an elevated PSA.

A variation on this theme, PSA transitional zone (TZ) density, is also worthy of mention. PSA TZ density is defined as the total PSA (ng/ml)/TZ volume (cc), as measured by TRUS. Reissigl *et al.* concluded that PSA TZ density is an important diagnostic tool for calculating the probability of prostate cancer, and that the combination of per cent free PSA (see 'Free PSA' below) and PSA TZ density was superior to free PSA alone (10). They also found a significant proportion of cancers (29%) arising from the TZ in their study, only detectable on their two additional TZ biopsies, providing another compelling reason to look at the TZ during TRUS (10). This needs to be further investigated, as many authorities believe these TZ tumors have a much lower biologic potential (which explains some good outcomes of patients treated by 'watchful waiting')

than the peripheral tumors that have greater access to adjacent routes of spread (25).

Age-specific PSA

Age-specific PSA attempts to account for prostatic hyperplasia, which increases PSA as men age. It improves sensitivity in younger patients who may benefit most from screening, while also improving specificity in older patients who will benefit less (26). As with PSAD, it is based on the premise that since prostatic volume and BPH increase with age, the normal 4 ng/ml cut-off may be too high for young men (40–50 years) and too low for older men. Oesterling initially suggested that the PSA cut-off for biopsies should change based on age, with 2.5 ng/ml for men aged 40–49, 3.5 ng/ml for 50–59-year-olds, 4.5 ng/ml for 60–69-year-olds, and 6.5 ng/ml for 70–79-year-olds (27). However, Catalona *et al.* reported that decreasing the PSA cut-offs in younger men resulted in a significant increase in biopsies with only a minimal increase in cancer detection (28). Additionally, higher cut-offs in older men resulted in fewer biopsies but missed many organ-confined cancers. In one series comparing age-specific reference ranges for total PSA to total PSA plus DRE, a 30% decrease in biopsies was found, but 18% of the cancers in men with a PSA of 4–10 ng/ml were missed (29). In this study, age-specific PSA ranges did not preferentially select younger men for biopsy, while the missed cancers were distributed evenly for all age groups. Of course, missing organ-confined cancers may be regarded as favorable when they are of small volume and biologically insignificant. However, if they were to grow there is no certainty that PSA screening would detect them before they escaped the gland.

Another matter is that age-specific PSA ranges have varied with different races; the original age-specific PSA ranges were determined from the almost exclusively Caucasian, mostly northern European population that inhabits Olmsted County, MN (27). These ranges cannot be readily extrapolated to non-Caucasians or Caucasians of other ethnic backgrounds. Despite the problems, age-specific PSA is a cost-effective approach to improve the specificity of PSA, and as such may have value in larger population-based screening efforts. Perhaps the best arguments for the use of age-specific PSA are clinical, not statistical, however, as the detection of cancer in a individual patient must be suited to his needs, and tailored to his expected life-span and overall health. It is logical to try to increase sensitivity in younger men and decrease invasive biopsies in older patients who are poorer candidates for aggressive management.

PSA velocity

Another measurement for selecting men to biopsy is the rate of change of an individual's PSA over time (PSA velocity). Sudden increases in PSA value from an established baseline or slope, are suggestive of neoplastic change, and biopsies might be taken at that time. Carter and colleagues, utilizing the Baltimore Longitudinal Study of Aging data, found that in contrast to men with no prostatic disease or with BPH only, prostate carcinoma patients exhibited an early linear phase followed by an exponential phase of PSA velocity prior to diagnosis (30). On average, the exponential phase began 7–9 years before clinical detection. However, changes found at intervals shorter than 12 months are usually unreliable to extrapolate to a rate of change over 12–24 months, hence, limiting the utility of PSA velocity to individuals with numerous PSA determinations over several years. However, because of inter-assay variability, to be interpretable, these multiple determinations must be performed by the same laboratory, something that is often not controllable in clinical situations. Additionally, this criterion is not useful in large mass screenings that are one-time events with poor continuity. One obvious benefit, however, is that men found to have little or no change in PSA over time, may not need to be tested every year, reducing costs.

Free PSA

The most promising development to improve PSA's specificity in detecting early prostate cancer has been the recognition that most PSA in the serum is bound by several proteins (protease inhibitors); the amounts bound, and by which proteins, differ in various disease and normal states. To date, three forms of PSA have been identified: PSA complexed to α1-antichymotrypsin (ACT, the predominant form), PSA complexed with β2-macroglobulin, and PSA not bound to any protease inhibitor ('free PSA'). β2-Macroglobulin encapsulates the PSA and makes that form unrecognizable by monoclonal and polyclonal antibodies prepared against PSA. Therefore only two of these forms, PSA complexed with α1-antichymotrypsin and free PSA, are actually immuno-detectable by today's avail-

able assays. Assays that can measure unbound and total PSA, will then permit the calculation of the proportion of all *detectable* PSA (total PSA) that is not bound, or the proportion of free PSA (free PSA/total PSA). For unknown reasons, the α1-ACT bound form is preferentially elevated in prostatic cancer cases. Therefore, the percentage of free PSA is lower in serum samples from patients with prostate cancer than in serum samples from patients with benign disease particularly (BPH) or normal prostates. It is thought that enzymatic activity is required for the PSA to complex with ACT, and thus some believe the low percentage free PSA seen with cancer is a result of tumor cells preferentially secreting enzymatically active PSA (20). Another explanation, offered by Lilja *et al.*, who found expression of ACT in tumor cells, is that complex formation with ACT is initiated within the tumor cell and the whole complex is secreted instead of PSA alone being secreted (31). Regardless of the actual mechanisms, data using the percentage free PSA are quite encouraging.

Evidence has shown that the percentage of free PSA increases the specificity of the PSA alone in distinguishing BPH from cancer from 25% to 37% (32). In the intermediate PSA range of 4.0–10.0 ng./ml, a diagnostic 'gray zone', free/total PSA ratios improve the specificity of total serum PSA significantly (32). Several groups have tried to calculate the trade-off of improving specificity with reducing sensitivity by advocating biopsies not be performed on men whose total PSAs are between 4.0 and 10.0 ng./ml, and whose percentage of free PSAs are above various cut-offs. For example, Catalona *et al.*, using a free PSA cut-off of 25% in a man with a palpably benign gland and total PSA between 4.0 and 10.0 ng/dl, detected 95% of the cancers and spared 20% of those with BPH from undergoing biopsy (19). Because BPH is found in most men with a total PSA in this 'gray zone', this represents a substantial number of individuals who would avoid an unnecessary biopsy.

Catalona *et al.* also have attempted to use free PSA alone to detect cancer even earlier, without increasing the number of negative biopsies performed (33). Using 4.0 ng/ml as a cut-off for PSA alone, 20% of men would have had their tumors missed were it not for the use of a percentage of free PSA cut-off of 27% (below which all men have undergone biopsy regardless of how low total PSA is). Additionally, with this new cut-off, 80% of the cancers were organ-confined as compared to 70% by using the 4 ng/ml total PSA cut-off alone. While these data are promising, there are several concerns about relying too heavily on free/total PSA. First, while little is understood about PSA's role in the serum (if any) in general, less is known about the mechanisms regulating its binding by globular proteins. Perhaps of even more concern, from a screening perspective, is that only a relatively small number of subjects without cancer have been used to calculate the appropriate cut-off percentages, and almost no men with prostatitis or prostate diseases other than BPH (let alone not knowing if the BPH values were in men with primarily glandular or stromal hyperplasia), have been studied to know their effects on this ratio. Until these studies are undertaken, a more appropriate way to use free PSA to increase sensitivity (cancer detection) may be in patients who have already undergone a biopsy with negative findings. If a free PSA ratio is low in these men, indicating high risk, a second biopsy may be advised, as approximately 20% of cancers are missed on the first biopsy (33).

Another possible use for free PSA may be in predicting prognostic features of prostate cancer. Catalona *et al.* have reported that a lower pre-operative percentage of free PSA was significantly associated with the presence of capsular penetration, positive surgical margins, a higher Gleason score, an increased percentage of the gland-containing cancer, and an increased tumor volume (34). Other researchers have not found free PSA to significantly contribute to the pre-operative prediction of pathologic features, and more work needs to be done in the group of men with a PSA in the grey zone of 4.0–10.0 ng./ml. It was in this range that Catalona *et al.* found prognostic utility for percentage free PSA (34). In the future, clinicians and patients may be able to use this information to make informed decisions about prostate cancer management.

Not only may percentage free PSA enhance early prostate cancer detection and decrease the number of unnecessary biopsies, but also it is suitable for screening a large population, in that it and the standard PSA can be done from the same blood draw. Also, the free PSA ratio is less expensive and unpleasant for subjects than measurement of PSA density.

Research is still ongoing to find even more specific markers for prostate cancer screening. Complexed PSA (cPSA) refers to PSA complexed with α1-antichymotrypsin. A new test named the Immuno 1 cPSA assay is reportedly specific for the E-epitope on the free PSA molecule, the site normally bound by α1-antichymotrypsin (35). By directly measuring complexed PSA, advocates of this assay propose that it is more specific for cancer than the percentage of free PSA, perhaps because it is the PSA complexed to α1-antichymotrypsin that is preferentially increased in prostate cancer. Another marker, human glandular kallikrein-2 (hK2), is a gene with 80% homology to the PSA gene in sequence and structure, as well as having similar enzymatic activity, localization to the prostate, and factors that regulate production (35). Immunoassays are now available for research protocols and suggest that hK2 may have value as a clinical marker for prostate cancer diagnosis. Complexed PSA and/or hK2 may further optimize earlier detection in the future. Additionally, if used with other experimental markers such as N-telopeptide and prostate-specific membrane antigen (PSMA), better molecular staging may be feasible (35, 36). For now, more research is needed to determine the best combinations for a safe (sensitive) and cost-effective (specific) way to incorporate PSA density, PSA velocity, age-specific PSA, percentage of free PSA, and total serum PSA into screening algorithms.

Populations at risk

One way to improve the predictive value of a screening test is to increase the prevalence of the disease by modifying the population to be screened. The only well-established risk factors for prostate cancer are increased age, African-American race, and family history. Screening is not recommended below age 50 because of the low prevalence of prostate cancer in younger men. Race also plays a role in prostate cancer. Reports have shown a 30% higher incidence and 120% higher mortality rate in black than white men in the United States (5). The higher mortality rate in this group may be due to the relative increase in the number of high-grade cases among African-Americans, along with their persistently lower age at diagnosis (37). While a 25–30% PPV for total PSA values greater than 4.0 ng/ml apply for the general public, a higher estimate of 36–60% may occur in African-Americans (37). Since PPV depends on the prevalence rate of a population, the higher cancer rate in African Americans explains the higher PPV for PSA. The higher PPV in African-American men suggests that lowering total PSA cut-offs may be a strategy to optimize cancer detection in this group, realizing that it will also increase the number of negative biopsies (37). On the other hand, Asians have a much lower incidence of prostate cancer and may not be as appropriate as subjects for screening.

Walsh and Partin have reported that a positive family history increases the relative risk of prostate cancer in male first-degree relatives (fathers, brothers, or sons) approximately two-fold, and this increases with multiple affected relatives (38). It is believed that a type of familial prostate cancer is passed on as an autosomal dominant trait, particularly if the proband was young when first diagnosed. While 25% of men with prostate cancer have a family history of it, only 9% have a hereditary form of the disease (38). Yet, they have estimated 'hereditary prostate carcinoma' to be associated with 43% of cancer patients who were diagnosed below age 55 years, 34% of men diagnosed at < 70 years, and only 9% of men diagnosed at age 85 (38). They concluded that first-degree relatives in high-risk families should start screening before 50 years of age, as the hereditary prostate cancer is characterized by an early age at onset (38). Because age, race, and family history are the only known risk factors, earlier detection through screening these men represents one promising option for further reducing prostate cancer morbidity and mortality.

General population screening practices

The 1993 recommendations of the American Cancer Society (ACS) and the American Urological Association (AUA) for prostate cancer screening are as follows (39):

- men 50 years of age or older, with an average risk for prostate cancerm should undergo an annual of developing DRE and PSA measurement;
- screening of higher risk groups (African-Americans and first-degree relatives of prostate cancer patients) should start earlier;
- TRUS should only be used in patients with abnormal DRE and/or PSAs;
- screening will only benefit men with a life expectancy of 10 years or longer.

These recommendations are not shared by the American College of Physicians, the US Preventative Services Task Force, the Australian Cancer Society, several European countries including the United Kingdom, France, and the Scandinavian countries, and many more. Some of these groups follow much less aggressive guidelines, while others strongly disagree with the practice of most

prostate cancer screening (with the exception of men with strong family histories). Reasons for this will be discussed later in the chapter.

While total PSA and DRE are the major screening tools, the previously discussed modifications of PSA are also being used more and more by urologists to improve the PPV of their screening efforts. PSA velocities in men with no prostatic malignancy show a linear phase increase in PSA of < 0.04 ng/ml per year, and if a more rapid sustained rise in of PSA is seen, it usually begins 7–9 years before clinical detection (40). This indicates that men with little or no change in PSA over time may not need to be tested every year. Similarly, Carter *et al.* show that a 2-year PSA testing interval is not likely to miss a curable lesion when the initial PSA level is less than 2.0 ng/ml and the DRE is normal (41). Also, in a man with an elevated total PSA who has undergone a negative biopsy, the percentage of free PSA can strongly influence the decision of whether to repeat the biopsy.

Over the past several years, public awareness of prostate cancer has increased considerably (42). At times, concerns about the disease have been based upon bleak assumptions and have led to unbounded confusion about the value of screening. For example, in a study from Australia, Ward *et al.* found more than 33% of respondents thought that at least one in five men would develop prostate cancer before age 74 years, and 11% thought that one in five would actually die from the disease before that age (42). In the United States, DeAntoni *et al.* found that of 3001 men undergoing screening, 84% believed prostate cancer screening was proven to save lives (43). Men and their family members are often the ones requesting prostate cancer screening (44), and primary care physicians must familiarize themselves with controversies surrounding routine screening and counsel their patients in this regard. Such discussions must take into considerations, risks, and morbidities of the disease and its treatments, in the context of the patient's co-morbidities, lifestyle, inheritance, and priorities in terms of longevity and quality of life. These sessions may often consume more time than a busy PCP wishes to spend, or gives more responsibility to patients than they want to assume for their own care. However, it is time and effort best spent before hand, because once the PSA test is performed and is elevated, it is much more difficult for either the patient or his physician to ignore the value and forego biopsy (45). It is their beliefs about the risks and benefits of the available treatments that will in turn affect their patients' choices.

Since the progression rates of moderately differentiated prostate cancer to metastatic disease, if left untreated, was found to be 42% at 10 years, and if subsequent life expectancy is estimated at 3 more years, it can be assumed that only men with a 10–15 year life expectancy could benefit from early detection and treatment (23). In the US, the average male life expectancy decreases below 10 years at approximately the age of 73. If one includes those men with poorly differentiated tumors, to possibly improve the survival of *all* patients with localized cancer, then one could argue that screening should include individuals whose life expectancies are 5–10 years or longer.

Problems with prostate cancer screening

The value of prostate cancer screening continues to be debated. Often quoted are the remarks of Dr. Willet Whitmore: 'Is cure possible in those in whom it is necessary? Is cure necessary in those in whom it is possible?' (46). Many governmental health agencies and medical organizations throughout the world recommend against the use of routine prostate cancer screening, since its early detection has no proven benefit as of yet. Specifically there are no longitudinal studies that demonstrate reduced prostate cancer mortality in screening compared with prospectively randomized controls. Such trials are needed to overcome the biases discussed earlier, which occur in less well-designed studies. It should be understood, however, that no studies so designed using repetitive PSA and DRE screening have yet been completed, and because of difficulties with early cross-overs on the unscreened arm, it is uncertain whether trials underway can be completed.

A second factor is that because prostate cancer is often a disease of elderly men who have competing causes of demise, it is widely recognized that individuals with prostate cancer often die *with* their disease rather than *of* it. Groups that do not support screening say that even though the malignancy is extremely common, it is the actual cause of death in only a small proportion of patients who have histologic evidence of prostate cancer (if one includes autopsy cancers) (47). With only 20–25% of patients clinically diagnosed with prostate cancer actually dying from the cancer itself, it is considered by some to be a 'low-risk disease'.

A corollary to these considerations is that prostate cancer is a relatively slow-growing malignancy, often taking 10 years or longer to progress from localized to metastatic disease, and even at advanced stages, responding dramatically to very low morbidity therapy (9). Given that many of the patients are already in their last few decades of life, a disease that is this indolent often will never affect the patient

Moreover, while microscopic, latent cancers have been found on autopsy in 50–70% of older men, even if only 10–25% of these 'autopsy cancers' ever become clinically diagnosed and are not recognized for what they are, many men will undergo morbid, expensive, and necessary treatments for a condition that would never harm them (9, 48, 49). While estimates are that approximately 10% of what appear to be organ-confined tumors from radical prostatectomy specimens, might be considered clinically irrelevant based on grade of differentiation and tumor volume (5). This, along with failure to see a major shift in tumor grade at diagnosis with wide-scale PSA testing, would confirm that PSA screening is not detecting a large number of 'autopsy cancers'.

Additional arguments against general screening revolve around the low specificity of PSA (or its modifications), and the morbidity, rare mortality, and considerable expense of the evaluation it leads to. Even the biopsy, the part of the screening procedure with the highest risks, can cause problems such as febrile reactions, hemorrhagic complications, urinary retention, trauma to structures such as the ureter, pubic bone, terminal ileum, and finally, death (50). While no more than 2–3% of men under going TRUS-guided biopsy experience any complications, if 600 000–800 000 biopsies are performed each year in the United States to diagnose 179 000 new cases, then 12 000–24 000 men will experience complications of those biopsies, often cancer being present. Indeed, pessimists argue that PSA only increases the expenses of the disease, increases the number of invasive prostatic biopsies, and increases the stress and anxiety of older men as they fret about this lab value (51).

Since for screening to be valuable there must also be effective treatment for early-stage disease at diagnosis, a final reservation is that available therapies are not always effective, yet they are associated with considerable morbidity and expense. Expectant management of clinically localized prostate cancers has been embraced by many, but the majority of men who have life expectancies over 10 years are likely to die from prostate cancer with such strategies (25). Perhaps this is why Sweden has one of the highest prostate cancer death rates in the world (2). It is beyond the scope of this chapter to discuss in depth the therapies for localized prostate cancers and their associated morbidities.

Benefits of prostate cancer screening

Outcome data that benefit in a survival from the disease in favor of screening truly defines success for a screening program. We do not have the data yet for prostate cancer. If one accepts 10 years as an average time course for prostate cancer to become a problem in men diagnosed with localized disease, and PSA testing is thought to provide a lead-time of approximately 5 years (23), it is likely to be up to 15 years after widespread PSA testing became popular for one to assess the effects of PSA screening on mortality. However, there are already a few early indicators for effectiveness of a screening program. With screening one should see disease incidence increasing at first with detection of the backlog of clinically occult cases, then leveling off at a 'steady state' rate higher than the pre-screening incidence. Also, there should be a downward shift in age and stage at diagnosis. Indeed these expected events have each been seen. The rapid escalation in the incidence of prostate cancer from 1988 to 1992 was probably due to PSA screening. After the peak in 1992, it has been progressively declining to near the baseline levels. Mortality has also recently begun to decline as well, reaching a peak of 44 000 deaths in 1997 in the USA, and subsequently dropping by 12% over the next 2 years (3). This decline, occurring 8–9 years after *ad lib* screening became widely practiced, follows closely the predicted time course if early detection and therapy are to be effective. In one of the first prospective, randomized, large-scale trials (and somewhat controversial), more than 46 000 men were randomly allocated to be screened or to receive no screening. Labrie found a highly significant three-fold reduction in prostate cancer death over an 8-year period, in favor of men who were screened. In most European countries, one in two patients with prostate cancer will succumb to the disease itself; yet in the US, where screening is much more common, the ratio is reduced to one in five (2).

It is true that earlier detection will incur a certain amount of lead-time bias in survival statistics. However, the shift in age and stage should be viewed as a sign of screening effectiveness, in that the disease is being detected sooner. For any chance of a higher cure rate or increased survival, stage migration must occur to a more curable stage for treatment to be effective. It has been shown that the likelihood of a progression-free course after radical prostatectomy was increased for patients with PSA-detected cancers (T1c) in comparison with those who had palpable cancers (T2) (52, 53, 54). The combination of expected increased incidence, decrease in age at diagnosis, and downward stage migration, seen in an effective screening program, should result in an increased detection of organ-confined disease, when the hope for cure is realistic.

There are concerns that prostate cancer screening with PSA is disproportionately finding and treating insignificant cancers, also called over-diagnosis. Current data indicates that not more than 8–10% of surgical specimens subsequently have the pathological appearance of being a non-lethal form of prostate cancer (49). In general, US prostate cancer detection rates in first-round screening have been found in the range of 2.5–5%, compared to breast cancer screening detection rates of 0.2–0.5%. PSA appears to have a 10-fold greater detection rate than mammography for a disease with similar incidence and mortality rates (55). However, as appropriate, after 1, 2, and 3 years the detection rate drops significantly to about 0.5%. In this case it is the lower sensitivity that precludes finding the insignificant tumors, and is desirable in that it reduces risk of over-diagnosis, and possible resulting over-treatment.

Some contend that the sharp rise in prostate cancer detection that accompanied the advent of PSA testing caused a shift in tumor grade to less aggressive tumors that may not be clinically significant. Instead, about 75% of the increase was found to be due to moderate tumors of a Gleason score 5–7, and only an 8% rise in lower grade tumors (9). This and other evidence confirms that screening programs based on PSA testing will detect mainly clinically significant malignancies that are likely to progress. Although length-time bias may theoretically be a confounding factor in prostate cancer, the biological characteristics of the disease suggest this is unlikely (9). It has been found through serum PSA values that even the higher grade tumors themselves have doubling times that exceed 2 years (56, 57). Therefore it is unlikely that annual screening is 'missing' the aggressive tumors. In summary, it appears that PSA-based community screening is markedly increasing the percentage of clinically localized cancers at diagnosis without a significant concomitant rise in detection of clinically unimportant cancers.

If assessing the effectiveness of prostate cancer screening is complex, estimating cost-effectiveness is even more difficult. While an individual PSA test is relatively inexpensive at about $30, the expenses seem to multiply in the next step if the PSA value is abnormal. The TRUS, random biopsy, and pathological interpretation cost between $500 and $1500. This, coupled with the high incidence of prostate cancer and that there are three negative biopsies for every one diagnosis of cancer, has led to estimates of nationwide prostate cancer screening costing $8.5–25.7 billion for the first year. While these costs do appear exorbitant when taken at face value, when compared to other screening practices directly, they are less worrisome. The cost of diagnosing one case of prostate cancer at the first visit has been evaluated at $3000, well below the costs of diagnosing one case of breast or cervical cancer, malignancies for which regular screening is widely advocated. Prostate cancer screening costs per quality-adjusted life-year saved of $14 200–51 267 appear compatible to those of other diseases such as breast cancer screening (55). The costs of treating a localized cancer is less now than previously, because of mandates of American health economics. However, further studies are needed to clarify the costs of treating late stage disease and patients dying from prostate cancer.

Is prostate cancer really a low-risk disease? Issues are changing as the demographics of the worlds population is changing. A 67-year old man diagnosed with localized prostate cancer in the US now has an average life expectancy that exceeds 15 years, tremendously increasing his risk of eventually suffering from metastatic prostate cancer. The best available population-based cohort study of conservative management, done by Albertson *et al.*, shows that prostate cancer is not as indolent as suggested (23). Men with moderately differentiated tumors (75% of all tumors) lost 4–5 years of life and those with poorly differentiated tumors lose 6–8 years of life. In Sweden, records showed the relative survival of the men with prostate cancer was only 45% of controls at 10 years, or in other words men with prostate cancer lost an average of 40% of the remainder of their lives (58). Half of the men dying with prostate cancer are under 75 years of age, and a considerable proportion is under 65. Obviously none of these men want to hear that prostate cancer only kills a 'small proportion' of men with the disease. Even if prostate cancer is racing with co-morbidity for cause of death of the patient, a 50% death rate for one of the most prevalent cancers in men in the world is still a considerable number of deaths. As Charles R. Smart said (48):

... Because a patient dies of a heart attack does not mean that he would not have died of prostate carcinoma had he lived longer, nor does it mean that his malignancy is any less virulent. ...

Conclusions

Currently, no unequivocal recommendation can be made for prostate cancer screening. However, were it to be carried out, it would likely be restricted to men with at least an 8–10-year life expectancy, who would be willing to accept the morbidities of curative treatment, were prostate cancer diagnosed. Randomized prospective studies are underway to evaluate the efficacy of PSA/DRE screening, which should address lead-time bias and length-bias sampling issues. However, it will be another decade before results are in from such trials in terms of screening's impact on prostate cancer mortality. In the absence of such data, it must be recognized that since PSA screening became popular around 1988–90, reductions in mortality from this disease should become apparent 10 years later, if screening is effective. This has been seen. While there are other explanations for these reductions in disease-specific mortality, certainly the impact of wide-scale screening has to be strongly suspected, particularly in the absence of significant advances in the efficacy of curative therapies.

References

1. Goldstein MM, Messing EM. Prostate and bladder screening. *J Am Coll Surg* 1998, **186**, 63–74.
2. Parkin DM, Pisani P, Ferlay J. Global cancer statistics. *CA Cancer J Clin* 1999, **49**, 33–64.
3. Landis SH, Murray T, Bolden S *et al.* Cancer Statistics, 1999. *CA Cancer J Clin* 1999, **49**, 8–31.
4. Scardino PT. Early detection of prostate cancer. *Urol Clin North Am* 1989, **16**, 635–55.
5. Catalona WJ, Richie JP, Ahmann FR *et al.* Comparison of digital rectal examinations in serum prostate specific antigen in the early detection of prostate cancer: Results of a multi-center clinical trial of 6630 men. *J Urol* 1994, **151**, 1283–90.
6. Richie JP, Catalona WJ, Ahmann FR *et al.* Effect of patient age on early detection of prostate cancer with serum prostate specific antigen and digital rectal examination. *Urology* 1993, **42**, 365–74.
7. Roberts RO, Bergstralh EJ, Katusic SK. Decline in prostate cancer mortality from 1980 to 1997, and an

update on incidence trends in Olmsted County, Minnesota. *J Urol* 1999, **161**, 529–33.

8. Gann PH, Hennekens CH, Stampfer MJ. A prospective evaluation of plasma prostate-specific antigen for detection of prostatic cancer. *JAMA* 1995, **273**, 289–94.

9. Rosen MA. Impact of PSA screening on the natural history of prostate cancer. *Urology* 1995, **46**, 757–68.

10. Reissigl A, Horninger W, Fink K *et al*. Prostate carcinoma screening in the County of Tyrol, Austria. *Cancer* 1997, **80**, 1818–29.

11. Gerber GS, Thompson IM, Thisted R *et al*. Disease specific survival following routine prostate cancer screening by digital rectal examination. *JAMA* 1993, **269**, 61–4

12. Imai K, Ichinose Y, Kubota Y *et al*. Diagnostic significance of PSA and the development of a mass screening system for prostate cancer. *J Urol* 1995, **154**, 1085–9.

13. Bangma CH, Kranse R, Blijenberg BG *et al*. The value of screening tests in the detection of prostate cancer. Part II: Retrospective analysis of free/total prostate-specific analysis ratio, age-specific reference ranges, and PSA density. *Urology* 1995, **46**, 779–84.

14. Hara M, Koyanagi Y, Fukuyama T *et al*. Some physico-chemical characteristics of gammaseminoprotein, an antigenic component specific for human seminal plasma. *Nippon Hoigaku Zasshi* 1971, **25**, 322–4.

15. Wang MC, Valenzuela LA, Murphy GP *et al*. Purification of a human prostate-specific antigen. *Invest Urol* 1979, **17**, 159–63.

16. Catalona WJ, Smith DS, Ratliff TL *et al*. Detection of organ confined prostate cancer is increased through prostate specific antigen based screening. *JAMA* 1993, **270**, 948–54.

17. Oesterling JE. Prostate specific antigen: a critical assessment of the most useful tumor marker for adenocarcinoma of the prostate. *J Urol* 1991, **145**, 907–23.

18. Brawer MK, Chetner MP, Beatie J *et al*. Screening for prostatic carcinoma with prostate specific antigen. *J Urol* 1992, **147**, 841–5.

19. Catalona WJ, Partin AW, Slawin KM *et al*. Use of the percentage of free serum prostate specific antigen to enhance differentiation of prostate cancer from benign prostatic disease. *JAMA* 1998, **279**, 1542–7.

20. Reissigl A, Klocker H, Pointer J *et al*. Usefulness of the ratio free/total PSA in addition to total PSA levels in prostate cancer screening. *Urology* 1996, **48** (6a), 62–6.

21. Jacobsen SJ, Katusic SK, Bergstralh EJ *et al*. Incidence of prostate cancer diagnosis in the eras before and after serum prostate specific antigen testing. *JAMA* 1985, **274**, 1445–9.

22. Smith DS, Catalona WJ, Hersaschman JD. Longitudinal screening for prostate cancer with prostate specific antigen. *JAMA* 1996, **276**, 1309–15.

23. Albertson PC, Fryback DG, Storer BE *et al*. Long-term survival among men with conservatively treated localized prostate cancer. *JAMA* 1995, **274**, 626–31.

24. Benson MC, Whang IS, Pantuck A *et al*. Prostate specific antigen density: a means of distinguishing benign prostatic hypertrophy and prostatic cancer. *J Urol* 1992, **147**, 815–6.

25. Johansson JE, Holmberg L, Johansson S *et al*. Fifteen-year survival in prostate cancer. A prospective, population based study in Sweden. *JAMA* 1977, **277**, 467–71.

26. El-Galley RES, Petros JA, Graham Jr SD *et al*. Normal range PSA versus age-specific PSA in screening prostate adenocarcinoma. *Urology* 1995, **46**, 200–4.

27. Oesterling JE, Jacobsen SJ, Schute CG *et al*. Serum specific antigen in the community based population of healthy men: Establishment of age specific reference ranges. *JAMA* 1992, **270**, 860–64.

28. Catalona WJ, Hudson MA, Scardino PT *et al*. Selection of optimal prostate specific antigen (PSA) cut-offs for early detection of prostate cancer: Receiver operating characteristics (ROC) curves. *J Urol* 1994, **152**, 2037–42.

29. Bangma CH, Kranse R, Blijenberg BG *et al*. The free-to-total prostate-specific analysis ratio improves the specificity of PSA in screening for prostate cancer in the general population. *J Urol* 1997, **157**, 2191–6.

30. Carter HB, Pearson JD, Mettler EJ *et al*. Longitudinal evaluation of PSA levels in men with and without prostate disease. *JAMA* 1992, **267**, 2215–20.

31. Lilja H, Christensson A, Dahlen W *et al*. Prostate-specific antigen in serum occurs predominantly in complex with α1- antichymotrypsin. *Clin Chem* 1991, **37**, 1618–25.

32. Reissigl A, Klocker H, Pointer J *et al*. Improvement of prostate cancer screening by determination of the ratio free/total PSA in addition to PSA levels. *Prostate* 1997, **30**, 243–7.

33. Catalona WJ, Smith DS, Ornstein DK. Prostate cancer detection in men with serum PSA concentrations of 2.6–4.0 ng/ml and benign prostate examination: enhancement of specificity with free PSA measurements. *JAMA* 1997, **277**, 1452–5.

34. Archangeli CG, Humphrey PA, Catalona WJ *et al*. Percentage of free PSA as a predictor of pathologic features of prostate cancer in a screening population. *Urology* 1998, **51**, 558–65.

35. Brawer MK, Partin AW. The promise of new serum markers for prostate cancer. *Contemp Urol* 1999, **11**, 44–70.

36. Nejat RJ, Katz AE, Olsson CA. The role of reverse transcriptase-polymerase chain reaction for staging patients with clinically localized prostate cancer. *Semin Urol Oncol* 1998, **16**, 40–5.

37. Smith DS, Bullock AD, Catalona WJ. Racial differences in operating characteristics of prostate cancer screening tests. *J Urol* 1997, **158**, 1861–6.

38. Walsh PC, Partin AW. Family history facilitates the early diagnosis of prostate carcinoma. *Cancer* 1997, **80**, 1871–1874.

39. Von Eschenbach A, Ho R, Murphy GP *et al*. American Cancer Society guidelines for the early detection of prostate cancer: update 1997. *CA Cancer J Clin* 1997, **47**, 261–4.

40. Carter HB, Morrell CH, Pearson JD *et al*. Estimation of prostatic growth using serial PSA measurements in men with and without prostate disease. *Cancer Res* 1992, **52**, 3323–8.

41. Carter HB, Epstein JI, Pearson JD *et al.* Recommended PSA testing intervals for the detection of curable prostate cancer. *JAMA* 1997, **277**, 1456–60.

42. Ward JE, Hughes AM, Hirst GHL *et al.* Men's estimates of prostate cancer risk and self-reported rates of screening. *Med J Aust* 1997, **167**, 250–3.

43. DeAntoni EP, Glode LM, Crawford ED *et al.* Knowledge, attitudes and health behaviors in a prostate cancer screening program: exhibiting the need for informed consent. *Psycho-Oncology* 1996, **5**, 154.

44. Ward JE, Gupta L, Taylor NJ *et al.* Do general practitioners use PSA as a screening test for early prostate cancer? *Med J Aust* 1998, **169**, 29–31.

45. Fowler FJ, Bin L, Barry MJ *et al.* Prostate cancer screening and beliefs about treatment efficacy: a national survey of primary care physicians and urologists. *Am J Med* 1998, **104**, 526–31.

46. Consensus development conference on the management of clinically localized prostate cancer.1988.

47. Naitoh J, Zeiner RL, DeKernion JB. Diagnosis and treatment of prostate cancer. *Am Fam Phys* 1998, **57**, 1531–9.

48. Smart CR. The results of prostate carcinoma screening in the U.S. as reflected in the surveillance, epidemiology, and end results program. *Cancer* 1997, **80**, 1835–44.

49. Schroder FH. Screening, early detection, and treatment of prostate cancer: a European view. *Urology* 1995, **46** (Suppl), 62–70.

50. Reitbergen JB, Kruger AE, Kranse R *et al.* Complications of transrectal ultrasound-guided systematic sextant biopsies of the prostate: evaluation of complication rates and risk factors within a population-based screening program. *Urology* 1997, **49**, 875–80.

51. Whelan PC. Are we promoting stress and anxiety? *BMJ* 1997, **315**, 1549–50.

52. Humphrey PA. Prostate cancer in the serum PSA era. *Mayo Clin Proc* 1998, **73**, 489–90.

53. Pound CR, Partin AW, Walsh PC *et al.* PSA after anatomic radical retropubic prostatectomy: patterns of recurrence and cancer control. *Urol Clin North Am* 1997, **24**, 395–406.

54. Geary ES, Stamey TA. Pathological characteristics and prognosis of non-palpable and palpable prostate cancers with a Hyridtech PSA of 4 to 10 ng/ml. *J Urol* 1996, **156**, 1056–8.

55. Littrup PJ. Future benefits and cost-effectiveness of prostate carcinoma screening. *Cancer* 1997, **80**, 1864–70.

56. Carter HB, Morrell CH, Walsh PJ *et al.* Estimation of prostatic growth using serial PSA measurements in men with and without prostate disease. *Cancer Res* 1992, **52**, 3323–8.

57. Schmid HP, McNeal JE, Stamey TA. Clinical observations on the doubling time of prostate cancer. *Eur Urol* 1993, **2**, 60–3.

58. Greenberg H, Damber J, Jonsson H *et al.* Patient age as a prognostic factor in prostate cancer. *J Urol* 1994, **152**, 892–5.

Pre-clinical models of prostate cancer

Pamela J. Russell, Dale J. Voeks, and Rosetta Martiniello-Wilks

Introduction

Prostate cancer is now the most common malignancy and the second highest cause of cancer death of men in Western society. Because the disease is very heterogeneous in terms of grade, genetics, ploidy, and oncogene expression, its biological and molecular characteristics are complex and no ideal single model for its study exists. Such a model would have a reasonably slow doubling time, be androgen-dependent (AD) or androgen-sensitive (AS), produce prostate-specific antigen (PSA), metastasize to lymph nodes and bone, and progress to an androgen-independent (AI) state after castration (1). Prostate cancer rarely arises spontaneously in animals, and the human cancer cells are particularly difficult to grow in culture or as xenografts in immune-deprived mice, even short term. Moreover, human and animal prostates differ in their anatomy, cellular content, and in the development of spontaneous benign hyperplasia, which commonly occurs in men as they age but rarely in other species. Existing prostate cancer models include rodent models, human cell lines (in the main derived from metastatic deposits), gene transfer, and transgenic models. Only the transgenic models provide the spectrum of disease as it occurs in men, with progression from prostate intra-epithelial neoplasia (PIN) through AD to AI disease with metastases. Other systems have been devised to study phenomena such as bony metastases of prostate cancer cells. The *in vivo* systems provide the appropriate cellular milieu allowing for epithelial cell–stromal cell interactions that are crucial to the behavior of prostate cancer cells. This chapter provides a critical appraisal of the models and their use in studies of disease progression, and for testing new therapeutic strategies.

The normal prostate elements

Human prostate

Although universal in mammals, the prostate differs among species by anatomy, biochemistry, and pathology (Table 8.1). The human prostate comprises 70% glandular elements and 30% fibromuscular stroma; it develops from the urogenital sinus by stimulation with dihydroxytestesterone (DHT) (2). McNeal (3) replaced the lobular view of the prostate with the concept of concentric zones, the prostate having four zones, each in contact with a different area of the urethra. The peripheral zone contains 75% of the glandular content of the prostate and is the predominant site for adenocarcinomas, while the transition zone contains < 5% of the glandular content but is the predominant site of benign prostatic hyperplasia (BPH) (4). In human BPH, both glandular and stromal overproliferation occur resulting in clinical symptoms related to pressure on the urethra (5).

Rodent prostates

Unlike the 'merged' prostate structure that occurs in man, the rodent prostate consists of anatomically distinct lobes. The dorsal or dorsolateral lobe of the mouse, rat, and guinea-pig prostate shows histologic and biochemical homology to the human prostate peripheral zone (6, 7). The epithelial to stroma ratio in the mouse and rat prostate is ~5:1, but increased growth shifts the ratio towards the stromal component (8). The epithelial to stroma ratio in the guinea-pig prostate decreases during adulthood until the prostate becomes ~75% stroma at 2 years of age, the equivalent of 70 years of age in humans (9).

Table 8.1 Characteristics of the prostate gland among species

Species	Lobes zones	BPH (Spon)	BPH site (Predominant)	BPH Epithelium/stroma involvement	CaP (Spon)	CaP site (Predominant)	Other properties
Human	– Peripheral – Transition – Central – Anterior fibromuscular stroma	Yes	Transition	Epithelium & stroma	Frequent	Peripheral	– Peripheral contains 75% of prostate glandular content
Mouse	– Dorsolateral* (dorsal + lateral) – Ventral – Anterior	No	–	–	No	–	– Induced BPH & CaP
Rat	– Dorsal (dorsolateral)* – Lateral – Ventral – Anterior	Yes	Dorsal Lateral	Epithelium	Rare	Dorsolateral	– Induced BPH & CaP
Guinea-pig pig	– Dorsal* – Lateral – Anterior	Yes	Dorsal	Stroma	No	–	– Smooth muscle component of human BPH
Canine	– Homogenous epithelium*	Yes	Homogenous epithelium	Epithelium	Frequent	Homogenous epithelium	– Spon PIN – Induced BPH – Minimal stroma present
Primate	– Caudal* – Cranial	Yes	Caudal	Epithelium & stroma	Rare	Caudal	– Spon BPH in chimpanzees – Induced BPH in baboons – Chimpanzee & cynomolgus monkey are most similar to human

* Homologue to human peripheral zone.
BPH, benign prostatic hyperplasia; CaP, prostate cancer; Spon, spontaneous; PIN, prostatic intraepithelial neoplasia.

Spontaneous and induced hyperplasia and adenocarcinoma has been observed in the rat dorsal prostate in several studies. Despite the anatomical differences from the human prostate, tumors induced in rat models have provided valuable models for the study of prostate cancer due to their dependence on androgen as a tumor promoter (10). Spontaneous hyperplasia occurs as a result of aging in Brown Norway rats (11) and can be induced in rats by hormone or carcinogen treatment (10). Rat BPH is characterized by mainly epithelial hyperplasia (11). In contrast, age-related spontaneous BPH in the guinea-pig prostate is characterized by stromal hyperplasia similar to the human but with no epithelial component (9). The lobes of the mouse prostate rarely show spontaneous pathologic change with age although prostate hyperplasia and cancer has been induced in several lines of transgenic mice.

Canine prostate

The canine prostate does not display distinct lobular structure but is histologically homogenous consisting predominantly of epithelium with minimal stromal elements. Whilst the epithelium resembles that of the human prostate peripheral zone, there is no surrounding fibromuscular stroma (12). The canine prostate serves as a model for BPH, PIN, and adenocarcinoma (13–15). The dog is the most widely used model of BPH, but it correlates poorly with the human condition, since induced and spontaneous canine BPH contain diffuse epithelial proliferation but no stromal hyperplasia, and there are no clinical symptoms of BPH (16). However, the canine is the only non-human species where prostate cancer occurs frequently. Clinically aggressive disease with metastases arises spontaneously with age, and high-grade PIN is often present in older dogs (14, 15).

Primate prostates

Primate prostates consist of cranial and caudal lobes with the cranial similar to the central zone of the human prostate and the caudal homologous to the transition and peripheral zones (17). Spontaneous and induced hyperplasia is predominantly found in the caudal zone, and sporadic cases of prostate cancer have also been documented (18). The human and chimpanzee prostates show particular anatomic and physiologic similarity: the chimpanzee prostate is histologically heterogeneous with ducts and acini surrounded by stroma, has poor lobal separation, utilizes DHT for growth and development, and produces many of the same proteins as the human prostate (17). The chimpanzee develops spontaneous BPH similar to human BPH in pathologic and clinical variables including prostate volume, PSA, histologic BPH, and urodynamics (16). The baboon also develops BPH: hormonal stimulation causes glandular and stromal hyperplasia in the caudal zone (19). Among the monkey species, the cynomologus monkey prostate is the most similar to the human prostate. Unlike other monkey species, the cranial lobe is partly incorporated into the dorsal area of the caudal lobe creating a transition zone, and considerable stroma is present (20).

Prostate cancer in rodents

Different models mimic various aspects of the clinical disease. Rodent models are popular because they are relatively easy to use and economical in large numbers. Differences exist regarding the site of origin in spontaneous and induced transplantable models depending on the strain of rat and the protocol or carcinogen used. A recent workshop on animal models of prostate cancer (10) lists the characteristics and perceived strengths and limitations of rodent models of prostate cancer.

Spontaneous

Spontaneous tumors include the Pollard rat tumors in Lobund–Wistar (L–W) and Sprague–Dawley rats (21, 22), and ACI/Seg rat prostate cancers in aging August × Copenhagen hybrids (23, 24). Low tumor incidence and long latency periods, as well as a lack of metastases, limit the practicality of these models, which have been described elsewhere in detail (10, 25, 26). The best known model is the Dunning R-3327 rat prostatic adenocarcinoma model derived by the passage of a spontaneous prostate tumor discovered at autopsy in a Copenhagen rat (27). Subcutaneously (sc) implanted tumors become palpable in ~60 days and histologically are well-differentiated adenocarcinomas with both glandular and stromal elements. Multiple well-characterized sublines indicative of cancer progression have been developed (28), including AS lines (H) and AI tumors (A subline), which lack 5α-reductase and androgen receptors (29) and metastatic (30) sublines. Cell lines derived from the models are transfectable, transplantable, and produce reproducible metastases. A limitation of this model is the expression of non-prostatic proteins by the H subline (31). Nevertheless, the Dunning model has demonstrated utility by identifying genes important in the prostate, such as KAI-1, CD44 and beta-thymosin (32).

The Shionogi mouse mammary carcinoma (SC-115) was established from a mammary adenocarcinoma but after passage in male DD/S mice was found to be AD. Serial passage has generated variant lines, which include AI lines, as well as those sensitive to estrogens and glucocorticoids. These lines are useful for studies of intermittent androgen therapy and for analysis of the mechanisms involved in the generation of androgen independence (25, 33).

Induced

Prostate tumors have been induced by chronic administration of testosterone in Lobund–Wistar (34), and Noble rats (35, 36), illustrating the critical role of androgens as promoters in the pathogenesis of prostate cancer. Chemical carcinogens have also been used to induce prostate cancers in Fischer F344 and Wistar (37) rats. The features of these models have been summarized elsewhere (10). Recently, studies of hormone-induced tumors in Noble rats indicated that insulin-like growth factor-1 (IGF-1) changed from paracrine production by stromal cells to an autocrine loop in prostate epithelial cells during cancer induction (38).

The use of intraprostatic rather than intravenous (iv) administration of N-methyl-N-nitrosurea to Wistar rats increased the incidence and decreased the latency of prostate neoplasms and prevented the formation of tumors in other organs typically found after iv injection (39). Whilst induced prostate tumors show differences in their location in regions of the rat prostate–seminal vesicle complex (40) depending on the agent used for induction and the strain of rats, they are particularly useful for studies of chemoprevention and dietary modulation, and most develop a high incidence of invasive carcinomas, although bony metastases are rare. They do allow studies of the progression of disease. Cell lines have been derived from spontaneous ACI/Seg rat tumors, from Lobund–Wistar and from chemically induced Wistar rat tumors (10).

Human prostate cancer cell lines

Lines derived from human tumors

Most human prostate cancer cell lines (Table 8.2) have been established from metastatic deposits with the exception of PC-93 (41), grown from an AD primary tumor (43). However, PC-93 and other widely used lines, including PC-3 (43, 44, 45), DU-145 (46), and TSU-PR1 (47), are all AI; all lack androgen receptors (with the possible exception of PC-93), PSA and 5α-reductase; and all produce poorly differentiated tumors if inoculated into nude mice (48–51). Until very recently, the paucity of AD cell lines has made studies of the early progression of prostate cancer using human material very difficult. However, metastatic sublines of PC-3 have been developed by injection of cells into nude mice via different routes, especially orthotopically (52).

Until recently, the LNCaP cell line, established from a metastatic deposit in a lymph node (49) was the only human prostate cancer cell line to demonstrate androgen sensitivity. After its initial characterization, several laboratories found LNCaP cells to be poorly tumorigenic in nude mice (53–60) unless co-inoculated with tissue-specific mesenchymal or stromal cells (61) or Matrigel (62), emphasizing the importance of extracellular matrix and paracrine-mediated growth factor in prostate cancer growth and site-specific metastasis (63). New lines were obtained by culturing LNCaP cells that had been grown in castrated mice (49). The C-4 LNCaP line is AI, produces PSA and a factor that stimulates PSA production, and the C4–2 and C4–2B lines metastasize to lymph nodes and bone after subcuta-

neous or orthotopic inoculation (49, 50). Others have also selected more highly metastatic cells (52) by serial reinjection into the prostate of prostate cancer cell lines. The LN-3 cells derived from the LNCaP line by this method are more metastatic to liver, less sensitive to androgen, and produce high levels of both PSA and prostate specific membrane antigen (PSMA). The LNCaP line expresses a mutated androgen receptor (AR). Some mutations of the AR are associated with stimulation of the cells by antiandrogens, causing concern over the use of drugs such as finasteride for the treatment of late stage prostate cancer. The subline, LNCaP 104-R2, manifests this phenomenon (51).

Recently, new androgen-responsive lines have been established. The MDA PCa 2a and MDA PCa 2b lines were both isolated from a single bone metastasis from a black American who had AI prostate cancer. They both express PSA (MDA PCa 2a produces 0.43 and MDA PCa 2b, 0.67 ng/ml of PSA/g of tumor), are AS and both grow in nude mice; they differ in their morphology *in vitro* and in their karyotypes, and are thought to represent distinct clones from the same tumor (53). The ALVA101 (54) line is also AS; these cells respond to 5α-DHT by up-regulating an autocrine loop involving epidermal growth factor receptors (EGFR) and their ligand, transforming growth factor-α (TGFα) (64). Other ALVA lines have also been used (ALVA-34 and ALVA-41, 65) but information about them is scarce.

An unusual cell line, ARCaP (55), was derived from prostate cancer cells in ascites fluid of a man with metastatic disease, and exhibits androgen- and estrogen-repressed growth and tumor formation in hormone-deficient or castrated mice. These cells express low levels of AR and PSA and are highly metastatic when inoculated orthotopically. Androgen-repressed prostate cancers are thought to occur only very late in the progression of the disease. Other human prostate cancer cell lines used in research include CRL-1740 (66), PPC-1 (which is AI) (67), and CPA (68), but there is little information about these lines and their properties.

Molecular analyses have shown that many of the cell lines contain p53 mutations (Table 8.2), consistent with the finding that p53 mutations occur in late stage prostate cancer. In some cases, alterations of other oncogenes/suppressor genes have been observed. The DU-145 line shows a mutation in the p16 gene, involved in cell-cycle control (45). Relatively few of the lines express PSA, or prostate-specific membrane antigen (PSMA), which has been shown to be overexpressed in late-stage prostate cancers in man (69).

Table 8.2   Characteristics of malignant human prostate epithelial cell lines

Cell line	Origin	Androgen receptor	Androgen sensitivity	5α-reductase	PSA	PSMA	p53/other features	Ref
PC-93	AD primary prostate cancer	?	AI	–	–	NR	NR	41
PC-3	Lumbar metastasis	–	AI	–	–	–	Deletion mutation of p53 (42)	43
DU-145	Central nervous system metastasis	–	AI	–	–	–	Mutated p53, pro to leu codon 223; val to phe codon 274 (44) Has mutated p16 codon 84 (45)	46
TSU-PR1	Cervical lymph node metastasis in Japanese man	–	AI	NR	–	NR	Mutated p53 (42) (has mutated H-ras)	47
LNCaP	Lymph node metastasis in white male	+ mutated	AS	–	+	+	Silent mutation of p53 (42)	48
Sublines:								
C4			AI		++	+		49
C4-2B			AI + mets		+++	+	Low levels of functional p53	50
C4-2B P104-R2			AI + mets Stimulated by finasteride		+++	+	p53	51
LN-3			Less sensitive than LNCaP		+++	++		52
MDA PCa 2a	AI bone metastasis from black American	+	AS		+	NR	NR	53
MDA PCa 2b	AI bone metastasis from black American	+	AS		+	NR	NR	53
ALVA101	Bone metastasis	+	AS	+	+	NR	NR	54
ARCaP	Ascites from man with metastases	+	Androgen repressed	NR	+	NR	NR	55
LACP-4	Grown from xenograft from advanced prostate cancer	+	AS	NR	+	NR	AI sublines express high levels of HER/2-neu (56)	57

Table 8.2 Characteristics of malignant human prostate epithelial cell lines *continued*

Cell Line	Origin	Androgen receptor	Androgen sensitivity	5α-reductase	PSA	PSMA	p53/other features	Ref
Immortalized cell lines:								
P69SV40T	Immortalized by transfection with SV40large T	NR	NR	NR	NR	NR	Express EGFR and TGFα	58
RWPE-2	RWPE-1 cells immortalized by HPV-18, then infected with Ki-MuSV to induce tumorigenicity	+	+	NR	+	NR	Express HPV-18 E7 protein; mutated Ki-ras	59
CA-HPV-10 10	Immortalized using HPV-18	NR	NR	NR	NR	NR	Cytogenetic abnormalities	60

Immortalized cell lines

Several new immortalized non-tumorigenic, as well as tumorigenic, adult human prostatic epithelial cell lines, which express functional characteristics of prostatic epithelial cells, provide additional *in vitro* cell models for studies on prostatic neoplasia. Researchers have immortalized cells (Table 8.2) by transfection with an SV40 construct containing the SV40 large-T antigen gene (58) or by transfection with plasmids containing a single copy of the HPV-18 genome (59, 70, 71). In each case, the viral proteins used interact with p53, indicating that loss of p53 function may be extremely important for the growth of prostate cancer cells. The use of HPVs for immortalization is based on observations that around 40% of prostate cancers contain DNA from either HPV-16, -18, or -33 (72, 73), suggesting a possible role for HPV in prostate cancer. Further transformation of immortalized cells with the Ki-ras, based on observations of Ki-ras mutations in prostate cancer (73), was performed in order to make the cells tumorigenic (59). In addition, a stromal myofibroblast line has been established for studies of epithelial-stromal interactions. This line, WPMY-1, immortalized with SV40largeT, expresses smooth muscle alpha-actin and vimentin, is positive for AR, large-T Ag, heterogeneous for p53 and pRb, and grows in serum-free medium (74). Conditioned medium from WPMY-1 cells causes marked inhibition of growth of WPE1–10 epithelial cells, immortalized from the same prostate. Other lines immortalized using HPV-18 include PZ-HPV-7 (normal prostate) and CA-HPV-10 (primary prostate cancer), which show multiple cytoge-

netic changes (60). E7 and E7-transforming proteins of HPV-16 have been used to establish 14 immortal benign or malignant prostate epithelial cell cultures from primary adenocarcinomas (75), and these lines have used to study allelic loss of heterozygosity (LOH). LOH at chromosome 8p was seen in tumor-derived lines, but not those from autologous benign prostatic epithelium.

In a similar fashion, normal rat prostate epithelial cells immortalized with SV-40 large T antigen have been used to study the progression to AI and malignancy in Copenhagen rats (76). The immortalized cells were transfected with v-H-ras and c-myc to create invasive cancer lines.

Primary cultures

Stromal–epithelial interactions are pivotal in many aspects of prostatic biology. The investigation of factors that regulate these interactions, and the growth and differentiation of human prostatic cells, has been carried out using defined culture systems for both epithelial and stromal cells from primary prostate cancers (77–79). Using such systems, fibroblastic or smooth muscle cells can be promoted, maintained and investigated in a defined manner (80).

Xenografts

Xenografts provide the opportunity to study the expression of human genes within an *in vivo* context and within the particular organ environment of interest. They also allow an assessment of organ-preferred metastasis, and the evaluation of important principles such as reciprocal stromal cell/epithelial interactions in association with altered hormonal status (81). The limitations of these models include a poor take rate from fresh operation material, relatively poor metastatic potential when implanted sc and potential species–species interactions, which may influence tumor growth and progression (82). Apart from the growth of established cell lines in immune-deficient mice, other xenograft lines, which may or may not grow in tissue culture, have also been established. The CWR22 xenograft line is highly AD *in vivo* and relapses to an AI line, CWR22R, after androgen withdrawal (83), thus providing a useful model for studies of the progression of human prostate cancer. PC-82 is one of several xenograft lines established in Rotterdam. PC-82 and PC-EW are AD prostate cancer xenograft lines (84, 85) useful for studies of androgen-receptor regulation (86). Honda and LuCap xenografts are also both AS (87, 88). A series of xenograft lines established in nude mice from prostate cancer metastases, DUKAP-1 and DUKAP-2 (AS) and DU9479 (AI), have been used to confirm the alternative splicing of the fibroblast growth factor receptor 2 (FGF-R2), which has been shown to change from the FGF-R2 (IIIb) isoform (which has high affinity for keratinocyte growth factor) to the FGF-R2(IIIc) isoform (with a high affinity for basic and acidic fibroblast growth factors). The above progression of prostate cancer in rats (89, 90) also occurs in human prostate cancer (91). The LuCaP23 xenograft series was established from different prostate metastases, two from lymph nodes (LuCaP 23.1 and 23.8) and one from a liver metastasis (LuCaP 23.12) (92). The xenografts show glandular differentiation, are AS, express PSA, and show decreased PSA expression after androgen withdrawal. Two populations of cells are represented in LuCaP xenografts: a neurone-specific enolase (NSE)-positive population, which is also positive for Bcl-2, emerges after castration; whilst the other population is NSE-negative (93). FISH analysis indicates differences in chromosomal rearrangements between LuCaP 23 and another xenografted line, RP22090, about which there is little information (94). The UCRU-PR-2 xenograft line, established from a patient with primary prostatic adenocarcinoma, is a small cell carcinoma of the prostate that is NSE-positive and secretes pro-opiomelano-corticotropin-derived peptides (95, 96). Cell lines have not been established *in vitro* from these lines. Xenografts propogated in SCID mice appear to grow more easily than those grown in nude mice. Six of eight explants from locally advanced or metastatic prostate cancer tissue were established (57) and grew in a manner that recapitulates the clinical transition from AS to AI growth, accompanied by micro-metastases. Four of these were PSA-positive and two, LAPC-3 and LAPC-4, showed chromosomal abnormalities and expressed wild-type ARs. LAPC-3 is AI, whilst LAPC-4 is AS. The LAPC-4 xenograft has been propogated as a continuous cell line (Table 8.2), which retains its hormone-responsive characteristics, but the xenografted line can progress to androgen-independence when grown in female or castrated male mice. In this model, the AI sublines express higher levels of HER-2/neu than the AS cells. Forced over-expression of HER-2/neu in AD cells allowed ligand-independent growth. HER-2/neu activated the AR pathway in the absence of ligand and synergized with low levels of androgen to 'superactivate' the pathway (56). As in human prostate cancer, prostate cancer xenografts secrete PSA, which is complexed with a murine protease inhibitor with high homology to murine alpha1-P1, and the percentage of free PSA is a characteristic of each xenograft line tested, in agreement with patient values at the time of tumor harvest (97).

Models for bone metastases

Prostate cancer is unique in that it is osteogenic, resulting in the formation of dense sclerotic bone with high levels of osteoblastic activity. A potential regulator of the tropism of prostate cancer to bone is a family of proteins that belong to the transforming growth factor β (TGF-β) family called bone morphogenetic protein (BMP), which is involved in stimulating bone formation *in vivo*. Some BMPs and their receptors are expressed on prostate cancer cells. These receptors are regulated by androgen and can differentially modulate prostate cancer cell growth in response to BMP under different hormonal conditions (98). As xenografts grown sc in nude mice rarely metastasize, special methods have been developed to study bony metastases from human prostate cancers in experimental models. As mentioned previously, the C4-2 and C4-2B sublines, which were developed from LNCaP cells by co-inoculation with tissue specific or bone derived mesenchymal or stromal cells in castrated mice, metastasize to lymph nodes and bone after subcutaneous or orthotopic inoculation (49, 50). Intrafemoral injection has been used to establish osteoblastic bone lesions of PC-3, LNCaP, C4-2 and C4-2B4 in athymic (99) and SCID/bg mice. In the latter, osteoblastic tumors occurred in the bone marrow space within 3–5 weeks, and serum PSA showed a stepwise elevation with tumor growth (100).

Transgenic and reconstitution models

The combination of advances in the hormonal control of reproduction, the harvest/manipulation and reimplantation of fertilized embryos, and recombinant DNA techniques led to the advent of transgenic technology nearly 20 years ago (reviewed in ref.101). The ability to stably introduce foreign genetic information into the mammalian cell line has been a landmark development in molecular biology shifting emphasis back to the whole animal as an experimental-model system. Transgenics offer a unique opportunity to study the effects of altered gene expression and ultimately carcinogenesis in the proper biologic milieu. The potential exists to create an animal model that faithfully represents the broad spectrum of human prostate cancer from early to late stages allowing insight into key genetic events in tumor initiation and promotion and also serving as a tool to evaluate therapeutics. The majority of transgenic studies involve restricted transcription of various genes with oncogenic potential through the use of tissue-specific promoters. In prostate-directed transgenics (Table 8.3), a number of promoter elements have been investigated (102–108).

Rat probasin is largely found in the dorsolateral region of the rodent prostate (109). Transcriptional activity is hormonally-regulated and begins in the prostate at sexual maturity (110). Transgenic mice bearing the minimal rat probasin promoter region (–426 to +28) (PB) driving a chloramphenicol acetyltransferase (CAT) reporter construct, displayed highly restricted expression to the prostate with the most pronounced activity in the dorsolateral prostate (111). In subsequent research, a large 11.5-kb fragment of the probasin promoter (LPB), containing upstream androgen and zinc regulatory regions, was able to direct high levels of reporter expression specifically to prostate epithelial cells in transgenic mice (112).

Recent interest has focused on PSA, a serine protease with nearly exclusive production by normal and, in most cases, neoplastic luminal prostatic epithelial cells (reviewed in ref.113). Its androgen-regulated promoter region has been isolated and characterized (114). Transgenic mice were generated bearing a reporter construct under the transcriptional control of the 632bp proximal PSA promoter or the 6 kb PSA promoter containing an upstream enhancer region (115). Transgene expression was not detected with the 632bp promoter. Mice bearing the 6-kb promoter demonstrated prostate-specific expression mirroring that seen in humans (115). In further research, transgenic mice harboring a 14-kb

genomic sequence, which encompassed the entire gene and adjacent flanking sequences, had similar PSA expression patterns to those of humans (116).

Several transgenic models have generated hyperplasia in the prostate. The apoptosis suppressing oncogene, bcl-2, under transcriptional control of the C3(1) promoter resulted in increased cell numbers in the prostatic stroma and epithelium (117). In related models, MMTV-int-2/Fgf-3 (fibroblast growth factor member) and MMTV-kgf (keratinocyte growth factor, which is up-regulated in int-2 derived mammary tumors) caused prostate gland enlargement in transgenic mice (118, 119). Transgenic mice over-expressing the prolactin gene, also displayed dramatically enlarged prostates (120). Other transgenic models bearing MMTV-WAP (whey acidic protein) and metallothionine-TGF-α (transforming growth factor) developed hyperplasia of the coagulating gland epithelium (121, 122).

The current transgenic models of prostate cancer that display the most potential utilize tissue-specific regulatory regions to target expression of the SV40 large tumor antigen (Tag), which functions as an oncogene by binding to, and interfering with, the p53 and Rb tumor suppressor genes (123). Losses of wild-type p53 and pRb function are considered to be critical events in prostate cancer progression (124). Separate models have been created employing the 5′ flanking region of the prostate steroid binding protein C3(1) gene (102), the human fetal globin promoter (103), a region of the mouse cryptdin-2 gene (104), the long PB promoter (105), or the minimal PB promoter (106) to drive the expression of Tag.

In the C3(1)-Tag model, male mice develop prostatic hyperplasia that progresses to adenocarcinoma in most animals by 7 months of age in the ventral lobe and 11 months of age in the dorsolateral lobe, with occasional metastasis to lung (102, 125). The mice display a progression from low- to high-grade PIN precursor lesions histologically resembling that found in humans (125). Female mice develop mammary adenocarcinoma in 100% of the animals by 6 months of age (102).

Transgenic mice from the fetal globin-Tag lines somewhat unexpectedly developed prostate tumors, brown adipose tumors, and adrenocortical tumors (103). In the line with prostate involvement, tumors originating from ventral and dorsal lobes showed mixed epithelial and neuroendocrine features and metastasized to lymph nodes and distant sites (126).

The cryptdin-2 gene was able to direct Tag expression to neuroendocrine cells in the prostate. Transgene expression begins between 7 and 8 weeks of age resulting in PIN within a week (104). Androgen-independent prostate cancer with local invasion develops rapidly with

Prostate cancer

Table 8.3   Characteristics of transgenic mouse models of prostate cancer

Model	Tissues involved	PIN–CaP Progression	Metastasis (age of onset)	Androgen status	Reference
C3(1)-Tag	Prostate—ventral most affected Urethra Mammary gland Salivary gland	8–≥ 28 weeks	No	Not Determined	102
FG-Tag	Prostate Adrenals Adipose	16–20 weeks	Lymph Adrenals Kidney Lung Bone Thymus (20 weeks)	Androgen-independent	103
Cryptdin-2-Tag	Prostate–neuroendocrine cells	8–≥ 12 weeks	Lymph Liver Lung Bone (24 weeks)	Androgen-independent	104
LPB-Tag*	Prostate—dorsolateral most affected	10–≥ 22 weeks	No	Androgen-dependent	105
PB-Tag (TRAMP)	Prostate—dorsolateral most affected	7–≥ 12 weeks	Lymph Lung Kidney Bone Adrenals (28 weeks)	Variable	106
C3(1)-Py-MT	Prostate—ventral most affected Lung Vas deferens Epididymus Mammary gland Salivary gland Urethra	11 weeks (CaP)	No	Not determined	107

Tag, SV40 large T and small t antigen; Tag*, SV40 large T antigen; C3(1), prostate steroid binding protein promoter; FG, human fetal globin promoter; LPB, 11.5 kb probasin promoter; PB, 454 bp probasin promoter; Py-MT, polyomavirus middle T; PIN, prostatic intraepithelial neoplasia; CaP, prostate cancer.

eventual metastasis to lymph nodes, liver, lung, and bone by 6 months (104). This model demonstrates that prostate neuroendocrine cells are sensitive to transformation and resulting cancer is highly aggressive (104).

In the LPB model, a tag-deletion mutant (without expression of the small t antigen) was able to transform prostate epithelial cells of transgenic mice with an incidence of 100% by 10 weeks of age (105). Progression typically proceeds through hyperplasia, low- and high-grade dysplasia, carcinoma *in situ*, adenocarcinoma, and local invasion in a manner similar to the human condition but without evidence of metastasis (105). The model also exhibits multi-focality, reactive stromal proliferation, and androgen-dependent growth of the primary tumor.

The PB-Tag (TRAMP, transgenic adenocarcinoma mouse prostate) model appears to closely mimic the human disease. Mice show highly specific prostate expression of the transgene by 8 weeks of age leading to the development of adenocarcinoma in the dorsolateral region as early as 10–12 weeks of age (106). Metastasis to the lymph nodes and lungs is present in 100% of mice by 28 weeks of age (127). A longitudinal cohort analysis of prostate cancer progression in this line showed that primary tumors became palpable by 10–38 weeks of age, with cancer death occurring between 24 and 39 weeks of age (128). Castration studies demonstrated that prostate cancer is variable in androgen-dependence as early as 12 weeks of age (129). The TRAMP model reliably develops prostate adenocarcinoma that resembles the disease progression of human prostate cancer. This model already is serving as a tool to investigate the basic science of prostate cancer initiation and progression (130), and to evaluate the efficacy of potential therapeutics (131).

In a different model of prostate cancer, the role of signal transduction in prostatic epithelium transformation was investigated through the generation of transgenic mice bearing the polyomavirus middle T gene under transcriptional control of the C3(1) gene (107). Androgen-responsive urogenital tissues expressing the transgene showed disrupted growth and development with the presence of hyperplasia, dysplasia, and invasive carcinoma (107). Expression of the transgene was detected in the ventral and dorsal prostate, epididymis, parotid gland, seminal vesicles, coagulating gland, and also in unexpected sites like the lung where endogenous C3(1) is not detected in the rat (107).

Thompson *et al.* (132) developed a transgenic gland model of prostate cancer (MPR, mouse prostate reconstitution) by utilizing the ability of mesenchyme and epithelium from fetal urogenital sinus to form a mature prostate when grafted into the renal capsule of an adult mouse (133). Introduction of candidate genes into separate compartments allows for the study of stromal and epithelial interactions in carcinogenesis. Following retroviral transfer of ras and myc to the dissociated urogenital sinus, the reconstituted prostate develops adenocarcinoma in a reproducible manner; while transfection with either ras or myc alone results in dysplasia or focal epithelial hyperplasia, respectively (132). Transfection of the urogenital epithelium with both ras and myc results in the development of carcinoma in 80% of animals after 8 weeks when combined with the mesenchyme component. When urogenital mesenchyme is transfected with ras and myc and combined with the epithelium component, the reconstituted prostate develops dysplasia in 100% of animals (134). Numerous studies of prostate carcinogenesis have been carried out in the MPR model, and resulting cell lines have been extensively utilized for basic and applied prostate cancer research (135, 136).

Uses of pre-clinical models of prostate cancer

The comparative utility of rodent models of prostate cancer was summarized in a recent workshop (10). Rat species that develop spontaneous prostate tumors are particularly useful for studies on mechanisms or enhancement of carcinogenesis and latency. In contrast, the biology of progression of prostate cancer can be studied in induced models that tend to become AI and show invasion and metastases. Experimental therapies

for prostate cancer that metastasizes to the bone have used either Copenhagen rats, inoculated with R3327-MATLyLu (Dunning) prostate tumor cells with concomitant clamping of the inferior caval vein, which results in bony metastases (137), or the SCID models injected intrafemorally with prostate cancer cell lines (100). Biodistribution studies in the rat model have indicated preferential uptake of ^{186}Rhenium-hydroxyethylidene diphosphonate (^{186}Re-HEDP) in bone tissue, particularly in areas of bone formation and turnover, suggesting that such treatment has potential for treatment of prostate cancer that has disseminated to the skeleton. Problems of myelotoxicity would need to be carefully considered (137). Subsequent studies in Chacma baboons, prior to clinical trials, indicated that the radiation dose delivered to the bone marrow by ^{186}Re-HEDP did not cause detrimental effects in baboons (138). Other researchers have used promoters from osteocalcin to drive expression of gene therapy in bony metastases (55).

Hormone therapy

One of the mainstays of treatment for prostate cancer is androgen ablation, which can inhibit tumor growth when the cancer is AD or AS. However, prostate tumors can adapt to an environment with low androgen supply by using a hyperactive AR; the mechanisms involve mutations of the AR, generating receptors with broadened activation spectra, increased receptor expression and activation by interaction with other signaling pathways (26, 139). For these reasons, prostate cancer models have been widely used to study a variety of experimental hormonal manipulations, including those possibly suitable for AI disease. Intermittent use of hormone ablation in the LNCaP model prolonged the time until AI PSA production began (140). In LNCaP cells, an interaction occurs between the DNA- and ligand-binding domains of AR and the leucine zipper region of c-Jun. This association provides a link between the transcription factor, AP-1, and AR signal transduction pathways in the regulation of the PSA gene (141). Both LH-RH and GH-RH analogs have proved useful for treating PC-3 or DU-145 AI xenografts, and both appear to invoke increased expression of mRNA for IGF-II in the tumors (142–145). LH-RH vaccines have also been used to induce atrophy of the prostate in rat models (146) and may provide a cheap alternative to the use of LH-RH analogs. Photodynamic therapy given *in vitro* was more effective in LNCaP cells when pretreated with

DHT, suggesting an androgen-modulated effect on both uptake and phototoxicity (147). This effect was not observed in AI PC-3 cells *in vitro*. However, subsequent studies *in vivo* using R3327-MatLyLu Dunning cells grown orthotopically in the ventral prostate, indicated that benzoporphyrin derivative monoacid ring A, combined with surgery, could inhibit both local primary tumor growth as well as reduce distant metastases (148).

Novel therapies

Metastatic human prostate cancer requires novel therapeutic strategies in order to overcome its low proliferative rate and its resistance to conventional chemotherapeutic agents. Some new approaches, which have been tested in pre-clinical models of prostate cancer, include interruption of angiogenesis, generation of apoptosis, the use of targeted toxins, targeted using antibodies or growth factors, and transcriptionally targeted gene therapy. Many other prospective treatments have also been used but are outside the scope of this review.

The use of antibodies either to target therapy to prostate cancer, or to inhibit prostate cancer cell function, is returning to favor. An iodine (I) labeled monoclonal antibody, ^{125}I-E4, shows good localization to DU145 cells grown sc in nude mice, with an average radiation dose of 0.08 Gy/MBq after intraperitoneal injection (149). In other studies, based on the high expression of vascular endothelial growth factor (VEGF) by highly metastatic human prostate cancers growing orthotopically in athymic mice (150), a neutralizing antibody to VEGF (A4.6.1) has been shown to inhibit angiogenesis and to prevent tumor growth beyond the initial prevascular growth phase of DU145 spheroids implanted sc (151). Others have inhibited angiogenesis and tumorigenicity of prostate cancer cells by inducing interferon β (IFN-β) expression in the tumor cells before implantation in nude mice (152). Toxins have been targeted to prostate cancer cells by using antibodies or ligands for receptors expressed by prostate cancer cells. Tumor sublines derived from DU-145 cells treated *in vivo* with a basic fibroblast growth factor-saporin toxin chimera (bFGF-SAP) were able to modify the ligand-targeted receptor in order to generate resistance indicating how to better design chimeric toxins (153). Of a series of toxins tested against prostate cancer cell lines using a clonogenic assay only

diphtheria toxin (DT) and ricin had highly potent cytotoxic activity. DT-mediated cell death was found to be both cell cycle and p53 independent, providing a good candidate for antibody-mediated application (154).

Gene therapy for prostate cancer

The pre-clinical models have been extensively used for a variety of studies of gene therapy for prostate cancer. These include corrective gene replacement to restore suppressor gene activity or to abrogate oncogene activity, immunotherapy to augment the immune response against prostate cancer *ex vivo* or *in vivo*, and cytotoxic reduction of prostate cancer using enzyme-directed pro-drug therapy (EPT) or specific approaches for the induction of apoptosis. Different viral delivery systems or naked DNA with liposomes and molecular conjugates have been used for these studies; their advantages and disadvantages have been reviewed elsewhere (155).

Corrective gene therapy

Numerous strategies to replace disabled tumor suppressor genes or inhibit aberrant expression of oncogenes are under investigation. As previously mentioned, p53 mutations appear to play a significant role in prostate cancer, especially in aggressive human tumors (124). The p53 target gene, p21/WAF1, is a cyclin-dependent kinase inhibitor (156) involved in cell-cycle arrest at the G1 checkpoint. Transduction of AI human prostate cancer cell lines, with deleted p53 (human PC-3, TSU-PR) or which express mutated (DU-145, C4–2) p53 (Table 8.2), with recombinant adenoviruses expressing wild-type p53 under the control of a CMV promoter (Ad-p53), caused growth inhibition *in vitro* and when injected into BALB/c nude male mice following transduction *ex vivo* (157, 158). A similar viral construct expressing p21/WAF1 inhibited the growth of a pre-established tumors of a p53-negative mouse prostate cancer cell line, 148–1PA, in 129/Sv mice (159) to a greater extent than Ad-p53. Based on the finding that Ad-p53 could inhibit the growth of pre-established DU145 tumors grown intraperitoneally (ip) in male SCID mice (160), phase I clinical trials of p53 gene replacement for advanced prostate cancer have been initiated (161).

Similar experiments have been performed to successfully suppress the growth of DU-145 and PC-3 human tumor xenografts in BALB/c nude mice using recombinant adenoviruses expressing other putative suppressor genes under the control of a CMV promoter, including the progressive multi-focal leucoencephalopathy (PML) gene (162) and the cell-adhesion molecule, C-CAM1 (163).

Anti-sense strategies have been used to inhibit translation (164) of oncogenes, which are over-expressed in prostate cancer. Such experiments, involving transfection of MatLyLu cells prior to *in vivo* growth in rats, have indicated that TGF-β1 can promote prostate cancer growth and aggressiveness (165), and should be a target for therapeutic intervention. Successful inhibition of growth of cell lines and xenografts of DU-145 cells has been obtained using anti-sense c-myc (166, 167) leading to a clinical trial (161), as well as with anti-sense bcl-2 in LNCaP cells (168). The induced expression of bcl-2 allows the prostate cells to undergo apoptosis.

Cytotoxic-reduction gene therapy

Because the prostate gland can be surgically removed without killing the patient, it is possible to 'target' therapy to the prostate. This can be done in two ways. A recombinant replication-competent virus, which is targeted using a PSA promoter to replicate only in prostate cells, was tested using LNCaP cells and xenografts (169); a clinical trial based on this work showed success in some patients. More recently, an enhancer element from the PSA (human glandular kallekrein, hK2) gene, or the prostate-specific antigen enhancer, together with the hK2 enhancer/promoter, were used to create variant Calydon viruses (CV763, CV764, respectively), which replicate in prostate tumor cells but are attenuated in non-prostate tumor cells creating a high therapeutic index in LNCaP cells (170). Based on animal studies, this work has proceeded to clinical trial. Alternatively, enzyme-directed pro-drug therapy (EPT) can be used. For EPT, replication incompetent viruses are used to deliver a gene that expresses a 'toxin-producing enzyme'. A pro-drug delivered systemically is converted to a toxic metabolite, which both kills the cells expressing the enzyme and diffuses between cells to produce a local bystander effect (171, 172), obviating the need to target every cell. Three such

systems are currently under investigation for prostate cancer using pre-clinical models.

Using herpes virus thymidine kinase (HSVTK) that phorphorylates the pro-drug, ganciclovir (GCV), that then interferes with DNA synthesis, significant cytotoxicity against mouse and human prostate cancer cell lines *in vitro* and the mouse RM-1 line *in vivo* has been demonstrated (173). Pre-established RM-1 tumors in C57BL/6 mice could be growth inhibited by administration of Ad-TK with an RSV promoter when grown sc (174) or orthotopically (174). Moreover, experimental lung metastases induced by intravenous injection in the same model were also inhibited indicating that this treatment may cause an immune response that may be useful for targeting metastases. This 'distant bystander effect' was mediated largely by natural killer cells (NK) (175). A phase I clinical study using Ad-TK with an RSV promoter has recently been performed at Baylor College of Medicine, Houston (176) with promising results.

Mammalian cells do not produce the bacterial enzyme, cytosine deaminase (CD), which can convert 5-fluorocytosine (5-FC) to the cytotoxic agent, 5-fluorouracil (5-FU) (177, 178). Using a CMV promoter, adenoviruses expressing both HSVTK and CD have been used to transduce PC-3 cells that became sensitized to killing by GCV and 5-FC; radiation sensitivity was also increased by treatment with this EPT and pro-drug combination (179).

The *E. coli* DeoD gene product, purine nucleoside phosphorylase (PNP), can metabolize adenine-based nucleotides (180, 181) to toxic non-phosphorylated purines, which because of their small molecular weight can diffuse readily within tissues creating an extensive bystander effect (182, 183). Moreover, drugs produced by PNP are effective against quiescent and proliferating cells as they are incorporated into both RNA and DNA. They are thus very suitable for prostate cancer, which has a low proliferative index. Recent studies have indicated that tumor cells expressing PNP require only low pro-drug concentrations compared to 5-FU to inhibit cell growth, and this could offer advantages over the HSVTK or CD EPT systems (184). Using a 630bp promoter from PSA to achieve tissue specificity, we have compared recombinant adenoviruses expressing HSVTK/GCV and PNP/6 methyl-purine deoxyriboside (6MPDR; which is converted to 6 methyl purine by PNP) for their ability to kill PC-3 tumor cells *in vitro* (185) and *in vivo* (186). The Ad-PSA-PNP virus/6MPDR system was far more efficient than Ad-PSA-HSVTK/GCV *in vitro* (185), but both systems inhibited growth of pre-established PC-3 xenografts in nude mice by around 75–80% with a 20% cure rate and with enhancement of host survival (186).

Immunotherapy for prostate cancer

Prostate cancer is poorly immunogenic, possibly due to its ability to modulate expression of the major histocompatibility class I (MHC class I) antigens, which are required for cytotoxic T cell responses (187). Some potential prostate cancer specific antigens that may be targets for immune therapies have been identified. These include PSA, PSMA, prostate carcinoma associated sialoglycoprotein complex (PAC), TAG-72, GAGE-7 and PAGE (188–191). A potential way to stimulate an immune response against prostate cancer is to express cytokines, such as interleukin-2 (IL-2), granulocyte-macrophage colony stimulating factor (GM-CSF) or interferon-gamma (IFN-γ), each of which can up-regulate the immune response (155). Such approaches have used irradiated, *ex vivo* transduced prostate cancer cells, which are then injected into tumor-bearing animals to study their effects. When Dunning rat MatLyLu tumor cells were used, expression of IL-2 was found to be more effective than GM-CSF in reducing tumor growth and in inhibiting metastases. IFN-γ was not particularly effective. IL-2 also provided protection against subsequent challenge (192). When MatLyLu cells were grown orthotopically, IL-2 prolonged survival (193), but there were no cures. These studies emphasize the importance of the orthotopic model, since local immune influences in the prostate may differ substantially from those in the sc environment. When RM-1 mouse prostate cancer cells transduced *ex vivo* with a novel canarypox virus, ALVAC, were used for vaccination, of several cytokines, only TNF-α alone delayed tumor growth, whilst a combination of IL-2 and TNF- inhibited growth in C57BL/6 mice and SCID mice (194). These rodent experiments have led to several clinical trials of cytokine therapy for patients with prostate cancer.

The cytokine, interleukin-12 (IL-12), has also been tested against prostate cancer. Both tumor growth and experimental lung metastases of RM9 tumors in C57BL/6 mice were inhibited by administration of Ad-CMV-IL-12; the anti-tumor effect appeared to be mediated by macrophages and T cells, whilst the anti-metastatic activity was due to natural killer cells (195). In the more aggressive RM1 model, Ad-IL12 (with an RSV promoter) decreased prostate tumor weights and the numbers of lung metastases were observed within a week of treatment; the activity was mediated through host-induced IFN-γ resulting in Fas up-regulation and tumor cell death (196). A combination of HSVTK/GCV EPT therapy with IL-12 therapy, both delivered by an adenovirus, was more effective than either alone against RM-1 tumors grown orthotopically in mice (197). Other combination therapies may provide a better attack against metastatic as well as local cancer growth.

A study of seven human prostate cancer cell lines, three from primary tumors and four from distant metastases, has shown that Fas cell surface expression, and thus sensitivity to Fas ligand (FasL), induced apoptosis decreases with increased prostate cancer tumor stage (198). Tissue specimens from radical prostatectomies were found to have reduced expression of interleukin-1β converting enzyme (ICE), which plays a central role in the apoptotic pathway (199), suggesting a disruption of the apoptotic signalling pathway. The importance of this pathway for the growth of prostate cancer cells has been supported by gene therapy using Ad-FasL, which prevented growth and induced regression of two human prostate cancer cell lines implanted in nude mice (200).

Concluding remarks

Research into the development of models of prostate cancer representative of the heterogeneity of the disease in humans has yielded numerous breakthroughs in recent years. The combination of pre-neoplastic prostate models, early rodent models, human prostate cancer cell lines, xenografts with particular emphasis on distant site metastasis, and transgenics provides a great diversity of tools for the examination of prostate cancer and prostate cancer metastasis. Knowledge of the molecular mechanisms involved in the shift to invasive disease allows for the development of new treatment strategies. Existing models also serve to evaluate novel therapeutics in multiple stages of the disease encompassing AD and AI growth and the targeting of metastatic deposits.

References

1. Coffey DS, Isaacs JT. Requirement for an idealized animal model of prostatic cancer. *Prog Clin Biol Res* 1980, **37**, 379–88.

2. Brooks JD. Anatomy of the lower urinary tract and male genitalia. In: *Campbell's urology* (ed. PC Walsh). WB Saunders, Philadelphia 1998, 89–128.

3. McNeal JE. The zonal anatomy of the prostate. *Prostate* 1981, **2**, 35–49.

4. Partin AW, Coffey DS. The molecular biology, endocrinology, and physiology of the prostate and seminal vesicles. In: *Campbell's urology* (ed. PC Walsh). WB Saunders, Philadelphia 1998, 1381–428.

5. Shapiro E, Becich MJ, Hartanto V *et al.* The relative proportion of stromal and epithelial hyperplasia is related to the development of symptomatic benign prostate hyperplasia. *J Urol* 1992, 147, 1293–1297.

6. Price D. Comparative aspects of development and structure in the prostate. *Monogr Natl Cancer Inst* 1963, **12**, 2–25.

7. Zhau CY, Tam CC, Wong YC. Morphogenesis and ductal development of the prostatic complex of the guinea pig. *J Morphol* 1993, **217**, 219–27.

8. Hayashi N, Sugimura Y, Kawamura J *et al.* Morphological and functional heterogeneity in the rat prostatic gland. *Biol Repro* 1991, **45**, 308–21.

9. Horsfall DJ, Mayne K, Ricciardelli C *et al.* Age-related changes in guinea pig prostatic stroma. *Lab Invest* 1994, **70**, 753–63.

10. Lucia MS, Bostwick DG, Bosland M *et al.* Workgroup 1: Rodent models of prostate cancer. *Prostate* 1998, **36**, 49–55.

11. Banerjee PP, Banerjee S, Lai JM *et al.* Age-dependent and lobe-specific spontaneous hyperplasia in the brown norway rat. *Biol Repro* 1998, **59**, 1163–70.

12. McNeal JE. Anatomy of the prostate and morphogenesis of BPH. In: *New approaches to the study of benign prostatic hyperplasia* (ed. FA Kimball). Alan R Liss, New York 1984, 27–43.

13. Berry SJ, Strandberg JD, Saunders WJ *et al.* Development of canine benign prostatic hyperplasia with age. *Prostate* 1986, **9**, 363–73.

14. Waters DJ, Bostwick DG. Prostatic intraepithelial neoplasia occurs spontaneously in the canine prostate. *J Urol* 1997, 157, 713–6.

15. Leav I, Ling GV. Adenocarcinoma of the canine prostate. *Cancer* 1968, **22**, 1329–45.

16. Steiner MS, Couch RC, Raghow S *et al.* The chimpanzee as a model of human benign prostatic hyperplasia. *J Urol* 1999, **162**, 1454–61.

17. Lewis RW. Benign prostatic hyperplasia in the nonhuman primate. In: *New approaches to the study of benign prostatic hyperplasia* (ed. FA Kimball). Alan R Liss, New York 1984, 235–55.

18. Lewis RW, Kim JCS, Irani D *et al.* The prostate of the nonhuman primate: normal anatomy and pathology. *Prostate* 1981, **2**, 51–70.

19. Karr JP, Kim U, Resko JA *et al.* Induction of benign prostatic hypertrophy in baboons. *Invest Urol* 1984, **23**, 276–89.

20. Kamischke A, Behre HM, Weinbauer GF *et al.* The cynomolgus monkey prostate under physiological and hypogonadal conditions: an ultrasonographic study. *J Urol* 1997, **157**, 2340–4.

21. Pollard M. Spontaneous prostate adenocarcinomas in aged germfree Wistar rats. *J Natl Cancer Inst* 1973, **51**, 1235–41.

22. Pollard M, Luckert P. Prostate cancer in a Sprague-Dawley rat. *Prostate* 1985, **6**, 389–93.

23. Shain SA, McCullough B, Segaloff A. Spontaneous adenocarcinomas of the ventral prostate of aged AXC rats. *J Natl Cancer Inst* 1975, **55**, 177–80.

24. Shain SA, Boesel RW, Kalter SS *et al.* AXC rat prostatic adenocarcinoma: initial characterization of testosterone regulation of hormone receptors of cultured cancer cells and derived tumors. *J Natl Cancer Inst* 1981, **66**, 565–74.

25. Gleave ME, Hsieh JT. Animal models in prostate cancer. In: *Principles and practice of genitourinary oncology* (ed. D Raghavan, HI Scher, SA Leibel *et al.*). Lippincott-Raven Publishers, Philadelphia 1997, 367–78.

26. Russell PJ, Bennett S, Stricker P. Growth factor involvement in progression of prostate cancer. *Clin Chem* 1998, **44**, 705–23.

27. Dunning WR. Prostate cancer in the rat. *Natl Cancer Inst Monogr* 1963, **12**, 351–69.

28. Isaacs JT. Development and characteristics of the available animal models for the study of prostate cancer. In: *Current approaches to the study of prostate cancer* (ed. DS Coffey, N Bruchovsky, WH Gardner *et al.*). Alan R.Liss, New York 1987, 513–75.

29. Voigt W, Feldman M, Dunning WF. 5α-Dihydrotestosterone-binding proteins and androgen sensitivity in prostatic cancer of Copenhagen rats. *Cancer Res* 1975, **35**, 1840–6.

30. Isaacs JT, Isaacs WB, Feitz WFJ *et al.* Establishment and characterization of seven Dunning rat prostatic cancer cell lines and their use in developing methods for predicting metastatic abilities of prostatic cancers. *Prostate* 1986, **9**, 261–81.

31. Goebel HW, Rausch U, Steinhoff M *et al.* Arguments against the prostatic origin of the R-3327 Dunning H Tumor. *Virchows Arch [B]* 1992, **62**, 9–18.

32. Bao L, Loda M, Janmey PA *et al.* Thymosin beta 15: A novel regulator of tumor cell motility upredulated in metastatic prostate cancer. *Nat Med* 1996, **2**, 1322–8.

33. Rennie PS, Bruchovsky N, Coldman AJ. Loss of androgen-dependence is associated with an increase in tumorigenic stem cells and resistance to cell-death genes. *J Steroid Biochem Mol Biol* 1990, **37**, 843–7.

34. Pollard M, Luckert PH, Schmidt MA. Introduction of prostatic adenocarcinomas in Lobund-Wister rats by testosterone. *Prostate* 1982, **3**, 563–8.

35. Noble RL, Hoover L. The classification of transplantable tumors in Nb rats controlled by estrogen from dormancy to autonomy. *Cancer Res* 1975, **35**, 2935–41.

36. Noble RL. The development of prostatic adenocarcinoma in the Nb rat following prolonged sex hormone administration. *Cancer Res* 1977, **37**, 1929–33.

37. Shirai T, Nakamura A, Fukushima S *et al*. Different carcinogenic responses in a variety of organs, including the prostate, of five different rat strains given 3,2'-dimethyl-4-aminobiphenyl. *Carcinogenesis* 1990, **11**, 793–7.

38. Wang YZ, Wong YC. Sex hormone-induced prostatic carcinogenesis in the noble rat: the role of insulin-like growth factor-I (IGF-I) and vascular endothelial growth factor (VEGF) in the development of prostate cancer. *Prostate* 1998, **35**, 165–77.

39. Schleicher RL, Fallon MT, Austin GE *et al*. Intravenous vs intraprostatic administration of N-methyl-N-nitrosourea to induce prostate cancer in rats. *Prostate* 1996, **28**, 32–43.

40. Bosland MC, Chung LWK, Greenberg NM *et al*. Recent advances in the development of animal and cellculture models for prostate cancer research. A minireview. *Urol Oncol* 1996, **2**, 99–128.

41. Claas FHJ, van Steenbrugge GJ. Expression of HLA-like structures on a permanent human tumor line PC-93. *Tissue Antigens* 1983, **21**, 227–32.

42. Carroll AG, Voeller JH, Sugars L *et al*. p53 oncogene mutation in three human prostate cancer cell lines. *Prostate* 1993, **23**, 123–34.

43. Kaighn M, Shakar, Narayan K *et al*. Establishment and characterization of a human prostatic carcinoma cell line (PC-3). *Invest Urol* 1979, **17**, 16–23.

44. Isaacs WB, Carter RS, Ewing CM. Wild-type p53 suppresses growth of human prostate cancer cells containing mutant p53 alleles. *Cancer Res* 1991, **51**, 4716–20.

45. Gaddipatti JP, McLeod DG, Sesterhenn IA *et al*. Mutations of the p16 gene product are rare in prostate cancer. *Prostate* 1997, **30**, 188–94.

46. Mickey D, Sone K, Wunderli H *et al*. Hetero-transplantation of a human prostatic adenocarcinoma cell line in nude mice. *Cancer Res* 1977, **37**, 4049–58.

47. Iizumi T, Yazaki T, Kanoh S *et al*. Establishment of a new prostatic carcinoma cell (TSU-PR1). *J Urol* 1987, **137**, 1304–6.

48. Horoszewicz J, Leong S, Chu T *et al*. The LNCaP cell line: a new model for studies on human prostatic carcinoma. *Prog Clin Biol Res* 1980, **37**, 115–32.

49. Wu H-C, Hsieh JT, Gleave ME *et al*. Derivation of androgen-independent LNCaP prostate cancer sublines: role of bone stromal cells. *Int J Cancer* 1994, **57**, 406–12.

50. Thalmann GN, Anezinis PE, Chang SH *et al*. Androgen-independent cancer progresion and bone metastasis in the LNCaP model of human prostate cancer. *Cancer Res* 1994, **54**, 2577–81.

51. Umekita Y, Hiipakka RA, Kokontis JM *et al*. Human prostate tumor growth in athymic mice: inhibition by androgens and stimulation by finasteride. *Proc Natl Acad Sci USA* 1996, **93**, 11802–7.

52. Pettaway CA, Pathak S, Greene G *et al*. Selection of highly metastatic variants of different human prostatic carcinomas using orthotopic implantation in nude mice. *Clin Cancer Res* 1996, **1**, 1627–36.

53. Navone NM, Olive M, Ozen M *et al*. Establishment of two human prostate cancer cell lines derived from a single bone metastasis. *Clin Cancer Res* 1997, **3**, 2493–500.

54. Plymate SR, Loop SM, Hoop RC *et al*. Effects of sex hormone binding globulin (SHBG) on human prostatic carcinoma. *J Steroid Biochem Mol Biol* 1991, **40**, 833–9.

55. Chung LW, Kao C, Sikes RA *et al*. Human prostate cancer progression models and therapeutic intervention. *Kinyokika Kiyo—Acta Urologica Japonica* 1997, **43**, 815–20.

56. Craft N, Shostak Y, Carey M *et al*. A mechanism for hormone-independent prostate cancer through modulation of androgen receptor signaling by the HER-2/neu tyrosine kinase. *Nature Medicine* 1999, **5**, 280–5.

57. Klein KA, Reiter RE, Redula J *et al*. Progression of metastatic human prostate cancer to androgen independence in immunodeficient SCID mice. *Nature Medicine* 1997, **3**, 402–8.

58. Bae VL, Jackson-Cook CK, Brothman AR *et al*. Tumorigenicity of SV40 T antigen immortalized human prostate epithelial cells: Association with decreased epidermal growth factor receptor (EGFR) expression. *Int J Cancer* 1994, **58**, 721–9.

59. Bello D, Webber MM, Kleinman HK *et al*. Androgen responsive adult human prostatic epithelial cell lines immortalized by human papilloma-virus 18. *Carcinogenesis* 1997, **18**, 1215–23.

60. Weijerman PC, van Drunen E, Konig JJ *et al*. Specific cytogeneitc aberrations in two novel human prostatic cell lines immortalized by human papillomavirus type 18 DNA. *Cancer Genetics & Cytogenetics* 1997, **99**, 108–15.

61. Gleave ME, Hsieh JT, Gao CA *et al*. Acceleration of human prostate cancer growth *in vivo* by factors produced by prostate and bone fibroblasts. *Cancer Res* 1991, **51**, 3753–61.

62. Gleave ME, Hsieh JT, von Eschenbach AC *et al*. Prostate and bone fibroblasts induce human prostate cancer growth *in vivo*: implications for bidirectional stromal-epithelial interactions in prostate carcinoma growth and metastasis. *J Urol* 1992, **147**, 1151–9.

63. Chung LWK, Gleave ME, Hsieh JT *et al*. Reciprocal mesenchymal-epithelial interaction affecting prostate cancer growth and hormonal responsiveness. *Cancer Surv* 1991, **11**, 91–121.

64. Liu XH, Wiley HS, Meikle AW. Androgens regulate proliferation of human prostate cancer cells in cultures by increasing transforming growth factor-α (TGF-α) and epidermal growth factor (EGF)/TGF-α rectpor. *J Clin Endocrinol Metab* 1993, **77**, 1472–8.

65. Zhuang SH, Schwartz GG, Cameron D *et al*. Vitamin D receptor content and transcriptional activity do not fully predict antiproliferative effects of vitamin D in human prostate cancer cell lines. *Mol Cell Endocrinol* 1997, **126**, 83–90.

66. Sigounas G, Anagnostou A, Steiner M. dl-alpha-tocopherol induces apoptosis in erythroleukemia, prostate and breast cancer cells. *Nutrition and Cancer* 1997, **28**, 30–5.

67. Brothman AR, Lesho LJ, Somers KD *et al*. Phenotypic and cytogenetic characterization of a cell line derived from a primary prostate carcinoma. *Int J Cancer* 1989, **44**, 898–903.

68. Jones HE, Eaton CL, Barrow D *et al.* Comparative studies of the mitogenic effects of epidermal growth factor and transforming growth factor-alpha and the expression of various growth factors in neoplastic and non-neoplastic prostatic cell lines. *Prostate* 1997, **30**, 219–31.

69. Wright GLJr, Grob M, Haley C *et al.* Up-regulation of prostate-specific membrane antigen after androgen-deprivation therapy. *Urology* 1996, **48**, 326–34.

70. Rhim JS, Webber MM, Bello D *et al.* Stepwise immortalization and transformation of adult huiman prostate epithelial cells by a combination of HPV-18 and v-Ki-ras. *Proc Natl Acad Sci USA* 1994, **91**, 11874–8.

71. Webber MM, Bello D, Kleinman HK *et al.* Prostate specific antigen and androgen receptor induction and characterization of an immortalized adult human prostatic epithelial cell lines. *Carcinogenesis* 1996, **17**, 1641–6.

72. McNicol I'J, Dodd JG. High prevalence of human papillomavirus in prostate tissues. *J Urol* 1991, **145**, 850–3.

73. Anwar K, Nakakuki K, Shiraishi T *et al.* Presence of ras oncogene mutations and human papillomavirus DNA in human prostate carcinomas. *Cancer Res* 1992, **52**, 5991–6.

74. Webber MM, Trakul N, Thraves PS *et al.* A human prostatic stromal myofibroblast cell line WPMY-1: a model for stromal-epithelial interactions in prostatic neoplasia. *Carcinogenesis* 1999, **20**, 1185–92.

75. Bright RK, Vocke CD, Emmert-Buck MR *et al.* Generation and genetic characterization of immortal human prostate epithelial cell lines derived from primary cancer specimens. *Cancer Res* 1997, **57**, 995–1002.

76. Lehr JE, Pienta KJ, Yamazaki K *et al.* A model to study c-myc and v-H-ras induced prostate cancer progression in the Copenhagen rat. *Cell Mol Biol* 1998, **44**, 949–59.

77. Peehl DM, Sellers RG, Wong ST. Defined medium for normal adult human prostatic stromal cells. *In Vitro Cell & Developmental Biol Animal* 1998, **34**, 555–60.

78. Wang Q, Tabatabaei S, Planz B *et al.* Identification of an activin-follistatin growth modulatory system in the human prostate: secretion and biological activity in primary cultures of prostatic epithelial cells. *J Urol* 1999, **61**, 1378–84.

79. Dahiya R, Lee C, Haughney PC *et al.* Differential gene expression of transforming growth factors alpha and beta, epidermal growth factor, keratinocyte growth factor, and their receptors in fetal and adult human prostatic tissues and cancer cell lines. *Urology* 1996, **48**, 963–70.

80. Peehl DM, Sellers RG. Basic FGF, EGF and PDGF modify TGFbeta-induction of smooth muscle cell phenotype in human prostatic stromal cells. *Prostate* 1998, **35**, 125–34.

81. Stearns ME, Ware JL, Agus DB *et al.* Workgroup 2: Human xenograft models of prostate cancer. *Prostate* 1998, **36**, 56–68.

82. Russell PJ, Brown J, Grimmond S *et al.* Tumour-induced host stromal-cell transformation: induction of mouse spindle-cell fibrosarcoma not mediated by gene transfer. *Int J Cancer* 1990, **46**, 299–309.

83. Nagabhushan M, Miller CM, Pretlow TP *et al.* CWR22: the first human prostate cancer xenograft with strongly androgen-dependent and relapsed strains both *in vivo* and in soft agar. *Cancer Res* 1996, **56**, 3042–6.

84. Hoehn W, Schroeder F, Riemann J *et al.* Human prostatic adenocarcinoma; some characteristics of serially transplantable line in nude mice (PC-82). *Prostate* 1980, **1**, 95–104.

85. Van Weerden WM, van Kreuningen A, Elissen NM *et al.* Castration induced changes in morphology, androgen levels and proliferation activity of human prostate tissue grown in athymic nude mice. *Prostate* 1993, **23**, 149–63.

86. Ruizeveld de Winter JA, van Weerden WM *et al.* Regulation of androgen receptor expression in the human heterotransplantable prostate carcinoma PC-82. *Endocrinology* 1992, **131**, 3045–50.

87. Ito Y, Nakazato Y. A new serially transplantable human prostatic cancer (Honda) in nude mice. *J Urol* 1984, **132**, 384–7.

88. Bladou F, Vessella RL, Buhler KR *et al.* Cell proliferation and apoptosis during prostatic tumor xenograft involution and regrowth after castration. *Int J Cancer* 1996, **67**, 785–90.

89. Yan G, Fukabori Y, McBride G *et al.* Exon switching and activation of stromal and embryonic fibroblast growth factor (FGF)-FGF receptor genes in prostate epithelial cells accompany stromal independence and malignancy. *Mol Cell Biol* 1993, **13**, 4513–22.

90. Carstens RP, McKeehan WL, Garcia-Blanco MA. An intronic sequence element mediates both activation and repression of rat fibroblast growth factor receptor 2 pre-mRNA splicing. *Mol & Cell Biol* 1998, **18**, 2205–17.

91. Carstens RP, Eaton JV, Krigman HR *et al.* Alternative splicing of fibroblast growth factor receptor 2 (FGF-R-2) in human prostate cancer. *Oncogene* 1997, **15**, 3059–65.

92. Ellis WJ, Vessella RL, Buhler KR *et al.* Characterization of a novel androgen-sensitive prostate-specific antigen-producing prostatic carcinoma xenograft: LuCaP 23. *Clin Cancer Res* 1996, **2**, 1039–48.

93. Liu AY, Corey E, Bladou F *et al.* Prostatic cell lineage markers: emergence of BCL2+ cells of human prostate cancer xenograft LuCaP 23 following castration. *Int J Cancer* 1996, **65**, 85–9.

94. Williams BJ, Jones E, Kozlowski JM *et al.* Comparative genomic hybridization and molecular cytogenetic characterization of two prostate cancer xenografts. *Genes, Chromosomes & Cancer* 1997, **18**, 299–304.

95. Pittman S, Russell PJ, Jelbart ME *et al.* Flow cytometric and karyotypic analysis of a primary small cell carcinoma of the prostate: a xenografted cell line. *Cancer Genet Cytogenet* 1987, **26**, 165–9.

96. Jelbart M, Russell PJ, Fullerton M *et al.* Ectopic hormone production by a prostatic small cell carcinoma xenograft line. *Mol Cell Endocrinol* 1988, **55**, 167–72.

97. Buhler KR, Corey E, Stray JE *et al.* Study of free and complexed prostate-specific antigen in mice bearing

human prostate cancer xenografts. *Prostate* 1998, **36**, 194–299.

98. Ide H, Yoshida T, Matsumoto N *et al.* Growth regulation of human prostate cancer cells by bone morphogenetic protein-2. *Cancer Res* 1997, **57**, 5022–7.

99. Soos G, Jones FT, Haas GP *et al.* Comparative intraosseal growth of human prostate cancer cell lines LNCaP and PC-3 in the nude mouse. *Anticancer Res* 1997, **17**, 4253–8.

100. Wu TT, Sikes RA, Ciu Q *et al.* Establishing human prostate cancer cell xenografts in bone: induction of osteoblastic reaction by prostate-specific antigen-producing tumors in athymic and SCID/bg mice using LNCaP and lineage-derived metastatic sublines. *Int J Cancer* 1998, **77**, 887–94.

101. Shuldiner AR. Transgenic animals. *Mol Med* 1996, **334**, 653–5.

102. Maroulakou IG, Anver M, Garrett L *et al.* Prostate and mammary adenocarcinoma in transgenic mice carrying a rat C3(1) simian virus 40 large tumor antigen fusion gene. *Proc Natl Acad Sci USA* 1994, **91**, 11236–40.

103. Perez-Stable C, Altman NH, Brown J *et al.* Prostate, adrenocortical, and brown adipose tumors in fetal globin/T antigen transgenic mice. *Lab Invest* 1996, **74**, 363–73.

104. Garabedian EM, Humphrey PA and Gordon JI. A trangenic mouse model of metastatic prostate cancer originating from neuroendocrine cells. *Proc Natl Acad Sci USA* 1998, **95**, 15382–7.

105. Kasper S, Sheppard PC, Yan Y *et al.* Development, progression, and androgen-dependence of prostate tumors in probasin-large T antigen transgenic mice: a model for prostate cancer. *Lab Invest* 1998, **78**, i–xv.

106. Greenberg NM, DeMayo F, Finegold MJ *et al.* Prostate cancer in a transgenic mouse. *Proc Natl Acad Sci USA* 1995, **92**, 3439–43.

107. Tehranian A, Morris DW, Min BH *et al.* Neoplastic transformation of prostatic and urogenital epithelium by polyoma virus middle T gene. *Amer J Pathol* 1996, **149**, 1177–91.

108. Green JE, Greenberg NM, Ashendel CL *et al.* Workgroup 3: Transgenic and reconstitution models of prostate cancer. *Prostate* 1998, **36**, 59–63.

109. Spence AM, Sheppard PC, Davie JR *et al.* Regulation of a bifunctional mRNA results in synthesis of secreted and nuclear probasin. *Proc Natl Acad Sci USA* 1989, **86**, 7843–7.

110. Matusik RJ, Kreis C, McNichol P *et al.* Regulation of prostatic genes: roles of androgens and zinc in expression. *J Biochem Cell Biol* 1986, **64**, 601–7.

111. Greenberg NM, DeMayo FJ, Sheppard PC *et al.* The rat probasin gene promoter directs hormonally and developmentally regulation of a heterologous gene specifically to the prostate in transgenic mice. *Mol Endocrinol* 1994, **8**, 230–9.

112. Yan Y, Sheppard PC, Kasper S *et al.* A large fragment of the probasin promoter targets high levels of transgene expression to the prostate of transgenic mice. *Prostate* 1997, **32**, 129–39.

113. Peehl DM. Prostate specific antigen role and function. *Cancer Suppl* 1995, **75**, 2021–6.

114. Lundwall A. Characterization of the gene for prostate-specific antigen, a human glandular kallikrein. *Biochem Biophys Res Commun* 1989, **161**, 1151–6.

115. Cleutjens KB, van der Korput HA, van Eekelen CC *et al.* A 6-kb promoter fragment mimics in transgenic mice the prostate-specific and androgen-regulated expression of the endogenous prostate-specific antigen gene in humans. *Mol Endocrinol* 1997, **11**, 1256–64.

116. Wei C, Willis RA, Tilton BR *et al.* Tissue-specific expression of the human prostate-specific antigen gene in transgenic mice: implications for tolerance and immuno therapy. *Proc Natl Acad Sci USA* 1997, **94**, 6369–74.

117. Zhang X, Chen MW, Ng A *et al.* Abnormal prostate development in C3(1)-bcl-2 transgenic mice. *Prostate* 1997, **32**, 16–26.

118. Tutrone RF Jr, Ball RA, Ornitz DM *et al.* Benign prostatic hyperplasia in a transgenic mouse: a new hormonally sensitive investigatory model. *J Urol* 1993, **149**, 633–9.

119. Kitsberg DI, Leder P. Keratinocyte growth factor induces mammary and prostatic hyperplasia and mammary adenocarcinoma in transgenic mice. *Oncogene* 1996, **13**, 2507–15.

120. Wennbo H, Kindblom J, Isaksson OG *et al.* Transgenic mice overexpressing the prolactin gene develop dramatic enlargement of the prostate gland. *Endocrinol* 1997, **138**, 4410–15.

121. Hennighausen L, McKnight R, Burdon T *et al.* Whey acidic protein extrinsically expressed from the mouse mammary tumor virus long terminal repeat results in hyperplasia of the coagulation gland epithelium and impaired mammary development. *Cell Growth Diff* 1994, **5**, 607–13.

122. Sandgren EP, Leuttke NC, Palmiter RD *et al.* Overexpression of TGFalpha in transgenic mice: induction of epithelial hyperplasia, pancreatic metaplasia, and carcinoma of the breast. *Cell* 1990, **61**, 1121–35.

123. Ludlow JW. Interactions between SV40 large-tumor antigen and the growth suppressor proteins pRB and p53. *FASEB J* 1993, **7**, 866–71.

124. MacGrogan D, Bookstein R. Tumour suppressor genes in prostate cancer. *Semin Cancer Biol* 1997, **8**, 11–9.

125. Shibata MA, Ward JM, Devor DE *et al.* Progression of prostatic intaepithelial neoplasia to invasive carcinoma in C3(1)/SV40 large T antigen transgenic mice: histopathological and molecular biological alterations. *Cancer Res* 1996, **56**, 4894–903.

126. Perez-Stable C, Altman NH, Mehta PP *et al.* Prostate cancer progression, metastasis, and gene expression in transgenic mice. *Cancer Res* 1997, **57**, 900–6.

127. Gingrich JR, Barrios RJ, Morton RA *et al.* Metastatic prostate cancer in a transgenic mouse. *Cancer Res* 1996, **56**, 4096–4102.

128. Hsu CX, Ross BD, Chrisp CE *et al.* Longitudinal cohort analysis of lethal prostate cancer progression in transgenic mice. *J Urol* 1998, **160**, 1500–05.

129. Gingrich JR, Barrios RJ, Kattan MW *et al.* Androgen-independent prostate cancer progression in the TRAMP model. *Cancer Res* 1997, **57**, 4687–91.

130. Kaplan PJ, Mohan S, Cohen P *et al.* The insulin-like growth factor axis and prostate cancer: lessons from the

transgenic adenocarcinoma of mouse prostate (TRAMP) model. *Cancer Res* 1999, **59**, 2203–9.

131. Granziero L, Krajewski S, Farness P *et al.* Adoptive immunotherapy prevents prostate cancer in a transgenic animal model. *Euro J Immunol* 1999, **29**, 1127–38.

132. Thompson TC, Southgate J, Kitchener G *et al.* Multistage carcinogenesis induced by ras and myc oncogenes in a reconstituted organ. *Cell* 1989, **56**, 917–30.

133. Cuhna GR, Fujii H, Neubauer BL *et al.* Epithelial-mesenchymal interactions in prostate development. I, Morphological observations of prostatic induction by urogenital sinus mesenchyme I epithelium of adult rodent urinary bladder. *J Cell Biol* 1983, **96**, 1662–70.

134. Royai R, Lange PH, Vessella R. Pre-clinical models of prostate cancer. *Sem Oncol* 1996, **23**, 35–40.

135. Thompson TC, Kadmon D, Timme TL *et al.* Experimental oncogene induced prostate cancer. *Cancer Surveys* 1991, **11**, 55–71.

136. Nasu Y, Bangma CH, Hall GW *et al.* Adenovirus-mediated interleukin-12 gene therapy for prostate cancer: suppression of orthotopic tumor growth and pre-established lung metastases in an orthotopic model. *Gene Ther* 1999, **6**, 338–49.

137. Geldof AA, van den Tillaar PL, Newling DW *et al.* Radionuclide therapy for prostate cancer lumbar metastasis prolongs symptom-free survival in a rat model. *Urology* 1997, **49**, 795–801.

138. Van Aswegen A, Roodt A, Marais J *et al.* Radiation dose estimates of 186Re-hydroxyethylidene diphosphonate for palliation of metastatic osseous lesions: an animal model study. *Nuclear Medicine Communications* 1997, **18**, 582–8.

139. Culig Z, Hobisch A, Hittmair A *et al.* Expression, structure and function of androgen receptor in advanced prostatic carcinoma. *Prostate* 1998, **35**, 63–70.

140. Gleave M, Santo N, Rennie PS *et al.* Hormone release and intermittent hormonal therapy in the LNCaP model of human prostate cancer. *Progres en Urologie* 1996, **6**, 375–85.

141. Sato N, Sadar MD, Bruchovsky N *et al.* Androgenic induction of prostate-specific antigen gene is repressed by protein-protein interaction between the androgen receptor and AP-1/c-Jun in the human prostate cancer cell line, LNCaP. *J Biol Chem* 1997, **272**, 17485–94.

142. Jungwirth A, Galvan G, Pinski J *et al.* Luteinizing hormone-releasing hormone antagonist Cetrorelix (SB-75) and bombesin antagonist RC-3940-II inhibit the grwoth of androgen-independent PC-3 prostate cancer in nude mice. *Prostate* 1997, **32**, 164–72.

143. Lamharzi N, Schally AV, Koppan M. Luteinizing hormone-releasing hormone (LH-RH) antagonist Cetrorelix inhibits growth of DU-145 human androgen-independent prostate carcinoma in nude mice and suppresses the levels and mRNA expression of IGF-II in tumors. *Regulatory Peptides* 1998, **77**, 185–92.

144. Sica G, Iacopino F, Settesoldi D *et al.* Effect of leuprorelin acetate on cell growth and prostate-specific antigen gene expression in human prostatic cancer cells. *European Urol* 1999, **35** (Suppl 1), 2–8.

145. Lamharzi N, Schally AV, Koppan M *et al.* Growth hormone-releasing hormone antagonist MZ-5-156 inhibits growth of DU-145 human androgen-independent prostate carcinoma in nude mice and suppresses the levels and mRNA expression of insulin-like growth factor II in tumors. *Proc Natl Acad Sci USA* 1998, **95**, 8864–8.

146. Diwan M, Dawar H, Talwar GP. Induction of early and bioeffective antibody response in rodents with the luteinizing hormone-releasing hormone vaccine given as a single dose in biodegradable microspheres along with alum. *Prostate* 1998, **35**, 279–84.

147. Momma T, Hamblin MR, Hasan T. Hormonal modulation of the accumulation of 5-aminolevulinic acid-induced protoporphyrin and phototoxicity in prostate cancer cells. *Int J Cancer* 1997, **72**, 1062–9.

148. Momma T, Hamblin MR, Wu HC *et al.* Photodynamic therapy of orthotopic prostate cancer with benzoporphyrin derivative: Local control and distant metastasis. *Cancer Res* 1998, **58**, 5425–31.

149. Rydh A, Ahlstrom KR, Widmark A *et al.* Radioimmunoscintigraphy with a novel monoclonal antiprostate antibody (E4). *Cancer* 1997, **80**, 2398–403.

150. Balbay MD, Pettaway CA, Kuniyasu H *et al.* Highly metastatic human prostate cancer growing within the prostate of athymic mice overexpresses vascular endothelial growth factor. *Clin Cancer Res* 1999, **5**, 783–9.

151. Borgstrom P, Bourdon MA, Hillan KJ *et al.* Neutralizing anti-vascular endothelial growth factor antibody completely inhibits angiogenesis and growth of human prostate carcinoma micro tumors *in vivo*. *Prostate* 1998, **35**, 1–10.

152. Dong Z, Greene G, Pettaway C *et al.* Suppression of angiogenesis, tumorigenicity, and metastasis by human prostate cancer cells engineered to produce interferon-beta. *Cancer Res* 1999, **59**, 872–9.

153. Davol PA, Frackelton AR Jr. Targeting human prostatic carcinoma through basic fibrlblast growth factor receptors in an animal model: Characterizing and circumventing mechanisms of tumor resistance. *Prostate* 1999, **40**, 178–91.

154. Rodriquez R, Lim HY, Bartkowski LM *et al.* Identification of diphtheria toxin via screening as a potent cell cycle and p53-independent cytotoxin for human prostate cancer therapeutics. *Prostate* 1998, **34**, 259–69.

155. Malkowicz SB, Johnson JO. Gene Therapy for prostate cancer [Review]. *Haematology-Oncology Clinics of North America* 1998, **12**, 649–64.

156. El-Deiry WS, Tokino T, Velculescu VE *et al.* WAF1, a potential mediator of p53 tumor suppression. *Cell* 1993, **75**, 817–25.

157. Ko SC, Gotoh A, Thalmann GN *et al.* Molecular therapy with recombinant p53 adenovirus in an androgen-independent, metastatic human prostate cancer model. *Hum Gene Ther* 1996, **7**, 1638–91.

158. Yang C, Cirelli C, Capogrossi MC *et al.* Adenovirus-mediated wild-type p53 expression induces apoptosis and suppresses tumourigenesis of prostatic tumour cells. *Cancer Res* 1995, **55**, 4210–3.

159. Eastham JA, Hall SJ, Sehgal I *et al. In vivo* gene therapy with p53 or adenovirus for prostate cancer. *Cancer Res* 1995, **55**, 5151–55.

160. Neilsen LL, Gurnani M, Syed J *et al.* Recombinant E1-deleted adenovirus-mediated gene therapy for cancer: efficacy studies with p53 tumour suppressor gene and liver histology in tumour xenograft models. *Hum Gene Ther* 1998, **9**, 681–94.

161. Human gene marker/therapy clinical protocols. *Human Gene Ther* 1997, **8**, 2301–38.

162. He D, Mu ZM, Le X *et al.* Adenovirus- mediated expression of PML suppresses g1rowth and tumorigenicity of prostate cancer cells. *Cancer Res* 1997, **57**, 1868–72.

163. Lin SH, Pu YS, Luo W *et al.* Schedule dependence of C-CAM1 adenovirus gene therapy in a prostate cancer model. *Anticancer Res* 1999, **19**, 337–40.

164. Zheng RQ, Kemeny DM. Inhibition of gene expression by anti-sense oligodeoxynucleotides. *Clin Exp Immunol* 1995, **100**, 380–2.

165. Steiner MS, Barrack ER. Transforming growth factor beta 1 overproduction in prostate cancer: Effects on growth *in vivo* and *in vitro. Mol Endocrinol* 1995, **6**, 15–25.

166. Steiner MS, Satterwhite DJ, Moses HL. Molecular rights into altered cell cycle regulation and genitourinary malignancy. *Urol Oncol* 1995, **1**, 3–7.

167. Steiner MS, Anthony CT, Lu Y *et al.* Anti-sense c-myc retroviral vector suppresses established human prostate cancer. *Hum Gene Ther* 1998, **9**, 747–55.

168. Raffo AJ, Perlman H, Chen MW *et al.* Overexpression of bcl-2 protects prostate cancer cells from apoptosis *in vitro* and confers resistance to androgen depletion *in vitro. Cancer Res* 1995, **55**, 4438–45.

169. Rodriquez R, Schuur ER, Lim HY *et al. Prostate* attenuated replication competent adenovirus (ARCA) CN706: a selective cytotoxic for prostate-specific antigen-positive prostate cancer cells. *Cancer Res* 1997, **57**, 2559–63.

170. Yu DC, Sakamoto GT, Henderson DR. Identification of the transcriptional regulatory sequences of human kallikrein 2 and their use in the construction of calydon virus 764, an attenuated replication competent adenovirus for prostate cancer therapy. *Cancer Res* 1999, **59**, 1498–504.

171. Freeman SM, Abboud CN, Wartenby KA *et al.* The 'bystander effect': tumour regression when a fraction of the tumour mass is genetically modified. *Cancer Res* 1993, **53**, 5274–83.

172. Oldfield EH, Ram Z, Culver KW *et al.* Gene therapy for the treatment of brain tumours using intra-tumoral transduction with the thymidine kinase gene and intravenous ganciclovir. *Hum Gene Ther* 1993, **4**, 39–69.

173. Eastham JA, Chen SH, Seghal I *et al.* Prostate cancer gene therapy: herpes simplex virus thymidine kinase gene transduction followed by ganciclovir in mouse and human prostate cancer models. *Hum Gene Ther* 1996, **7**, 515–23.

174. Hall SJ, Mutchnik SE, Chen SH *et al.* Adenovirus-mediated herpes simplex virus thymidine kinase gene and ganciclovir therapy leads to systematic activity against spontaneous and induced metastasis in an orthotopic

175. mouse model of prostate cancer. *Int J Cancer* 1997, **70**, 183–7.

176. Hall SJ, Sanford MA, Atkinson G *et al.* Induction of potent antitumor natural killer cell activity by herpes simplex virus-thymidine kinase and ganciclovir therapy in an orthotopic mouse model for prostate cancer. *Cancer Res* 1998, **58**, 3221–5.

176. Hermann JR, Adler HL, Aguilar-Cordova E *et al. In situ* gene therapy for adenocarcinoma of the prostate: a phase I clinical trial. *Hum Gene Ther* 1999, **10**, 1239–49.

177. Trinh T, Austin EA, Murray DM *et al.* Enzyme/prodrug gene therapy: comparison of cytosine deaminase/5-flurocytosine versus thymidine kinase/ganciclovir enzyme/prodrug systems in a human colorectal carcinoma cell line. *Cancer Res* 1995, **55**, 4808–12.

178. Hirschowitz EA, Ohwada A, Pascal WR *et al. In vivo* adenovirus mediated gene transfer of E. coli cytocine deaminase gene to human colon carcinoma derived tumours indused chemosensitization to 5-flurocytosine. *Hum Gene Ther* 1995, **6**, 1055–63.

179. Blackburn RV, Galoforo SS, Corry PM *et al.* Adenoviral transduction of a cytosine deaminase/thymidine kinase fusion gene into prostate carcinoma cells enhances prodrug and radiation sensitivity. *Int J Cancer* 1999, **82**, 293–7.

180. Zimmerman TP, Gerstein NB, Ross AF *et al.* Adenine as substrate for purine nucleoside phosphorylase. *Can J Biochem* 1971, **49**, 1050–4.

181. Jensen KF, Nygaard P. Purine nucleoside phosphorylase from *Escherichia coli* and *Salmonella typhimurium*. Purification and some properties. *Eur J Biochem* 1975, **51**, 253–65.

182. Sorscher EJ, Peng S, Bebok Z, *et al.* Tumour cell bystander killing in colonic carcinoma utilizing the *Escherichia coli* DeoD gene to generate toxic purines. *Gene Ther* 1994, **1**, 233–8.

183. Hughes BW, King SA, Allan PW *et al.* Cell to cell contact is not required for bystander cell killing by Echerichia coli purine nucleoside phosphorylase. *J Biol Chem* 1998, **273**, 2322–8.

184. Parker WB, Allan PW, Shaddix SC *et al.* Metabolism and metabolic actions of 6-methylpurine and 2-fluoroadenine in human cells. *Biochem Pharmacol* 1998, **55**, 1673–81.

185. Lockett LJ, Molloy PL, Russell PJ *et al.* Relative efficiency of tumour cell killing *in vitro* by two enzyme-prodrug systems delivered by identical adenovirus vectors. *Clinical Cancer Research* 1997, **3**, 2075–80.

186. Martiniello-Wilks R, Garcia-Aragon J, Daja M *et al. In vivo* gene therapy for prostate cancer: pre-clinical evaluation of two different enzyme-prodrug systems delivered by identical adenovirus vectors. *Human Gene Therapy* 1998, **9**, 1617–26.

187. Sanda MG, Restifo NP, Walsh JC *et al.* Molecular charcterisation of defective antigen processing in human prostate cancer. *J Natl Cancer Inst* 1995, **87**, 280–85.

188. Beckett M, Wright G. Characterization of a prostate carcinoma mucin-like antigen (PMA). *Int J Cancer* 1995, **62**, 703–10.

189. Wright G, Beckett M, Lipford G *et al.* A novel prostate carcinoma-associated glycoprotein complex (PAC) rec-

ognized by monoclonal antibody TURP-27. *Intl J Cancer* 1991, **47**, 717–25.

190. Brenner P, Rettig W, Sanz-Moncasi M *et al.* TAG-72 expression in primary, metastatic and hormonally treated prostate cancer as defined by monoclonal antibody CC49. *J Urol* 1995, **153**, 1575–79.

191. Chen M, Sikes R, Troncoso P *et al.* PAGE and GAGE-7 in the LNCaP prostatic carcinogenesis model that share homology with melanoma associated antigens. *J Urol* 1996, **155**, 264a.

192. Viewcg J, Rosenthal FM, Bannerji R *et al.* Immunotherapy of prostate cancer in the Dunning rat model: use of cytokine gene modified tumour vaccines. *Cancer Res* 1994, **54**, 1760–65.

193. Vieweg J, Heston WD, Gilboa E *et al.* An experimental model simulating local recurrence and pelvic lymph node metastasis following orthotopic induction of prostate cancer. *Prostate* 1994, **24**, 291–8.

194. Kawakita M, Rao GS, Ritchey JK *et al.* Effect of canarypox virus (ALVAC)-mediated cytokine expression on murine prostate tumour growth. *J Nat Cancer Inst* 1997, **89**, 428–36.

195. Nasu Y, Bangma CH, Hull GW *et al.* Adenovirus mediated interlukin-12 gene therapy for prostate cancer: suppression of orthotopic tumour growth and pre-established lung metastases in an orthotopic model. *Gene Therapy* 1999, **6**, 338–49.

196. Sanford MA, Hassen WA, Atkinson G *et al.* Interleukin-12 gene therapy induces cell death through induction of Fas/Fas-Ligand mediated death in metastatic mouse prostate cancer. *J Urol* 1999, **161** (Suppl 4), abstract 211.

197. Hassen WA, Sanford MA, Atkinson G *et al.* Natural killer cells induce by herpes simplex virus thymidine kinase gene transduction and ganciclovir therapy are enhanced by interleukin-12 gene therapy in an orthotopic model of mouse prostate cancer. *J Urol* 1999, **161** (Suppl 4), abstract 198.

198. Hedlund TE, Duke RC, Schleicher MS *et al.* Fas-mediated apoptosis in seven human prostate cancer cell lines: correlation with tumor stage. *Prostate* 1998, **36**, 92–101.

199. Sasaki Y, Ahme H, Takeuchi T *et al.* Immunohistochemical study of Fas, Fas ligand and interleukin-1 beta converting enzyme expression in human prostatic cancer. *Br J Urol* 1998, **81**, 852–5.

200. Hedlund TE, Meech SJ, Srikanth S *et al.* Adenovirus-mediated expression of Fas ligand induces apoptosis of human prostate cancer cells. *Cell Death and Differentiation* 1999, **6**, 175–82.

9 Pre-malignant lesions of the prostate

Ximing J. Yang and Charles B. Brendler

Prostatic intra-epithelial neoplasia

Introduction

Prostatic intra-epithelial neoplasia (PIN) is defined as neoplastic growth of epithelial cells within pre-existing prostatic ducts or acini. High-grade PIN is considered most likely to be a precursor of prostate cancer. This lesion was first described by McNeal in 1969 (1), and a precise characterization and the term intraductal dysplasia were introduced by McNeal and Bostwick in 1986 (2). Later, the term prostatic intra-epithelial neoplasia was proposed by Bostwick and Brawer in 1987 (3) and endorsed by consensus in 1989 (4). Other terms used in the past for this entity include large acinar atypical hyperplasia, atypical hyperplasia, atypical primary hyperplasia, and hyperplasia with malignant change (5–7). The term carcinoma *in situ* of the prostate is not recommended for this entity because of the uncertain natural history and behavior of this lesion.

Pathology of PIN

Architectural and cytologic features

Prostatic parenchyma is composed of epithelium and fibromuscular stroma. The prostatic epithelial cells form glands normally consisting of acini, ductules, and ducts that are often difficult to distinguish on H&E sections. There are at least three types of epithelial cells in a normal prostatic gland: secretory cells, basal cells, and neuroendocrine cells. Most prostatic neoplasms, including adenocarcinoma and PIN, demonstrate the phenotype of secretory cells.

In PIN, the epithelial cells proliferate in the ducts and acini, and become piled up and crowded forming pseudostratified layers (Fig. 9.1(a)). Enlargement, elongation, irregularity, and hyperchromasia of the nuclei

are present, less notable in low-grade PIN (Fig. 9.1(b)) than in high-grade PIN (Fig. 9.1(c)). Mitotic figures can be seen occasionally (Fig. 9.2(a) arrows). Partial involvement of a duct or acinus by neoplastic cells is also common (Fig. 9.2(b)). Usually there is a maturation gradient from the periphery to the center of the gland with the more mature epithelial cells in the center (Figs 9.1(b) and 9.2(a)). A thin layer of basal cells can be recognized in the periphery (base) of the ducts or acini (Figs 9.1(c) and 9.2(a), arrowheads). The ducts and acini demonstrating PIN are often large and branching with a convoluted inner contour. The nuclei are often ovoid or cigar-shaped with the long axis perpendicular to the basement membrane. The presence of prominent nucleoli, very similar to those seen in prostatic adenocarcinoma cells, is typical of high-grade PIN (Figs 9.1(c) and 9.2(a)) but not of low-grade PIN (Fig. 9.1(b)).

Presence of basal cells in PIN

A thin layer of basal cells, sometimes discontinuous, is present in PIN. Loss of basal cells is considered to be a hallmark of invasive prostatic adenocarcinoma (Fig. 9.3(a)) (8). The basal cells can be recognized by routine hemotoxylin and eosin (H&E) stain as a layer of flat or cuboidal cells at the base of a prostatic gland (Figs 9.1(c) and 9.2(a)). They often have clear cytoplasmic halos around nuclei, which are especially obvious in tissue preserved in certain fixatives such as Bouin's solution. Immunohistochemical staining with an antibody for high molecular cytokeratins (34βE12) can be used to identify the presence of prostatic basal cells in PIN and absence of basal cells in adenocarcinoma (Fig. 9.3(b)), which may be helpful in distinguishing PIN from invasive prostatic adenocarcinoma (8–10). Sometimes, the transformation between high-grade PIN and an early invasive adenocarcinoma can be high-

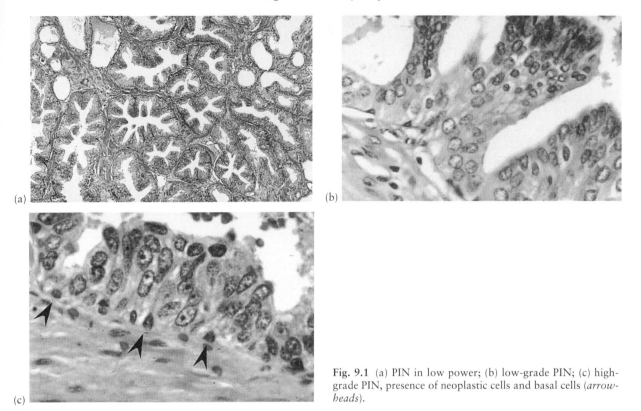

Fig. 9.1 (a) PIN in low power; (b) low-grade PIN; (c) high-grade PIN, presence of neoplastic cells and basal cells (*arrowheads*).

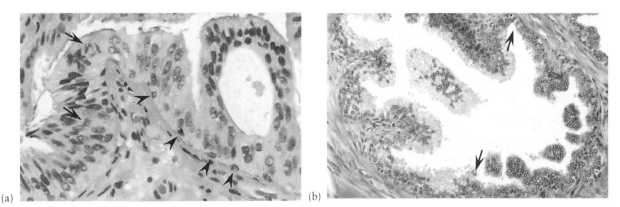

Fig. 9.2 (a) High-grade PIN with mitoses (*arrows*) and basal cells (*arrowheads*); (b) partial involvement of a gland by PIN (*right*) indicated by *arrows*.

lighted with immunostaining specific for prostatic basal cells (Fig. 9.3(c)).

High-grade versus low-grade PIN

Originally, McNeal and Bostwick proposed a three-grade system, in which PIN was divided into PIN-1, PIN-2 and PIN-3 (2). In a consensus meeting in 1989, a two-grade system for PIN was recommended to replace this three-grade system because of its poor reproducibility (4). In the two-grade system, PIN is divided into low grade (PIN-1), and high grade (PIN-2 and PIN-3). The major histologic difference between high-grade PIN and low-grade PIN is the presence of multi-

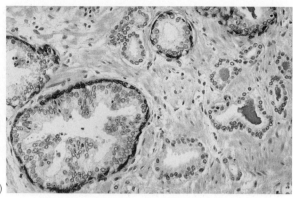

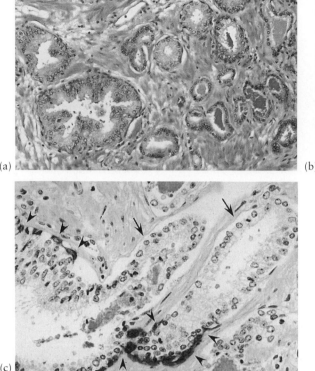

Fig. 9.3 (a) Comparison of high-grade PIN (*left*) with adenocarcinoma (*right*); (b) comparison of high-grade PIN with adenocarcinoma, basal cell specific immunostaining (34βE12) showing the presence of basal cells in PIN (*left*) and the absence of basal cells in adenocarcinoma (*right*); (c) early invasion of high-grade PIN (budding of PIN), basal cell specific immunostaining (34βE12) showing basal cells (*arrowheads*) in PIN and loss of basal cell in several atypical small glands (*arrows*).

ple prominent nucleoli in high-grade PIN (Fig. 9.1(c)). However, there remain considerable intra-observer and inter-observer variations even when this system is used (11).

In this chapter, the term PIN, unless specified otherwise, is used strictly to refer to high-grade PIN. Most pathologists in practice, including us, do not use the term low-grade PIN as a pathologic diagnosis because of the lack of clinical significance of this entity (12–15) and a possible resultant clinical confusion with high-grade PIN, which does have significant relationship to prostatic cancer.

Histologic patterns

There are several histologic patterns of PIN (16): tufting, micropapillary, flat, and cribriform are common forms (Fig. 9.4(a)–(d)). PIN is often multifocal and different histologic patterns may be observed in the same prostate (17). Rare patterns of PIN include mucinous, signet-ring cell, small cell (18), and a more recently described foamy-gland PIN (19). These rare types of PIN have a stronger association with invasive

adenocarcinoma because most cases have been identified in prostates also containing carcinoma. Some pathologists argue that these patterns may represent intraductal spread of prostatic cancer (20). This issued will be discussed in the section addressing intraductal spread of prostatic cancer.

Diagnosis

PIN is cytologically atypical but architecturally benign. The nuclear features of PIN, particularly high-grade PIN, are very similar or essentially identical to adenocarcinoma of the prostate by routine histologic examination or by morphometric measurements (21–23). In some countries, fine-needle aspiration (FNA) is used as a means of establishing a diagnosis of prostatic cancer. We believe this will over-diagnose prostatic cancer, because FNA does not provide architectural features and PIN cannot be distinguished from adenocarcinoma of the prostate by cytology alone. A diagnosis of prostatic cancer established by using FNA cytology is generally not accepted in the United States.

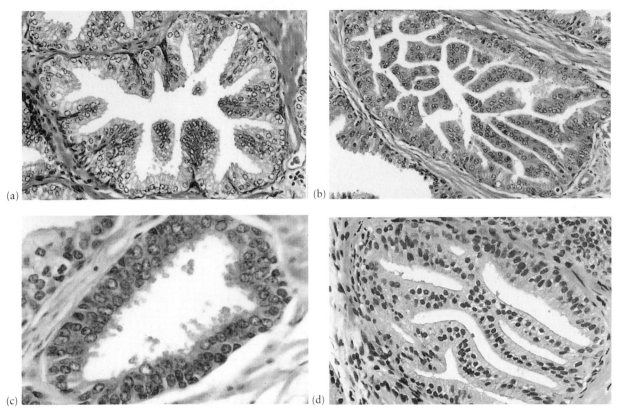

Fig. 9.4 Histologic forms of high-grade PIN: (a) tufting; (b) micropapillary; (c) flat; (d) cribriform.

PIN is a microscopic finding, and the diagnosis can be made reliably only by histologic examination of a prostate needle core biopsy or transurethral resection of the prostate in addition to examination of the whole prostate. Neither digital examination or transrectal ultrasonography can be reliably used to diagnose PIN because of its architectural similarity to benign prostatic hyperplasia (BPH). There is no specific clinical finding associated with the presence of PIN. One report suggested that the presence of PIN might result in an elevation of PSA (24), but this finding has not been substantiated by others (25). In general, PIN in itself does not result in an elevated PSA. Therefore, if a patient with an elevated PSA is found to have high-grade PIN on prostate needle biopsy, a repeat biopsy is indicated to rule out prostatic cancer.

Differential diagnosis

The histologic features of prostatic adenocarcinoma are complex and discussed in other chapters. The major histologic difference between PIN and adenocarcinoma is the presence of invasion and/or architectural atypia in adenocarcinoma. In addition, basal cells are present in PIN but not in adenocarcinoma, a distinction that can be confirmed by using immunohistochemistry with antibodies specific for prostatic basal cells. Other lesions that should be distinguished from PIN are BPH, basal-cell hyperplasia, adenosis, urothelial (transitional cell) metaplasia and neoplasia.

Incidence

The incidence of PIN is difficult to ascertain. Based on published reports, the incidence of isolated PIN (PIN without associated cancer) on needle core biopsies ranges from 0.7% to 20% at different institutions (26–34) (Table 9.1). Most European studies report a higher incidence of PIN than American studies (12.3% versus 6.5%) except for one large European screening study of 1824 patients from The Netherlands (35), in which a reported incidence of 0.7% is much lower than

Table 9.1 Incidence of high grade PIN in prostate needle (14 gauge or 18 gauge) core biopsies.

	Year (ref.no.)	No. patients	Cases with PIN-incidence (%)
US Studies			
Lee *et al.*	1989 (26)	256	28 (11)
Mettlin *et al.*	1991 (27)	330	17 (5.2)
Richie *et al.*	1994 (28)	163	14 (8.6)
Bostwick *et al.*	1995 (29)	200	27 (13.5)
Bostwick *et al.*	1995 (29)	200	21 (10.5)
Langer *et al.*	1996 (30)	1275	56 (4.4)
Wills *et al.*	1997 (31)	439	24 (5.5)
Total (US)	2863	187	6.5
European studies			
Feneley *et al.*	1997 (32)	212	42 (20)
Feneley *et al.*	1997 (32)	1205	133 (11)
Skjorten *et al.*	1997 (33)	79	6 (7.6)
Perachino *et al.*	1997 (34)	148	21 (14.1)
Total (European)	1644	202	12.3

that from other studies. If this large European study is included, the incidence of PIN in European studies is 6.2% (215/3468), which is very similar to that in American studies. The incidence calculated from all these studies listed is 6.4% (402/6331).

The variability in the incidence of PIN on needle biopsies may be related to different patient populations, the methods used to prepare the specimens, or, most likely, the variability in the pathologic criteria used to diagnose this condition (11). Compared to needle biopsy specimens, the incidence of isolated PIN from TUR specimens is slightly lower, ranging from 3.2% at Johns Hopkins to 2.8% at the Mayo Clinic (36, 37). This is consistent with the finding that PIN is more frequently found in the peripheral zone than in the transition zone of the prostate (17).

PIN and prostate cancer

Extension and early invasion of PIN

The most common way by which PIN spreads is within pre-existing ducts and acini (38, 20). Sometimes a single benign gland can be identified, which is partially replaced by neoplastic cells. It is possible that this is a field effect with change from benign cells to neoplastic cells. The other way PIN spreads is by a pagetoid process that is observed only in rare cases. When the neoplastic cells of PIN start to penetrate the basement membrane, that is an indication of the development of micro-invasive or early invasive carcinoma (39, 40).

Early invasion or progression from PIN to adenocarcinoma is a dynamic process, and it is often difficult to draw a precise line between high-grade PIN and early invasive cancer. Sometimes, a few atypical small glands with features of adenocarcinoma may be seen adjacent to PIN. The question is whether this represents invasive cancer or, out-pouching (budding) of PIN. To answer this question, multiple levels of tissue section should be prepared and examined to exclude tangential sectioning of PIN. Immunostaining for basal cells may also be helpful to identify the presence of basal cells. If these atypical glands contain discontinuous basal cells and are connected to PIN, they are probably out-pouching or budding of PIN (41). If these atypical glands are numerous and crowded without basal cells, a diagnosis of malignancy can be made (Figs 9.3(a)–(c)) (42). In uncertain situations, we employ the diagnostic term 'high-grade PIN with adjacent atypical small glands suspicious for invasive adenocarcinoma' or 'high-grade PIN with adjacent atypical small glands, invasive adenocarcinoma cannot be excluded'. We believe that the risk of having invasive prostatic cancer in these patients is high and that re-biopsy is strongly recommended.

Distinction of PIN from intraductal spread of prostatic carcinoma

Intraductal spread of prostatic carcinoma (IDSPC) was first described by Kovi in 1985 (20) and is characterized by invasion and growth of prostatic adenocarcinoma cells into prostatic ducts and replacing the benign epithelial cells. The involved prostatic ducts may retain their basal cells. IDSPC usually bears a close histologic resemblance to and is often found in close proximity to invasive cancer.

PIN and IDSPC are conceptually different processes; PIN is a pre-malignant lesion with a tendency to grow from inside a prostatic duct or acinus to the outside to become invasive cancer; IDSPC is a lesion of cancer progression that infiltrates from the outside to the inside of a prostatic duct. PIN has been observed in otherwise benign prostates, and it is common to find PIN separated from areas of infiltrating adenocarcinoma. Furthermore, some of the architectural patterns of PIN such as micropapillary and tufting are so complex that they are unlikely to represent infiltrating cancer. In practice, however, it is often difficult to distinguish PIN from IDSPC. Particular patterns of PIN, such as cribriform or foamy gland PIN, usually found in prostates with invasive adenocarcinoma, are considered to be IDSPC by some pathologists. Inability to distinguish PIN from IDSPC may hamper our understanding of prostatic carcinogenesis and additional studies are necessary to clarify this issue. It is possible that molecular markers will assist us in distinguishing pre-malignant PIN from fully malignant IDSPC.

Evidence linking PIN to cancer

In addition to the histologic similarities between the two entities, both PIN and adenocarcinoma are more commonly identified in the peripheral zones of the prostate (43, 44, 17). It has been shown that both low-grade and high-grade PIN can be first seen in men in their twenties, and that the grade and volume of PIN increase with age. The onset of PIN precedes the onset of carcinoma by more than 10 years (15). In men over 50 years of age, the frequency of PIN in prostates with cancer is greater than in prostates without cancer (82% versus 43%) (2).

Clinical significance

Several studies have shown that approximately 40% of patients with isolated high-grade PIN on initial biopsy are found to have prostatic cancer on a repeat biopsy (Table 9.2) (13, 14, 45–49). When carcinoma is found on repeat biopsy, it is not necessarily at the site where the PIN was found. Therefore, it is recommended that the technique of an optimal repeat biopsy for patients with high-grade PIN should include systematic sextant biopsies (14). Recently, however, several reports have indicated that the frequency of detecting cancer on a second biopsy in men found to have PIN on their first biopsy is no greater than the frequency of detecting cancer in men whose initial biopsy was benign (34% versus 25%) (50). It is important to point out that the detection rate of prostatic cancer on initial prostate needle biopsies is approximately 30–40% in many academic institutions in the United States, including our own institution, because we are dealing with a high-risk population for prostate cancer in a referral practice. Additional studies with better controls and strict diagnostic criteria for high-grade PIN are necessary to resolve this issue.

Basic research

Molecular basis of PIN

In recent years, many studies have been carried out to search for molecular changes in PIN (51). It has been reported that, in PIN, there is a progressive loss of biomarkers such as PSA, blood group antigens, cytoskeletal proteins and other secretory proteins (52–54). These changes may be related to the loss of normal secretory function and neoplastic transformation.

GST-pi is one of the major cellular antioxidant enzymes with an important function of inactivation of carcinogens. GST-pi expression is markedly reduced or

Table 9.2 Detection of cancer in patients with high-grade PIN on repeat biopsy

Authors	Year (ref.no.)	No. patients with PIN	% Patients with cancer (on repeat biopsy)
Brawer *et al.*	1991 (13)	10	100%
Berner *et al.*	1993 (45)	37	38%
Weinstein and Epstein	1993 (46)	19	53%
Davidson *et al.*	1995 (47)	100	35%
Keetch *et al.*	1995 (48)	37	51%
Langer *et al.*	1996 (30)	53	27%
Raviv *et al.*	1996 (49)	48	48%
Total		304	41% (126/304)

absent in PIN, as well as in prostatic adenocarcinoma (55). It has been hypothesized that the inability of prostatic cells to inactivate carcinogens may be an early event in prostatic carcinogenesis.

Similar to prostatic carcinoma, other proteins related to cell growth are progressingly increased as PIN develops. These include c-erb-2, bcl-2, epidermal growth factor, and proliferative markers (56–61). The frequency of DNA aneuploidy is also increased in PIN (62, 63). However, most of these molecular alterations are present in both PIN and cancer, and there is at present no distinct molecular marker that can be used to distinguish PIN from prostatic cancer. With advances in knowledge and technology, it is likely that we will learn more about the molecular events leading to the development of PIN and the progression from PIN to prostatic cancer in the near future.

Research implication

In the prostate, cancer cells, PIN, and benign glands are often intermingled so that they cannot easily be distinguished. Furthermore, it seems likely that the molecular abnormalities characteristic of pre-malignant PIN may be intermediate between those characteristic of cancer and benign lesions such as BPH. Thus, it is possible that neoplastic cells in PIN may contain the genetic alterations of both malignant and benign lesions of the prostate. Unfortunately, a molecular or biochemical study comparing differences between PIN, cancer, and benign cells using homogenized prostatic tissue may not be worthwhile without knowing the exact location of each cell type. Micro-dissection of prostatic tissue to separate PIN and cancer is necessary to achieve this goal because it will allow precise correlation between histologic and molecular differences.

Chemoprevention

If PIN is a precursor of prostatic cancer, can cancer be prevented reducing or eliminating PIN? It is known that androgen deprivation produces both marked atrophy of prostatic cancer cells and also a prominent regression of PIN (64, 65). Androgen deprivation, however, is obviously unacceptable to patients as a means of chemoprevention. Some investigators have proposed using finasteride, an inhibitor of 5α-reductase, for chemoprevention of prostatic cancer (66). Finasteride blocks the production of more potent dihydrotestosterone from testosterone and, therefore, reduces the androgen effect on the prostate. The histo-

logic effects of this agent on PIN are unclear. In our own study of needle biopsy specimens, finasteride had minimal histologic effect on both benign and malignant prostatic cells, suggesting that finasteride might not have much effect on PIN (67). It will be interesting to learn the outcome of a large, on-going national study to determine whether finasteride can inhibit the development of PIN and prevent prostatic cancer.

Clinical management

We believe those patients with high-grade PIN, but without definite evidence of adenocarcinoma on needle biopsy, should be re-biopsied but not treated unless a diagnosis of prostatic carcinoma is established. Repeat biopsy is especially indicated if the patient has an elevated PSA. As discussed earlier, PIN is a microscopic finding and, in general, does not cause an elevation of PSA.

The natural history of PIN is unclear. Evidence indicates that PIN can sometimes progress to prostatic cancer, but whether and how often it can regresses or remain unchanged is unclear. Although men with PIN have an increased risk of developing prostatic cancer, it is not known how often this happens or in whom it will occur. Men with isolated high-grade PIN should be re-biopsied once immediately, especially when they have elevated PSA, and then followed closely if the second biopsy is negative for cancer. However, at present we do not know how closely they should be followed or how many of these men will ultimately develop prostatic cancer. Each patient should be managed based on the individual clinical situation.

Adenosis (atypical adenomatous hyperplasia): a lesion of questionable pre-malignant potential

Introduction

Adenosis is defined as a well-circumscribed proliferation of small closely packed glands (acini) most commonly identified in the transition zone of the prostate. The term atypical adenomatous hyperplasia was first used by Baron in 1941 (68) and characterized by McNeal in 1965 (69). The term adenosis was used to describe this entity by Brawn in 1986 (70). Recently the term atypical adenomatous hyperplasia was advocated in a consensus meeting (71). Other synonyms used in the are atypical small acinar hyperplasia, small gland hyperplasia, and glandular hyperplasia with atypia (72–74). We still prefer the term adenosis, because any pathologic entity using the word 'atypical' may imply a relationship to cancer, and many experts regard adenosis of the prostate as a benign lesion.

Depending on variable diagnostic criteria, sources of specimens and different institutions, the prevalence of adenosis of the prostate ranges from 1.6% to 19.6% in transurethral resection specimens to 23% in radical prostatectomy specimens (75–77). Adenosis can be multi-focal and is often identified in the transition zone. Adenosis is more often seen in prostatectomy and transurethral resection specimens than in prostatic needle biopsies sampled mostly from the peripheral zone (78).

Pathology

At low power, a lobular growth of small crowded glands can be appreciated (Fig. 9.5(a)). Adenosis has architectural patterns similar to low-grade prostatic adenocarcinoma (Gleason patterns 1 and 2) of the transition zone (79–81), but without irregular borders frequently seen in carcinoma. Cytologically, however, there is minimal atypia, and nuclear enlargement and hyperchromasia are uncommon (Fig. 9.5(b)). Nucleoli can be seen in adenosis but smaller than those observed in cancer cells. Presence of crystalloids is a frequent finding and has been described in up to 24% of the cases of adenosis (75, 78, 82). Pink amorphous secretion and blue mucin, frequent findings in adenocarcinoma, can be also seen in adenosis but at a lower frequency. A patchy distribution of basal cells (disrupted basal cell layers) is characteristic of adenosis, and immunostaining for basal cells can be helpful to confirm the diagnosis (Fig. 9.5(c)). The distinction between adenosis and adenocarcinoma of the transition zone can sometimes be difficult, because of the morphologic similarities of these two entities (71). The histologic features most helpful in distinguishing adenosis from adenocarcinoma are:

(1) minimal cytologic atypia and lack of prominent large nucleoli;

(2) similarity of nuclear and cytoplasmic characteristics in small (atypical) and admixed larger (benign) glands;

(3) presence of patchy basal cells in the lobule.

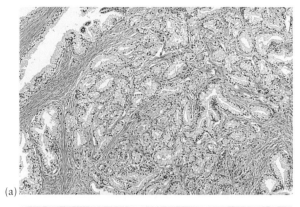

(a)

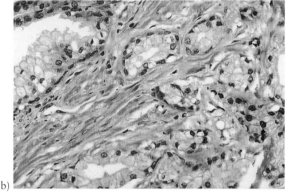

(b)

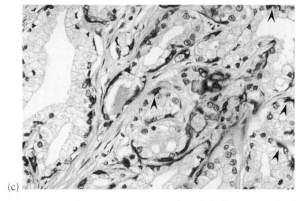

(c)

Fig. 9.5 (a) Adenosis appearing to be a lobule composed of small acini at low power; (b) adenosis showing lack of cytologic atypia; (c) adenosis, basal cell-specific immunostaining (34βE12) showing the presence of basal cells (*arrowheads, color*).

Adenosis has many histologic features common to BPH and is possibly a histologic variant of this disease.

Relationship to adenocarcinoma

It is controversial whether adenosis has a pre-malignant potential. It has been hypothesized that there is a relationship between adenosis and low-grade adenocarcinoma because of the location and histologic similarities of these two lesions. Molecular and biochemical studies of adenosis are inclusive or contradictory. As determined by Ki67 staining, the proliferation rate of adenosis was either intermediate between BPH and prostatic carcinoma, or more closely similar to that of BPH (83). Recently, it was shown that 47% of cases of adenosis contain similar genetic alterations commonly found in early prostatic carcinoma (84). Another study, however, showed allelic loss of 8p22 in 6% cases of adenosis and 56% of cases of adenocarinomas studied (85). To date there is insufficient evidence to substantiate the hypothesis that adenosis is a pre-malignant lesion. Unlike PIN, adenosis, in most cases, is present without adenocarcinoma. In addition, it is rare to find low-grade adenocarcinoma in close proximity to adenosis. Finally, the finding of adenosis is not associated with an increased risk of adenocarcinoma, and unlike PIN, adenosis appears to have no prognostic significance for developing of adenocarcinoma (70).

Management

Regardless of the relationship between adenosis and low-grade adenocarcinoma, the presence of adenosis does not warrant an immediate repeat biopsy unless there is a clinical indication. Low-grade adenocarcinoma (Gleason pattern 1 or 2) of the transition zone of the prostate is extremely unlikely to develop into significant prostate cancer (86, 87). In a series we studied of 100 cases of metastatic prostatic adenocarcinoma, none of the cases was derived from low-grade carcinoma (41). Even though it is possible that adenosis might be a precursor of low-grade adenocarcinoma, the latent period and frequency of malignant transformation are uncertain. At the present time, we regard adenosis as a benign condition, and patients with a diagnosis of adenosis should be followed accordingly.

Benign lesions of the prostate: conditions not considered to be pre-malignant

Atrophy

Atrophy refers to a spectrum of common prostatic lesions characterized by atrophic changes of prostatic acini (88). Atrophy has been observed in 40% of prostatic needle biopsy specimens from patients with BPH

(67). Interestingly, it has been shown that atrophy is a proliferative process (89). Lesions such as postatrophic hyperplasia (90) and partial atrophy are similar to typical atrophy but have an even greater proliferative appearance (91). Occasionally, atrophy can be seen adjacent to adenocarcinoma. However, there is insufficient evidence to link atrophy to the development of carcinoma.

Basal-cell hyperplasia

The term atypical basal-cell hyperplasia has been used to describe a benign proliferative process of basal cells (92, 93). The proliferating basal cells may demonstrate cytologic atypia (94, 95). This lesion can be difficult to distinguish from adenocarcinoma or basaloid carcinoma of the prostate (96). There is no evidence that basal-cell hyperplasia has any relationship to adenocarcinoma of the prostate. Nevertheless, it should not be mistaken for adenocarcinoma (94).

Atypical glands suspicious for adenocarcinoma

Sometimes there is a small focus of atypical prostatic glands or acini suspicious for, but not diagnostic of, adenocarcinoma. This is often due to the small size of the biopsy with scant glands that lack all the malignant cytological and architectural features necessary to establish a diagnosis of carcinoma. It is important to realize that this is a diagnostic term and not a pathologic entity or pre-malignant lesion. A diagnosis of atypical glands suspicious for adenocarcinoma of the prostate indicates that the likelihood of prostatic cancer being present is high, but the pathologist cannot make a definitive diagnosis of malignancy because of insufficient histologic evidence. Based on several recent studies, patients with a diagnosis of atypical glands suspicious for adenocarcinoma have more than a 50% probability of having prostatic cancer on a repeat biopsy (97).

Conclusions

The histologic features and management of adenocarcinoma, PIN and adenosis are summarized in Table 9.3. Adenocarcinoma has both cytological and architectural atypia, and basal cells are absent in the malignant prostatic acini or ducts. In PIN, the glandular architecture remains intact, but adenosis has architectural

Table 9.3 Comparison of common prostatic lesions

Lesions	Adenocarcinoma	PIN	Adenosis
Cytology	atypical	atypical	benign
Architecture	atypical	benign	atypical
Basal cells	absent	present	present
Management	treatment	re-biopsy	follow

patterns similar to low-grade adenocarcinoma. Cytologically, PIN has features similar or identical to adenocarcinoma, while adenosis lacks cytologic atypia. Both PIN and adenosis contain basal cell layers, whereas adenocarcinoma does not.

PIN is a microscopic finding and can be diagnosed only by histopathologic examination. There is steadily increasing evidence that PIN is a precursor for prostate cancer. Based on current studies, the molecular alterations of PIN are similar to those occurring in prostate cancer. However, the natural history, molecular basis and pathogenesis of PIN are unknown. We agree with the majority of experts who believe that men with high-grade PIN diagnosed on needle biopsy should be followed closely and undergo at least one additional biopsy, particularly those with an elevated PSA. Chemoprevention of prostatic cancer using finasteride to inhibit PIN is currently being investigated. Treatment for prostatic cancer is not indicated in men with high-grade PIN unless an unequivocal diagnosis of cancer is established.

It is controversial whether adenosis is a precursor of prostate cancer. Currently, there is insufficient evidence to support this hypothesis. And further studies are necessary to clarify this issue. It is possible that some cases of adenosis might be related to low grade adenocarcinoma arising in the transition zone of the prostate, which has a low risk of progression. We believe that it is unnecessary for men with a diagnosis of adenosis to undergo a repeat biopsy unless there are other clinical indications such as an elevated PSA.

Both atrophy and basal-cell hyperplasia are benign lesions of the prostate. Although they can be confused with prostate cancer because of histologic similarities, these two entities are considered 'benign mimickers of prostate cancer' and not pre-malignant lesions.

Acknowledgement

We are grateful to Dr Cyril Abrahams for his critical review of the manuscript.

References

1. McNeal JE. Origin and development of carcinoma in the prostate. *Cancer* 1969, **23**, 24–34.
2. McNeal JE, Bostwick DG. Intraductal dysplasia: a pre-malignant lesion of the prostate. *Hum Pathol* 1986, **17**, 64–71.
3. Bostwick DG, Brawer MK. Prostatic intra-epithelial neoplasia and early invasion in prostate cancer. *Cancer* 1987, **59**, 788–94.
4. Drago JR, Mostofi FK, Lee F. Introductory remarks and workshop summary. *Urology* 1989, **34** (Suppl), 2–3.
5. Kovi J, Mostofi FK, Heshmat MY *et al.* Large acinar atypical hyperplasia and carcinoma of the prostate. *Cancer* 1988, **61**, 555–61.
6. McNeal JE, Villers A, Redwine EA *et al.* Microcarcinoma in the prostate: its association with duct-acinar dysplasia. *Hum Pathol* 1991, **22**, 644–52.
7. Kastendieck, H. Correlations between atypical primary hyperplasia and carcinoma of the prostate. *Pathol Res Pract* 1980, **169**, 366–70.
8. Brawer MK, Peehl DM, Stamey TA *et al.* Keratin immunoreactivity in benign and neoplastic human prostate. *Cancer* Res 1985, **45**, 3665–9.
9. O'Malley FP, Grignon DJ, Shum DT. Usefulness of immunoperoxidase staining with high-molecular-weight cytokeratin in the differential diagnosis of small-acinar lesions of the prostate gland. *Virchows Arch A Pathol Histopathol* 1990, **417**, 191–6.
10. Hedrick L, Epstein JI. Use of keratin 903 as an adjunct in the diagnosis of prostate carcinoma. *Am J Surg Pathol* 1989, **13**, 389–96.
11. Epstein JI, Grignon DJ, Humphrey PA *et al.* Interobserver reproducibility in the diagnosis of prostatic intra-epithelial neoplasia. *Am J Surg Pathol* 1995, **19**, 873–86.
12. McNeal JE. Significance of duct-acinar dysplasia in prostatic carcinogenesis. *Urology* 1989, **34** (Suppl), 9–15.
13. Brawer MK, Bigler SA, Sohlberg OE *et al.* Significance of prostatic intra-epithelial neoplasia on prostate needle biopsy. *Urology* 1991, **38**, 103–107.
14. Shepherd D, Keetch D, Humphrey PA *et al.* Isolated prostatic intra-epithelial neoplasia in needle biopsy as a marker for detection of adenocarcinoma on re-biopsy. *J Urol* 1996, **156**, 460–3.
15. Sakr WA, Haas GP, Cassin BJ *et al.* The frequency of carcinoma and intra-epithelial neoplasia of the prostate in young male patients. *J Urol* 1993, **150**, 379–85.
16. Bostwick DG, Amin MB, Dundore P *et al.* Architectural patterns of high-grade prostatic intra-epithelial neoplasia. *Hum Pathol* 1993, **24**, 298–310.
17. Qian J, Wollan P, Bostwick DG. The extent and multicentricity of high-grade prostatic intra-epithelial neoplasia in clinically localized prostatic adenocarcinoma. *Hum Pathol* 1997, **28**, 143–8.
18. Reyes AO, Swanson PE, Carbone JM *et al.* Unusual histologic types of high-grade prostatic intra-epithiel neoplasia. *Am J Surg Pathol* 1997, **21**, 1215–22.
19. Berman DM, Yang XJ, Epstein JI. Foamy gland high grade prostatic intra-epithelial neoplasia. *Am J Surg Pathol*, 2000, **24**, 140–4.
20. Kovi J, Jackson MA, Heshmat MY. Ductal spread in prostatic carcinoma. *Cancer* 1985, **56**, 1566–73.

21. Montironi R, Searpelli M, Sisti S *et al.* Quantitative analysis of prostatic intra-epithelial neoplasia on tissue sections. *Anal Quani Cytot Histot* 1990, **12**, 366–72.

22. Montironi R, Braccischi A, Matera G *et al.* Quantitation of the prostatic intra-epithelial neoplasia. Analysis of the nuclear size, number and location. *Pathol Res Pract* 1991, **187**, 307–14.

23. Petein M, Michel P, Van Velthoven R *et al.* Morphonuclear relationship between prostatic intra-epithelial neoplasia and cancers as assessed by digital cell image analysis. *Am J Clin Pathol* 1991, **96**, 628–34.

24. Brawer MK, Lange PH. Prostate-specific antigen and pre-malignant change. Implications for early detection. *CA Cancer J Clin* 1989, **39**, 361–75.

25. Ronnett BM, Carmichael MJ, Carter HB *et al.* Does high-grade prostatic intra-epithelial neoplasia result in elevated serum prostate specific antigen levels? *J Urol* 1993, **150**, 386–9.

26. Lee F, Torp-Pedersen ST, Carroll JT *et al.* Use of transrectal ultrasound and prostate-specific antigen in diagnosis of pro-static intra-epithelial neoplasia. *Urology* 1989, **24** (Suppl), 4–8.

27. Mettlin C, Lee F, Drago J *et al.* The American Cancer Society National Prostate Cancer Detection Project. Findings on the detection of early prostate cancer in 2425 men. *Cancer* 1991, **67**, 2949–59.

28. Richie JP, Kavoussi LR, Ho GT *et al.* Prostate cancer screening: role of digital rectal examination and prostate-specific antigen. *Ann Surg Oncol* 1994, **1**, 117–20

29. Bostwick DG, Qian J, Frankel K. The incidence of high grade prostatic intra-epithelial neoplasia in needle biopsies. *J Urol* 1995, **154**, 1791–4.

30. Langer JE, Rovner ES, Coleman BG *et al.* Strategy for repeat biopsy of patients with prostatic intra-epithelial neoplasia detected by prostate needle biopsy. *J Urol* 1996, **155**, 228–31.

31. Wills ML, Hamper UM, Partin AW *et al.* Incidence of high grade prostatic intra-epithelial neoplasia in sextant needle biopsy specimens. *Urology* 1997, **49**, 367–73.

32. Feneley MR, Green JSA, Young NVA *et al.* Prevalence of prostatic intra-epithelial neoplasia (PIN) in biopsies from hospital practice and pilot screening: clinical implications. *Prostate Cancer and Prostatic Diseases* 1997, **1**, 79–83.

33. Skjorten Fl, Berner A, Harvei S *et al.* Prostatic intra-epithelial neoplasia in surgical resections. Relationship to coexistent adenocarcinoma and atypical adenomatous hyperplasia of the prostate. *Cancer* 1997, **79**, 1172–9.

34. Perachino M, Diciolo L, Barbetti V *et al.* Results of rebiopsy for suspected prostate cancer in symptomatic men with elevated PSA levels. *Euro Urol* 1997, **32**, 155–9.

35. Hoedemaeker RF, Kranse R, Rietbergen JB *et al.* Evaluation of prostate needle biopsies in a population-based screening study: the impact of borderline lesions. *Cancer* 1999, **85**, 145–52.

36. Gaudin PB, Sesterhenn IA, Wojno KJ *et al.* Incidence and clinical significance of high-grade prostatic intra-epithelial neoplasia in TURP specimens. *Urology* 1997, **49**, 558–63.

37. Pacelli A, Bostwick DG. The clinical significance of high-grade prostatic intra-epithelial neoplasia in transurethral resection specimens. *Urology* 1997, **50**, 355–9.

38. Bostwick DG, Srigley J. Pre-malignant lesions. In: *Pathology of the prostate* (ed. DG Bostwick). Churchill-Livingston, New York 1990, 37–55.

39. Quinn BD, Cho KR, Epstein JI. Relationship of severe dysplasia to stage B adenocarcinoma of the prostate. *Cancer* 1990, **65**, 2328–37.

40. McNeal JE, Villers A, Redwine EA *et al.* Microcarcinoma in the prostate: its association with duct-acinar dysplasia. *Hum Pathol* 1991, **22**, 644–52.

41. Yang XJ, Lecksell K, Gaudin P *et al.* Rare expression of high molecular weight cytokeratin in adenocarcinoma of the prostate: a study of 110 cases of metastatic and locally advanced prostate cancer. *Am J Surg Pathol* 1999, **23**, 147–52.

42. Epstein JI. Prostate biopsy interpretation (2nd edn). Lippincott-Raven, New York 1995, 57.

43. Epstein JI, Cho KR, Quinn BD. Relationship of severe dysplasia to stage A (incidental) adenocarcinoma of the prostate. *Cancer* 1990, **65**, 2321–7.

44. Quinn BD, Cho KR, Epstein JI. Relationship of severe dysplasia to stage B adenocarcinoma of the prostate. *Cancer* 1990, **65**, 2328–37.

45. Berner A, Danielsen HE, Pettersen EO *et al.* DNA distribution in the prostate. Normal gland, benign and pre-malignant lesions, and subsequent adenocarcinomas. *Anal Quant Cytol Histol* 1993, **15**, 247–52.

46. Weinstein MH, Epstein JI. Significance of high grade prostatic intra-epithelial neoplasia (PIN) on needle biopsy. *Hum Pathol* 1993, **24**, 624–9.

47. Davidson D, Bostwick DG, Qian J *et al.* Prostatic intra-epithelial neoplasia is a risk factor for adenocarcinoma: predictive accuracy in needle biopsies. *J Urol* 1995, **154**, 1295–9.

48. Keetch DW, Humphrey P, Stahl D *et al.* Morphometric analysis and clinical follow-up of isolated prostatic intra-epithelial neoplasia in needle biopsy of the prostate. *J Urol* 1995, **154**, 347–51.

49. Raviv G, Janssen TH, Ziotta AR *et al.* Prostatic intra-epithelial neoplasia: Influence of clinical and pathological data on the detection of prostate cancer. *J Urol* 1996, **156**, 1050–5.

50. Bigler SA, Fowler JE Jr, Kilambi N *et al.* High grade prostatic intra-epithelial neoplasia and subsequent diagnosis of carcinoma in patients with two prostate needle biopsy procedures. *Mod Pathol* 1999, **12**, 94A, 515.

51. Bostwick DG, Pacelli A, Lopez-Beltran A. Molecular biology of prostatic intra-epithelial neoplasia. *Prostate* 1996, **29**, 117–34.

52. McNeal JE, Alroy J, Leav 1 *et al.* Imrnunohistochemical evidence of impaired cell differentiation in the pre-malignant phase of prostate carcinogenesis. *Am J Clin Pathol* 1988, **90**, 23–32.

53. Perlman E, Epstein JI. Blood Group Antigen Expression in Dysplasia and Adenocarcinoma of the prostate. *Am J Surg Pathol* 1990, **14**, 810–8.

54. Nagle RB, Brawer MK, Kittelson J *et al.* Phenotypic relationships of prostatic intra-epithelial neoplasia to invasive prostatic carcinoma. *Am J Pathol* 1991, **138**, 119–28.

55. Lee WH, Morton RA, Epstein JI *et al.* Cytidine methylation of regulatory sequences near the pi-class glutathione S-transferase gene accompanies human prostatic carcinogenesis. *Proc Natl Acad Sci* 1994, **91**, 11733–7.

56. Myers RB, Srivastava S, Oelsehlager DK *et al.* Expression of pl60 erbB-3 and pl85erbB-2 in prostatic intra-epithelial neoplasia and prostatic adenocarcinoma. *J Nat Cancer Inst* 1994, **86**, 1140–4.

57. Colombel M, Syminans F, Gil S *et al.* Detection of the apoptosis-suppressing oncoprotein bcl-2 in hormone-refractory human prostate cancers. *Am J Pathol* 1993, **143**, 390–400.

58. Maygarden SJ, Strom S, Ware JL. Localization of epidermal growth factor receptor by immunohistochemical methods in human prostatic carcinoma, prostatic intra-epithelial neoplasia, and benign hyperplasia. *Arch Pathol Lab Med* 1992, **116**, 269–73.

59. Montironi R, Magi Galluzzi C, Searpelli M *et al.* Occurrence of cell death (apoptosis) in prostatic intra-epithelial neoplasia. *Virch Arch (A) Pathol Anat* 1993, **423**, 351–7.

60. Gainnulis 1, Montironi R,Galluzzi CM *et al.* Frequency and location of mitoses in prostatic intra-epithelial neoplasia (PIN). *Anticancer Res* 1993, **13**, 2447–52.

61. Montironi R, Magi Galluzzi C, Diamanti L *et al.* Prostatic intra-epithelial neoplasia. Expression and location of proliferating cell nuclear antigen (PCNA) in epithelial, endothelial and stromal nuclei. *Virchow Arch [A] Pathol Anat* 1993, **422**, 185–92.

62. Amin MM, Schultz DS, Zarbo RJ *et al.* Computerized Static DNA Ploidy analysis of prostatic intra-epithelial neoplasia. *Arch Pathol Lab Med* 1993, **117**, 794–8.

63. Baretton GB, Vogt T, Blasenbreu S *et al.* Comparison of DNA ploidy in prostatic intra-epithelial neoplasia and invasive carcinoma of the prostate: an image cytometric study. *Hum Pathol* 1994, 25, 506–13.

64. Ferguson J, Zincke H, Ellison E *et al.* Decrease of prostatic intra-epithelial neoplasia following deprivation therapy in patients with stage T3 carcinoma treated by radical prostatectomy. *Urology* 1994, **44**, 91–5.

65. Brawley OW, Thompson IM. Chemoprevention of prostate cancer. *Urology* 1994, **43**, 594–9.

66. Yang XJ. Lecksell K, Epstein JI. Does long-term finasteride (Proscar) affect the histology of benign prostate tissue and prostate cancer on needle biopsy? *Urology* 1999, **53**, 686–700.

67. Baron E, Angrist A. Incidence of occult adenocarcinoma of the prostate after 50 years of age. *Arch Pathol* 1941, **32**, 787–93.

68. McNeal JE. Morphogenesis of prostatic carcinoma. *Cancer* 1965, **18**, 1659–66.

69. Brawn PN. Adenosis of the prostate: a dysplastic lesion that can be confused with prostate adenocarcinoma. *Cancer* 1992, **49**, 826–33.

70. Bostwick DG, Algaba F, Amin MB *et al.* Consensus on terminology: recommendation to use atypical adenomatous hyperplasia in place of adenosis of the prostate. *Am J Surg Pathol* 1994, **18**, 1069–72.

71. Kovi J. Microscopic differential diagnosis of small acinar adenocarcinoma. *Pathol Annu* 1985, **20**, 157–96.

72. Harbitz TB, Haugen OA. Histology of the prostate in elderly men: a study in an autopsy series. *Acta Pathol Scand [A]* 1972, **80**, 756–68.

73. Gleason DF. Atypical hyperplasia, benign hyperplasia and well-differentiated adenocarcinoma of the prostate. *Am J Surg Pathol* 1985, **9** (Suppl), 53–67.

74. Gaudin P, Epstein JI. Adenosis of the prostate: histologic features in transurethral resection specimens. *Am J Surg Pathol* 1994, **18**, 863–70.

75. Srigley JR, Toth P, Hartwick RWJ. Atypical histologic patterns in cases of benign prostatic hyperplasia. *Lab Invest* 1989, **60**, 90A.

76. Qian J, Bostwick DG. The extent and zonal location of prostatic intra-epithelial neoplasia and atypical adenomatous hyperplasia: Relationship with carcinoma in radical prostatectomy specimens. *Pathol Res Pract* 1995, **191**, 860–7.

77. Gaudin P, Epstein JI. Adenosis of the prostate: histologic features in needle biopsy specimens. *Am J Pathol* 1995, **19**, 737–47.

78. McNeal JE, Redwine, Freiha FS *et al.* Zonal distribution of prostatic adenocarcinoma. *Am J Surg Pathol* 1988, **12**, 897–906.

79. Bostwick DG, Srigley J, Grignon D *et al.* Atypical adenomatous hyperplasia of the prostate: morphologic criteria for its distinction from well-differentiated carcinoma. *Hum Pathol* 1993, **24**, 819–32.

80. Grignon DJ, Sakr WA. Zonal origin of prostatic adenocarcinoma: are there biologic differences between transition zone and peripheral zone adenocarcinoma of the prostate gland? *J Cell Biochem* 1994, **19**, 267–8.

81. Bennett BD, Gardner WA Jr. Crystalloids in prostatic hyperplasia. *Prostate* 1993, **22**, 309–15.

82. Helpap B. Cell kinetic studies on prostatic intra-epithelial neoplasia (PIN) and atypical adenomatous hyperplasia of the prostate. *Pathol Res Pract* 1995, **191**, 904–7.

83. Cheng L, Shan A, Cheville JC *et al.* Atypical adenomatous hyperplasia of the prostate: a pre-malignant lesion? *Cancer Res* 1998, **58**, 389–91.

84. Furman J, Zhu Z, Kaleen Z *et al.* Chromosome 8p22 allelic loss in atypical adenomatous hyperplasia (adenosis) and carcinoma in the prostate. *Mod Pathol* 1996, **9**, 73A.

85. McNeal JE, Villers AA, Redwine EA *et al.* Capsular penetration in prostate cancer. *Am J Surg Pathol* 1990, **14**, 240–7.

86. Green DR, Wheeler TM, Egawa S *et al.* A comparison of the morphological features of cancer arising in the transition zone and in the peripheral zone of the prostate. *J Urol* 1991, **146**, 1069–76.

87. Gardner WA Jr, Culberson DE. Atrophy and proliferation in young adult prostate. *J Urol* 1987, **137**, 56–67.

88. Ruska KM, Sauvageot J and Epstein JI. Histology and cellular kinetics of prostatic atrophy. *Am J Surg Pathol* 1998, **22**, 1073–7.

89. Cheville JC, Bostwick DG. Postatrophic hyperplasia of the prostate: a histologic mimic of prostatic adenocarcinoma. *Am J Surg Pathol* 1995, **19**, 1068–76.

90. Oppenheimer JR, Wills ML, Epstein JI. Partial atrophy in prostate needle cores-another diagnostic pitfall for

the surgical pathologists. *Am J Surg Pathol* 1998, **22**, 440–5.

91.   Cleary KR, Choi HY, Ayala AG. Basal-cell hyperplasia of the prostate. *Am J Clin Pathol* 1983, **80**, 850–4.

92.   Grignon DJ, Ro JY, Ordonez NG *et al*. Basal-cell hyperplasia, adenoid basal cell tumor, and adenoid cystic carcinoma of the prostate: an immunohistochemical study. *Hum Pathol* 1988, **19**, 1425–33.

93.   Epstein JI, Armas OA. Atypical basal-cell hyperplasia of the prostate. *Am J Surg Pathol* 1992, **16**, 1205–14.

94.   Devaraj LT, Bostwick DG. Atypical basal-cell hyperplasia of the prostate: immunophenotypic profile and pro-

posed classification of basal cell proliferations. *Am J Surg Pathol* 1993, **17**, 645–59.

95.   Yang XJ, McEntee M, Epstein JI. The distinction of basaloid carcinoma of the prostate from benign basal cell lesions by using immunohistochemistry for Bcl-2 and Ki-67. *Human Pathol* 1998, **29**, 1447–50.

96.   Chan TY, Epstein JI. Follow-up of atypical prostate needle biopsies. *Urology* 1997, **53**, 351–5.

97.   Iczkowski KA, Maclennan GT, Bostwick DG. Atypical small acinar proliferation suspicious for malignancy in prostate needle biopsies, clinical significance in 22 cases. *Am J Surg Pathol* 1997, **21**, 1489–95.

10 | Morphobiology of prostate cancer

F. Algaba

For a clear understanding of present knowledge about the pathology of prostate cancer, we need to know the basic structure of this gland and some morphologic features in close relation with cellular differentiation, physiology, and hormone sensitivity. Therefore, before addressing the pathologic aspects of prostate cancer, we will consider the normal structure of the gland.

Prostate microanatomy (sonographic correlation)

The prostate comprises a number of tubulo-alveolar glands (30–50), which drain directly into the urethra through 16–32 ducts (1), surrounded by stromal component with abundant smooth muscle.

The distribution of these glands has been debated ever since Lowsley's embryological studies (5-lobe distribution—anterior, middle, left and right lateral, and posterior lobes, with fetal involution of the anterior lobe) (2). Lowsley's concept was modified by LeDuc's anatomic studies (two lateral masses and a smaller median lobe) (3) and Franks' proposal (no lobes, only an 'inner gland' around the urethra and an 'outer gland' around it) (4). However, the present conception regarding the topographic anatomy of the prostate was introduced by Salvador Gil-Vernet, who clearly demonstrated that the prostate consists of two main parts (cranial and caudal), separated by an intermediate area. These regions were defined according to where their glandular ducts open into the urethra (5). Between 1968 and 1978, McNeal confirmed Gil-Vernet's model and added new aspects, enhancing our understanding of prostate anatomy with sonographic correlation.

McNeal model

McNeal divides the prostate into four zones (6), of which one is chiefly stromal and three are chiefly glandular (Fig. 10.1):

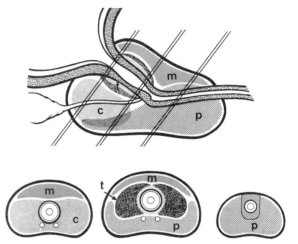

Fig. 10.1 McNeal model of zonal prostate distribution: anterior fibromuscular zone (m); central zone (c); transition zone (t);.peripheral zone (p).

- The *anterior fibromuscular zone*, which represents about 33% of the prostate volume and comprises stromal elements with minimal glandular representation. It extends downward from the bladder neck over the anteromedial surface of the organ, narrowing to join the urethra at the prostate apex, its lateral margins blending with the external fibromuscular prostate condensation ('capsule'). The deep surface is in contact with the sphincter and glandular transition zone (see below).
- The *central zone* (Fig. 10.2) (25% of the glandular component and 16.5% of the prostate). It is conically shaped, with its base at the neck of the bladder and vertex toward the urethra, surrounding part of the proximal urethra; it is crossed by the ejaculatory ducts.
- The *transition zone* (Fig. 10.3) (5% of the glandular component and 3.3% of the prostate). It is located around the proximal urethra up until the point where it angles upwards.

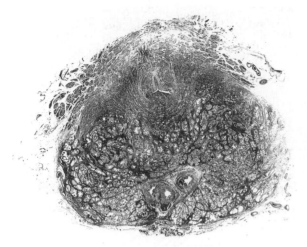

Fig. 10.2 Whole-mount section: central zone (with seminal way).

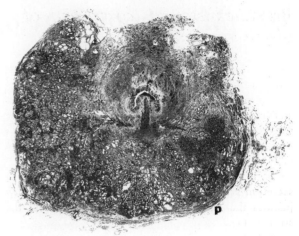

Fig. 10.4 Whole-mount section, peripheral zone (p): the urethra is in the anterior area of prostate.

● The *peripheral zone* (Figs 10.3 and 10.4) (70% of the glandular component and 46.2% of the prostate). It is pear-shaped and in contact with the central and transition zones. This zone constitutes the apex of the prostate and is therefore the area most accessible for digital rectal examination.

Glandular elements and stromal composition in the different zones differ (7):

● The *anterior fibromuscular zone* is composed of collagen and spindle-shaped smooth muscle cells that are proximally contiguous with the detrusor fibers of the anterior bladder wall.

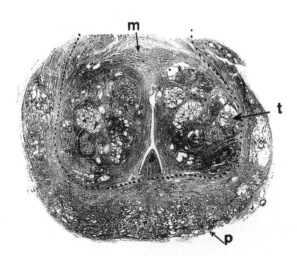

Fig. 10.3 Whole-mount section: peripheral zone (p) and transition zone (t). Note the nodular transformation of the transition zone (BPH) surrounding the urethra (m).

● In the *central zone*, the acini are large with irregular contours and branching is very elaborate, with prominent intraluminal ridges. Muscle bundles have a compact streaming arrangement.
● The *transition zone* has small, simple round glands with a stroma similar to those in the central zone.
● In the *peripheral zone*, the acini are either small and round or triangular, and the muscle bundles are multi-directional and loose.

The sonographic image results from the echo pattern created by reflections of the wave propagated from the interface between the stroma and the fluid-filled acinar lumina. Each zone therefore has its own specific ultrasound appearance (8):

● The *fibromuscular anterior zone*, with minimal glandular presence, has few interfaces and appears hypoechoic.
● The normal *transition zone*, because of its low stroma/glandular index, is more echoic that the fibromuscular zone, but less that the rest of the prostate.
● The *central and peripheral zones* have similar sonographic features, with relatively homogeneous texture and medium echogenicity (used as a pattern of normality and designated as isoechoic).

The importance of the McNeal model is not merely restricted to ultrasound-anatomic correlation; it also has a significant bearing on zonation of prostate pathology and on predicting the natural history of prostate cancer, which varies according to the zone of origin (see below).

Prostate histology (correlation of physiology and cell kinetics)

Classical glands have secretory and excretory areas, but the prostate is an organ with slow accumulation of secretion (0.5–2 cm^3/24 h) (9). Under these circumstances, specialization of ducts and acini would appear to be of limited value; morphology is thus identical in both parts, except in the para-urethral ductal portion (10), where we can see a very short area of transitional-cell-type mucosa (urothelium). The small volume of secretion is expelled occasionally and rapidly, which justifies the large amount of smooth muscle in the stroma (11).

With routine staining we can see two different cell types (basal cells and secretory or luminal cells, with a normal basal-secretory ratio of 1:3 in the normal prostate) (12) (Fig. 10.5). If we add some silver method (e.g. Gomori), a third type of cell can be observed (neuroendocrine cells), confirmed by the immunohistochemical method (chromogranin A) (Fig. 10.6). Yet with the introduction of the double-label procedure, simultaneous demonstration of cell-specific epithelial markers became possible, and some prostate cells are now known to have compound immunophenotypes. Thus, intermediate cells are now recognized, probably representing basal cells (stem cells) in the process of becoming terminal cells in a stem-cell model (12).

It must also be borne in mind that the prostate is a hormonal organ, with cells bearing different types of hormonal receptors or none at all. Therefore, physiologically, there are two functional compartments—the androgen-independent proliferative compartment and the secretory compartment, which is androgen-dependent and has limited proliferative capacity.

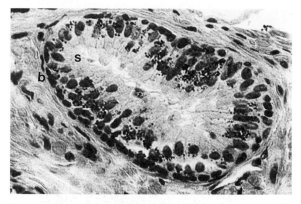

Fig. 10.5 Prostate acin. (H&E): basal (b) and secretory cells (s).

Putting together all these findings and opinions, we have a modern histological conception of the prostate that comprises the following cells:

- *Basal cells* are small cells with scant cytoplasm, located in the deep portion of the glands and arrayed parallel to the basal membrane. They have a specific high-molecular-weight cytokeratin (34-β-E12) (Fig. 10.7), and no PSA secretion. They express EGFR (erbB 2, erbB 3) and represent 70% of proliferating cells. The presence of estrogen and progestagen receptors, with no androgen receptors, means that continuous support by circulating androgens is not required for their maintenance. Bcl-2 (antiapoptotic gene) expression, which prevents androgen-dependent programmed cell death, confirms the androgen independence of the basal cells. However, a small population of basal cells does express androgen receptors (13), and for this reason can respond to androgenic stimulation by

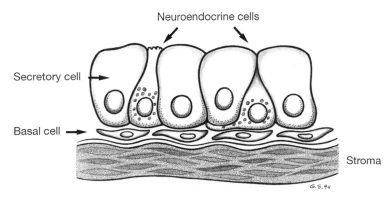

Fig. 10.6 Scheme of the cells of the prostate acini.

Prostate cancer

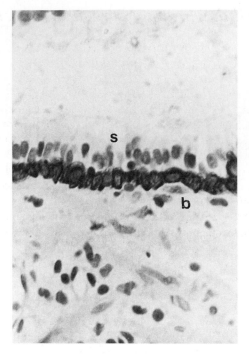

Fig. 10.7 High molecular-weight cytokeratin (34-β-E12)-positive expression in the basal cells (b), while the secretory cells (s) are cytokeratin-negative.

cells (16). They typically express cytokeratins 8 and 18, and secrete prostate-specific antigen (PSA) (Fig. 10.8), prostate acid phosphatase (PAP), and prostate-specific membrane antigen (PSMA) (17). Only 10% of proliferative activity is in this compartment. These are the cells containing the majority of androgen receptors, without Bcl-2 and with Bcl-x (apoptosis activator gene), meaning that they are sensitive to apoptosis (16).

- *Neuroendocrine cells* are usually located at the basal level, with or without communication with the luminal pole (i.e. open type or closed type); they have certain filiform 'dendritic' prolongations extending toward the surrounding cells (Fig. 10.9). Most of these cells express chromogranin A, synaptophysin, and serotonin, but it is also possible to find substances resembling calcitonin, bombesin, somatostatin, parathyroid-hormone-related protein, calcitonin gene products (18) (Fig. 10.10), etc., and cells can produce more that one of these peptides (16). Neuroendocrine cells were once thought to originate from the migratory neural crest but at present it is widely accepted that they originate from local stem cells, as previously discussed (12). For this reason, some open-type neuroendocrine

both differentiating into secretory cells (sustained activation), and maintaining proliferation (transient activation) (14). According to these findings, we may ascribe stem cells to the basal cell compartment.

- The proof of the stem-cell model was found when the existence of *intermediate cells* (also called amplifying cells) was demonstrated. These cells include different features of basal cells and terminal cells. Therefore, cells have been described (15) with simultaneous expression of: cytokeratin 34-β-E12 (basal phenotype) and PSA (secretory phenotype); cytokeratin 34-β-E12 (basal phenotype) and chromogranin A (neuroendocrine phenotype); PSA (secretory phenotype) and chromogranin (neuroendocrine phenotype). Hormonal receptors in these cells also vary.

The last group of cells is terminal cells, with two completely different phenotypes:

- *Secretory cells* are cylindrical and have clear and abundant cytoplasm; they lie perpendicular to the basal membrane and represent 75% of all epithelial

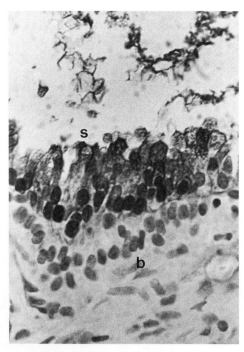

Fig. 10.8 PSA expression in the secretory cells (s), while the basal cells (b) are PSA-negative.

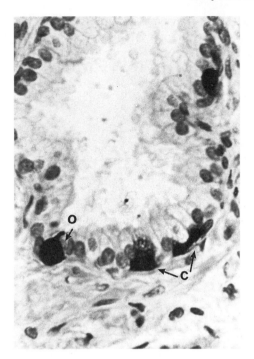

Fig. 10.9 Chromogranin A expression in the neuroendocrine cells. Open type (o) with minimal luminal extension and closed type (c).

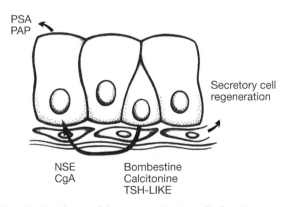

PSA
PAP

Secretory cell regeneration

NSE
CgA

Bombestine
Calcitonine
TSH-LIKE

Fig. 10.10 Scheme of the neuroendocrine cells function.

cells can express PSA focally, and some closed-type cells can express cytokeratin 34-β-E12 (12). No androgen receptors or proliferation activity have been demonstrated in these cells, but their proximity to proliferative cells suggests some type of proliferation control over them through serotonin and the other peptides (15).

Cellular origin of prostate cancer

The commonest prostate cancer cells (adenocarcinoma) have a phenotype similar to secretory cells (expression of cytokeratins 8 and 18, PSA production and generally expressed nuclear androgen receptors, and 5α-reductase 1 and 2) (19). This fact leads some authors to conclude that prostate cancer is derived from prostate luminal cells (20). But this hypothesis is not completely proven by the similarity between malignant cells and luminal cells, because the initial basal (stem) cells can lose their phenotype during transformation and acquire another (21).

Other phenotype chraracteristics of malignant cells include a high proliferation index, with inversion of the proliferative compartment, and expression of Bcl-2 (19). The prolonged life-span of cells due to aberrant expression of Bcl-2 may predispose these cells to accumulate genetic instability and progress in their aggressiveness.

The second malignant cell phenotype is the neuroendocrine cancer cell. Normal neuroendocrine cells show no evidence of proliferation (22), but in experimental castration studies, using sections of PC-295 xenografts (human prostate tumor model), researchers observed proliferation of malignant neuroendocrine cells shortly after androgen deprivation, the expression of a post-mitotic cell with neuroendocrine and exocrine (secretory) phenotype (23). These findings, together with the amphicrine characteristics of some of these cells, suggest that this phenotype derives from exocrine tumor cells that acquire endocrine features during tumor progression (15).

Therefore, the stem-cell model of normal prostate cell kinetics can explain the morphobiology of prostate cancer. Stem cells are transformed into different phenotypes, some of them combined in the same malignant cell, under a complex network of inductors (androgens, growth factors erbB2 and erbB3, oncogenes, and tumor suppressor genes) (13).

Morphobiological diagnostic basis of prostate cancer

So far, pathologists alone are able to recognize malignant cells. This is possible because genetic abnormalities accumulated in the nucleus can change the features of the nuclear matrix. It has become clear that the nuclear matrix not only provides the nuclear structure, but also plays a part in the regulatory nuclear function (24). Lamins are adjacent to the intermediate filaments and actin of the cytoskeleton, and these in turn are in contact with adhesion molecules (E-cadherin, α-catenin, integrins) (Fig. 10.11). Nucleolar size has been shown to correlate well with proliferative activity. The fibrillogranular network is involved in replication and transcription. Therefore, we can use anomalous nuclear and nucleolar morphology and the disarrangement of normal architecture (through the abnormal expression of adhesion molecules) as diagnostic criteria. Thus, we may consider cytological and architectural features for recognition of adenocarcinoma (25):

- *Cytological features* include nuclear and nucleolar enlargement and irregular chromatin distribution. Nucleoli are found in virtually all cells (Fig. 10.12).
- *Architectural features* can be observed under low magnification because malignant proliferation in the stroma is scattered in nodules or isolated elements. The acini are smaller that the normal glands, and are monolayer (Fig. 10.13).
- *Other features*: absence of basal cells is one of the best diagnostic criteria, which makes cytokeratin 34-β-E12 an important tool. Evidence of complete circumferential perineural growth and/or vascular/lymphatic invasion is very important in some cases with not completely atypical cells, but it is

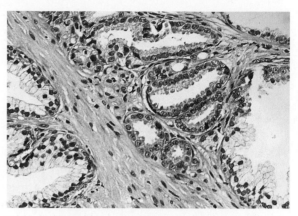

Fig. 10.12 Prostatic cancer (*right*). Note the nuclear and nucleolar prominence of the prostate cancer, in front of the normal prostate (*left*).

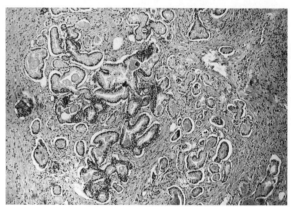

Fig. 10.13 Irregular architectural distribution of the prostate cancer.

necessary to be very strict in identifying these features. Luminal mucin, crystalloids, and collagenous micronodules can help, but they are only indirect features.

Pre-malignant prostate lesions

Use of new screening methods for the detection of prostate cancer has allowed detection of morphological changes with phenotypes intermediate between the normal and malignant cells; these lesions have been defined as 'pre-malignant'.

At present, two types of lesions have been considered: atypical adenomatous hyperplasia (AAH), and prostatic intra-epithelial neoplasia (PIN). Both lesions

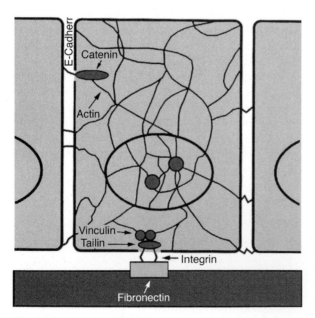

Fig. 10.11 Relationship of the nuclear matrix, cytoskeleton, and adhesion melecules.

lie on the continuum between normalcy and malignancy, posing pitfalls for diagnosis (26). Therefore, we shall consider the biology of these lesions, diagnostic issues and clinical attitude in the face of isolated pre-malignant changes.

Atypical adenomatous hyperplasia—AAH (Adenosis) (Fig. 10.14)

This lesion is characteristic of the transition zone, in other words, the BPH zone. BPH morphology is characterized by a nodular stromo-glandular transformation. Glandular proliferation can grow in a budding-in or budding-off pattern, and some budding-off proliferation develops microglandular areas. On some occasions, this microglandular growth can be quite exuberant, resembling well-differentiated adenocarcinoma. These are the lesions that can be included under AAH. Differential diagnosis must consider atrophy, post-atrophic hyperplasia, sclerosing adenosis and well-differentiated adenocarcinoma. The absence of a large nucleolus, lack of real infiltration of the stroma, and persistence of isolated basal cells can help towards recognition of AAH (26). Prevalence depends on the type of specimen; in BPH material it is around 7% and in needle biopsy material about 0.8% (27), signifying a clear preference of AAH for the transition zone.

The main problem in this lesion is to know whether AAH only mimics a low-grade adenocarcinoma or whether it is a pre-malignant lesion. Fourteen to seventeen percent of prostates with AAH have carcinoma areas (28, 29), with contiguity in 23–34% (29, 30). Our case follow-up has only revealed 2.3% subsequent carcinomas among patients who initially had AAH alone. The proliferation rate of this lesion lies halfway between benign and malignant lesions (27). DNA content is diploid and euploid (31). Loss of chromosome 8p22 (31, 32) is detected in 4–6% of AAH cases, while it is present in 56% of prostate cancers (32). In conclusion, we must be very strict in diagnosing AAH, and urologists should be notified in cases where AAH is observed with glandular aggregates presenting carcinoma features, though they should be aware that the presence of these small areas is seldom of any clinical significance for the patient.

Prostatic intra-epithelial neoplasia–PIN

PIN is characterized by nuclear and nucleolar changes with ductal and acinar architectural preservation. The nuclear atypia of the cells can be very similar to the atypia in malignant cells, though without complete loss of basal cells and stromal invasion. Proliferation compartment is inverted and shifts to secretory luminal cells (22). As a cellular lesion, it is graded as low-grade PIN (Fig. 10.15) or high-grade PIN (HGPIN) (Fig. 10.16). The present consensus is to report only high-grade PIN due to its good reproducibility, and to avoid mention of the low-grade PIN diagnosis in the pathology report. Differential diagnosis must include reactive proliferation lesions and papillary intraductal cancer (26).

With present knowledge, we can presume that HGPIN is located preferentially in the peripheral zone (68.8% of cases, with only 20% in the transition zone) (33), increases with age, and precedes cancer by decades (34). Adenocarcinoma was identified in 28.7% of subsequent biopsies from cases with isolated HGPIN (35). There is loss of 8p22 in 32–69% of PIN lesions, while allelic imbalance at 7q31 is present in 17% of PIN as opposed to 30% of cancers (36). Bcl-2 extends

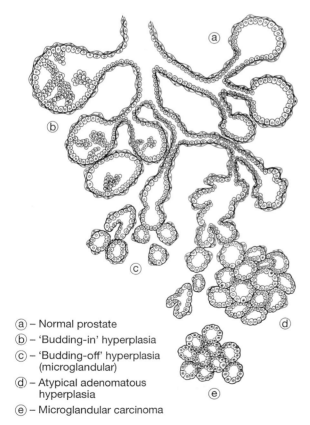

ⓐ – Normal prostate
ⓑ – 'Budding-in' hyperplasia
ⓒ – 'Budding-off' hyperplasia (microglandular)
ⓓ – Atypical adenomatous hyperplasia
ⓔ – Microglandular carcinoma

Fig. 10.14 Scheme of the different microglandular prostatic proliferation.

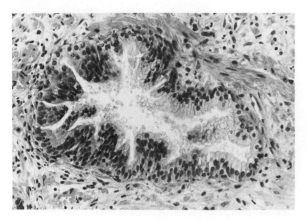

Fig. 10.15 Low-grade prostatic intra-epithelial neoplasia (*right*).

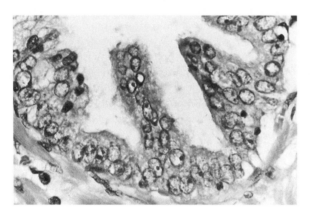

Fig. 10.16 High-grade prostatic intra-epithelial neoplasia.

up to secretory luminal cells, and its aberrant expression may predispose PIN to evolve into cancer (22). Other molecular features are the controversial expression of the c-erbB-2 gene product (analogous to EGFr), and the occasional over-expression of p53 (37). All these findings lead us to consider HGPIN the more favorable pre-malignant lesion in prostate cancer, but from a practical point of view it also must be considered a marker of concomitant cancer.

Morphobiology of stromal invasion

Stromal invasion requires cellular (cell–cell) detachment, basal membrane (basement membrane) degradation, and cellular capacity to grow in the stromal environment. All of these capabilities are acquired through different mechanisms:

Loss of cell–cell adhesion

A complex system of adhesion molecules in the cytoplasmatic membrane, including E-cadherin and α-catenin, mediates binding to the microfilaments (actin) of the cytoskeleton. Nuclear abnormalities cause downward regulation of the expression of these molecules, which correlates with grade and stage (38). Therefore we can observe, by immunohistochemical methods, a strong expression of E-cadherin in 64.7% of prostate cancers with Gleason score < 7, but only in 25% of cases with Gleason score > 7. α-Catenin expresses strongly in 88.2% of cases where Gleason score < 7, but 50% where Gleason score >7 (39) (Figs 10.17 and 10.18).

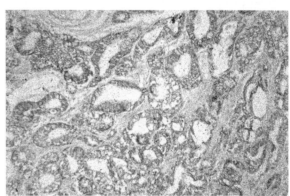

Fig. 10.17 Prostatic cancer with E-cadherin expression in a cellular membrane pattern.

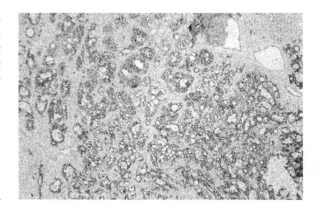

Fig. 10.18 Prostatic cancer with α-catenin expression in a cellular membrane pattern.

Loss of cell–stromal adhesion

Loss of basal cell differentiation is associated with loss of hemidesmosome-forming proteins and associated adhesive molecules, including collagen VII, laminin 5 and some integrins (40).

Overcoming the basal membrane barrier

Loss of the basal membrane correlates closely with cancer grade. Normal turnover in this membrane is regulated by metalloproteinases; proteolytic action is inactivated by some tissue inhibitors (TIMPs). Inappropriate TIMPs expression by malignant cells deregulates this system and permits access to the stroma (41).

Decreased cell–substrate normal attachment and neoplastic new attachment

Cells need an attachment to the basal membrane to proliferate, but cancer cells continue to proliferate when unattached; this phenomenon is known as anchorage independence (42). Such independence requires some false message to the nucleus that the cell is properly attached when actually it is not; this message is probably sent through the synthesis of basal membrane material by the malignant cell, which lacks hemidesmosome-associated laminin 5, collagen VII and IV. (12). Prostate cancer produces distinct peri-acinar and peri-cellular basal membranes (43), with simultaneous expression of laminin receptors (VLA-6) and collagen receptors (VLA-2). Co-expression with their ligands in neoplastic basal membranes mediates the attachment of tumor cells to neoplastic new membrane, granting increased ability to invade the extracellular matrix (44). This new basal membrane increases with tumor progression, and this fact probably explains why over-expression of some adhesion molecules, such as tailin, correlates to grade (Gleason score < 7, only 25% of cases; Gleason score > 7, 57.9%) (39). However, for cancer to expand beyond 2 mm, new capillaries seem to be necessary; angiogenic factors are therefore crucial for stromal invasion.

Angiogenesis

Angiogenic factors are secreted by malignant cells, adjacent tissues and macrophages (histiocytes) mobilized by various stimuli. There are activators, such as vascular endothelial growth factor (VEGF), basic fibroblastic growth factor, and thymidine phosphorylase, and inhibitors, such as thrombospondin and angiostatin (from plasminogen) (45). Prostate cancer produces angiostatin, which explains the indolent evolution of some patients, and neuroendocrine malignant cells can activate VEGF, explaining the aggressiveness of this neuroendocrine differentiation.

Morphobiology of cancer progression

Cancer progression is defined as the acquisition of metastatic capacity and subsequently of androgen independence in prostate cancer.

Metastatic capacity

The present hypothesis of cancer progression considers it secondary to the accumulation of chromosomal alterations (46), which means progressive nuclear atypia with abnormal intercellular communication expressed by architectural atypia. These morphologic anomalies are considered under *grading*, now improved with molecular evaluation of cell-cycle control, proliferation activity, and apoptosis. Another morphological marker of the metastatic capacity of prostate cancer is the amount of tumor, local extension, and vascular permeation, evaluated under *local staging*. Recently, new aspects regarding the 'area code' of metastatic sites have been included in the morphobiologic evaluation of cancer progression.

Grading

Still a gold standard in the evaluation of the aggressiveness of malignant neoplasias. This does not mean that evaluation is not subjective, although it is statistically valid. Grade is based on the idea of cell differentiation. Differentiation refers to the extent to which neoplastic cells resemble comparable normal cells. Well-differentiated tumors are thus composed of cells resembling the mature normal cells, poorly differentiated or undifferentiated tumors have unspecialized cells. Evaluating the degree of differentiation is a difficult task, not only because of subjectivity (present in all evaluation methods) but also because of the problems in defining precise criteria. Therefore, some classifications are based on cellular pleomorphism; others take into account only the anomalous glandular proliferation;

126   *Prostate cancer*

and others combine both criteria. At present, the most widely known classification is the Gleason system (47) (Fig. 10.19), which evaluates the architecture of the neoplasia and its relation with the stroma. It defines five patterns and considers a primary (or predominant) and a secondary (or least-abundant) pattern, thereby defining a total score or sum ranging from 2 to 10.

Some morphologic subtypes are assimilated to some Gleason patterns; thus, endometrioid prostate cancer is considered pattern 3, mucinous cancer is pattern 4, and cases with central necrosis (comedo-type) are pattern 5, which also includes sarcomatoid carcinoma and signet-ring cell carcinoma (48). By means of this system, correlation can be established with pathological extension (tumor volume) (49), and metastatic capacity (score 2–5, 14% metastasis; score 6, 32%; score 7, 50%; score 8, 75%; and score 9–10, 100%) (50). Numerous modifications have been proposed for the Gleason grading system to improve its power of discrimination; the most important is the inclusion of nuclear grading, as in the WHO classification.

Molecular cell-cycle control (Fig. 10.20)

As previously discussed, the crucial event in cancer progression is the accumulation of DNA abnormalities, but such accumulation fundamentally requires escape from cell-cycle control. Among the different controllers, Tp53 (17p13.1) and p21WAF1 (6p21.2) are the most studied in relation with prostate cancer (51). Wild-type p53 (protein) has a short half-life (4–45 min) and is not detectable by immunohistochemical methods, but the mutated form (incapable of normal cell-cycle control) stabilizes the protein and is detectable

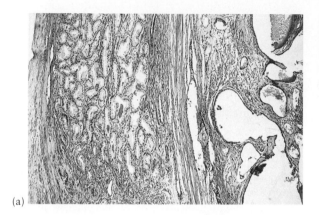
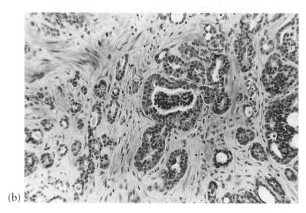
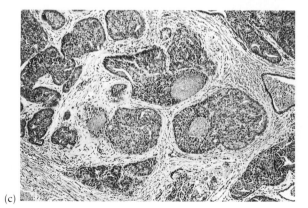

Fig. 10.19 (a) Gleason pattern 1–2;.(b) Gleason pattern 3; (c) Gleason pattern 5.

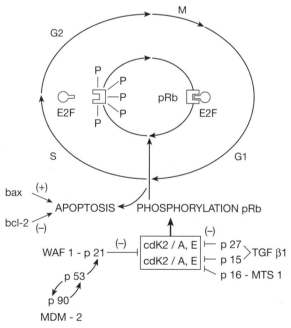

Fig. 10.20 Scheme of the basic molecular cell-cycle control.

with different antibodies, so the gene mutation can be recognized. Over-expression of p53 is irregular and increases in metastatic and hormone-independent patients (52). The controlling action of Tp53 is exerted through the activation of gene p21WAF1, but only wild-type p53 can perform this activation, therefore tumors that are p53-positive and p21-negative have a poor prognosis compared with those that are p53-negative and p21-positive (53).

Proliferation activity and apoptosis control

As a consequence of oncogenes expression, such as H-rasp21 (54) or HER-2/neu (p185 erbB-2) (55), the action of TGF-β 1 and 2 (with activator action instead of inhibition, probably caused by modified expression of the TGF-β receptor) (56), and abnormal cell-cycle control, malignant cells are characterized by a high proliferation capacity, increased by the blocking of apoptosis. The classical method of identifying a proliferating cell is to observe it while it is undergoing mitosis, but this is a very subjective method, difficult to apply, and with variations depending on the fixation process. With new immunohistochemical methods and the identification of proliferating antigens (Ki67), some of which are used in paraffin tissues (PCNA, Mib-1), certain types of patients with significantly lower survival rates can now be identified (PCNA 15%) (57), (Mib-1 high index) (58). Within all normal tissues, cell number homeostasis is achieved by balancing cell growth and cell death; apoptosis is the genetically programmed active mode of cell death. It is widely believed that apoptosis is an effective intrinsic anti-cancer mechanism (59); thus, its suppression may favor accumulation of abnormalities in the cell. Apoptosis is regulated by a complex molecular system. Bcl-2 (18q21.3) was the first described suppressor oncoprotein, and its over-expression in cancer cells may block or delay onset of apoptosis, selecting and maintaining long-living cells. Bcl-2 is over-expressed in 32–41% of prostate cancers (60); 67% of patients with bcl-2 over-expression recur at 5 years, versus 30.5% of those without bcl-2 expression (61); in irradiated patients, bcl-2 expression is a marker of aggressiveness (62); and all patients with over-expression of bcl-2 and p53 recur at 6 years.

Local staging

The most common clinical factor still associated with prognosis is the stage or level of extension of the carci-noma. Following the UICC (T category) classification of 1992, we note that rates of lymph node metastasis for incidental localized carcinoma are, respectively, 2% (T1a), 26% (T1b), and 4% (T1c), while the rates for clinically localized carcinomas are 1% (T2a) and 25% (T2b) (63, 64). This confirms that tumor volume remains quite reliable in terms of prognostic value (incidence of lymph node metastases is the same in T1b tumors—involving more than 5% of the tissue—and T2b tumors—extensive clinical tumors). For this reason, one of the primary roles of the pathologist is to determine extension (T stage) according to the sample.

Refinement of local extension evaluation

Microvascular invasion is present in 38% of radical prostatectomy specimens. It is commonly associated with extra-prostatic extension (62%) and lymph node metastases (67%), and correlates with grade and progression (65). Intraprostatic perineural invasion indicates tumor spread along the path of least resistance; only 50% of these patients have extra-prostatic extension, so it is not as useful (66).

Genes controlling metastatic phenotype

For a long time, the bone metastatic preference of prostate cancer was thought to be caused by a retrograde flow from the Batson plexus into the pelvic area during the Valsalva maneuver, but other factors now seem more important to metastasis. Among them, the expression of adhesion molecules with an 'area code' for bone marrow (OB-cadherin and α-2 β-1 integrin) is the most studied. Other metastasis-associated genes are the KAI1 (11p11.2), loss of which is associated with greater metastasis (67); protein p9Ka, located in cytoskeletal components in a pattern identical to actin filaments, which changes normal Ca++ metabolism (68); and the bone morphogenetic proteins that induce bone morphogenesis in vivo and are involved in the skeletal metastases of advanced prostate cancer. Nm23-H1 and CD44 are less consistent factors (69).

Androgen independence

All prostate carcinomas are initially androgen-dependent, but become independent from this hormone in the long term. However, even in this situation, malignant cells have androgen receptors though they do not imply androgen dependence. The exact mechanism of independence is unknown, but it seems to require the development of new clones needing no androgen stimulation. Androgen-deprivation therapy increases the estrogen/androgen ratio; androgen-independent cells express estrogen receptors at a high level, the cells become estrogen-responsive and may survive (40). Hormone-refractory tumors, in 30% of cases, have amplification of androgen receptor Xq11-q13, in 80% amplification of 8q24 (through c-myc amplification?), and changes in chromosome 7 (46, 70). Bcl-2 can play some role in the hormonal independence mechanism because it is more frequent in these tumors than in hormone-sensitive tumors (71). Finally, the extensive and multifocal neuroendocrine differentiation of prostate adenocarcinoma may represent a different path to androgen independence, because these cells can maintain cell proliferation through a paracrine androgen-independent pathway (72).

Translational approach to clinical practice

Pathologists can receive different types of specimens, taken for diagnostic purposes (needle biopsies), or for treatment (radical prostatectomies); but incidental prostate cancer may be found in BPH-treatment surgical specimens. Clinical requirements are different for each different type of surgical sample; we shall therefore consider the application of all morphobiologic aspects to the different pathologic specimens.

Needle core biopsy

Diagnostic approach

The majority of biopsies are performed for elevated serum PSA with no other clinical evidence of cancer, so with more specimens being generated there is a greater risk of encountering rare lesions, atypical small acinar proliferations (ASAP) (73), or other small glandular lesions, recently described, that can mimic cancer. For this reason, one of the most important tasks for pathologists is the diagnosis of carcinoma (see Morphobiological diagnosis basis), a subject that goes beyond the aim of this chapter and is addressed in general papers (25). From a clinical point of view, the diagnostic yield of sextant prostate biopsies is as much as 43% higher than the yield from two or fewer biopsies (74, 75), but in some cases of small tumor volume (less than 5.1 cm^3) and/or large prostate, more cores may be necessary (76). Pathologists need to handle

cylinders correctly, laying them flat to avoid excluding any part because of bending in the paraffin block (77). In case of isolated high-grade PIN or ASAP, a complete and serial sectioning is not cost-effective and only three slides are recommended (78).

Prognostic approach

The best marker to determine extra-prostatic invasion in needle biopsy is demonstration of peri-prostatic fat and/or seminal vesicle infiltration (Fig. 10.21), but the presence of fatty tissue is infrequent, except in some centers where urologists actively try to obtain it (79). The percentage of positive cores is the next-best prognostic marker of pathologic stage (28.6% in confined tumors—T2—and 50% in non-confined tumors—T3— $P < 0.0001$), with similar prognostic value to the rate of tumor surface area involvement (49).

It is widely accepted that the Gleason grading system has prognostic value (49, 50), but the problem with core biopsies is correlating the biopsy Gleason score with the final Gleason score in radical prostatectomy. Exact correlation may range from 28% to 68%; 26% to 60% of biopsies are under-graded and 5% to 32% over-graded (80), but the exact correlation rate can be about 68%, or 97% within one grade, as long as a minimal protocol is observed (80). In our laboratory, only 8% of cases diagnosed with a score of less than 8 turned out to have a higher score after radical prostatectomy. Thus, Gleason-score evaluation is useful in needle biopsy, though it should be avoided in case of minimal cancer representation. Combining the percentage of positive cores and the Gleason score can be helpful, because some authors have found that 15–50% of patients with a Gleason pattern –4 or –5

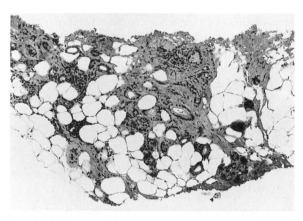

Fig. 10.21 Fine-needle biopsy; prostatic carcinoma in the fat.

carcinoma and/or neoplasia in more than three core biopsies, or one cylinder with over 50%, show progression after 8–10 years (63). Microvessel invasion can also be useful to predict extra-prostatic extension (62%) or lymph node invasion (67%) (65).

Peri-neural invasion has contradictory results in literature, with sensitivity only 51%, specificity 71% and a positive predictive value of 49% (66). Neuroendocrine expression has some correlation with extra-prostatic extension (82.3% cases with neuroendocrine differentiation progress, in front of only 26% without this differentiation), and lymph node metastases (53.8% with neuroendocrine, an any case without neuroendocrine cells), but it is not an independent factor (81). Finally, molecular parameters such as waf-p21, bcl-2, p53 are very promising, but the focality of their expression and the need for a standardized methodology represent a difficulty in routine studies (82).

BPH samples

In treating BPH, tissue is only obtained from the transition zone, thereby detecting only stage-T1 carcinomas. The pathologist is faced with two different problems with this sort of material: the first is to distinguish AAH from well-differentiated adenocarcinoma (see previous discussion of pre-malignant lesions); the second is to evaluate tumor volume in order to distinguish T1a from T1b, as only 8% of T1a cases progress, versus 63% of the T1b cases. Thus, the debate centers on how much tissue should be included. At present, it seems to have been established that all fragments should be included up to 10 g, adding a block per each additional 5 g (83). If fewer than 5% of the chips are found to have cancer, all the remaining tissue should be included. If more than 5% are found to be cancerous, inclusion of the remaining material will not alter or vary the stage (84). For open-surgery specimens, at least six sections are mandatory (85). For incidental prostate cancer, the percentage of affected tissue and the Gleason score (4 or lower versus more that 4) is a further prognostic factor (86).

Radical prostatectomy

All the information offered by radical prostatectomy offers begins with processing (87, 88). The specimen must be transported fresh to the pathology laboratory.

Fresh tissue sampling is only indicated in case of molecular or genetic studies. Fixation must be done in a 10% neutral-buffered formalin solution during 24–48 h (some authors recommend injecting this solution in multiple sites by hypodermic needle). After fixation, and prior to sectioning, surgical margins are inked. Many authors recommend using different colors for each side or zone, but it is possible to use only one color (black) and make the slightest incision (without tissue removal) on one of the sides; with this procedure, damage to the prostate 'capsule' is minimal and does not affect pathological evaluation (Fig. 10.22). Sampling depends on laboratory guidelines. Only 12% of laboratories process the entire gland (89), but it is not mandatory for a correct evaluation. Any partial sampling method for radical prostatectomy specimens should not be purely mechanical, several factors can contribute to sampling and at least must include:

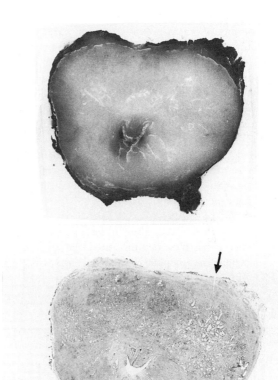

Fig. 10.22 Whole-mount section (paraffin block and microscopic section). Note the indian ink in the periphery of the specimen and the minimal section in the left side of the rectal surface (*arrow*).

- apical and bladder neck margins must be entirely embedded;
- portion of seminal vesicles where the vesicle joins the prostate gland;
- at least one-third of the gland, with special attention to the large peripheral nerve tracts of the neurovascular bundles (posterolateral, close to seminal vesicles);
- selected areas with grossly identifiable abnormalities (88, 89).

The staging in radical prostatectomy specimens is critical to determine the prognosis (Table 10.1). The prostatic capsule is a peripheral layer of fibromuscular stroma, which borders the periprostatic fat, the capsule is incomplete in some parts of the prostate (around the seminal vesicles, and apex), but it is still an important boundary to evaluate. Following the UICC (TNM) classification, the capsular invasion without extension to periprostatic fat tissue is considered a pT2 tumor. The volume of extra-prostatic tumor extension is important, some authors recommend distinguishing focal (tumor not exceeding two high-power microscopic fields or not present in more than two separate sections on any amount) versus non-focal (88). In relation to the seminal vesicles, the pathologist must distinguish microscopic tumor invasion into the muscularis of the seminal vesicle (pT3b), from involvement of the peri-vesicle tissue; the last situation is equivalent to the extra-prostatic fat invasion (pT3a). In the staging of radical prostatectomy specimens we must consider two interesting aspects:

(a) The infiltration according to zonal distribution, because it has been demonstrated that, depending on where the neoplasia is located, it will have a greater or lesser capacity to reach the capsule and seminal vesicles throughout its course of development: carcinomas in the peripheral zone usually invade the seminal vesicles (24%) much more frequently that carcinomas in the transition zone (13%) (90).

(b) The 'black holes' in TNM classification, become evident in the moment to interpret the following situations:

(i)   Is the fibromuscular zone invasion intra or extra-positive extension?

(ii) Is the ejaculator invasion a pT2 or a pT3 tumor?

(iii) Has the isolated bladder neck invasion ominous prognosis?

(iv) Has the same bad prognosis a minimal or extensive seminal vesicle invasion?

Finally be must remember that categories T1 a, b and c have no pathologic equivalents, and the TNM classification no consider the margins status.

The margins were considered positive when the prostate cancer extended to the inked margin of resection. We can consider three different type of positive margins:

1. Prostate cancer may extend to the inked margin of resection of an intact gland, the tumor follows the curve of the organ (smooth surface). This is a category pT2, and some consensus meetings recomended the use of + (pT2+) (91).

2. With irregular surface.

3. With extra-prostatic positive margin.

Table 10.1   Pathological staging of prostate cancer

Any radical prostatectomy from a T1 prostatic cancer is at least a pT2a	
No pT1 category:	Because there is insufficient tissue to assess the highest pT category
PT2: Tumor confined within the prostate	
	pT2a Tumor involves one lobe
	pT2b Tumor involves both lobes
pT3: Tumor extends through the prostate capsule*	
	pT3a Extra-capsular extension (unilateral or bilateral)
	pT3b Tumor invades seminal vesicle(s)
pT4: Tumor invades adjacent structures other than seminal vesicles: bladder neck, external spincter, rectum, levator muscles, and/or pelvic wall	

(*) Invasion into the prostatic apex or into (but not beyond) the prostatic capsule is not classified pT3, but as pT2.

All of them unifocal o multi-focal. The clinical significance is different according the type (is worse in the extra-prostatic positive margin) (92), multi-focal in 21.7% of cases (93). In spite of the prognosis importance of positive margins, only 30–40% of patients with focally positive margins progress at 5 years because, despite the margins being called positive by the pathologist, there is no residual left within the patient, or the granulation tissue and local isquemia destroyed the few cells left; for this situation it is recommended a complete prognosis evaluation to look for regular versus irregular surface, uni-focal versus multi-focal lesion, intra versus extra-prostatic extension, and Gleason score (94).

The neuroendocrine differentiation (Figs 10.23 and 10.24) has some bad prognosis implication, and explains the hormono-independence in some cases (95),

probably for the correlation with the VEFF and TGF-α (angiogenic factors) (96), and the absence of androgenic receptors, respectively. Among the molecular markers the p53 mutation is the most studied in clinical practice (97, 98), but the criteria of positive/negative is not yet standardize.

Future trends

The complexity of all these prognostic factors led to a definition of prognostic equation of recurrences. Partin *et al.* (99) were the first investigators who developed a biostatistical model equation that categorized post-radical prostatectomy patients into different risk groups. After multivariate regression analysis, only three variables were included:

- a sigmoidal transformation of PSA;
- prostatectomy Gleason score;
- margin status.

Recently a new proposition of prognostic equation has been presented including, race, PSA, margin status, p53, and bcl-2 (60). At present this new equation is an example of how molecular markers could be used in the future, but it is very important to remember that the classical markers are still useful, and that any approach to the true is just an approach.

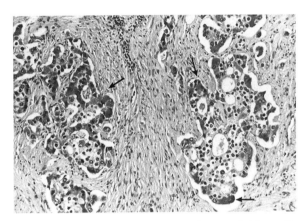

Fig. 10.23 Prostatic carcinoma with Paneth-like cells (*arrows*). These cells are neuroendocrine cells (H&E).

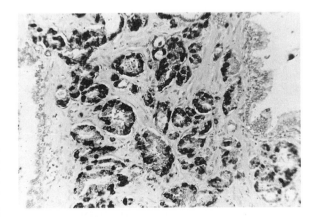

Fig. 10.24 Prostatic adenocarcinoma with wide neuroendocrione differentiation, with chromogranin A expression.

References

1. Herbut PA. *Urological pathology*, Vol II. Lea & Febiger, Philadelphia 1952, Ch.IX, 888.
2. Lowsley OS. The development of human prostate gland with reference to the development of other structures at the neck of the urinary bladder. *Am. J Anat* 1912, **13**, 299–349.
3. LeDuc IE. The anatomy of the prostate and the pathology of early benign hypertrophy. *J Urol* 1939, **42**, 1217–41.
4. Franks LM. Benign hyperplasia of the prostate. A review. *Ann R Coll Surg* 1954, **14**, 92–106.
5. Gil-Vernet S. Patología Urogenital: biología y patología de la próstata. *Madrid, Editorial Paz Montalvo* 1953, **1** (2), 1–72.
6. McNeal JE. Regional morphology and pathology of the prostate. *Am J Clin Pathol* 1968, **49**, 347–57.
7. McNeal JE, Bostwick DG. Anatomy of the prostate: Implications for disease. In: *Pathology of the prostate* (ed. DG Bostwick). Churchill Livingstone, New York 1990, 1–14.

8. Shinohara K, Scardino PT, Carter SSC *et al.* Pathologic basis of the sonographic appearance of the normal and malignant prostate. *Urol Clin N Amer* 1989, **16**, 675–91.

9. Huggins C. Physiology of the prostate gland. *Physiol Rev* 1945, **25**, 281–94.

10. McNeal JE. Prostate. In: *Histology for pathologists* (ed. SS Sternberg). Raven Press Ltd, New York 1992, Ch.40, 749–763.

11. McNeal. Normal histology of the prostate. *Am J Surg Pathol* 1988, **12**, 619–33.

12. Bonkhoff H, Remberger K. Differentiation pathways and histogenetic aspects of normal and abnormal prostatic growth: a stem cell model. *Prostate* 1996, **28**, 98–106.

13. Magi-Galluzi C, Loda M. Molecular events in the early phases of prostate carcinogenesis. *Eur Urol* 1996, **30**, 167–76.

14. Bonkhoff H, Stein U, Remberger K. Widespread distribution of nuclear androgen receptors in the basal cell layer of the normal and hyperplastic human prostate. *Wirchows Arch (A)* 1993, **422**, 35–8

15. Bonkhoff H, Stein U, Remberger K. Multidirectional differentiation in the normal, hyperplastic, and neoplastic human prostate. Simultaneous demonstration of cell specific epithelial markers. *Hum Pathol* 1994, **25**, 42–6.

16. Xue Y, Smedts F, Verhofstad A *et al.* Cell kinetics of prostate exocrine and neuroendocrine epithelium and their differential interrelationship: new perspectives. *Prostate* 1998, **S8**, 62–73.

17. Wright GL, Haley C, Beckett ML *et al.* Expression of prostate-specific membrane antigen in normal, benign, and malignant prostate tissues. *Urol Oncol* 1995, **1**, 18–28.

18. Deftos LJ. Granin-A, parathyroid hormone-related protein, and calcitonin gene products in neuroendocrine prostate cancer. *Prostate* 1998, **S8**, 23–31.

19. Bonkoff H. Role of the basal cells in pre-malignant changes of the human prostate: a stem cell concept for the development of prostate cancer. *Eur Urol* 1996, **30**, 201–5.

20. Nagle RB, Ahmann FR, McDaniel KM *et al.* Cytokeratin characterization of human prostatic carcinoma and its derived cell lines. *Cancer Res* 1987, **47**, 281–6.

21. Sherwood ER, Berg LA, Mitchell NJ *et al.* Differential cyttokeratin expression in normal, hyperplastic and malignant epithelial cells from human prostate. *J Urol* 1990, **143**, 167–71.

22. Bonkoff H, Stein U, Remberger K. The proliferative function of basal cells in the normal and hyperplastic human prostate. *Prostate* 1994, **24**, 114–8.

23. Noordzij MA, van Weerden WM, Ridder CH *et al.* Neuroendocrine differentiation in human prostatic tumor models. *Am J Pathol* 1996, **149**, 859–71.

24. Bosman FT. The nuclear matrix in pathology. *Virchows Arch* 1999, **435**, 391–9.

25. Algaba F, Epstein JI, Aldape HC *et al.* Assessment of prostate carcinoma in core needle biopsy: definition of minimal criteria for the diagnosis of cancer in biopsy material. *Cancer* 1996, **78**, 376–81.

26. Algaba F, Trias I. Diagnostic limits in precursor lesions of prostatic cancer. *Eur Urol* 1996, **30**, 212–21.

27. Grignon DJ, Sakr WA. Atypical adenomatous hyperplasia of the prstate: a critical review. *Eur Urol* 1996, **30**, 206–11.

28. Gaudin PB, Epstein JI. Adenosis of the prostate: Histologic features in needle biopsy specimens. *Am J Surg Pathol* 1995, **19**, 737–47.

29. Algaba F, Martínez-Hurtado J, Trias I *et al.* Significado biológico de la hiperplasia atípica adenomatosa prostática. *Act Urol Esp* 1994, **S43** (A).

30. Bostwick DG, Qian J. Atypical adenomatous hyperplasia of the prostate: Relationship with carcinoma in 217 whole-mount radical prostatectomies. *Am J Surg Pathol* 1995, **19**, 506–18.

31. López-Beltrán A, Pacelli A, Qian J *et al.* Atypical adenomatous hyperplasia of the prostate: immunophenotype, genotype and DNA ploidy analysis. *Mod Pathol* 1996, **9**, (A).

32. Furman J, Zhu X, Kaleem Z *et al.* Chromosome 8p22 allelic loss in atipical adenomatous hyperplasia (adenosis) and carcinoma in the prostate. *Mod Pathol* 1996, **9**, S73 (A).

33. Kovi J, Mostofi FK, Heshmat MY. Large acinar atypical hyperplasia and carcinoma of the prostate. *Cancer* 1988, **61**, 555–61.

34. Bostwick DG. Progression of prostatic intra-epithelial neoplasia to early invasive adenocarcinoma. *Eur Urol* 1996, **30**, 145–52.

35. Algaba F. Evolution of isolated high-grade prostatic intra-epitelial neoplasia in a Mediterranean patient population. *Eur Urol* 1999, **35**, 496–7.

36. Qian J, Jenkins RB, Bostwick DG. Genetic and chromosomal alterations in prostatic intra-epithelial neoplasia and carcinoma detected by fluorescence *in situ* hybridization. *Eur Urol* 1999, **35**, 479–83.

37. Myers RB, Grizzle WE. Biomarker expression in prostatic intra-epithelial neoplasia. *Eur Urol* 1996, **30**, 153–66.

38. Paul R, Ewing CM, Jarrad DF. The cadherin cell-cell adhesion pathway in prostate cancer progression. *Br J Urol* 1997, **79**, 37–41.

39. Rubio-Briones J, Pulymood A, Collett G *et al.* Expression and localization of talin in benign and malignant human prostate and its relation to E-cadherin and α-catenin. Int J Cancer (Submitted).

40. Bonkhoff H, Remberger K. Morphogenic concepts of normal and abnormal growth in the human prostate. Rev Esp Patol 1999, 32, 368–369.

41. Fuchs ME, Brawer MK and Reunels MA. The relationship of basement membrane to histologic grade of human prostatic carcinoma. Mod Pathol 1989, 2, 105–111.

42. Ruoslahti E, Reed JC. Anchorage dependence integrins, and apoptosis. Cell 1994, 77, 477–478.

43. Bonkhoff H, Wernert N, Dhom G *et al.* Distribution of basement membranes in primary and metastatic carcinomas of the prostate. *Hum Pathol* 1992, 23, 934–9.

44. Bonkhoff H, Stein U, Remberger K. Differential expression of α-6 and α-2 very late antigen integrins in the normal, hyperplastic, and neoplastic prostate: simultaneous demonstration of cell surface receptors

and their extracellular ligands. *Hum Pathol* 1993, **24**, 242–8.

45. Furusato M, Wakui S, Sasaki H. Tumour angiogenesis in latent prostatic carcinoma. *Br J Cancer* 1994, **70**, 1244–6.

46. Nupponen N, Visakorpi T. Molecular biology of progression of prostate cancer. *Eur Urol* 1999, **35**, 351–4.

47. Gleason DF. Histologic grading of prostate cancer: a perspective. *Hum Pathol* 1992, **23**, 273–9.

48. Bostwick DG. Pathology of prostate cancer. In: *Urologic cancer* (ed. MS Ernstoff, JA Heaney, RE Peschel). Blackwell Science, Cambridge 1997, 15–47.

49. Sebo TJ, Bock BJ, Cheville JC et al. The percent of cores positive for cancer in prostate needle biopsy specimens is strongly predictive of tumor stage and volume at radical prostatectomy. *J Urol* 2000, **163**, 174–8.

50. Paulson CF, Piserchia PV, Gardner W. Predictors of lymphatic spread in prostatic adenocarcinoma. *J Urol* 1980, **123**, 697–9.

51. Burton JL, Oakley N, Anderson JB. Recent advances in the histopathology and molecular biology of prostate cancer. *BJU International* 2000, **85**, 87–94.

52. Heindenberg HB, Sesterhenn I, Gaddipati J et al. Alteration of the tumor supressor gene p53 in a high fraction of treatment-resistant prostate cancer. *J Urol* 1995, **154**, 414–21.

53. Matsushima H, Sasaki T, Goto T et al. Immunohistochemical study of p21 WAF1 and p53 proteins in prostatic cancer and their prognostic significance. *Hum Pathol* 1998, **29**, 778–83.

54. Bos JL. Ras oncogenes in human cancer: a review. *Cancer Res* 1989, **49**, 4682–9.

55. Sadasivan R, Morgan R, Jennings S et al. Over-expression of HER-2/neu may be an indicator of poor prognosis in prostate cancer. *J Urol* 1993, **150**, 126–31.

56. Perry KT, Anthong CT, Steiner MS. Immunohistochemical localization of TGF-β 1, TGF-β 2, TGF-β 3 in normal and malignant human prostate. *Prostate* 1997, **33**, 133–40.

57. Naito S, Sakamoto N, Kotoh S. Proliferating cell nuclear antigen in needle biopsy specimens of prostatic carcinoma. *Eur Urol* 1994, **26**, 164–9.

58. López-Beltrán A, Algaba F, de Torres I et al. Cell proliferation and apoptosis in needle biopsy specimens with prostatic adenocarcinoma. *J Urol Pathol* (in press).

59. Thompson CB. Apoptosis in the pathogenesis and treatment of disease. *Science* 1995, **267**, 1456–62.

60. Moul JWE. Angiogenesis, p53, bcl-2 and Ki-67 in the progression of prostate cancer after radical prostatectomy. *Eur Urol* 1999, **35**, 399–407.

61. Bauer JJ, Sesterhenn IA, Mostofi FK et al. Elevated levels of apoptosis regulator proteins p53 and bcl-2 are independent prognostic biomarkers in surgically treated clinically localized prostate cancer patients. *J Urol* 1996, **156**, 1511–6.

62. Huang A, Gandour-Edwarda R, Rosenthal SA. P53 and bcl-2 immunohistochemical alterations in prostate cancer treated with radiation therapy. *Urology* 1998, **51**, 346–51.

63. Epstein JI, Walsh PC, Carmichae lM. Pathologic and clinical findings to predict tumor extent of non-palpable (Stage T1c) prostate cancer. *JAMA* 1994, **271**, 868–74.

64. Donohue RE, Mani JH, Whitesel JA. Pelvic lymph node dissection. Guide to patient management in clinically located confined adenocarcinoma of prostate. *Urology* 1982, **20**, 559–65.

65. Bahnson RR, Dresner SM, Gooding W et al. Incidence and prognostic significance of lymphatic and vascular invasion in radical prostatectomy specimens. *Prostate* 1989, **15**, 149–55.

66. Egan AJM, Bostwick DG. Prediction of extra-prostatic extension of prostate cancer based on needle biopsy findings: perineural invasion lacks independent significance. *Lab Invest* 1997, **76**, 421.

67. Isaacs JT. Molecular markers for prostate cancer metastasis. *Am J Pathol* 1997, **150**, 1511–21.

68. Gibbs FEM, Wilkinson MC, Rudland PS et al. Interaction in vitro of p9Ka, the rat S-100 related, metastasis-inducing, calcium-binding protein. *J Biol Chemistr* 1994, **269**, 18992–9.

69. Hrouda D. Mechanisms of metastasis in prostate cancer. Prospectives contemporary issues in managing prostatic disease. *Prostate* 1998, **7**, 5–8.

70. Bussemakers MJK, van Bokhoven A, Debruyne FMJ et al. A new prostate-specific markers, over-expressed in prostatic tumors. *J Urol* 1997, **157**, 21 (Abstract).

71. Isaacs JT. The biology of hormone refractory prostate cancer. Why does it develop? *Urol Clin N Amer* 1999, **26**, 263–73.

72. Cussenot O, Villette JM, Cochand-Priollet B et al. Evaluation and clinical value of neuroendocrine differentiation in human prostatic tumors. *Prostate* 1998, **S8**, 43–51.

73. Dundore PA. Atypical small acinar proliferations (ASAP) suspicious for malignancy in prostate needle biopsies. *J Urol Pathol* 1998, **8**, 21–9.

74. Shaw EB, Wofford ED, Carter J. Processing prostate needle biopsy specimens for 100% detection of carcinoma. *Am J Clin Pathol* 1995, **103**, 507–12.

75. Terris MK, McNeal JE, Stamey TA. Detection of clinically significant prostate cancer by transrectal ultrasound-guided systematic biopsies. *J Urol* 1992, **148**, 829–32.

76. Eskew LA, Bare RL, McCullough DL. Systematic 5 region prostate biopsy is superior to sextant method for diagnosing carcinoma of the prostate. *J Urol* 1997, **157**, 199–203.

77. Rogatsch H, Mairinger T, Horninger W et al. Optimized preembedding method improves the histologic yield of prostatic core needle biopsies. *Prostate* 2000, **42**, 124–9.

78. Reyes AO, Humphrey PA. Diagnostic effect of complete histological sampling of prostate needle biopsy specimens. *Am J Clin Pathol* 1998, **109**, 416–22.

79. Allepuz CA, Sanz JI, Gil MJ et al. Seminal vesicle biopsy in prostate cancer staging. *J Urol* 1995, **154**, 1407–11.

80. Carlson GD, Calvanese CB, Kahane H et al. Accuracy of biopsy Gleason scores from a large uropathology laboratory: use of a diagnostic protocol to minimize observer variability. *Urology* 1998, **51**, 525–9.

81. Algaba F, Trias I. Significance of neuroendocrine differentiation of prostatic cancer in needle biopsy samples. *Pathol Intern* 1996, **46** (Abstract), 800.

82. Van der Kwast TH, Houtsmuller AB. Accuracy of grading: can it be replaced by other prognostic tissue factors? Present and future. Progress and controversies in oncological. In: *Urology V* (ed. KH Kurth, GH Mickisch, FH Schröder). The Parthenon Publising Group, New York 1999, 119–30.

83. Murphy GP, Busch C, Abrahamsson PA. Histopathology of localized prostate cancer. *Scand J Urol Nephrol* 1994, **162** (Suppl), 7–42.

84. McDowell PR, Fox WM, Epstein JI. Is submission of remaining tissue necessary when incidental carcinoma of the prostate is found on transurethral resection? *Hum Pathol* 1994, **25**, 493–7.

85. Graham SD, Bostwick DG, Hoisaeter A *et al.* Report of the committee on staging and pathology. *Cancer* 1992, **70**, 359–61.

86. Caicedo PS, Chechile G, Featherston M *et al.* Determinación de factores pronósticos en el carcinoma prostático incidental. *Arch Esp de Urol* 1993, **46**, 868–74.

87. Hoedemaeker RF, Ruijter ETG, Ruizeveld-de Winter JA *et al.* Processing radical prostatectomy specimens. A comprehensive and standardized protocol. *J Urol Pathol* 1998, **9**, 211–22.

88. Sakr WA, Grignon DJ. Practice parameters, pathologic staging, and handling radical prostatectomy specimens. *Urol Clin N Amer* 1999, **26**, 453–63.

89. True LD. Surgical pathology examination of the prostate gland: Practice survey by American Society of Clinical Pathologists. *Am J Clin Pathol* 1994, **102**, 572–9.

90. Greene DR, Whecler TM, Egawa S *et al.* A comparison of the morphological features of cancer arising in the transition zone and in peripheral zone of the prostate. *J Urol* 1991, **146**, 1069–76.

91. Algaba F, Böcking A, Bono A *et al.* Prognostic markers in acinar prostate cancer. Proceedings First International Consultation on prostate cancer. *SCI* 1997, 415–423.

92. Wheeler TM, Dillioglugil Ö, Kattan MW *et al.* Clinical and pathological significance of the level and extent of capsular invasion in clinical stage T1–2 prostate cancer. *Hum Pathol* 1998, **29**, 856–62.

93. Musulén E, Algaba F. Prostatectomía radical con márgenes positivos. *Rev Esp Patol* 1997, **30** (Suppl), (Abstract 235).

94. Epstein JI, Carmichel M, Pizov G *et al.* Influence of capsular penetration on progression following radical prostatectomy. A study of 196 cases with long-term follow-up. *J Urol* 1993, **150**, 135–41.

95. Krijnen JLM, Bojdanowicz JFAT, Selderijk CA *et al.* The prognostic value of neuroendocrine differentiation in adenocarcinoma of the prostate in relation to progression of disease after endocrine therapy. *J Urol* 1997, **158**, 171–4.

96. Harper ME, Glyne-Jones E, Goddard L *et al.* Vascular endothelial growth factor (VEGF) expression in prostatic tumours and its relationship to neuroendocrine cells. *Br J Cancer* 1996, **74**, 910–6.

97. Stricker HJ, Kay JK, Linden MD *et al.* Determining prognosis of clinically localized prostate cancer by immunohistochemical detection of mutant p53. *Urology* 1996, **47**, 366–9.

98. Byrne RL, Wilson Horne CH, Robinson MC *et al.* The expression of Wf-1, p53, and bcl-2 in prostatic adenocarcinoma. *Br J Urol* 1997, **79**, 190–5.

99. Partin AW, Piantadosi S, Marshall FF *et al.* Selection of men at high risk for disease recurrence for experimental adjuvant therapy following radical prostatectomy. *Urology* 1995, **45**, 831–7.

11 | Biology of prostate cancer

Alexandra Giatromanolaki, Efthimios Sivridis, and Konstantinos Syrigos

Background

Prostate cancer is a serious public health problem in many industrialized countries. It is the most common malignant neoplasm of men in the United States (1) and the second most frequent type of cancer in the United Kingdom (2). This high incidence of prostate cancer is, probably, the result of an aging population and improved methods of detection. For there are, indeed, effective procedures today, like the assay for prostate-specific antigen (PSA), which conveniently detect the disease (3, 4). It is estimated that 1 in 10 American men will, eventually, develop prostate cancer in their lifetimes (1).

The etiology of prostate cancer is obscure, but the disease is known to occur in the presence of testosterone (T) and dehydrotestosterone (DHT) secretion (5). Many investigators attempted to show a difference in sex hormone levels in prostate cancer patients compared to controls, but their results have not been consistent (6–9). Race is an important risk factor, as black Americans have a higher incidence of prostate cancer (100 per 100 000) compared to white Americans (70.1 per 100 000) (10–12). Furthermore, black men tend to develop the disease at a younger age and have higher grade and stage tumors at diagnosis (13, 14). Not unexpectedly, survival is less favorable in black Americans (15). On the other hand, the incidence of prostate cancer is particularly low in American Indians, Hispanics, Asians, and Eskimos (16, 17). It was thought that increased serum 5α-reductase levels (converts T into DHT in peripheral tissues) in blacks might responsible for the racial differences but substantial evidence is lacking (18). The composition of the diet was also implicated, as high-fat diets, by increasing the levels of sex hormones, was thought to be responsible for the induction of prostate cancer (19, 20). Genetic factors may also play a role and some prostate cancers show a clear hereditary predisposition (21, 22).

Prostate cancer is, in general, a relatively slow-growing disease: it starts at 30 or 40 years of age and grows over a period of many years to invasive disease through precursor lesions (23, 24); prostate intra-epithelial neoplasia (PIN) and, probably, atypical adenomatous hyperplasia. Not all cases of prostate cancer, however, will develop symptoms during a man's lifetime (25, 26). In fact, the disease is characterized by three different types of clinical manifestations. Thus, most cases remain latent and will never progress to a clinically important disease (type I prostate cancer) (26). Survival rates of up to 87% at 10 years have been reported for untreated localized disease (27, 28). For those cases, however, that will manifest an overt clinical disease, the natural history is quite variable and prostate cancer may either grow slowly and remain localized for many years (type II prostate cancer) or may metastasize and follow a rapidly fetal course (type III prostate cancer) (26). The median survival for such patients with metastatic disease ranges from 24 to 36 months (29).

This unpredictable biological behavior of prostate cancer is probably due to its great heterogeneity in terms of histological Gleason's grade, stage of disease and genetic alterations. There is, therefore, a need to define reliable biological markers that would accurately predict the clinical behavior of the individual tumor and determine the appropriate treatment.

The genesis and progression of prostate cancer—growth kinetics

The currently accepted theory of carcinogenesis holds that multiple genetic alterations, both inherited and somatic, are important in the process of malignant transformation. Such alterations have been studied extensively in colorectal cancer and a model of multi-step tumor progression has been proposed in which the activation of oncogenes and the loss of function of tumor suppressor genes are of paramount importance (30). In this model, a variety of polypeptide growth factors and their receptors may also play a role. Cytogenetic information on prostate cancer has been sparse, however, a similar process of progressive genetic changes was thought to occur in prostate cancer cells (31–33).

In general, the time from tumor initiation and progression to invasive prostate cancer is long, beginning early in life, perhaps in the third or fourth decade of age, and extending over many years (23, 24). What causes irreversible changes in the genome of previously normal cells and renders them susceptible to malignant transformation is obscure but, certainly, prostate cancer cannot develop in the absence of hormones (5). Pathological changes preceding prostate cancer have long been recognized and have been associated with an increased risk of developing cancer. The earliest histologically detectable precursor lesions include prostatic intra-epithelial neoplasia (PIN) and, probably, atypical adenomatous hyperplasia. These are small acinar lesions, usually a few millimeters in diameter, showing a spectrum of atypical cytological features which are, however, surrounded by an intact basement membrane (34–36). It is assumed that at this *in situ* or pre-invasive stage, which may persist for years, the neoplastic lesion lacks its own capillary network, resulting in slow growth and a dormant state (37–39).

The critical events that trigger the evolution of a focal intra-epithelial lesion into a rapidly expanding invasive neoplasm (tumor progression) are not well understood. They, certainly, involve an uncontrolled proliferative activity of cells combined with prevention of cell death by inhibiting apoptosis and induction of tumor angiogenesis. Indeed, intratumoral angiogenesis is of fundamental importance in prostate cancer progression (40–44). Tumors cannot grow beyond the size of 1–2 mm unless they are supported by ingrowth of new capillaries (45). New blood-vessel formation is stimulated by a number of tumor angiogenesis factors (vascular endothelial growth factor, VEGF; basic fibroblast growth factor, bFGF; transforming growth factor β1, TGF-β1), which are released by the tumor itself, the tumor supporting stroma, or by macrophages and lymphocytes in the tumor stroma. The richly vascularized neoplasm begins to grow rapidly, invades the surrounding tissues, through ruptures of the basement membrane, and eventually metastasize (24, 38, 39, 46, 47). The metastatic potential of a prostatic tumor is determined by the size of the primary tumor, the Gleason's grade, the presence of genetic alterations

and, apparently, by an increased tumor angiogenesis (46, 47). The increased oxygen and nutrient supply results in an increased number of proliferating cells, which favor the appearance of new subclones of tumor cells with a more malignant phenotype (37).

The study of cell proliferation in tumors is of equal importance in understanding biological behavior. Tumor kinetics have been studied extensively by several methods based on mitotic counts (thymidine labeling, bromodeoxyuridine incorporation, AgNOR quantitation, and cytometric DNA analysis) (48–51) and, more recently, by using monoclonal antibodies (ki-67, proliferating cell nuclear antigen or PCNA) directed against nuclear antigens expressed in all phases of the cell cycle other than Go. Feneley *et al.* (52), using the antibody ki-67, found that the proliferation index for malignant acini is consistently higher (1.6–16%) than that of benign acini (0.19–4.0%) which, on average, show a volume increase of 1.6–2% per year (53, 54). Ruddon describes that during the latent phase of tumor growth, which may persist for up to 10 years, the neoplasm reaches a diameter of 1 or 2mm (10^6 tumor cells or 1mg tumor mass) (37). In the rapid phase of tumor growth, which follows an accelerated intratumoral angiogenesis (38, 39, 46, 47), the growth becomes rapid and a clinically detectable lesion of approximately 1 cm in diameter (10^9 tumor cells or 1 g tumor mass) may develop within a few months or years (37). A neoplasm of this size can be detected clinically by sensitive diagnostic methods. During the next few years, an untreated neoplasm could potentially approach a large size (10^{12} tumor cells or 1 kg tumor mass) (37) and metastasize (45). It is important to note, however, that the above growth kinetics represent only an approximation of the tumor burden for they do not take into account apoptosis. Tumor cell loss is dramatic in the central, less well-vascularised areas of the tumor, where there is deprivation of oxygen and nutrients. Furthermore, not all prostate tumors are equally vascularized, as some exhibit a higher microvessel density than others.

Such epithelial cell proliferation is stimulated by several polypeptide growth factors, which are synthesized and secreted by prostate cancer cells; these include the epidermal growth factor (EGF), the insulin-like growth factor (IGF), the fibroblast growth factor (FGF) (55, 56), the transforming growth factor-α (TGF-α) (57–59), and the transforming growth factor-β-1 (TGF-β1) and TGF-β2 (58, 60, 61). Growth factor receptors for these ligands are acting through a transmembrane glycoprotein receptor and tyrosine kinase and their expression is increased in prostate cancer. In this context,

Price *et al.* demonstrated a 15-fold increase in extracellular signal-regulated kinase activation in prostate cancer specimens compared with normal human prostate tissue (55). In addition, several neuropeptides, such as bombesin, calcitonin, parathyroid hormone related peptide, serotonin and endothelin, are potent mitogens for prostate cancer cells and induce epithelial cell proliferation, mainly through paracrine stimulatory mechanisms (62–65). These active agents are synthesized and secreted by the neuroendocrine cells (66), scattered as they are throughout the epithelial cells, and may also have a role in the genesis and progression of prostate cancer. Thus, an increase number of neuroendocrine cells are associated with progression towards an advanced or an androgen-independent tumor state (65, 67, 68) and with an increased detection of serum neuroendocrine markers (chromogranin A and NSE) (69).

Another factor that is important in determining tumor growth and the neoplastic phenotype of the initiated cells is the milieu in which tumor progression takes place. Stromal and epithelial cells both produce a great number of mitogenic and inhibitory substances, which react in an autocrine, paracrine, and/or intracrine manner, resulting in growth stimulation, inhibition, and apoptosis (70, 71). It is probable that imbalances in the stromal-epithelial interactions are important in the pathogenesis of prostate cancer (72, 73). Furthermore, the high proliferation rate, combined with the genomic liability of neoplastic cells, may generate a large number of phenotypic variants that are under the pressure of environmental selection (immune surveillance, nutrient supply, etc.) for survival (37). This view could explain, at least in part, the heterogeneity and karyotypic variability within the same tumor.

The aforementioned growth kinetics that occur in malignant tumors in general, and in prostate cancer in particular, are the immediate result of acquisition of the malignant phenotype after progressive accumulation of multiple genetic changes.

Prostatic intra-epithelial neoplasia and atypical adenomatous hyperplasia: relationship to prostate cancer

Prostatic intra-epithelial neoplasia (PIN) is the immediate precursor of invasive prostate cancer (24, 74, 75). It represents an atypical proliferation of secretary cells within pre-existing ducts and acini (74, 76, 77). The morphological continuum that merges into early invasive cancer is divided into low- and high-grade lesions (78).

Low-grade lesions (PIN 1) display crowding of the secretary cells, nuclear stratification, and variation in nuclear size. The nucleoli are inconspicuous. The basal cell layer is intact. High-grade lesions (PIN 2 and 3) are characterized by cytological features that are indistinguishable from those of malignant cells (75). Cellular crowding and nuclear stratification is exuberant. Hyperchromatism is distinct. Nucleoli are conspicuous and, often, multiple. The basal cell layer is retained, but it is usually incomplete. It is selectively demonstrated by monoclonal antibodies directed against high-molecular weight keratins (e.g. 34β-E12) (79). There is no stromal invasion.

The reported incidence of PIN in needle biopsy specimens varies from 8 to 31% (80–82). Data from the USA indicate that the prevalence of the lesion is higher in African-American men than in whites (83), following a similar trend with prostate cancer. It has been also postulated that PIN precedes the development of prostate cancer by several years (84) and, indeed, low-grade PIN first occurs in the third (85), fourth or fifth decade of life (24). Others found that its prevalence in prostates with cancer increases with age, predating the onset of carcinoma by more than 5 years (86, 87). Several other studies have demonstrated that patients whose initial biopsies reveal high-grade PIN, but not prostate cancer, have a 50% risk of prostate cancer on subsequent biopsies (81, 88–90).

As a direct pre-invasive lesion, high-grade PIN is significantly more common in prostates with cancer than in those without the disease (on average 67.7% versus 11.2%) (34, 84, 86, 91–93). Similarly, large and multiple foci of PIN (size greater than 4.5 mm, number more than 10) occur significantly more frequently in cancer specimens than in cancer-free prostates (33% versus 7%, and 71% versus 15%, respectively) (91). By contrast, the extent of PIN is inversely proportional to the stage of the invasive disease, as high-stage tumors tend to obliterate the co-existing foci of pre-invasive lesions (92–94). With regard to the site of development, low- and high-grade PINs show a close topographic relationship with prostate cancer (91, 93): 86% of PIN arise in the peripheral zone, 13% occur in the central zone, and only 1% of PIN originates in the transition zone of the prostate (91, 95).

Furthermore, PIN and prostate cancer share most measures of nuclear abnormality in common, i.e. nuclear area, nuclear perimeter, nuclear diameter, chromatin heterogeneity, and chromatin condensation

(96–98). The number, the size, and the location of nucleoli are also similar in PIN and in prostate cancer, and significantly different from those of the non-neoplastic epithelium (96, 99–101). Proliferating cell nuclear antigen (PCNA) immunoreactivity, mitoses, and apoptosis are higher in PIN lesions than are in benign prostatic hyperplasia or normal tissues (102, 103) and, in many cases, the number of proliferating cells in high-grade PIN exceeds that of well-differentiated invasive carcinomas (102, 104).

The transmembrane glycoprotein Ep-CAM is expressed strongly in both PIN and prostate cancer, in contrast to benign prostatic epithelium (105). Glycoprotein expression, on the other hand, is decreased in both conditions, as this is indicated by binding to a number of lectins (106–108). Other features in common include the loss of expression of blood groups A and B (106), alterations in acid mucin production (109), and a decreased expression of vimentin (108).

Cytoplasmic reactivity with PSA, PAP and Leu.7 show a progressive loss with increasing grades of PIN, indicating an impairment of cell differentiation with advancing grade of pre-invasive disease (106, 108–111). There is, however, an abrupt re-expression of these proteins at the invading tumor front, which is associated with an increase activity of type IV collagenase in both PIN and prostate cancer (112).

Further clues for an intimate relationship between PIN and prostate cancer are provided by the existence of common genetic alterations, including the loss of chromosomes 8p, 10q, 16q, 18q, and the gain of chromosomes 7 and 8q (113–122). The p27/Kip1 gene is widely expressed in normal and hyperplastic prostatic tissues, but it is down-regulated in high-grade PIN and invasive disease (123). The nm23-H1 gene product, a potential suppressor of metastasis, is consistently detected in both lesions (124), and PIN often shows non-diploid patterns as a sign of genetic instability (75, 96, 125–127). In fact, 30% of PINs are aneuploid and 70% of these were associated with aneuploid carcinomas (128).

The above data supports the concept that PIN is a true precursor of prostate cancer and its identification, therefore, in a biopsy specimen requires continuous observation (24). The detection of low-grade PIN is associated with an adjacent invasive carcinoma in 13–18% of cases, whereas high-grade PIN accompanies invasive carcinomas in 33–100% of cases (104).

With regard to atypical adenomatous hyperplasia (AAH), or adenosis, this is another prostatic lesion that has been proposed as a precursor of adenocarcinoma (129), although the evidence for this is not conclusive (104). The lesion has been identified in prostates from men under the age of 40 with an incidence of approximately 20% (130, 131, 132). It is characterized by small acinar proliferations, which may or may not accompanied by cytological atypia (129, 130). The acinar proliferations are usually multiple and vary in size from 2 to 7 mm (131). They form a spectrum of morphological changes ranging from minimal architectural and cytological atypia to those that are indistinguishable from a well-differentiated adenocarcinoma (25). AAH occurs more frequently in association with cancer (31% in prostates with cancer versus 15% in those without) and it usually arises in the peripheral zone of the prostate (131, 133).

Genetic alterations in prostate cancer cells

The molecular mechanisms responsible for the initiation and progression of prostate cancer are elusive, despite of voluminous research. There is, however, strong evidence that carcinogenesis proceeds through a series of genetic alterations, involving the activation of oncogenes and the loss of function (inactivation) of tumor-suppressor genes (134), and the inhibition of apoptosis. Growth factors and growth-factor receptors may also play a role. The tumor is characterized by widely heterogeneous growth patterns, ranging from slow indolent incidental lesions to rapidly progressive disease with a tendency for early metastasis. Not unexpectedly, prostate cancer is associated with a similar heterogeneity of genetic alterations (135).

Chromosomal abnormalities

Allelic loss

The most common genetic alterations identified in prostate cancer are loss of heterozygosity (LOH) of chromosome arms 7q, 8p, 10q, 16q, and 18q (21, 113–115, 136–138). The high frequency with which such allelic losses occur, at one or more chromosomal loci, suggest that these regions contain tumor-suppressor genes that are potentially important for the initiation and progression of prostate neoplasia (32, 135).

The deletion colon carcinoma (DCC) gene, a tumor-suppressor gene that is not restricted to colon cancer, shows allelic deletion and loss of expression more frequently in advanced prostate cancer compared with localized disease, indicating that inactivation of this gene is a late event in prostate cancer (139, 140).

Another tumor-suppressor gene that is important in tumor progression is the APC (adenomatous polyposis coli) gene (140). Inactivation of this molecule may also play a role in the progression of prostate cancer (140).

Recently, a region on the long arm of chromosome 1 (1q24–25) has been identified as containing a gene, the HPC1, which is responsible for the development of hereditary prostate cancer (22). This genetic defect occurs in approximately one-third of cases of hereditary prostate cancer (22).

Gain

Genetic alterations involving gains of chromosomes, particularly those of 7 and 8, have also been reported, and are thought as being markers of prostate tumor aggressiveness and prognosis (120).

Ploidy

DNA ploidy of prostate cancer is an important marker of tumor progression and patient's survival (141–144). This is not unexpected since the aneuploid status correlates well with high histological grade, high stage of disease and post-operative recurrence (145, 146). In fact, ploidy is more accurate than Gleason grade for predicting recurrence (145, 147). On the other hand, early hormonal therapy offers a survival advantage in patients with diploid tumors (148).

Apoptosis related genes

p53

The p53 gene is located on the short arm of chromosome 17, and p53 mutation in prostate cancer is related with tumor progression (149–153). This protein product of the p53 tumor-suppressor gene (154) is involved in the regulation of cell cycle (155) and the apoptosis pathway (156, 157). Mutations of the p53 gene have been found in many human tumors, including prostate cancer (158–160). They lead to a pro-

longed half-life of the protein, allowing nuclear accumulation of the p53 protein and its detection by immunohistochemical techniques. Positive immunostaininig varies widely, ranging from 4% (159) to 65% (161). This great variability in the reported incidence reflects the widespread heterogeneity of p53 mutations that exists from tumor to tumor and within individual tumors (162). Most investigators showed an increase in p53 mutations in advanced/metastatic lesions (163–167), suggesting that it may be a late event in the progression of prostate cancer (158, 165, 168–170). p53 mutation is associated with an increased proliferation rate, high grade and stage, and androgen independence (160, 168–170). Others failed to confirm these results (171, 172), and still others detected p53 nuclear accumulation in PIN lesions suggesting that it may be an early event in a subset of prostate cancers (173). The data on survival are conflicting, but many investigators correlated p53 immunohistochemical staining with poor prognosis (152, 160, 174–176). Similarly, the expression of p53 in prostate cancer may be associated with resistance to radiotherapy in much the same way as the expression of bcl-2.

bcl-2 and family

The proto-oncogene bcl-2 encodes a protein that inhibits apoptosis (177) and has been associated with progression (153, 178–180). Early studies suggested that this anti-apoptotic protein is often undetectable in hormone-dependent prostate cancers, but high levels are found in hormone-independent tumors (181, 182). It is also infrequent in localized malignant disease (159). Aberrant expression of bcl-2 has been correlated with reduced disease-free survival (175) and with cancer recurrences after radical prostatectomy (183) or external beam radiation therapy (149, 181, 184). This is because radiation therapy is particularly dependent on the induction of apoptotic cellular pathways and, therefore, it may depend on the expression of apoptotic regulator proteins bcl-2 and p53. Thus, pretreatment needle biopsy may serve as an independent prognostic marker for predicting response to radiotherapy.

Retinoblastoma gene

The retinoblastoma gene (RB) is located on the short arm of chromosome 13. It encodes a protein that has been implicated in the regulation of the cell cycle (185). In addition of being present in all cases of retinoblastoma, mutations of the RB gene have been identified in various human neoplasms, including prostate cancer (186–188). Inactivation at chromosome 13q of the retinoblastoma (RB) tumor-suppressor gene, seen only infrequently in prostate cancers, is associated with advance stage of disease (186).

Hormones and hormone receptors

It is generally accepted that androgens may play a critical role in the development of prostate cancer by acting as mitogens (5). The SRD5A2 locus, in particular, is a hot spot for somatic mutations, which can result in cytogenetic abnormalities on 2p23 chromosome, and alterations in the enzymatic activity of the 5α-reductase may initiate prostate cancer progression (189). Furthermore, androgens stimulate endothelial cell proliferation and ingrowth of new blood vessels (65, 190, 191) and loss of androgen regulation of VEGF synthesis is connected with progression of prostate cancer to an androgen independent state (190).

The androgen receptor (AR) acts as a hormone receptor complex that interacts with its target genes to regulate transcription. Mutations in the AR gene are not uncommon in metastatic prostate cancer (192, 193) and may increase the sensitivity of cells to androgens (193). However, androgen-receptor expression is not associated with tumor progression or patient survival in primary prostate cancer, but its expression in lymph node metastases appears to be an independent prognostic factor in men with advanced prostate cancer (194).

Another androgen-regulated protein, the apolipoprotein D (Apo-D), was shown to be a marker of malignant transformation in the prostate and may be involved in the initiation or maintenance of the transformed phenotype (195). Indeed, malignant transformation in the prostate is associated with increased cellular levels of Apo-D.

Growth factors and growth factor receptors

EGF and EGFR

A number of polypeptide growth hormones have been implicated in growth control of human prostate cancer (57, 196). Of these, three growth factor families have been the most extensively studied: the epidermal growth factor family (EGF), the transforming growth factor-α and -β (TGF-α, TGF-β), and the fibroblast growth factor family (FGF). Polypeptide growth factors

may influence prostate cancer cells by intracrine, paracrine and autocrine mechanisms (32).

The EGF and the TGF-α secreted by prostate cancer cells may interact with EGF-receptor in the formation of an autocrine loop of cell proliferation (57). Activation of the EGF-receptor in prostate cancer cells by EGF or TGF-α may cause mitogenesis, invasiveness, and regulation of specific cellular genes (197). Basic fibroblast growth factor (bFGF) has also been implicated as a mitogen for human prostate cancer cells (57, 198).

c-erbB-2

The c-erbB-2 oncogene encodes a transmembrane protein, with tyrosine-kinase activity, which shares structural and sequence homology with the epidermal growth factor receptor (EGFR) (199). c-erbB-2 oncoprotein blocks gap-junctional intercellular communication and disrupts the cadherin–catenin cell–cell adhesion system, facilitating tumor growth and metastasis (200, 201). Most studies on c-erbB-2 expression in the prostate found increased expression with cancer (202). Data are conflicting regarding its prognostic significance (202, 203), but it is generally believed that c-erb-B2 over-expression is associated with aggressive tumor behavior and a decreased survival in patients with prostate cancer (204).

Angiogenic factors and angiogenesis

Tumor growth beyond a certain size depends upon angiogenesis. New blood-vessel formation is a typical feature of aggressive tumors, including prostate cancer. Microvessel density (MVD) is significantly associated with nuclear grade, Gleason grade, and pathological stage (205–207). It is also related with time to recurrence (205) and with disease-specific survival (206). The 5-year recurrence-free survival is significantly lower for patients with a MVD 90 or greater than for those with a MVD less than 90 (205).

Tumor angiogenesis is controlled by chemical signals, known as angiogenic factors. Vascular endothelial growth factor (VEGF) is a cytokine that is most frequently associated with angiogenic activity (208, 209) in prostate cancer (210). Immunohistochemical studies revealed that increased levels of VEGF are present in prostate cancer but not in benign prostatic hyperplasia or normal prostate cells *in vivo* (209). Similarly, patients with metastatic prostate cancer have significantly higher plasma VEGF levels (28 pg/ml) than patients with localized disease (7.0 pg/ml) or healthy controls (0 pg/ml) (210). Interestingly, patients with serum PSA greater than 20 ng/ml have significantly higher plasma VEGF values than patients with serum PSA less than 20 ng/ml (210). Increased VEGF secretion contributes to the progression of prostate cancer by promoting angiogenesis (211).

Cell-adhesion molecules

The CD44, a transmembrane glycoprotein involved with cell adhesion, has recently been identified as a metastatic suppressor for prostate cancer (212–214). A decreased expression of CD44 is associated with increased histological Gleason's grade and metastases. The potential prognostic significance of CD44 has not been investigated sufficiently, but the loss of CD44 expression may signify an adverse prognostic behavior (215).

E-cadherin, a typical cell-adhesion molecule with invasion/metastasis suppressor activity, has been shown to be reduced in high-grade prostate tumors and to correlate with advanced stage, metastasis, and poor survival (21, 216). Similarly, LOH at chromosome 16q24, which harbors the E-cadherin gene, is significantly related with a high metastatic potential of prostate tumors (21).

C-CAM is another adhesion molecule the inactivation of which was associated with malignant transformation. It was thought to be a unique marker of early prostate carcinogenesis (33).

The transmembrane glycoprotein Ep-CAM, which is localized to the basal and lateral aspects of prostatic epithelial cells, is also involved in cell adhesion (217). Compared with benign prostatic epithelium, Ep-CAM is expressed strongly in both PIN and prostate cancer (105), representing an early event in the development of prostate cancer. This is somewhat contradictory since it is the loss of cellular adhesion that is generally considered as a hallmark in the neoplastic process. It has been suggested, however, that, in the case of Ep-CAM, an increased expression of the glycoprotein on the surface of tumor cells is associated with a reduced adhesiveness of other adhesion molecules, leading to an increased potential of tumor cell invasiveness (217).

Other cell-adhesion molecules include mucin genes and MUC1 protein epitopes. MUC1 epitopes are frequently expressed on the apical cell membranes, although neoplastic transformation may be associated with aberrant expression and, less frequently, with loss

of expression of membrane-bound mucins (218). It is assumed that such changes are, probably, the result of altered mucin mRNA levels and/or altered mucin glycosylation (218).

Tumor-suppressor genes

The nm23-H1 gene has been associated with suppressor of metastasis in many solid tumors, including prostate cancer (219, 220). The cellular mechanisms by which the nm23 protein modulate the metastatic phenotype are not yet known, but the protein was shown to be located on human chromosome 17 (221). All prostate cancer specimens and areas of prostatic intra-epithelial neoplasia (PIN) showed immunoreactivity with nm23-H1/NDPKA antibody, whilst normal prostatic tissues were unreactive (219). Comparable results have been reported for prostate carcinoma cell lines (221–223). It is believed that over-expression of nm23-H1/NDPKA gene occurs frequently in prostate cancer and may be an early event in prostate tumorigenesis (219). Other studies showed that an intense nm23-H1 staining of cells is significantly more frequent in primary sites of clinically malignant disease than in latent prostate cancers, indicating that there is a biologically different population of cells within the latent cancers (220). Furthermore, the nm23-H1 gene was related to cell proliferation and tumor metastatic potential (220).

The p27/kip1 gene, like other members of cyclin-dependent kinase inhibitors, encodes a small protein that has been postulated to be a possible tumor-suppressor gene. The down-regulation of p27/kip1 is a common phenomenon in prostate cancer, occurring in the early phases of neoplastic transformation (123). It is associated with an increased proliferation, and with a reduction in intercellular adhesion (224). Interestingly, the *in vitro* down-regulation of the p27/kip1 gene has a most important effect in sensitization against some chemotherapeutic agents (224). This possibility merits further investigation because of its possible therapeutic implications.

Another gene that has been implicated as a metastasis suppressor gene for prostate cancer is the KA11. This was isolated from chromosome 11p (225). An increased expression of KA11 in prostate cancer may be associated with restraint of tumor progression, whereas a decrease in KA11 gene expression may accompany aggressive cancers through loss of such restraint. It is suggested that KA11 gene expression may serve as a potential marker of metastatic prostate cancer (225).

Other oncogenes

Activated oncogenes, such as H-ras, K-ras, and N-ras are infrequent in prostate cancer and their significance remains uncertain (202, 226, 227). Some studies, however, suggested a correlation of ras oncogenes with higher grade and higher stage prostate cancer (228).

Alterations in c-myc expression in human prostate cancer have not been investigated extensively (229, 230) but, in general, higher levels of c-myc have been associated with prostate malignancy compared with benign prostatic hyperplasia. In one study, high c-myc expression was related with tumors of higher grade, suggesting a link between over-expression of c-myc transcripts and prognosis (230).

Proto-oncogene expression for H-ras, c-myc, and c-jun is significantly higher in drug-resistant than in drug-sensitive prostate cancer cells, indicating that the amplification of early response genes may play a role in the emergence of *de novo* resistance in prostate tumor cells (231). The expression of c-fos, but not of c-jun, oncogene is increased in prostate cancer as compared with benign prostatic hyperplasia and normal prostate (232). This differential expression of oncogenes could possibly be used as markers for progression in human prostate cancer (232). Other studies also indicated that jun/fos are possible markers for tumor progression, since they are present at low levels in organ-confined specimens but are at significantly increased levels in samples exhibiting capsular penetration and localized spread (233).

The oncogenic antigen 519 (OA-519), a molecule expressing haptoglobin-related protein epitopes, is expressed by some prostate cancers, but not by normal or hyperplastic prostate tissues. It is significantly associated with higher tumor grades, larger tumors, and with advancing clinical stage (234). Since high tumor grades, large tumor volumes, and advanced stage of disease are known indicators of poor prognosis, OA-519 expression is considered as being of potential prognostic value in prostate cancer.

Telomerases

Some molecular changes precede the development of prostate cancer or PIN and, therefore, they appear to act at the initiation stage (235). Such changes include an enhanced expression of telomerase activity (236–239).

Telomeres are terminal chromosomal structures that are composed of tandem repeats of the sequence TTAGGG and protein complexes (238). The loss of telomeres, which normally provide stability to chromosome ends, may initiate genomic instability resulting in abnormal chromosomes and uncontrolled proliferation of cells. It is presumed that the telomere length is maintained by telomerase, an unusual DNA polymerase. Telomerase is a ribonucleoprotein enzyme that adds telomeric sequences onto chromosome ends (240). Using the telomeric repeat amplification protocol (TRAP assay), telomerase activity was shown to be essential in the pathogenesis of many human malignancies (241), including prostate cancer (239–245).

Another factor associated with the pathogenesis of prostate cancer is the length of CAG repeats on the androgen receptor. Men with prostate cancer have shorter repeats than age-matched men with benign nodular hyperplasia, and the same applies to white men relative to Japanese who have a low incidence of prostate cancer (21).

References

1. Parker SL, Tong T, Bolden S et al. Cancer statistics, 1997. CA Cancer J Clin 1997, 47, 5–7.
2. OPCS (Office of Population Censuses and Surveys) Mortality statistics: causes. 1991. Monitor DH2. No 18. HMSO, London, 1993.
3. Smith DS, Humphrey PA, Catalona WJ. The early detection of prostate carcinoma with prostate specific antigen. Cancer 1997, 80, 1852–6.
4. Polascik TJ, Oesterling JE, Partin AW. Prostate specific antigen: a decade of discovery—what we have learned and where we are going. J Urol 1999, 162, 293–306.
5. Montie JE, Pienta KJ. Review of the role of androgenic hormone in the epidemiology of benign prostatic hyperplasia and prostate cancer. Urology 1994, 43, 892–9.
6. Andersson SO, Adami HO, Bergstrom WL. Serum pituitary and sex steroid hormone levels in the etiology of prostatic cancer—a population-based case-control study. Brit J Cancer 1993, 68, 97–102.
7. Hsing AW, Comstock GW. Serologic precursors of cancer: serum hormones and risk of subsequent prostate cancer. Cancer Epidemiol Biomarkers Prev 1993, 2, 27–32.
8. Gann PH, Hennekens CH, Ma J et al. Prospective study of sex hormone levels and risk of prostate cancer. J Natl Cancer Inst 1996, 88, 1118–26.
9. Signorello LB, Tzonou A, Mantzoros CS et al. Serum steroids in relation to prostate cancer risk on a case-control study (Greece). Cancer Causes Control 1997, 8, 632–6.
10. Seidman H, Mushinski MH, Gelb et al. Probabilities of eventually developing or dying of cancer—United States, 1985. CA Cancer J Clin 1985, 35, 36–56.
11. Nomura AMY, Kolonel LN. Prostate cancer: a current perspective. Epidemiol Rev 1991, 13, 200–27.

12. Morra MN, Das S. Prostate cancer: epidemiology and etiology. In: *Cancer of the prostate* (ed. S Das, ED Crawford). Marcel Dekker, New York, 1993, 1–12.

13. Morton RA Jr. Racial differences in adenocarcinoma of the prostate in North American men. *Urology* 1994, **44**, 637–45.

14. Sohayda CJ, Kupelian PA, Altsman KA *et al*. Race as an independent predictor of outcome after treatment for localized prostate cancer. *J Urol* 1999, **162**, 1331–6.

15. Fowler JE Jr, Bigler SA, Bowman G *et al*. Race and cause specific survival with prostate cancer: influence of clinical stage, Gleason score, age and treatment. *J Urol* 2000, **163**, 137–42.

16. Morra MN, Das S. Prostate cancer: epidemiology and etiology. In: *Cancer of the prostate* (ed. S Das, ED Crawford). Marcel Dekker, New York, 1993, 1–12.

17. Cook LS, Goldoft M, Schwartz SM *et al*. Incidence of adenocarcinoma of the prostate in Asian immigrants to the United States and their descendants. *J Urol* 1999, **161**, 152–5.

18. Ross RK, Bernstein L, Lobo RA *et al*. 5α-Reductase activity and risk of prostate cancer among Japanese and U.S. white and black males. *Lancet* 1992, **339**, 887–9.

19. Nelson PS, Gleason TP, Brawer MK. Chemoprevention for prostatic intra-epithelial neoplasia. *Eur Urol* 1996, **30**, 269–78.

20. Hayes RB, Ziegler RG, Gridley G *et al*. Dietary factors and risks for prostate cancer among blacks and whites in the United States. *Cancer Epidemiol Biomarkers Prev* 1999, **8**, 25–34.

21. Isaacs WB, Bova GS, Morton RA *et al*. Molecular genetics and chromosomal alterations in prostate cancer. *Cancer* 1995, **75**, 2004.

22. Smith JR, Carpten J, Kallioniemi O *et al*. Major susceptibility locus for prostate cancer on chromosome 1 revealed by a genome-wide search. *Science* 1996, **274**, 1371–4.

23. Sakr WA, Haas GP, Cassin BJ *et al*. The frequency of carcinoma and intra-epithelial neoplasia of the prostate in young male patients. *J Urol* 1993, **150**, 379–85.

24. Montironi R, Mazzucchelli R, Marshall JR *et al*. Prostate cancer prevention: review of target populations, pathological biomarkers, and chemopreventive agents. *J Clin Pathol* 1999, **52**, 793–803.

25. Bostwick DG. Pathology of prostate cancer. In: *Prostate cancer* (ed. MS Ernstoff, JA Heaney, RE Peschel). Blackwell Science, London, 1998, 15–47.

26. von Eschenbach EC. The biologic dilemma of early carcinoma of the prostate. *Cancer* 1996, **78**, 326–9.

27. Johansson JE, Adami HO, Andersson SO *et al*. High 10 year survival rate in patients with early, untreated prostatic cancer. *JAMA* 1992, **267**, 2191–6.

28. Chodak GW, Thisted RA, Gerber GS *et al*. Recent results of conservative management of clinically localized prostate cancer. *N Engl J Med* 1994, **330**, 242–8.

29. Prostate Cancer Trialists' Collaborative Group. Maximum androgen blockade in advanced prostate cancer: an overview of 22 randomised trials with 3283 deaths in 5710 patients. *Lancet* 1995, **346**, 265–9.

30. Fearon ER, Vogelstein B. A genetic model for colorectal tumorigenesis. *Cell* 1990, **61**, 759–67.

31. Isaacs WB, Carter BS. Genetic changes associated prostate cancer in humans. In: *Prostate cancer: cell and molecular mechanisms in diagnosis and treatment. cancer surveys, vol 11* (ed. JT Isaacs). Cold Spring Harbor, NY, Cold Spring Harbor Laboratory, 1991, 15–24.

32. Netto GJ, Humphrey PA. Molecular biologic aspects of human prostatic carcinoma. *Am J Clin Pathol* 1994, **102** (Suppl 1), S57–64.

33. Pu YS, Luo W, Lu HH *et al*. Differential expression of C-CAM cell-adhesion molecule in prostate carcinogenesis in a transgenic mouse model. *J Urol* 1999, **162**, 892–6.

34. McNeal JE, Bostwick DG. Intraductal dysplasia: a premalignant lesion of the prostate. *Hum Pathol* 1986, **17**, 64–71.

35. Bostwick DG, Brawer MK. Prostatic intra-epithelial neoplasia and early invasion in prostate cancer. *Cancer* 1987, **59**, 788–94.

36. Amin MB, Ro JY, Ayala AG. Prostatic intra-epithelial neoplasia. Relationship to adenocarcinoma of prostate. In: *Pathology annual: nineteen ninety-four. Part 2/Vol 29* (ed. PP Rosen, RE Fechner). Appleton & Lange. Norwalk, Connecticut, 1994, 1–30.

37. Ruddon RW. Biology of tumor metastasis. In: *Cancer biology* (3rd edn) (ed. RW Ruddon). Oxford University Press, New York, 1995, 402–427.

38. Siegal JA, Yu E, Brawer Mk. Topography of neovascularity in human prostate caricnoma. *Cancer* 1995, **75**, 2545–51.

39. Montironi R, Diamanti L, Thormpson D *et al*. Analysis of the capillary architecture in the precursors of prostate cancer: recent findings and new oncogens. *Eur Urol* 1996, **30**, 191–200.

40. Wakui S, Furasato M, Itoh T *et al*. Tumour angiogenesis in prostatic carcinoma with and without bone marrow metastasis: a morphometric study. *J Pathol* 1992, **168**, 257–62.

41. Brawer MK, Deering RE, Brown M *et al*. Predictors of pathologic stage in prostatic carcinoma. *Cancer* 1994, **73**, 678–87.

42. Furasato M, Wakui S, Sasaki H *et al*. Tumour angiogenesis in latent prostatic carcinoma. *Br J Cancer* 1994, **70**, 1244–6.

43. McNeal JE, Yemoto CEM. Significance of demonstrable vascular space invasion for the progression of prostatic adenocarcinoma. *Am J Surg Pathol* 1996, **20**, 1351–60.

44. Franck Lissbrant I, Stattin P, Damber JE *et al*. Vascular density is a predictor of Cancer specific survival in prostatic carcinoma. *Prostate* 1997, **33**, 38–45.

45. Folkman J. The role of angiogenesis in tumour growth. *Semin Cancer Biol* 1992, **3**, 65–71.

46. Weidner N, Caroll P, Flax J *et al*. Tumor angiogenesis correlates with metastasis in invasive prostate cancer. *Am J Pathol* 1993, **143**, 401–9.

47. Brawer M, Deering R, Brown M *et al*. Predictors of pathological stage in prostatic cancer—the role of neovascularity. *Cancer* 1994, **73**, 678–87.

48. Quinn CM, Wright NA. The clinical assessment of proliferation and growth of human tumours: evaluation of methods and applications as prognostic variables. *J Pathol* 1990, **160**, 93–102.

49. Hall PA, Levison DA. Review: assessment of cell proliferation in histological material. *J Clin Pathol* 1990, **43**, 184–92.

50. Yu CC, Filipe MI. Update on proliferation-associated antibodies applicable to formalin-fixed, paraffin embedded tissue and their clinical applications. *Histochem J* 1993, **25**, 843–53.

51. Hall PA, Coates PJ. Assessment of cell proliferation in pathology—what next? *Histopathology* 1995, **26**, 105–12.

52. Feneley MR, Young MPA, Chinyama C *et al.* Ki-67 expression in early prostate cancer and associated pathological lesions. *J Clin Pathol* 1996, **49**, 741–8.

53. Rhodes T, Girman CJ, Jacobsen SJ *et al.* Longitudinal prostate growth rates during 5 years in randomly selected community men 40 to 79 years old. *J Urol* 1999, **161**, 1174–9.

54. Bosch JLHR, Hop WCJ, Niemer AQHJ *et al.* Parameters of prostate volume and shape in a community based population of men 55 to 74 years old. *J Urol* 1994, **152**, 1501–5.

55. Price DT, Rocca GD, Guo C *et al.* Activation of extracellular-regulated kinase in human prostate cancer. *J Urol* 1999, **162**, 1537–42.

56. Maygarden SJ, Strom S, Ware JL. Localization of epidermal growth factor receptor by immunohistochemical methods in human prostatic carcinoma, prostatic intraepithelial neoplasia, and benign hyperplasia. *Arch Pathol Lab Med* 1992, **116**, 269–73.

57. Steiner MS. Role of peptide growth in the prostate: a review. *Urology* 1993, **42**, 99–110.

58. Myers RB, Kudlow JE, Grizzle WE. Expression of transforming growth factor-α, epidermal growth factor and the epidermal growth factor receptor in adenocarcinoma of the prostate and benign prostatic hyperplasia. *Mod Pathol* 1993, **6**, 733–7.

59. Harper ME, Goddard L, Glynne-Jones E *et al.* An immunocytochemical analysis of TGF-α expression in benign and malignant prostatic tumors. *Prostate* 1993, **23**, 9–23.

60. Thompson TC, Truong LD, Timme TL *et al.* Transforming growth factor *B*-1 as a biomarker for prostate cancer. *J Cell Biochem* 1992, **16H** (Suppl), 54–61.

61. Eklov S, Funa K, Nordgren H *et al.* Lack of the latent transforming growth factor β binding protein in malignant, but not benign prostatic tissue. *Cancer Res* 1993, **53**, 3193–7.

62. Di Sant'Agnese PA. Neuroendocrine differentiation in carcinoma of the prostate. Diagnostic, prognostic and therapeutic implications. *Cancer* 1992, **70** (1 Suppl), 254–68.

63. Di Sant'Agnese PA, Cockett AT. The prostatic endocrine-paracrine (neuroendocrine) regulatory system and neuroendocrine differentiation in prostatic carcinoma: a review and future directions in basic research. *J Urol* 1994, **152**, 1927–31.

64. Krijnen JL, Bogdanowicz JF, Seldenrijk CA *et al.* The prognostic value of neuroendocrine differentiation in adenocarcinoma of the prostate in relation to progression of disease after endocrine therapy. *J Urol* 1997, **158**, 171–4.

65. Burchardt T, Burchardt M, Chen MW *et al.* Transdifferentiation of prostate cancer cells to a neuroendocrine cell phenotype *in vitro* and *in vivo*. *J Urol* 1999, **162**, 1800–5.

66. Abrahamsson PA. Neuroendocrine differentiation in the human prostate gland. *Curr Trends Exp Endocrinol* 1994, **2**, 21.

67. Abrahamsson PA. Neuroendocrine differentiation and hormone-refractory prostate cancer. *Prostate* 1996, **6** (Suppl), 3–8.

68. Weinstein MH, Partin AW, Veltri RW *et al.* Neuroendocrine differentiation in prostate cancer: enhanced prediction of progression after radical prostatectomy. *Hum Pathol* 1996, **27**, 683–7.

69. Cussenot O, Villete JM, Cochand-Priollet B *et al.* Evaluation and clinical value of neuroendocrine differentiation in human prostatic tumours. *Prostate* 1998, **8** (Suppl), 43–51.

70. Planz B, Kirley SD, Wang Q *et al.* Characterization of a stromal cell model of the human benign and malignant prostate from explant culture. *J Urol* 1999, **161**, 1329–36.

71. Nemeth JA, Lee C. Prostatic ductal system in rats: regional variationin stromal organization. *Prostate* 1996, **28**, 124–8.

72. Chung LW, Gleave ME, Hsieh JT *et al.* Reciprocal mesenchymal-epithelial interaction affecting prostate tumour growth and hormonal responsiveness. *Cancer Surv* 1991, **11**, 91–121.

73. Cunha GR, Hayward SW, Dahiya R *et al.* Smooth muscle-epithelial interactions in normal and neoplastic prostatic development. *Acta Anat* 1996, **155**, 63–72.

74. Bostwick DG, Brawer MK. Prostatic intra-epithelial neoplasia and early invasion in prostate cancer. *Cancer* 1987, **59**, 788–94.

75. Bostwick DG. High grade prostatic intra-epithelial neoplasia: the most likely precursor of prostate cancer. *Cancer* 1995, **75**, 1823.

76. McNeal JE, Bostwick DG. Intraductal dysplasia: a premalignant lesion of the prostate. *Hum Pathol* 1986, **17**, 64–71.

77. Amin MB, Ro JY, Ayala AG. Prostatic intra-epithelial neoplasia. Relationship to adenocarcinoma of prostate. In: *Pathology annual: nineteen ninety-four. Part 2/Vol 29* (ed. PP Rosen, RE Fechner). Appleton & Lange. Norwalk, Connecticut, 1994, 1–30.

78. Epstein JI, Grignan DJ, Humphrey PA *et al.* Interobserver reproducibility in the diagnosis of prostatic intra-epithelial neoplasia. *Am J Surg Pathol* 1995, **19**, 873–86.

79. Brawer MK, Peehl DM, Stamey TA *et al.* Keratin immunoreactivity in benign and neoplastic human prostate. *Cancer Res* 1985, **45**, 3663–7.

80. Lee F, Torp-Pedersen ST, Carroll JT *et al.* Use of transrectal ultrasound and prostate-specific antigen in diagnosis of prostatic intra-epithelial neoplasia. *Urology* 1989, **34** (Suppl), 4–8.

81. Keetch DW, Humphrey P, Stahl D *et al.* Morphometric analysis and clinical follow up of isolated prostatic intra-epithelial neoplasia in needle biopsy of the prostate. *J Urol* 1995, **154**, 347–51.

82. Bostwick DG, Qian J, Frankel K. The incidence of high grade prostatic intra-epithelial neoplasia in needle biopsies. *J Urol* 1995, **154**, 1791–4.

83. Sakr WA, Grignon DJ, Haas GP *et al*. Age and racial discribution of prostatic intra-epithelial neoplasia. *Eur Urol* 1996, **30**, 138–44.

84. Haggman MJ, Macoska JA, Wojno KJ *et al*. The relationship between prostatic intra-epithelial neoplasia and prostate cancer: critical issues. *J Urol* 1997, **158**, 12–22.

85. Sakr WA, Haas GP, Cassin BJ *et al*. The frequency of carcinoma and intra-epithelial neoplasia of the prostate in young male patients. *J Urol* 1993, **150**, 379–85.

86. Kovi J, Mostofi FK, Heshmat MT *et al*. Large acinar atypical hyperplasia and carcinoma of the prostate. *Cancer* 1988, **61**, 555–61.

87. Lee F, Torp-Pedersen ST, Carroll JT *et al*. Use of transrectal ultrasound and prostate- specific antigen in diagnosis of prostatic intra-epithelial neoplasia. *Urology* 1989, 34 (Suppl), 4–8.

88. Brawer MK, Bigler SA, Sohlberg OE *et al*. Significance of prostatic intra-epithelial neoplasia on prostate needle biopsy. *Urology* 1991, **38**, 103–7.

89. Weinstein MH, Epstein JI. Significance of high grade prostatic intra-epithelial neoplasia (PIN) on needle biopsy. *Hum Pathol* 1993, **24**, 624–9.

90. Shepherd D, Keetch DW, Humphrey PA *et al*. Repeat biopsy strategy in men with isolated prostatic intra-epithelial neoplasia on prostate needle biopsy. *J Urol* 1996, **156**, 460–2.

91. Troncoso P, Babaian RJ, Ro JY *et al*. Prostatic intra-epithelial neoplasia and invasive prostatic adenocarcinoma in cystoprostatectomy specimens. *Urology* 1989, **34**, 52–6.

92. Quinn BD, Cho KR, Epstein JI. Relationship of severe dysplasia to stage B adenocarcinoma of prostate. *Cancer* 1990, **65**, 2328–37.

93. Epstein JI, Cho KR, Quinn BD. Relationship of severe dysplasia to stage A (incidental) adenocarcinoma of prostate. *Cancer* 1990, **65**, 2321–7.

94. Ronnett BM, Carmichael M, Epstein JI. Does prostatic intra-epithelial neoplasia (PIN) result in elevated serum PSA levels? *Mod Pathol* 1993, 6 (Abstract), 67A.

95. Srigley J, Toth P, Hartwick RWJ. Atypical histological patterns in cases of benign prostatic hyperplasia. *Lab Invest* 1989, 60 (Abstract), 90A.

96. Montironi R, Scarpelli M, Sisti S *et al*. Quantitative analysis of prostatic intra-epithelial neoplasia on tissue sections. *Anal Quant Cytol Histol* 1990, **12**, 366–72.

97. Montironi R, Braccischi A, Matera G *et al*. Quantitation of prostatic intra-epithelial neoplasia. Analysis of the nuclear size, number and location. *Path Res Pract* 1991, **187**, 307–14.

98. Petein M, Michel P, Van Velthoven R *et al*. Morphonuclear relationship between prostatic intra-epithelial neoplasia and cancers as assessed by digital cell image analysis. *Am J Clin Pathol* 1991, **96**, 628–34.

99. Helpap B. Observations on the number, size and location of nucleoli in hyperplastic and neoplastic prostatic disease. *Histopathology* 1988, **13**, 203–11.

100. Min KW, Jin JK, Blank J *et al*. AgNOR in the human prostate gland. *Am J Clin Pathol* 1990, **95**, 508.

101. Layfield LJ, Goldstein NS. Morphometric analysis of borderline atypia in prostatic aspiration biopsy specimen. *Anal Quant Cytol Histol* 1991, **13**, 288–92.

102. Montironi R, Galuzzi C, Diamanti L *et al*. Prostatic intra-epithelial neoplasia: expression and location of proliferating cell nuclear antigen (prostate carcinoma NA) in epithelial, endothelial and stromal nuclei. *Virchows Arch A Pathol Anat Histopathol* 1993, **422**, 185–92.

103. Giannulis I, Montironi R, Magi Galuzzi C *et al*. Frequency and location of mitoses in PIN. *AntiCancer Res* 1993, **13**, 2447–51.

104. Mikuz G. Pathology of prostate cancer. Old problems and new facts. *Adv Clin Pathol* 1997, **1**, 21–34.

105. Poczatek RB, Myers RB, Manne U *et al*. Ep-CAM levels in prostatic adenocarcinoma and prostatic intra-epithelial neoplasia. *J Urol* 1999, **162**, 1462–6.

106. Perlman EJ, Epstein JI. Blood group antigen expression in dysplasia and adenocarcinoma of the prostate. *Am J Surg Pathol* 1990, **14**, 810–8.

107. Doria M, Jin J, Wang H *et al*. Glycoconjugate expression in hyperplastic, dysplastic, and malignant prostatic epithelium. *Lab Invest* 1991, **4** (Abstract), 45A.

108. Nagle RB, Brawer MK, Kittelson J, Clark V. Phenotypic relationships of prostatic intra-epithelial neoplasia to invasive prostatic carcinoma. *Am J Pathol* 1991, **138**, 119–28.

109. Humphrey PA. Mucin in severe dysplasia in the prostate. *Surg Pathol* 1991, **4**, 137.

110. McNeal JE, Alroy J, Leav I *et al*. Immunohistochemical evidence for impaired cell differentiation in the premalignant phase of prostate carcinogenesis. *Am J Clin Pathol* 1988, **90**, 23–32.

111. McNeal JE, Leav I, Alroy J *et al*. Differential lectin staining of central and peripheral zones of the prostate and alterations in dysplasia. *Am J Clin Pathol* 1988, **89**, 41–8.

112. Boag AH, Young ID. Increased expression of the 72-kd type IV collagenase in prostatic adenocarcinoma. Demonstration by immunohistochemistry and in situ hybridization. *Am J Pathol* 1994, **144**, 585–91.

113. Bergerheim USR, Kunimi K, Collins VP *et al*. Deletion mapping of chromosomes 8, 10, and 16 in human prostatic carcinoma. *Genes Chromosome Cancer* 1991, **3**, 215–20.

114. Bova GS, Carter BS, Bussemakers MJG *et al*. Homozygours deletion and frequent allelic loss of chromosome 8p22 loci in human prostate cancer. *Cancer Res* 1993, **53**, 3869–73.

115. MacGrogan D, Levy A, Bostwick D *et al*. Loss of chromosome 8p loci in prostate cancer: mapping by quantitative allelic balance. *Genes Chromosome Cancer* 1994, **10**, 151–9.

116. Alers JC, Krijtenberg PJ, Vissers KJ *et al*. Interphase cytogenetics of prostatic adenocarcinoma and precursor lesions: analysis of 25 radical prostatectomies in 17 adjacent prostatic intra-epithelial neoplasia. *Genes Chromosomes Cancer* 1995, **12**, 241–50.

117. Emmert-Buck MR, Vocke CD, Pozzati RO *et al*. Allelic loss on chromosome 8p12–21 in microdissected prostatic intra-epithelial neoplasia (PIN). *Cancer Res* 1995, **55**, 2959–62.

118. Cunningham JM, Shan A, Wick MJ *et al*. Allelic imbalance and microsatellite instability in prostatic adenocarcinoma. *Cancer Res* 1996, **56**, 4475–82.

119. Sakr WA, Macoska JA, Benson P *et al.* Allelic loss in locally metastatic, multisampled prostate cancer. *Cancer Res* 1994, **54**, 3273–7.

120. Takahashi S, Qian J, Brown JA *et al.* Potential markers of prostate cancer aggressiveness detected by fluorescence *in situ* hybridization in needle biopsies. *Cancer Res* 1994, **54**, 3574–9.

121. Qian J, Bostwick DG, Takahashi S *et al.* Chromosomal anomalies in prostatic intra-epithelial neoplasia and carcinoma detected by fluorescence in situ hybridization. *Cancer Res* 1995, **55**, 5408–14.

122. Qian J, Jenkins RB, Bostwick DG. Potential markers of aggressiveness in prostatic intra-epithelial neoplasia detected by fluorescence in situ hybridization. *Eur Urol* 1996, **30**, 177–84.

123. Fernandez PL, Arce Y, Farre X *et al.* Expression of p27/kip1 is down-regulated in human prostate carcinoma progression. *J Pathol* 1999, **187**, 563–6.

124. Myers RB, Srivastava S, Oelschlager DK *et al.* Expression of nm23-H1 in prostatic intra-epithelial neoplasia and adenocarcinoma. *Hum Pathol* 1996, **27**, 1021–4.

125. Weinberg DS, Weidner N. Concodance of DNA content between prostatic intra-epithelial neoplasia and concomitant invasive carcinoma. Evidence that prostatic intra-epithelial neoplasia is a precursor of invasive prostatic carcinoma. *Arch Pathol Lab Med* 1993, **117**, 1132–7.

126. Crissman JD, Sakr WA, Hussein ME *et al.* DNA quantitation of intra-epithelial neoplasia and invasive carcinoma of the prostate. *Prostate* 1993, **22**, 155–62.

127. Amin MB, Schultz DS, Zarbo RJ *et al.* DNA ploidy analysis of prostatic intra-epithelial neoplasia. *Arch Pathol Lab Med* 1993, **117**, 794–8.

128. Baretton GB, Vogt T, Blassenbreu S *et al.* Comparison of DNA ploidy in prostatic intra-epithelial neoplasia and invasive carcinoma of the prostate: an image cytometric study. *Hum Pathol* 1994, **25**, 506–13.

129. Bostwick DG, Srigley J, Grignon D *et al.* Atypical adenomatous hyperplasia of the prostate: morphologic criteria for its distinction from well-differentiated carcinoma. *Hum Pathol* 1993, **24**, 819–32.

130. Bostwick DG, Qian J. Atypical adenomatous hyperplasia of the prostate: relatioship with carcinoma in 217 whole mount radical prostatectomies. *Am J Surg Pathol* 1995, **19**, 506–18.

131. Brawn PN, Speights VO, Contin JU *et al.* Atypical adenomatous hyperplasia in prostates of 20 to 40 year old men. *J Clin Pathol* 1989, **42**, 383–6.

132. Srigley J, Toth P, Hartwick RWJ. Atypical histologic patterns in cases of benign prostatic hyperplasia. *Lab Invest* 1989, **60**, 90A.

133. Kovi J. Microscopic differential diagnosis of small acinar adenocarcinoma of prostate. *Pathol Annu* 1985, **20**, 157–96.

134. Isaacs WB, Bova GS, Morton RA *et al.* Molecular biology of prostate cancer. *Semin Oncol* 1994, **21**, 514–21.

135. Bochner BH. Commentary: Genetic alterations in prostate cancer. *J Urol* 1999, **162**, 1543.

136. Carter BS, Ewing CM, Ward WS *et al.* Allelic loss of chromosomes 16q and 10q in human prostate cancer. *Proc Natl Acad Sci USA* 1990, **87**, 8751–5.

137. Sandberg AA. Chromosomal abnormalities and related events in prostate cancer. *Hum Pathol* 1992, **23**, 368–80.

138. Vocke CD, Pozzatti RO, Bostwick DG *et al.* Analysis of 99 microdissected prostate carcinomas reveals a high frequency of allelic loss on chromosome 8p12–21. *Cancer Res* 1996, **56**, 2411–6.

139. Gao X, Honn KV, Grignon D *et al.* Frequent loss of expression and loss of heterozygosity of the putative tumor-suppressor gene DCC in prostatic carcinomas. *Cancer Res* 1993, **53**, 2723–7.

140. Brewster SF, Browne S, Brown KW. Somatic allelic loss at the DCC, APC, nm23-HI and p53 tumor-suppressor gene loci in human prostatic carcinoma. *J Urol* 1994, **151**, 1073–7.

141. Carmichael MJ, Veltri RW, Partin AW *et al.* Deoxyribonucleic acid ploidy analysis as a predictor of recurrence following radical prostatectomy for stage T2 disease. *J Urol* 1995, **153**, 1015–9.

142. Borre M, Hoyer M, Nerstrom B *et al.* DNA ploidy and survival of patients with clinically localized prostate Cancer treated without intent to cure. *Prostate* 1998, **36**, 244–9.

143. Song J, Cheng WS, Cupps RE *et al.* Nuclear deoxyribonucleic acid content measured by static cytometry: important prognostic association for patients with clinically localized prostate carcinoma treated by external beam radiotherapy. *J Urol* 1992, **147**, 794–7.

144. van den Ouden D, Tribukait B, Blom JHM *et al.* Deoxyribonucleic acid ploidy of core biopsies and metastatic lymph nodes of prostate Cancer patients: impact on time to progression. The European Organization for Research and Treatment of Cancer Genitourinary Group. *J Urol* 1993, **150**, 400–6.

145. Ross JS, Figge H, Bui HX *et al.* Prediction of pathologic stage and postprostatectomy disease recurrence by DNA ploidy analysis of initial needle biopsy specimens of prostate cancer. *Cancer* 1994, **74**, 2811–8.

146. Brinker DA, Ross JS, Tran TA *et al.* Can ploidy of prostate carcinoma diagnosed on needle biopsy predict radical prostatectomy stage and grade? *J Urol* 1999, **162**, 2036–9.

147. Ross JS, Sheehan CE, Ambros RA *et al.* Needle biopsy DNA ploidy status predicts grade shifting in prostate cancer. *Am J Surg Pathol* 1999, **23**, 296–301.

148. Seay TM, Blute ML, Zincke H. Long-term outcome in patients with pTxN+ adenocarcinoma of prostate treated with radical prostatectomy and early androgen ablation. *J Urol* 1998, **159**, 357–64.

149. Bauer JJ, Sesterhenn IA, Mostofi FK *et al.* Elevated levels of apoptosis regulator proteins p53 and bcl-2 are independent prognostic biomarkers in surgically treated clinically localized prostate cancer. *J Urol* 1996, **156**, 1511–6.

150. Bubendorf L, Sauter G, Moch H *et al.* Prognostic significance of bcl-2 in clinically localized prostate cancer. *Am J Pathol* 1996, **148**, 1557–65.

151. Shurbaji MS, Kalbfleisch JH, Thurmond TS. Immunohistochemical detection of p53 protein as a

prognostic indicator in prostate cancer. *Hum Pathol* 1995, **26**, 106–9.

152. Grignon DJ, Caplan R, Sarkar FH *et al*. p53 status and prognosis of locally advanced prostatic adenocarcinoma: a study based on RTOG 8610. *J Natl Cancer Inst* 1997, **89**, 158–65.

153. Stackhouse GB, Sesterhenn IA, Bauer JJ *et al*. p53 and bcl-2 immunohistochemistry in pretreatment prostate needle biopsies to predict recurrence of prostate cancer after radical prostatectomy. *J Urol* 1999, **162**, 2040–5.

154. Baker SJ, Markowitz S, Fearon ER *et al*. Suppression of human colorectal carcinoma and growth by wild-type p53. *Science* 1990, **249**, 912–5.

155. Kastan MB, Onyekwere O, Sidransky D *et al*. Participation of p53 protein in the cellular response to DNA damage. *Cancer Res* 1991, **51**, 6304–11.

156. Lowe SW, Schmitt EM, Smith SW *et al*. p53 is required for radiation-induced apoptosis in mouse thymocytes. *Nature* 1993, **362**, 847–9.

157. Levine AJ, Momand J, Finlay CA. The p53 tumour suppressor gene. *Nature* 1991, **351**, 453–6.

158. Van Veldhuizen PJ, Sadasivan R, Garcia F *et al*. Mutant p53 expression in prostate carcinoma. *Prostate* 1993, **22**, 23–30.

159. Johnson MI, Robinson MC, Marsh C *et al*. Expression of Bcl-2, Bax, and p53 in high-grade prostatic intraepithelial neoplasia and localize prostate cancer: relationship with apoptosis and proliferation. *Prostate* 1998, **37**, 223–9.

160. Brewster SF, Oxley JD, Trivella M *et al*. Preoperative p53, bcl-2, CD44 and E-cadherin immunohistochemistry as predictors of biochemical relapse after radical prostatectomy. *J Urol* 1999, **161**, 1238–43.

161. McDonell TJ, Navone NM, Troncoso P *et al*. Expression of bcl-2 oncoprotein and p53 protein accumulation in bone marrow metastases of androgen independent prostate cancer. *J Urol* 1997, **157**, 569–74.

162. Mirchandani D, Zheng J, Miller GJ *et al*. Heterogeneity in intratumor distribution of p53 mutations in human prostate carcer. *Am J Pathol* 1995, **147**, 92–101.

163. Heidenberg HB, Sesterhenn IA, Gaddipati JP *et al*. Alteration of the tumour suppressor gene p53 in a high fraction of hormone refractory prostate cancer. *J Urol* 1995, **154**, 414–21.

164. Stapleton AM, Timme TL, Gousse AE *et al*. Primary human prostate cancer cells harboring p53 mutations are clonally expanded in metastases. *Clin Cancer Res* 1997, **3**, 1389–97.

165. Navone NM, Labate ME, Troncoso P *et al*. p53 mutations in prostate cancer bone metastases suggest that selected p53 mutants in the primary site define foci with metastatic potential. *J Urol* 1999, **161**, 304–8.

166. Meyers FJ, Gumerlock PH, Chi SG *et al*. Very frequent p53 mutations in metastatic prostate carcinoma and in matched primary tumours. *Cancer* 1998, **83**, 2534–9.

167. Cheng L, Leibovich BC, Bergstralh EJ *et al*. p53 alteration in regional lymph node metastases from prostate carcinoma: a marker for progression? *Cancer* 1999, **85**, 2455–9.

168. Navone NM, Troncoso P, Pisters LL *et al*. p53 protein accumulation and gene mutation in the progression of human prostate carcinoma. *J Natl Cancer Inst* 1993, **85**, 1657–69.

169. Bookstein R, MacGrogan D, Hilsenbeck SG *et al*. p53 is mutated in a subset of advanced-stage prostate cancers. *Cancer Res* 1993, **53**, 3369–73.

170. Effert PJ, McCoy RH, Walther PJ *et al*. p53 gene alterations in human prostate carcinoma. *J Urol* 1993, **150**, 257–61.

171. Stattin P, Bergh A, Karlberg L *et al*. p53 immunoreactivity as prognostic marker for cancer-specific survival in prostate cancer. *Eur Urol* 1996, **30**, 65–72.

172. Brooks JD, Bova GS, Ewing CM *et al*. An uncertain role for p53 gene alterations in human prostate cancers. *Cancer Res* 1996, **56**, 3814–22.

173. Salem CE, Tomasic NA, Elmajian DA *et al*. p53 protein and gene alterations in pathological stage C prostate carcinoma. *J Urol* 1997, **158**, 510–4.

174. Theodorescu D, Broder SR, Boyd JC *et al*. p53, bcl-2 and retinoblastoma proteins as long-term prognostic markers in localized carcinoma of the prostate. *J Urol* 1997, **158**, 131–7.

175. Matsushima H, Kitamura T, Goto T *et al*. Combined analysis with bcl-2 and p53 immunostaining predicts poorer prognosis in prostatic carcinoma. *J Urol* 1997, **158**, 2278–83.

176. Rakozy C, Grignon DJ, Li Y *et al*. p53 gene alterations in prostate cancer after radiation failure and their association with clinical outcome: a molecular and immunohistochemical analysis. *Pathol Res Pract* 1999, **195**, 129–35.

177. Sentman CL, Shutter JR, Hockenbery D *et al*. bcl-2 inhibits multiple forms of apoptosis but not negative selection in thymocytes. *Cell* 1991, **67**, 879–88.

178. McDonell TJ, Troncoso P, Brisbay SM *et al*. Expression of the protooncogene bcl-2 in the prostate and its association with emergence of androgen-independent prostate cancer. *Cancer Res* 1992, **52**, 6940–4.

179. McDonell TJ, Navone NM, Troncoso P *et al*. Expression of bcl-2 oncoprotein and p53 protein accumulation in bone marrow metastases of androgen independent prostate cancer. *J Urol* 1997, **157**, 569–74.

180. Raffo AJ, Perlman H, Chen MW *et al*. Over-expression of bcl-2 protects prostate cancer cells from apoptosis *in vitro* and confers resistance to androgen depletion *in vivo*. *Cancer Res* 1995, **55**, 4438–45.

181. McDormell TJ, Troncoso P, Brisbay SM *et al*. Expression of the protooncogene bcl-2 in the prostate and its association with emergence of androgen-independent prostate cancer. *Cancer Res* 1992, **52**, 6940–4.

182. Colombel M, Symmans F, Gil S *et al*. Detection of the apoptosis-suppressing oncoprotein bcl-2 in hormone refractory human prostate cancers. *Am J Pathol* 1993, **143**, 390–400.

183. Moul JW. Angiogenesis, p53, bcl-2 and ki-67 in progression of prostate cancer after radical prostatectomy. *Eur Urol* 1999, **35**, 399–407.

184. Scherr DS, Vaughan ED Jr, Wei J *et al*. Bcl-2 and p53 expression in clinically localized prostate cancer predicts response to external beam radiotherapy. *J Urol* 1999, **162**, 12–16.

185. Gooddrich DW, Wang NP, Qian YW *et al*. The retinoblastoma gene product regulates progression through the G1 phase of the cell cycle. *Cell* 1991, **67**, 293–302.

186. Bookstein R, Rio P, Madreperla S *et al*. Promoter deletion and loss of retinoblastoma gene expression in human prostate carcinoma. *Proc Natl Acad Sci USA* 1990, **87**, 7762–6.

187. Sarkar FH, Sakr W, Li YW *et al*. Analysis of retinoblastoma (RB) gene deletion in human prostatic carcinomas. *Prostate* 1992, **21**, 145–52.

188. Afonso A, Emmert-Buck MR, Duray PH *et al*. Loss of heterozygosity on chromosome 13 is associated with advanced stage prostate cancer. *J Urol* 1999, **162**, 922–6.

189. Akalu A, Elmajian DA, Highshaw RA *et al*. Somatic mutations at the SRD5A2 locus encoding prostatic steroid 5α-reductase during prostate cancer progression. *J Urol* 1999, **161**, 1355–8.

190. Haggstrom S, Lissbrant IF, Bergh A *et al*. Testosterone induces vascular endothelial growth factor synthesis in the ventral prostate in castrated rats. *J Urol* 1999, **161**, 1620–5.

191. Franck Lissbrant I, Haggstrom S, Damber JE *et al*. Testosterone stimulates angiogenesis and vascular regrowth in the ventral prostate in castrated adult rats. *Endocrinology* 1998, **139**, 451–6.

192. Tilley WD, Buchanan G, Hickey TE *et al*. Mutations in the androgen receptor gene are associated with progression of human prostate cancer to androgen independence. *Clin Cancer Res* 1996, **2**, 277–85.

193. Taplin ME, Bubley GJ, Shuster TD *et al*. Mutation of the androgen-receptor gene in metastatic androgen-independent prostate cancer. *N Engl J Med* 1995, **332**, 1393–8.

194. Sweat SD, Pacelli A, Bergstralh EJ *et al*. Androgen receptor expression in prostate cancer lymph node metastases is predictive of outcome after surgery. *J Urol* 1999, **161**, 1233–7.

195. Zhang SXD, Bentel JM, Ricciardelli C *et al*. Immunolocalization of apolipoprotein D, androgen receptor and prostate specific antigen in early stage prostate cancers. *J Urol* 1998, **159**, 548–54.

196. Koutsilieris M. Osteoblastic metastasis in advanced prostate cancer. *AntiCancer Res* 1993, **13**, 443–9.

197. Hofer DR, Sherwood ER, Bromber WD *et al*. Autonomous growth of androgen-independent human prostatic carcinoma cells: role of transforming growth factor. *Cancer Res* 1991, **51**, 2780–5.

198. Nakamoto T, Chang C, Li A *et al*. Basic fibroblast growth factor in human prostate cancer cells. *Cancer Res* 1992, **52**, 571–7.

199. Yamamoto TM, Ikawa S, Akiyama T *et al*. Similarity of protein encoded by the human c-erbB-2 gene to epidermal growth factor receptor. *Nature* 1986, **319**, 230–4.

200. Ochiai A, Akimoto S, Kanai Y *et al*. c-erbB-2 gene product associates with catenins in human cancer cells. *Biochem Biophys Res Commun* 1994, **205**, 73–78.

201. Yu D, Wang SS, Dulski KM *et al*. c-erbB-2/neu overexpression enhances metastatic potential of human lung Cancer cells by induction of metastasis-associated properties. *Cancer Res* 1994, **54**, 3260–6.

202. Kuhn EJ, Kurnot RA, Sesterhenn IA *et al*. Expression of the c-erbB-2 (HER-2/neu) oncoprotein in human prostatic carcinoma. *J Urol* 1993, **150**, 1427–33.

203. Ware J, Maygarden SJ, Kooniz WW *et al*. Immunohistochemical detection of c-erb-B2 protein in human benign and neoplastic prostse. *Hum Pathol* 1991, **22**, 254–8.

204. Fox SB, Persad SA, Coleman N *et al*. Prognostic value of c-erb-B2 and epidermal growth factor receptor in stage A1 (T1a) prostatic adenocarcinoma. *Br J Urol* 1994, **74**, 214–20.

205. Bettencourt MC, Bauer JJ, Sesterhenn IA *et al*. CD34 immunohistochemical assessment of angiogenesis as a prognostic marker for prostate cancer recurrence after radical prostatectomy. *J Urol* 1998, **160**, 459–65.

206. Borre M, Offersen BV and Overgaard J. Microvessel density predicts survival in prostate cancer patients subjected to watchful waiting. *Br J Cancer* 1998, **78**, 940–4.

207. Mydlo JH, Kral JG, Volpe M *et al*. An analysis of microvessel density, androgen receptor, p53 and HER-2/neu expression and Gleason score in prostate cancer: preliminary results and therapeutic implications. *Eur Urol* 1998, **34**, 426–32.

208. Connolly JM, Rose DP. Angiogenesis in two human prostate cancer cell lines with differing metastatic potential when growing as solid tumors in nude mice. *J Urol* 1998, **160**, 932–6.

209. Ferrer FA, Miller LJ, Andrawis RI *et al*. Angiogenesis and prostate cancer: *in vivo* and *in vitro* expression of angiogenesis factors by prostate cancer cells. *Urology* 1998, **51**, 161–7.

210. Duque JL, Loughlin KR, Adam RM *et al*. Plasma levels of vascular endothelial growth factor are increased in patients with metastatic prostate cancer. *Urology* 1999, **54**, 523–7.

211. Joseph IB, Nelson JB, Denmeade SR *et al*. Androgens regulate vascular endothelial growth factor content in normal and malignant prostate tissue. *Clin Cancer Res* 1997, **3**, 2507–11.

212. Gao AC, Lou W, Dong JT *et al*. CD44 is a metastasis suppressor gene for prostatic cancer located on human chromosome 11p13. *Cancer Res* 1997, **57**, 846–9.

213. Kallakury BV, Yang F, Figge J *et al*. Decreased levels of CD44 protein and mRNA in prostate carcinoma: correlation with tumour grade and ploidy. *Cancer* 1996, **78**, 1461–9.

214. Nagabhushan M, Pretlow TG, Guo YJ *et al*. Altered expression of CD44 in human prostate cancer during progression. *Am J Clin Pathol* 1996, **106**, 647–51.

215. Noordzij MA, van Steenbrugge GJ, Verkaik NS *et al*. The prognostic value of CD44 isoforms in prostate cancer patients treated by radical prostatectomy. *Clin Cancer Res* 1997, **3**, 805–15.

216. Umbas R, Isaacs WB, Bringuier PP *et al*. Decreased E-cadherin expression is associated with poor prognosis in patients with prostate cancer. *Cancer Res* 1994, **54**, 3929–33.

217. Litvinov SV, Velders MP, Bakker CM *et al*. Ep-CAM: a human epithelial antigen is a homophilic cell-cell-adhesion molecule. *J Cell Biol* 1994, **125**, 437–46.

218. Ho SB, Niehans GA, Lyftogt C *et al.* Heterogeneity of mucin gene expression in normal and neoplastic tissues. *Cancer Res* 1993, **53**, 641–51.

219. Jensen SL, Wood DP, Jr, Banks ER *et al.* Increased levels of nm23 H1/nucleoside diphosphate kinase A mRNA associated with adenocarcinoma of the prostate. *World J Urol* 1996, **14** (Suppl 1), S21–25.

220. Igawa M, Urakami S, Shiina H *et al.* Association of nm23 protein levels in human prostates with proliferating cell nuclear antigen expression at autopsy. *Eur Urol* 1996, **30**, 383–7.

221. Chekmareva MA, Hollowell CM, Smith RC *et al.* Localization of prostate cancer metastasis—suppressor activity on human chromosome 17. *Prostate* 1997, **33**, 271–80.

222. Chekmareva MA, Kadkhodaian MM, Hollowell CM *et al.* Chromosome 17-mediated dormancy of AT6.1 prostate cancer micrometastases. *Cancer Res* 1998, **58**, 4963–9.

223. Lim S, Lee HY, Lee H. Inhibition of colonization and cell matrix adhesion after nm23-H1 transfection of human prostate carcinoma cells. *Cancer Lett* 1998, **133**, 143–9.

224. St Croix B, Florenes VA, Rak JW *et al.* Impact of the cyclin-dependent kinase inhibitor p27kip1 on resistance of tumor cells to antiCancer agents. *Nature Med* 1996, **2**, 1204–10.

225. Bouras T, Frauman AG. Expression of the prostate cancer metastasis suppressor gene KA11 in primary prostate cancers: a biphasic relationship with tumour grade. *J Pathol* 1999, **188**, 382–8.

226. Moul JW, Friedrichs PA, Lance RS *et al.* Infrequent RAS oncogene mutations in human prostate cancer. *Prostate* 1992, **20**, 327–38.

227. Kiaris H, Eliopoulos AG, Sivridis E *et al.* Activating mutations of ras family genes in prostatic cancer. *Oncol Rep* 1995, **2**, 427.

228. Sumiya H, Masai M, Akimoto S *et al.* Histochemical examination of ras p21 protein and R 1881-binding protein in human prostatic cancers. *Eur J Cancer* 1990, **26**, 786–9.

229. Fleming WH, Hamel A, MacDonald R *et al.* Expression of the c-myc protooncogene in human prostatic carcinoma and benign prostatic hyperplasia. *Cancer Res* 1986, **46**, 1535–8.

230. Buttyan R, Sawczuk IS, Benson MC *et al.* Enhanced expression of the c-myc protooncogene in high-grade human prostate cancers. *Prostate* 1987, **11**, 327–37.

231. Yamazaki H, Schneider E, Myers CE *et al.* Oncogene over-expression and de novo drug-resistance in human prostate cancer cells. *Biochim Biophys Acta* 1994, **1226**, 89–96.

232. Merz VW, Arnold AM and Studer UE. Differential expression of transforming growth factor-β 1 and β 3 as well as c-fos mRNA in normal human prostate, benign prostatic hyperplasia and prostatic cancer. *World J Urol* 1994, **12**, 96–98.

233. Aoyagi K, Shima I, Wang M *et al.* Specific transcription factors prognostic for prostate cancer progression. *Clin Cancer Res* 1998, **4**, 2153–60.

234. Shurbaji MS, Kuhajda FP, Pasternack GR *et al.* Expression of oncogenic antigen 519 (OA-519) in prostate cancer is a potential prognostic indicator. *Am J Clin Pathol* 1992, **97**, 686–91.

235. Montironi R, Schulman CC. Precursor of prostatic cancer: progression, regression and chemoprevention. *Eur Urol* 1996, **30**, 133–7.

236. Brooks JD, Weistein M, Lin X *et al.* CG island methylation changes near the GSTP1 gene in prostatic intraepithelial neoplasia. *Cancer Epidemiol Biomarkers Prev* 1998, **7**, 531–6.

237. Kim NW, Piatyszek MA, Prose KR *et al.* Specific association of human telomerase activity with immortal cell and cancer. *Science* 1994, **266**, 2011–5.

238. Rhyu MS. Telomeres, telomerase and immortality. *J Natl Cancer Inst* 1995, **87**, 884–94.

239. Scates DK, Muir GH, Venitt S *et al.* Detection of telomerase activity in human prostate: a diagnostic marker for prostatic cancer. *Br J Urol* 1997, **80**, 263–8.

240. Wullich B, Rohde V, Oehlenschlager B *et al.* Focal intratumoral heterogeneity for telomerase activity in human prostate cancer. *J Urol* 1999, **161**, 1997–2001.

241. Sommerfeld HJ, Meeker AK, Piatyszek MA *et al.* Telomerase activity: a prevalent marker of malignant human prostate tissue. *Cancer Res* 1996, **56**, 218–22.

242. de Lange T. Telomeres and senescence: ending the debate. *Science* 1998, **279**, 334–5.

243. Lin Y, Uemura H, Fujinami K *et al.* Telomerase activity in primary prostate cancer. *J Urol* 1997, **157**, 1161–5.

244. Takahashi C, Miyagawa I, Kumano S *et al.* Detection of telomerase activity in prostate cancer by needle biopsy. *Eur Urol* 1997, **32**, 494–8.

245. Zhang W, Kapusta LR, Slingerland JM *et al.* Telomerase activity in prostate cancer, prostatic intraepithelial neoplasia, and benign prostatic epithelium. *Cancer Res* 1998, **58**, 619–21.

Section III

The employment of transrectal ultrasound (TRUS) and TRUS-guided needle biopsies have significantly con-... related to the better clinical evaluation of prostate

12 | Clinical presentation and investigation of prostate cancer

Stavros A. Gravas, Konstantinos N. Syrigos, and Platon Kehayas

Introduction

Prostate cancer is indisputably a major clinical problem for the male population, due to its increasing incidence. Continuous efforts towards a better understanding of prostate cancer has shed some light into the genetic and molecular basis of the disease. Despite significant scientific progress, the natural history, diagnosis, staging, and treatment of prostate carcinoma still raises more questions than answers, and clinicians face a new dilemma in every step.

Diagnosis of prostate carcinoma is determined finally by histologic examination of tissue taken either by needle biopsy, in the case of clinical suspicion, or by transurethral resection of the prostate, for presumed benign disease (10%). As prostate carcinoma is characterized by the initial absence of any specific or warning symptoms, an abnormal digital rectal examination and elevated serum prostate-specific antigen (PSA) levels are the main indications for performing prostate biopsy. The employment of transrectal ultrasound (TRUS) and TRUS-guided needle biopsies have significantly contributed to the better clinical investigation of prostate cancer.

In this chapter, our aim is to present the clinical manifestations of prostate cancer and review the diagnostic approach and investigation of patients suspected to have the disease.

Clinical manifestations

Prostate cancer is a heterogeneous disease, but even biologically aggressive tumors remain silent for years. As a result, the first manifestation of prostate cancer could be symptoms of metastatic disease. On the other hand, any obstructive and irritative voiding dysfunction symptoms are the most common manifestations of localized prostate carcinoma.

Local disease

In most cases, development of prostate cancer does not present typical clinical symptoms that would result in referral immediately to a urologist. This general lack of symptoms is demonstrated by the finding that the prevalence of histologic cancer exceeds that of clinical prostate cancer by as much as eight times (1). Prostate carcinoma is typically presented as a peripherally located multi-focal lesion in 75–80% of patients (2). A small-volume tumor, arising from the peripheral zone away from the urethra and bladder neck, is not able to cause symptoms related to the voiding. Voiding symptoms, including dysuria, urinary frequency, nocturia, urgency, slow urinary stream, decrease in the caliber of the stream, intermittency, and acute urinary retention, could be presented in with a peri-urethrally located transition zone carcinoma (15–20% of patients), or a tumor of significant mass.

Unfortunately none of these symptoms are specific to prostate cancer. Benign prostatic hyperplasia (BPH) and chronic prostatitis are also clinically presented with dysfunctional voiding. It is estimated that approximately 50% of men have prostatic symptoms due to prostatitis at some time (3). Patients suffering from chronic prostatitis are convinced that their disease is recurrent and very difficult to be treated. They consider it unnecessary to seek additional consultation by a specialist. Additionally, BPH is common in men older than 50 years. Mild symptoms are not properly evaluated by most of those men, and are generally attributed to 'prostate'. It is noteworthy that incidental carcinoma of the prostate is found in 10% of prostatectomies performed for BPH (4). The only sign that could be indicative of prostate cancer development is the sudden appearance and rapid progression of bladder outlet obstruction, but this has not been documented.

Hematuria and hematospermia are infrequent, non-specific symptoms occurring in prostate cancer patients (5, 6). Therefore, prostate cancer should be included in the differential diagnosis and considered during further investigation of these patients.

Locally advanced disease

The invasion of bladder trigone due to the extension of prostatic malignancy causes distal ureteral obstruction. Established renal failure and azotemia will cause weakness, anemia, fluid retention, and electrolyte-imbalance related symptoms. These symptoms, without the presence of significant urine residual, might raise suspicions to the clinicians of the existence of locally advanced prostate cancer. Priapism is rarely associated with prostate cancer as a result of invasion of the corporeal bodies (7).

Systemic disease

Lymph nodes and bone are the most common sites of metastasis of prostate carcinoma. Involvement of the lymph nodes runs without symptoms until a significant tumor burden causes venous and lymphatics compression, resulting in peripheral edema of the lower extremities and scrotum. Bone pain due to skeletal metastases is often the initial complaint that lead patients with disseminated prostate cancer to seek medical assistance. Pathologic fractures most commonly of the femur, the humerus, and the vertebral bodies may also occur.

Neurologic symptoms due to epidural cord compression will occur in the one-third of patients with advanced prostate carcinoma (8). Neurologic manifestations include local pain in radicular distribution, weakness of lower extremities, and numbness. Symptoms coming from involvement of other organs are extremely rare and have only been reported on the basis of case reports.

Digital rectal examination

Digital rectal examination (DRE) has been the cornerstone in the initial evaluation of prostate carcinoma. Before the widespread use of serum PSA in the early 1980s, an abnormal DRE was the only sign suggestive for the presence of prostate cancer. As most prostate cancers originate from the peripheral zone, DRE provides the examiner with the ability to palpate them. In contrast, transition zone cancers are not detected on DRE, at least in initial stages. Advantages of DRE include speed of performance and the relatively low cost of the method. However, reported positive predictive values of DRE ranged from 17% to 43.2% (9–13). This variability probably mirrors the subjectivity of the method. It is true that DRE is highly dependant on the experience of the examiner and with patient compliance. Although experienced examiners could detect cancers as small as 0.3–1.3 ml (14), the method in general may not be sensitive enough to detect the small-volume tumors that are the most likely to be cured. The overall sensitivity and specificity of the method have been reported to be 57.9% and 77.2%, respectively (15), but in the detection of organ-confined disease, sensitivity and specificity are dramatically lower (approximately 30% and 40%, respectively).

DRE should complete a thorough physical examination. Prior to DRE, the clinician should explain the method to the patient, outlining the significance of DRE. The examination can be made with the patient in one of the following positions: the left lateral position, the knee–elbow position, the standing and bent over the examining table position, and the lithotomy position. The position most familiar to the clinician should be chosen. Inspection of the anus for pathology, such as hemorrhoids, fissures, or a carcinoma, must never be omitted. The gloved finger should be adequately lubricated. Attention must be paid to the method of introducing the finger in order to avoid causing pain to the patient. The examiner should lay the pulp of the index finger flat upon the anal verge, and exert firm pressure until the sphincter is felt to relax. Then the finger is introduced slowly. Palpation of the prostate should be very careful and systematic. The index finger sweeps over the prostate from the base to the apex and the entire posterior surface of the gland can usually be palpated. Palpation should be very gently for the best evaluation of the surface and the landmarks of the prostate. Increasing pressure on the prostate may be helpful to identify firm or hard areas deeper in the gland. A normal prostate has a consistency similar to the contracted thenar eminence of the thumb (with the thumb opposed to the little finger) (16). Any area of the prostate with altered consistency such as firm, hard (wood-like), or very hard (stone-like) should be considered suspicious for the presence of prostate cancer. Other abnormalities detected on DRE including nodules, irregular surface, obliteration of the normal landmarks, and asymmetry of the gland could also be associated with prostate carcinoma. However, differential diagnosis of an abnormal DRE should include benign prostatic hyperplasia, prostatitis, prostatic calculi, infarcts, tuberculosis, post-surgical and biopsy changes, that present similar findings on DRE (1) and may puzzle even very experienced urologists.

All findings should be noted and recorded in details. A diagram of DRE findings is strongly suggested because it will be very helpful in many cases including:

- serial re-examinations of the patient;
- performance of TRUS by another examiner;
- comparison of DRE findings with those of TRUS to achieve more precise clinical staging;
- follow-up of patients who will undergo treatment other than radical prostatectomy.

A limitation of DRE is the lack of accuracy for predicting the location and extent of cancer. Patients with a unilateral suspicious lesion on DRE had a pathologically confined cancer to the same lobe in 11–69% of the reported cases, whereas in 31–89% of the cases, the pathological examination revealed bilateral tumor (17–20). Fixation of the gland on DRE or obliteration of the normal prostate landmarks by an induration, are suggestive of an extension of the pathologic process beyond the prostate. However, it is well-documented that DRE underestimates disease stage, as only 40–60% of the tumors detected on DRE and considered to be clinically localized, should prove to be organ confined after pathological staging (1).

A key in early diagnosis of prostate carcinoma may be the active involvement of general practitioners. General practitioners could offer opportunistic screening in all men older than 50 years seeking for medical assistance for any reason, by performing DRE in those men.

PSA

Prostate-specific antigen (PSA) is a single-chain glycoprotein, consisting of 237 amino acids (21). Recently, using ion spray mass spectroscopy, glycosylated PSA was found to have a molecular weight of 28 430 d (22). PSA is synthesized in the prostatic epithelium and the epithelium lining the peri-urethral glands and its function is to liquefy the seminal coagulum (23). It was first purified from prostate tissue by Wang in 1979 (24). PSA is a member of the human tissue kallikrein gene family. It is a serine protease with primarily chymotrypsin-like catalytic activity. Another member of this family is hK2 that shares an 80% sequence homology with PSA but has primarily trypsin-like activity. PSA has a half-life of 2.2 ±0.8 days (25).

PSA is the most important and widely used tumor marker in urologic oncology. The application of PSA to clinical practice includes early diagnosis, staging, and monitoring of prostate cancer. However, PSA presents limitations in sensitivity and specificity especially for high normal and mildly elevated levels, because PSA is organ- but not cancer-specific to the prostate gland. The traditional cut-off value for serum PSA of 4.0 ng/ml provides a severe overlap in serum PSA between patients with prostate cancer and BPH. Approximately 80% of men with prostate cancer and 25–30% of men with BPH have serum PSA levels greater than 4.0 ng/ml. and 20% of men with prostate cancer have serum PSA levels below 4.0 ng/ml (25–27).

Serum PSA level can be influenced by various factors, including:

- *Benign prostatic diseases*. The overlap in serum PSA between patients with benign prostatic hyperplasia (BPH) and those with prostate cancer has been already outlined. In their classical study, Stamey and colleagues estimated that each gram of hyperplastic tissue causes a PSA elevation of about 0.3 ng/ml (25). In addition, acute prostatitis (28), subclinical prostatitis (29), and urinary retention (30) have been found to be responsible to varying degrees for an increase in serum PSA levels of patients.
- *Medical manipulations*. Prostate needle biopsy (25, 31), transurethral resection of prostate (initially) (25, 31, 32), and vigorous prostatic massage (25) have been reported to be associated with a clinically significant elevation in serum PSA concentration.
- *Medication*. Following a 6-month treatment with finasteride, men without prostate cancer, were found to have decreased PSA levels by approximately 50% (33). Correction of PSA concentration was suggested by multiplying the post-treatment PSA values by a factor of 2 (34).
- *Ejaculation*. Recently, ejaculation has been shown to have a significant impact on serum PSA level. In 87% of men, Tchentgen *et al.* found an increase in serum PSA, with a peak 1 h after ejaculation (35).

Serum PSA concentration seems not to be affected by factors such as: digital rectal examination (31, 32), cystoscopy (31, 32) catheterization (36), transrectal ultrasound (31, 37), and exercise (38).

The appearance of PSA in the early 1980s, has revolutionized the diagnosis and management of prostate cancer. Increased public awareness for PSA leads a significant number of men to seek urological consultation. However, PSA still stands far from the definition of the ideal tumor marker. Efforts have been made to improve the clinical utility of PSA, and achieve optimal differentiation between men with and without prostate cancer, especially for those men who have serum PSA levels between 4.0 and 10.0 ng/ml. In attempt to enhance the sensitivity and specificity of PSA, various parameters have been developed and evaluated—these are discussed below.

PSA density

In order to distinguish men with PSA elevations due to prostate enlargement from those with prostate carcinoma, Benson *et al.* in 1992 suggested the use of PSA density to improve PSA specificity (39). PSA density (PSAD) is defined as total serum PSA (in ng/ml) divided by the transrectal ultrasound-determined volume of the prostate gland (in cm^3). The introduction of PSAD was based on the observation that prostate cancer causes a higher increase of PSA values (approximately 3.5 ng/ml/g of tumor) than BPH (0.3 ng/ml/g of hyperplastic tissue) (25).

Seaman *et al.* recommended a PSAD cut-off value of 0.15 ng/ml/ cm^3, in order to increase the prostate cancer detection for men with normal digital rectal examination and serum PSA levels between 4 and 10 ng/ml (40). Since these initial studies on the clinical use of PSAD, conflicting results have been reported by several authors (41–44). In the largest multi center study investigating the efficacy of PSAD for the early diagnosis of prostate cancer, it was reported that nearly half of prostate cancers would have been missed if the PSAD cut-off of 0.15 had been used to determine the subpopulation to be biopsied (41). On the other hand, Epstein *et al.* found that PSAD improved the detection of prostate cancer and was associated with the biologic behavior of the detected carcinomas (44).

The variability in PSAD reported results is probably related to several factors such as:

- the experience of the TRUS examiner;
- the diversity in prostate shape that makes the accurate calculation of prostate volume difficult;
- the variation in epithelium to stroma ratio between individuals that limits the correlation between the estimated BPH volume and serum PSA concentration, since PSA is produced only by the epithelium (45).

The reported results from the application of PSAD to prostate cancer diagnosis indicate that its effectiveness in identifying men who need to be biopsied remains debatable.

PSA age-specific reference ranges

Oesterling *et al.*, in attempt to improve the sensitivity of PSA in prostate cancer detection in younger men and its specificity in older men, suggested age-related PSA reference ranges (46). The predominant factor that is responsible for the increase in serum PSA concentration with advancing age is the concomitant increase of prostate volume. The proposed age-specific PSA reference ranges were 0.0–2.5 ng/ml for men aged 40–49 years, 0.0–3.5 ng/ml for men aged 50–59 years, 0.0–4.5 ng/ml for men aged 60–69 years, and 0.0–6.5 ng/ml for men aged 70–79 years (46). Race was reported to influence the age-specific PSA reference ranges. Therefore, the recommended age-specific PSA reference ranges for African-Americans were 0.0–2.0 ng/ml for men aged 40–49 years, 0.0–4.0 ng/ml for men aged 50–59 years, 0.0–4.5 ng/ml for men aged 60–69 years, and 0.0–5.5 ng/ml for men aged 70–79 years (47); whereas for Japanese men the recommended ranges were 0.0–2.0 ng/ml, 0.0–3.0 ng/ml, 0.0–4.0 ng/ml, and 0.0–5.0 ng/ml, respectively (48). Partin *et al.* showed that the potential detection of prostate cancer using age-specific PSA reference ranges increased by 18% in younger men and decreased by 22% in older men (49). Reissigl *et al.* conducted a mass-screening project in Tirol using the standard and age-adjusted PSA levels. They found an 8% (66 of 778) increase in the biopsy rate and number of the cancers detected (16 of 197). Cancers detected in men younger than 60 years were organ-confined and clinically significant. In men older than 60 years, 21% fewer biopsies were performed (205 of 983) and 12% (23 of 197) cancers were missed, but only eight of these proved to be organ-confined (50).

However, the superiority of the recommended age-specific PSA reference ranges to the standard cut-off point of 4 ng/ml was debated. Catalona *et al.*, in order to select the optimal cut-off value, evaluated different PSA values in a population of 6630 men. The authors showed that using the age-specific PSA reference ranges in men older than 60 years, detection rate of organ-confined cancers was decreased by 22.5% (9 of 40). This led to the conclusion that a serum PSA cut-off of 4.0 ng/ml should be appropriate for older men (26).

In clinical practice, the use of age-specific PSA reference ranges may increase the detection of potential curable prostate cancers in younger men (< 60 years), but may also result in a greater number of negative biopsies in this group. Furthermore, specificity may increased in older men (> 60 years) possibly at the expense of a greater number of undetected cancers. The important question that remains to be answered is whether and how many clinically significant cancers are missed by the use of age-specific PSA reference ranges. It is noteworthy that age-specific PSA reference ranges are not Food and Drug Administration approved or recommended by PSA assay manufacturers (51). Thus, urologists should use PSA values adjusted for patient age and race very cautiously in daily practice, bearing in mind the risks and benefits of these ranges when counseling patients.

PSA velocity

It is well documented that prostate cancer increases PSA levels more than BPH (25). Carter *et al.* confirmed the hypothesis that men with prostate cancer might have a faster rise of PSA levels compared to men without cancer (52). They found that the median annual increase of PSA in patients with prostate cancer, men with BPH, and healthy men was 0.88 ng/ml, 0.12 ng/ml, and 0.03 ng/ml, respectively. Based on the above observations, they suggested the use of PSA velocity (PSAV) that represents the rate of PSA change over time, as a method for assessing the risk of the presence of prostate cancer. PSAV is calculated by the following equation:

$$\text{PSA velocity (ng/ml/year)} = 1/2\{[\text{PSA2} - \text{PSA1/time1 in years}] + [\text{PSA3} - \text{PSA2/time2 in years}]\}, \qquad (12.1)$$

where PSA1 = first PSA measurement, PSA2 = second PSA measurement, PSA3 = third PSA measurement..

Carter *et al.* showed that, by using a PSAV cut-off value of 0.75 ng/ml/year, a sensitivity of 72% and a specificity of 95% in distinguishing men with from those without prostate cancer, were achieved (52). They also demonstrated that the optimal requirements for maintaining sensitivity and specificity are three PSA measurements taken during a period of at least 1.5–2 years.

Limitations of the method include:

- the variation of PSA measurements with time and different assays;

- the effect on PSA levels of several factors (such as prostatitis, pharmacological therapies), that may appear in the interval between PSA measurements;
- the necessity to monitor PSA changes for at least over a period of 1.5–2 years in order to obtain reliable PSAV results (53).

With the increasing numbers of men who systematically undergo annual serum PSA measurements for preventive reasons, PSA velocity seems to be an ideal method for optimizing surveillance. Therefore the most important application of PSA velocity is to follow men with normal but rising serum PSA levels, and younger men (<50years) belonging to high risk groups (positive family history, race). Moreover for men with PSA levels between 4.0 and 10.0 ng/ml, who have already undergone a prostate biopsy that disclosed no evidence of cancer, PSA velocity could be a useful adjunctive measure to determine the need for repeating prostate biopsy at a latter time.

%-Free PSA

In vitro, PSA has been shown to form sodium dodecyl sulfate stable complexes with two of the major extracellular, mainly liver-derived, proteinase inhibitors in blood, namely a1-antichymotrypsin (ACT) and a2-macroglobulin (AMG). In addition to ACT, other inhibitors—members of the serpin superfamily of serine protease inhibitors—are reported to form covalent complexes with PSA, such as a1-antitrypsin (a1-protease inhibitor, a1-PI) and the protein C inhibitor (PCI) (54–56). PSA circulates in the serum in both the complexed (bound) and uncomplexed (unbound or free) form. The existence of multiple molecular forms of PSA in serum was first reported in 1991 (55, 56). Free PSA and the PSA a1-antichymotrypsin complex (PSA–ACT) have been demonstrated to be enzymatically inactive, whilst the PSA a2-macroglobulin complex seems not to completely inactivate the PSA protease (57). Complex formation with a1-antichymotrypsin results in exposure of a limited number of the antigenic epitopes of PSA, whereas complex formation with a2-macroglobulin completely encapsulates the PSA molecule and blocks the epitopes sites (57). Therefore commercial PSA assays are capable of detecting total PSA, free PSA, and PSA a1-antichymotrypsin.

The free, unbound form of PSA ranges between 5% and 50% (with typical values of less than 30%) of the total measure of PSA. The PSA–ACT complex represents the major molecular form of PSA in the serum (with an average of about 70–85%) (57)

In the two pioneering studies on the molecular forms of PSA, Stenman *et al.* and Lilja *et al.* found that the percentage of free PSA decreases as the probability of the presence of prostate cancer increases (55, 56). This observation has been investigated and confirmed by several authors (58–66).

It still remains unclear why men with prostate cancer have a lower proportion of free-to-total PSA compared to men suffering from benign disease. Oesterling and Lilja have hypothesized that this difference might be due to mechanisms used by prostatic cells to prevent PSA from escaping the prostate ductal system into the general circulation (67). These mechanisms are better preserved in normal than in cancerous tissues. Bjork *et al.* noted that prostate cancer cells expressed not only PSA but also ACT. In contrast there was lack of ACT production in BPH areas (68). Similar observations in prostate cancer cell lines and prostate-cancer tissues have been reported by Vessella and Lange (57). The production of both PSA and ACT by most prostate cancers may facilitate the formation of PSA–ACT complexes and possibly result in lower free PSA levels in sera of men with prostate cancer.

The impressive number of studies that have been published since 1991 underlines the existing intensified demand to find a new improved, more helpful marker than total PSA in distinguishing men with prostate cancer from those without malignancy. It also explains the growing enthusiasm for free PSA being able to play this role successfully. However, differences in design of the reported studies and patient selection make comparison of the results a difficult task. Moreover there are many factors that might influence

the results and conclusions of the free-PSA clinical studies, such as: total PSA, prostate volume, age, race, biopsy verified diagnosis, digital rectal examination findings, pathological features, surgical history, drug treatment history, biopsy and prostate manipulation, sample stability, assay methods, interpretation of ROC curves, sample size, and calculation of prostate cancer risk (69). The variability in %-free PSA cut-off values used (ranging from 14% to 28%), resulted in a wide variation of sensitivity and specificity, which ranged from 305 to 1005, and from 13% to 95%, respectively (58–66). The lack of a commonly approved cut-off value of %-free PSA is therefore obvious (Table 12.1).

Another issue that needs to be determined, is the optimal range of total PSA levels for the use of the percentage of free PSA. This range is known as the 'reflex-range'.

While most investigators agree that the upper limit of the reflex range should be 10.0 ng/ml, controversy surrounds the determination of the lower limit (Table 12.1). In the literature, it is reported that prostate cancer can be detected within 3–5 years in approximately 13–20% of men with present total PSA levels of 2.6–4.0 ng/ml (70, 71). Based on the above, Vashi *et al.* suggested a reflex-range of total PSA from 3.0 to 10.0 ng/ml for calculation of free PSA. They studied 413 cases and found that in order to improve sensitivity, different cut points of %-free PSA should be used for men with total PSA levels between 3.0 and 4.0 ng/ml and men with PSA levels in the range of 4.1–10 ng/ml (19% and 24%, respectively) (64). Catalona *et al.* reported that the use of a %-free PSA cut point of 27% enabled the detection of 90% of cancers (20 of 22) and elimination of 18% of negative biopsies in

Table 12.1 Evaluation of free PSA cut-off values in men with total PSA less than 10 ng/ml

Reference	PSA (ng/m)	%-Free PSA cut-off	Sensitivity (%)	Specificity (%)
Luderer *et al.* (58)	4–10	25	100	31
Catalona *et al.* (59)	4–10	20	90	38
Prestigiacomo *et al.* (60)	4–10	14	95	64
Partin *et al.* (61)	4–10	20	95	29
Bangma *et al.* (62)	4–10	28	91	19
Catalona *et al.* (63)	2.6–4	27	90	18
Vashi *et al.* (64)	3–4	19	90	48
	4–10	24	95	13
Catalona *et al.* (65)	2.5–4	15	54	67
	2.5–4	10	30	94
van Cangh *et al.* (66)	1.8–10	25	92	32

332 men with total PSA levels between 2.6 and 4.0 ng/ml and a normal digital rectal examination (63).

The clinical utility of %-free PSA cut-off value could be the elimination of a number of unnecessary biopsies in men with PSA levels lower than 10.0 ng/ml and the possibility to indicate the development of an aggressive tumor several years before the clinical diagnosis (72).

New PSA derivatives

PSA transitional zone density

Kalish *et al.* introduced the term PSA transitional zone density (PSA-TZ), defined as the ratio of total serum PSA (in ng/ml) and transrectal ultrasound-determined transitional zone volume (in cm^3) (73). This concept is based on the knowledge that BPH is almost exclusively developed from the transitional zone of the prostate (74). Therefore PSA changes due to BPH should come almost exclusively from the inner gland elements, principally the TZ, whereas outer gland production of PSA should remain relatively constant as the gland enlarges due to BPH (73). A PSA-TZ cut-off value of 0.35 ng/ml/cm^3, suggested by Djavan *et al.*, provided the highest positive predictive value (74%) for prostate cancer detection (75).

Kurita *et al.* using a PSA transitional zone threshold of 0.17 in patients with prostate volume larger than 40 cm^3, reported that 88% of the cancers were detected, the number of biopsies was reduced by 56%, and the positive predictive value was 30%; with a threshold of 0.30 the sensitivity, the specificity, and the positive predictive value of PSA-TZ for detecting prostate cancer were 48%, 92%, and 55%, respectively (76). The same authors also concluded that PSA transitional zone seems to be more useful for selection of patients who should undergo prostate biopsy when the prostate volume is larger than 40 cm^3. Horninger *et al.*, using as the unique biopsy criterion a cut-off of 0.22 for PSA-TZ, demonstrated that 24.4% of unnecessary negative biopsies could be avoided while no case of prostate cancer was missed (100% sensitivity) (77).

It is obvious that the most significant limitation of PSA-TZ is the difficulty to calculate precisely the TZ volume using transrectal ultrasound. Establishment of a standard voluming technique among the many TRUS performers should facilitate the output of comparable data. Further data are needed to confirm the validity of PSA-TZ in distinguishing between men with and without prostate cancer.

Complexed PSA

It was reasonable to expect that the next concept to be investigated would be the potential role of complexed PSA (PSA–ACT) as a tumor marker for cancer detection. Progress in the standardization of complexed PSA assays allowed the development of clinical studies for the evaluation of the clinical usefulness of the complexed PSA. Initial reported results showed that specificity of complexed PSA was higher than that of total and free PSA in cancer detection (55, 78, 79). The completion of the ongoing studies will provide more information about the possible use of complexed PSA as an alternative serum tumor marker.

The ProstAsure Index

A new test, the ProstAsure Index, has been developed (80). This index is serum-based and is determined from several input variables (age, total PSA, prostatic acid phosphatase, and creatinine phosphokinase) using an artificial neural network-derived, non-linear algorithmic procedure. The ProstAsure Index results vary from less than 0.0 to greater than 1.0, and are given in terms of four zones (1–4). Zone 1 includes values less than 0.0, zone 2 from 0.0 to 0.5, zone 3 from 0.5 to 1.0, and zone 4 greater than 1.0. It has been suggested that normal values are less than 0.5, therefore a man classified as belonging in either zone 3 or 4 should undergo a prostate biopsy. The Index provides diagnostic improvement in men with serum PSA levels of 4.0 ng/ml or less.

Stamey *et al.*, studying 298 men with normal PSA levels, found that the Index exhibits a 71% sensitivity and a 86% specificity in detecting prostate cancer (80). Babaian *et al.* compared retrospectively the ProstAsure Index to %-free PSA for the diagnosis of prostate cancer in 225 men. They reported that the sensitivity and the specificity using the ProstAsure Index were 93% and 81%, respectively. Using a %-free PSA cut-off value of 15%, the sensitivity and the specificity were 80% and 74%, respectively; whilst for %-free PSA at 19%, sensitivity increased to 93% and specificity reduced to 59% (81). The authors concluded that the Index achieved statistically significant better results than the %-free PSA in detecting prostate cancer in men with normal DRE and a total PSA value of 4.0 ng/ml or less. It is clear that these yet preliminary, but promising observations should be validated by further prospective studies.

Other serum tumor markers

Human glandular kallikrein

The human glandular kallikrein, or hK2 protein, belongs to the kallikreins that are a multigene family of serine proteases (82). The hK2 product was first described in 1987 (83) and the primary structure of the hK2 protein is a 237 amino acids protein with an 80% sequence homology with PSA (83,84). However, in contrast to PSA, which has a chymotrypsin-like protease activity, hK2 is a trypsin-like protease (83). Preliminary studies on the biologic function of hK2 suggest that it might be involved in the activation of proPSA. The hK2 protein has been suggested as a new prostate cancer marker (85). Darson *et al.* evaluated the immunoreactivity for hK2 in 257 radical prostatectomy specimens. It was reported that hk2 was expressed in every cancer and the expression increased from benign prostatic tissue, to high-grade PIN and prostate cancer (86). It is noted that the hK2 expression is increased as the grading of the tumor increases. Furthermore, hK2 can be detected in the serum of patients with BPH or prostate cancer (87, 88). Kwiatkowski *et al.* demonstrated that the hk2/free PSA ratio had better specificity for prostate cancer at all sensitivity levels than total PSA or free/total PSA ratio within the range of 4.0–10.0 ng/ml (89). Further studies are required in order to investigate the potential clinical utility of hK2 as a new tumor marker.

Prostatic acid phosphatase (PAP)

The acid phosphatases are non-specific enzymes that hydrolyze phosphate esters in acidic conditions. Prostatic acid phosphatase is an isoenzyme found in greatest concentration in the prostate. This protein of molecular weight 100 000 is composed of two identical subunits. In 1938, Gutman and Gutman demonstrated elevated serum acid phosphatase levels in 11–15% of patients with metastatic prostate cancer (90) and 3 years later, Huggins and Hodges introduced PAP as a measure of response to bilateral orchiectomy or estrogen administration (91). PAP was the first widely used clinical tumor marker. However, PAP presented instability, low sensitivity, and specificity, thus it has been replaced by PSA.

Transrectal ultrasound

Transrectal ultrasound (TRUS) is currently the most common imaging modality for the prostate, and has become a daily routine procedure in almost any urological department. Since 1955, when Wild and Reid (92) first presented a transrectal scanner, important progress in imaging quality has been achieved with the employment of high-resolution, high-frequency (5–7 MHz) transducers in two planes. The use of TRUS includes the measurement of gland volume, definition of the anatomy and the margins of the prostate, identification of suspicious lesions of the prostate, evaluation of the seminal vesicles and the base of the bladder, and guidance of the puncture biopsy needle (53). During the last decade, TRUS has been proved to significantly increase the detection of prostate carcinoma in comparison with digital rectal examination (DRE) (93–95).

Transducer probe is prepared for the endorectal examination by using either the single-cover technique or the double-cover technique. In the single-cover technique a disposal latex or rubber cover is placed over the part of the transducer that will be placed into the rectum. Two types of probes can be used. With the first type after the insertion of the probe into the rectum, the cover is inflated with 50–100 ml of water through a specially designed opening in the external part of the probe. This distends the cover, and provides an airtight fit against the rectal mucosa placing the prostate in the sharpest focal zone of the probe. With the second type of probe, an acoustic gel is used instead of the water path. The gel is placed between the cover and the probe and complete acoustic contact is achieved.

In the double-cover technique (same with both types of probes), after placing the first or inner cover over the probe, gel is placed over the tip followed by the second cover. After completion of each examination the probe can be reused with its inner cover, while the outer one is removed. Slight image degradation may be the result of the use of double covers. Patient's preparation involves a cleansing, self-administered fleet-enema 2–4 h prior to the examination, so as to induce evacuation of the rectum. If the examination is to be followed by TRUS-guided biopsy, the patient's preparation also involves administration of antibiotics and cessation of aspirin or anticoagulants (see below). All steps of the procedure are explained to the patient prior to the examination.

As mentioned above, a methodical DRE must be performed before the TRUS, not only to provide the examiner with a diagram of irregularities and indurations of the prostate, but also to exclude any anal and rectal pathology (hemorrhoids, narrowed anus, rectal tumor). A Tran abdominal ultrasound scanning of the gland with longitudinal and transverse sections must also be performed and the volume of the gland should be estimated. TRUS can be performed with the patient in chest–knee, lateral decubitus, or dorsal lithotomy position. The tip of the covered probe and the anus are lubricated with gel and the probe is inserted into the rectum at a depth of 8–9 cm. Optimal TRUS imaging of the prostate requires examination of the gland from the base to the apex with both longitudinal and transverse sections. Once the transducer is placed into the rectum, the entire gland is usually seen in longitudinal section from base to the apex, including portion of the seminal vesicles (SV). The midline is usually imaged first with small movements of the probe towards the patient's back or abdomen and slight rotations clockwise or counterclockwise. The right side of the gland and the right SV are seen in counterclockwise rotation whilst the left side and the left SV in clockwise rotation. Transverse scanning is possible with 90^0 rotation of the probe. Primarily both SV are studied and then the probe is slightly withdrawn to study first the base and then the body and the apex of the gland. When water path probes are used, better visualization of the prostate is achieved by increasing the amount of water between cover and probe or by changing its distribution with movements of the probe towards patient's back or abdomen.

The normal central zone (CZ) and peripheral zone (PZ) have a similar and uniform echogenicity and usually are not distinguished. In patients where differentiation is possible, CZ appears more echogenic than PZ. The transitional zone (TZ) has usually a mixed echogenicity with hyperechoic and hypoechoic nodules, which create a heterogeneous appearance with distortions of the outline of the gland. As the prostate increases in size with age, the TZ, site of BPH origin, becomes the dominant zone. The bladder base is elevated and the PZ is compressed and becomes more echogenic than normal. The seminal vesicles are slightly less echogenic than the prostate. They appear smaller in the midline than in the lateral aspect. They have a variable appearance, and whether large or small, bilateral symmetry should be present in size, shape and echogenicity.

Lee *et al.* reported that typical prostate cancers are generally hypoechoic areas in the peripheral zone (96) (Fig. 12.1). However hypoechogenicity is non-specific to prostate cancer. At most only one of three hypoechoic areas will prove to be cancer, whilst carcinoma can be also found in normal echoic areas of the prostate (97). Similar observations on the appearance of prostate cancer on TRUS have been reported by

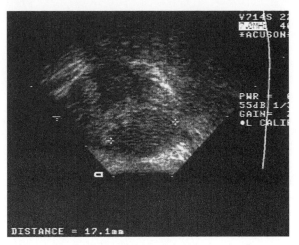

Fig. 12.1 Longitudinal image: an hypoechoic prostate cancer in the peripheral zone (cursors).

several investigators who indicated that 16.5–39.0% of cancers were detected only in isoechoic sectors (98–102). Melchior and Brower, comparing TRUS and biopsy results of 2231 patients, found that more than 70% had hypoechoic lesions on TRUS. However, a carcinoma was detected in only 30% of these cases. Moreover, carcinoma was also diagnosed in 18.4% of men with a normal appearance of the prostate on TRUS (102). Ellis *et al.* (98) evaluated the results of 6-sector prostate biopsies in 1001 men. It was reported that only 17% of the hypoechoic sectors demonstrated carcinoma on biopsy, whereas positive biopsy was found in 6,1% of isoechoic sectors and 25% of patients had cancer detected only in isoechoic sectors.

Moreover, small (< 5 mm) foci of prostate carcinoma are rarely detected by TRUS. Extensive tumors involving the entire PZ are sometimes difficult to be identified because comparison with normal PZ is not possible. Likewise, isoechoic tumors are usually not detected and tumors in the TZ, are difficult to be identified by TRUS, especially if BPH is very prominent. An hypoechoic lesion in PZ found by TRUS could also be the result of acute or chronic prostatitis, prostatic intra-epithelial neoplasia (PIN), atrophy, and prostate infarct, which all limit the specificity of TRUS (103).

Aarnink and colleagues reported that TRUS, in a select group of 717 patients suspected for prostate cancer, had 84% sensitivity, 67% specificity, 52% positive predictive value, and 91% negative predictive value (104). The limited sensitivity and low specificity of TRUS has not become higher with the evolution in technology. High-resolution transrectal ultrasound scanners have not substantially improved the localization of prostate cancer (104) and 3-dimensional TRUS images enhance the staging but not the diagnostic ability of the 2-dimensional ultrasonography (105). These studies demonstrate low sensitivity and specificity in prostate cancer detection by TRUS, therefore TRUS as a 'stand-alone' screening tool, is not convincing. Furthermore, the essential question it does raise is whether a TRUS-detected, impalpable prostate carcinoma with normal serum PSA concentration, particularly in older men, is clinically significant. TRUS could be used in combination with PSA and DRE as a method for the detection of prostate cancer.

New imaging techniques

The need for improved tumor-localizing modalities is apparent. Computer analysis of ultrasound images of the prostate aims to enhance diagnostic accuracy using an automated, and not eye-dependent, interpretation (104). Further evaluation of this technique is still needed. As cancer, in general, grows faster than normal tissue and requires increased blood supply, Color Doppler provides visualization of local changes in tissue blood supply and vascularization. However, early results of the method are not yet satisfactory (106). New imaging techniques using contrast agents to enhance the Doppler display of the vessels are also under investigation (104).

Prostate cancer appears on magnetic resonance imaging (MRI) as a low signal intensity focus discrete from normal tissue. Endorectal MRI was reported to have a 61% accuracy of detecting cancer localization with 60% sensitivity and 63% specificity. Furthermore, detection rate for cancer foci less than 5 mm was 5%, whereas that for foci greater than 10 mm it was 89% (107). Perrotti *et al.* demonstrated that tumor localization by endorectal MRI in men with prior negative prostate biopsy, was superior to that by TRUS. In addition, they reported that the overall diagnostic rates of MRI were 69.7% in accuracy, 85.7% in sensitivity, 64.5% in specificity, 40% in positive predictive value, and 94.4% in negative predictive value (108). The validity of endorectal MRI in guiding repeat prostate biopsies is now investigated. In addition, the application of proton spectroscopic MRI for cancer localization and evaluation of tumor aggressiveness by assessing the prostatic metabolites choline and citrate, is in the frame of future perspectives (109).

Combination of diagnostic modalities

As discussed previously, all the diagnostic modalities have several limitations that decrease their sensitivity and specificity for detecting prostate cancer. Thus, combination of the tests seems an appropriate method for achieving increased cancer detection. In Table 12.2, we demonstrate the results of several studies of diagnostic investigations with PSA, DRE, and TRUS. The positive predictive value (PPV) of these tests (as a percentage of recommendations for biopsy pathologically confirmed as cancer) provide useful information regarding the selection of patients who need to be biopsied.

As expected, the best PPV was obtained with the combination of all three tests (range from 45.2% to 75%), resulting in increased probability of discovering cancer on biopsy. It is noteworthy that elevated PSA is the best predictive test on individual basis (PPV ranged from 30% to 43%), for detection of prostate cancer. Moreover, the association of PSA results with PPV was significant. The combinations of PSA with either TRUS or DRE are superior to the combination of DRE and TRUS. This data support the need for multimodality investigation for early diagnosis of prostate cancer in urological practice (110–111).

Prostatic biopsy

A prostate carcinoma is definitively diagnosed only by tissue histologic confirmation. Today the most widely used method for obtaining prostate tissue specimens is the transrectal ultrasound guided needle biopsy. In daily practice, ultrasound-guided biopsy is indicated by an abnormal digital rectal examination (DRE) or elevated serum prostate-specific antigen (PSA) concentration. Indeed, the most important role of transrectal ultrasound (TRUS) in the diagnosis of prostate cancer is that it aids the precise placement of the biopsy needle, based on the visualization of the biopsy trajectory on ultrasound (Fig. 12.2). The transperineal biopsy, much less tolerated by the patient, is not in routine use, with the exception of men who underwent abdomino-perineal resection for anal or rectal carcinoma (112). Ultrasound-guided biopsies have also replaced digitally guided biopsies of palpable lesions in current practice due to the superior accuracy of the sonographic guidance, as was documented by several studies (113–115).

Table 12.2   Positive predictive value of cancer for combinations of digital rectal examination (DRE), prostate-specific antigen (PSA), and transrectal ultrasound (TRUS)

	Positive predictive value (No. of cancers/no. of biopsies)				
References	Ellis *et al.* (98)	Rietbergen *et al.* (110)	Catalona *et al.* (11)	Mettlin *et al.* (15)	Schröder *et al.* (111)
Population	Mixed	Screening	Screening	Screening	Screening
DRE(+)	27.4%	27.3%	21.4%	28.0%	36.7%
irrespective	213/777	265/972	146/683	33/118	54/147
PSA, TRUS					
PSA(+)	36.8%	29.8%	31.5%	NA	43.0%
irrespective	199/541	351/1176	216/686		43/100
DRE, TRUS					
TRUS(+)	28.8%	26.8%	NA	15.2%	24.9%
irrespective	230/797	257/958		44/290	54/217
DRE, PSA					
DRE (−)	0%	NB	NB	NB	NB
PSA (−)	0/24				
TRUS(−)					
DRE (+)	6.4%	10.1%	6.9%	16.7%	*13.6%
PSA (−)	5/78	45/444	16/233	5/30	3/22
TRUS(−)					
DRE (+)	19.6%	17.4%	20.7%	NB	19.0%
PSA (+)	10/51	124/711	57/276		8/42
TRUS(−)					
DRE (−)	9.1%	9.0%	NB	5.5%	5.5%
PSA (−)	5/55	40/442		9/164	5/91
TRUS(+)					
DRE (+)	15.7%	32.2%	41.3%	37.5%	63.6%
PSA (+)	8/51	48/149	26/63	3/8	7/11
TRUS(−)					
DRE (+)	14.5%	19.0	13.8%	14.6%	26.6%
PSA (−)	44/303	38/200	32/232	7/48	21/79
TRUS(+)					
DRE (−)	26.6%	32.8%	29.8%	24.3%	41.7%
PSA (+)	25/94	45/137	57/191	9/37	5/12
TRUS(+)					
DRE (+)	45.2%	74.8%	54.7%	68.0%	65.7%
PSA (+)	156/345	134/179	64/117	17/25	23/35
TRUS(+)					

PSA(+): greater than 4.0 ng/ml; **PSA(−):** less than 4.0 ng/ml; **DRE(+):** abnormal as described in the text; **DRE(−):** normal including benign prostatic hyperplasia; **TRUS(+):** any hypoechoic sector noted; **TRUS(−):** no hypoechoic sector noted; **NA:** non available; **NB:** no biopsies according to the study protocol.
* Different PSA cut-off values.

In order to minimize the patient's discomfort, TRUS examination should be performed when the clinical and biochemical investigation of the patient is completed and the results are known. Combining these results with the findings of TRUS, we will be able to decide if a prostate biopsy is required and repeat TRUS examination will be avoided. Using this approach, it is indispensable to prepare the patient for an eventual biopsy. It is prudent to investigate any history for bleeding diathesis. A fleet enema 2–4 h before biopsy, is also necessary. The patient should receive antibiotic prophylaxis (i.e. fluoroquinolone) 1 h before the procedure. In patients with subacute bacterial endocarditis, mitral valve prolapsis, cardiac valve, or prosthetic implants, treatment with stronger antibiotics (combination of vancomycin and gentamycin), half an hour before biopsy and 8 h after the initial dose is recommended. Anticoagulants and antiplatelet agents, such as aspirin and non-steroid anti-inflammatory agents, must be discontinued 5 days before the procedure.

The invention of spring-firing biopsy instruments made prostate biopsy possible without any kind of

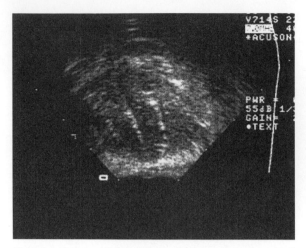

Fig. 12.2 Biopsy of the lesion of Fig. 12.1. Three needle tracks containing air inside the lesion.

anesthesia for the majority of patients. The apparatus employs an 18-gauge tru-cut type biopsy needle with a 17-mm sample notch near its tip (5 mm from the tip). The trigger produces an abrupt advancement of the outer cutting element. This results in the safe and less traumatic extraction of a tissue core adequate for the histologic diagnosis of the disease and, in case of cancer, for the grading of the malignancy. There is a wide range in size, shape, and length of the biopsy needles and trigger type devices available in the market.

A guide instrument for the needle, specially designed for each type of endorectal probe, is placed in position over the probe that is covered with the inner cover. Following application of gel over the tip of the probe, and placement of the second cover, the probe is positioned within the rectum and the TRUS study is performed. The needle with the trigger device is inserted through the biopsy guide, until the line of sight of needle insertion is displayed on the screen and then is placed to biopsy the abnormality. The trigger is released and the needle is automatically advanced about 20 mm (depending on the trigger device used) to obtain a core sample. Biopsies are performed in longitudinal images. The prostatic urethra is easily seen with TRUS and should be avoided.

Transrectal ultrasound-guided prostate biopsy is considered safe. The main complications of TRUS-guided biopsy are hematuria, hematospermia, rectal bleeding, urinary infections, vasovagal reactions, and peri-prostatic hematoma causing pain and discomfort to the patient (116). The most common complication is hematuria with a reported incidence varying from 20%

to 50%, and duration of 3–7 days, but significant hematuria with clots occurs in only 1–2% of patients biopsied (112, 116–118). However, complications are generally minor and self-limited. In only 0.4–1.2% of patients, severe complications requiring hospitalization, may be appeared (116–118) Proper patient preparation and good examination technique by an experienced examiner can reduce the number and severity of complications. In our series, urinary infection occurred in 27 of the 537 patients biopsied (5%), and 5 patients experienced significant hematuria (0.8%). However no patient required hospitalization (119).

An important concern of the urologist is the determination of the sampling regions of the prostate, as well as the adequate number of cores required for optimal results. Unfortunately, no information on tumor localization is provided by PSA levels, and it seems that DRE and TRUS have limited accuracy in localizing prostate cancer. Flanigan and colleagues (120), in a multicenter prostate cancer screening study, performed quadrant biopsies in 1086 men with PSA levels > 4.0 ng/ml, and/or abnormal DRE. Cancer was found in only 11% (110 from 1002) of the prostatic quadrants suspicious on DRE, and 9% (308 from 3342) of those quadrants that were not suspicious. Consequently, 74% of quadrants with cancer (308 from 418) or 61% of patients (137 from 225) would have been missed if only the exact site of the palpable induration had been biopsied. They also showed that cancer was detected in 18% (153 from 855) of the sonographically suspicious quadrants, and 8% (282 from 3581) of those that were sonographically normal. Therefore, 65% (282 from 435) of quadrants harboring cancer or 52% of patients (131 from 251) would have been missed if only the hypoechoic areas had been biopsied.

The limited value of directed ultrasound-guided biopsies of specific hypoechoic areas was first demonstrated by Hodge *et al.* (113). The authors introduced the systematic six transrectal core biopsies of the prostate compared to directed biopsies in 136 men with abnormal DRE. Nine per cent of cancers detected by systematic biopsies were missed by directed biopsies. According to the authors, the six systematic biopsies should be spaced at the apex, mid gland, and base of each lobe. This technique was also analyzed by Hammerer and colleagues (99). The systematic sextant biopsies and additional biopsy of any hypoechoic area or palpable abnormality remain the gold standard for the histological sampling of the prostate. Nevertheless, alternative biopsy schemes for optimal sampling of the prostate, have been evaluated by a number of investigators, with emphasis on the potential effect of prostate volume on the cancer detection by systematic sextant biopsy (121–127). The seemingly reasonable concept is that the chance for sampling error increases as the prostate enlarges. Eskew *et al.* suggested the 'five-region prostate biopsy' scheme that calls, in addition to sextant biopsies, for cores obtained from the far lateral and mid regions of the gland. A total of 13 cores in prostates smaller than 50 g, and 18 cores in those larger than 50 g, were sampled. The authors found this technique superior to the sextant biopsy; 17 from the 48 prostate cancers (35%) were detected only by the additional biopsies (121). Norberg *et al.* compared the standard sextant ultrasound-guided prostate biopsy with different biopsy models provided by combinations of 8–10 standardized samples with or without targeted biopsies in 512 men. A total of 276 cancers were identified but sextant biopsy missed 15% of them (122). Uzzo *et al.* analyzed 1021 sextant biopsies and showed that positive biopsy yield increased significantly in prostates smaller than 50 cm^3 than in those larger than 50 cm^3 (reported cancer detection was 38% and 23%, respectively) (123). Letran *et al.* reported similar results with 1057 men who underwent ultrasound-guided sextant biopsies. Cancer detection was significantly lower (22%) in prostates with volume greater than 55.6 cm^3 compared with those with volume less than 55.6 cm^3 (33.8%). It was concluded that 6 systematic biopsies are adequate for men with total prostate volume smaller than 55.6 cm^3; however, for larger prostates the optimal number of biopsies needs to be determined (124). Vashi *et al.* introduced a mathematical model to establish the number of cores required to detect life-hreatening prostate cancers, on the basis of patient age and prostate volume. Using this theoretical model, they show that sextant biopsy was adequate only for the few of prostate glands (125).

However, a number of studies failed to demonstrate any correlation between the TRUS-determined prostate volume and the number of needle biopsies required for detecting prostate carcinoma. Brown *et al.* performed two additional biopsies in the most suspicious areas (identified on TRUS or DRE) that resulted in only one additional case of cancer (1.1% of cancers). This data indicated that systematic sextant biopsy is adequate in most men (126). More recently, Ravery *et al.* evaluated an extensive biopsy protocol, consisting of four systematic biopsies in addition to the standard sextant biopsies. Only four cancers were detected by the additional biopsies alone in prostates smaller than 50 cm^3, resulting in a 4% increase in cancer detection rate.

Furthermore, in prostates larger than 40 cm^3, only one cancer was found by the additional biopsies, representing a 1.6% increase of detected cancers. The authors concluded that an increase in the number of cores has not a significant impact on cancer detection rate (127). Moreover, there is always the risk that the increasing number of sampled cores could result in identifying clinically insignificant prostate cancers. The problem could be solved by large series that will analyze the radical prostatectomy data of the patients who were found by the additional prostate biopsies only.

Routine transition zone (TZ) biopsy has also been a controversial issue. Since approximately 20% of prostate cancers originate from the transition zone a significant increase in cancer detection rate should be expected with additional transitional zone sampling. However, the reported proportion of prostate cancers detected exclusively in the transition zone biopsies was surprisingly low, ranging from 1.8 to 2.9% of total cancers (128, 129). Similarly, Fleshner and Fair performing 204 transition zone prostate biopsies in 185 men found eight isolated transition zone cancers only in the group of 156 patients who underwent a repeat biopsy, which represented 15.7% (8/51) of the cancers detected in this group. No sole transition zone carcinoma was detected among the seven cancers found in the group of 29 initially biopsied men (130). Chang *et al.* suggested that the discrepancy between the incidence of transition zone cancers and the results of the additional transitional zone biopsies could be the result of the sampling of transitional zone tissue by the peripheral zone (PZ) biopsy and the limited number of biopsy cores taken from the transitional zone. By performing systematic sextant biopsies of both the peripheral and transitional zone in 213 large prostates, the authors demonstrated that PZ biopsies detected significant number of TZ cancers, and 13% of the cancers were found by the additional TZ biopsies only (131). Nevertheless, patient discomfort, increased morbidity and cost of the additional biopsies cannot be ignored. It is therefore reasonable to suggest that routine TZ biopsies should be reserved only for patients with a previous ultrasound-guided negative PZ biopsy (128–132).

An interesting approach towards the identification of the adequate number and location of needle biopsies is the development of a computer simulation model of prostate biopsy (133, 134). Karalicwicz *et al.* simulated five 3-dimensional prostates ranging from 20 to 100 cm^3 in size and evaluated five different biopsy methods on all prostate models. They concluded that a gland volume-based biopsy algorithm was likely to improve detection of prostate cancer and recommended that one core for at least every 5 cm³ of prostatic tissue should be taken (133). More recently, Chen and colleagues digitally reconstructed 180 radical prostatectomy specimens and assessed 10 different biopsy schemes using a simulation system. They demonstrated that the detection rate of prostate cancer depended on both the numbers of biopsies and the sampled regions of the gland. A new 11-core multisite-directed scheme, consisting of sextant, two transition zone, one midline, and two anterior horn biopsies, proved to be most effective in this simulation study (134).

The use of numerous simulations in these experimental models allow the assessment of several parameters that may influence biopsy results (such parameters include prostate volume, gland shape, tumor volume, tumor localization, number of biopsy cores, and distribution of biopsy needles), otherwise difficult to investigate in clinical practice (135–139). Nevertheless, clinical studies are required in order to reproduce the simulation results and examine the applicability of the suggested biopsy techniques in daily practice.

In case of the histological examination of sampled tissue reveals the presence of prostate cancer, staging of the disease will follow and the appropriate treatment will be offered. If biopsy results are negative for cancer, the clinician will face a new dilemma, how to manage a patient who had a strong indication (clinical, biochemical, imaging) for biopsy, but a negative biopsy result. Recent studies are focused on the need to perform repeat biopsies to men with previous negative biopsies. The positive repeat biopsy rate in men with initial negative biopsy ranges from 11% to 38% (Table 12.3). Efforts have been made to identify patients who will need to be re-biopsied without submitting all patients to this invasive procedure (140–144).

A solid criterion for performing a repeat biopsy is the finding of isolated high-grade prostatic intra-epithelial neoplasia (PIN) in the first needle biopsy. PIN is considered to be a precursor of prostate carcinoma. The clinical significance of PIN is its high predictive value as a marker for prostate carcinoma (145) and its identification in 82% of step-sectioned autopsy prostrates with cancer (146). Thus, repeat biopsy is warranted either to identify a possible existing concurrent carcinoma missed by the first biopsy or to detect a subsequently developed prostate cancer. Several studies on the results of repeat biopsies for initial isolated high-grade PIN have been published (147–151). Cancer-

detection rate of repeat biopsy ranges from 35% to 100%. Most of the reports have an interval between initial and subsequent biopsy of less of than 1 year, indicating that the cancer was most probably co-existent. Patients with high-grade PIN should be re-biopsied after 3–6 months to exclude concomitant cancer. In the case of a negative repeat biopsy, patients should undergo the follow-up examinations, including PSA, DRE, TRUS, and repeat biopsy, biannually during the first 2 years and thereafter annually.

Persistently elevated PSA values, a rapidly increasing PSA value, and an abnormal DRE are the current indications for re-biopsy. Recent studies investigated the potential role of PSA derivatives in identifying patients at high risk, requiring repeat prostate biopsy. Conflicting results have been reported. There are studies that failed to demonstrate any superiority of PSA derivatives (PSA density, %-free PSA, PSA velocity, age-referenced PSA) to PSA cut-off value of 4.0 ng/ml (136, 152). Furthermore, Fleshner *et al.* defined a subgroup of patients who were considered to be at the lowest risk for a positive repeat biopsy. These patients fulfilled the following criteria: PSA less than 10 ng/ml, PSA density less than 0.15 ng/ml/cm³, PSA velocity less than 0.75 ng/ml/year, no PIN or atypia at the initial biopsy, negative DRE, negative TRUS, and no family history of prostate cancer. The positive repeat biopsy rate in this group was surprisingly high, 23.8% (5 of 21 patients) (135). In contrast, Morgan *et al.* demonstrated that a %-free PSA value less than 10%, which had 91% sensitivity and 86% specificity, in a selected group of men with persistently elevated serum PSA, a normal DRE, and two prior negative biopsies (138). Similarly, Catalona *et al.* evaluated 99 men who had PSA values of 4.01–10.0 ng/ml, a normal DRE, and prior negative biopsies. They detected 20 cancers on the repeat biopsy (20.2%) and found that both free PSA and PSA density were useful for predicting prostate cancer. Percentage free PSA cut-off values of 27.8% and 29.6% had 90% and 95% sensitivity and eliminated 13.4% and 11.9% of the unnecessary biopsies, respectively. The PSA density cut-off values that yielded 90% (0.1) and 95% (0.08) sensitivity avoided 31% and 12% of the negative biopsies, respectively (153). False-negative rate is present in repeat biopsy as well. A difference between the positive rate of first repeat biopsy and the positive rate of all repeat biopsies was observed in studies where patients underwent more than one repeat biopsy (Fig. 12.3). This difference mirrors the need for a certain number of patients to undergo serial prostate biopsies (154). However,

Table 12.3   Results of repeat prostate biopsies

Reference	First biopsy scheme	Indication for re-biopsy	Repeat biopsy scheme	Interval between initial and final biopsy	Positive rate of first repeat biopsy	Positive rate of all repeat biopsies
Fleshner *et al.* (135)	Sextant	PSA > 4 or DRE(+)	Sextant +TZbiopsies +suspicious	12.8 Months (mean)	30% (39/100)	*30% (39/130)
Ukimura *et al.* (136)	Directed or sextant or combined biopsies	No PIN and PSA > 4 or DRE(+) or TRUS(+)	Directed or sextant or combined biopsies	17 ± 16.1 Months	17% (33/193)	26% (51/193)
Ellis and Brawer (137)	Sextant	PIN or dPSA > 20% per year or PSA > 4 or DRE(+)	Sextant	15.0 Months (mean)	NA	21% (20/96)
Morgan *et al.* (138)	Sextant	PSA > 4 and DRE(−)	Sextant +TZ biopsies	NA	NA	16.4% (11/67)
Durcan and Greene (139)	NA	PSA > 4	Sextant +suspicious	NA	23% (11/48)	31% (15/48)
Rietbergen *et al.* (140)	Sextant +suspicious	PSA > 4 or DRE(+) or TRUS(+)	Sextant +suspicious	12 Months	11% (49/442)	*11% (49/442)
Keetch *et al.* (141)	4–6 Cores	PSA > 4 and DRE(+) or TRUS(+)	4–6 Cores	12 ± 8 Months	19% (82/427)	24.4% (104/427)
Rovner *et al.* (142)	Sextant	PSA > 4	9 Cores + suspicious +TZ biopsies (52/71)	8.4 Months (mean)	NA	24% (17/71)
Roehrborn *et al.* (143)	Sextant	PSA > 4 or DRE(+)	Sextant	NA	23% (28/123)	24% (30/123)
Lui *et al.* (144)	Sextant	PSA > 10 or dPSA > 20%/y DRE(+)	Sextant + TZ biopsies	NA	37.7% (17/47)	*37.7% 17/47

Positive rate of first repeat biopsy: cancer-detection rate of only the first repeat biopsy.
Positive rate of all repeat biopsies: cancer-detection rate of all repeat biopsies.
PSA: prostate–specific antigen; **DRE:** digital rectal examination; **TRUS:** transrectal ultrasound; **PIN:** prostatic intra-epithelial neoplasia; **dPSA:** % increase of PSA per year; **TZ:** transitional zone; **NA:** no available.
* Only one repeat biopsy was performed.

Keetch *et al.* found that 96% of cancers (473 of 495) were detected on the first two biopsies. Therefore, they suggested that a third biopsy should be reserved for men with strong clinical suspicion of carcinoma based on an abnormal DRE, and/or a high PSA level (141).

Rovner *et al.* evaluated the significance of transurethral prostate biopsy in 71 men with prior multiple negative transrectal biopsies due to elevated serum PSA levels. Four-quadrant transurethral prostate biopsy identified only 2 of 19 patients with cancer. In addition, both patients also had positive repeat transrectal ultrasound-guided biopsy. Therefore, transurethral prostate biopsy did not appear to yield a greater number of patients with prostate cancer than repeat sextant biopsies (142). Ornestein *et al.* found prostate cancer in 16% of men with symptomatic benign prostatic hyperplasia and at least one prior negative biopsy, undergoing transurethral resection of the prostate. In addition, 89% of the detected cancers were clinical stage T1b or greater. Using a theoretical model, they estimated that TURP might increase prostate cancer detection by 20% in men with symptomatic BPH, serum PSA greater than 4.0 ng/ml, and/or a suspicious DRE (155). Stamey reported that some of the transitional zone cancers are located anterior or just anterolateral to the urethra and thus, they are difficult

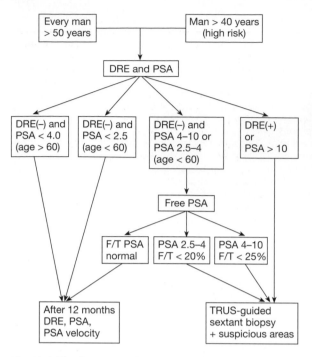

Fig. 12.3 The diagnostic algorithm for detection of prostate cancer. High risk: positive family history or black race; DRE: digital rectal examination; DRE(+): abnormal; DRE(−): normal including beign prostatic hyperplasia; PSA: prostate-sepcific antigen; F/T: free to total PSA ratio; TRUS: transrectal ultrasound.

to be sampled by transrectal biopsies (155). Transurethral resection of the prostate could be a way to diagnose cancer in some of these cases, when numerous prostate biopsies are negative but a high level of clinical suspicion exists. However, intentional transurethral resection of the prostate is rarely indicated to establish the diagnosis of a prostate carcinoma (112).

Recommendations

Following the updated guidelines of the American Cancer Society, beginning at age 50, annual PSA test and DRE are recommended to men who have at least a 10-year life expectancy and to younger men who are at high risk (156). Most urologists would not hesitate to recommend ultrasound-guided prostate biopsy to any patient with an abnormal DRE and/or elevated serum PSA concentration (greater than 10 ng/ml). The dilemma that clinicians often face is whether a man

with a normal DRE and serum PSA levels less than 10 ng/ml, should or should not be biopsied.

The decision for biopsy in this subpopulation of men with normal DRE and PSA levels between 4.0 and 10.0 ng/ml should be based on a balance between the need to detect all prostate cancers and the desire to prevent patients from undergoing unnecessary prostate biopsies, and consequently decrease the cost associated with TRUS and biopsy. Cooner showed that from every 18 men with PSA submitted to TRUS and 6.1 men to prostate biopsy, only 1 man with cancer should be detected. The necessity of such a decision is questionable, especially if we consider that we are not able to release the 12 men with negative TRUS and the 5 men with negative biopsy, by excluding the presence of an undetected cancer (157).

The controversy regarding the criteria that should be used to identify patients who are eligible for biopsy, still remains. In the gray-zone of 4.0–10.0 ng/ml of total PSA, there is not a definitive test for prostate cancer that could be used as the sole indication for a prostate biopsy. All suggested PSA derivatives have been presented in details and their limitations and potential applications have been discussed. It seems that %-free PSA should be considered as an adjunctive tool in distinguishing men with from those without prostate cancer. Unfortunately there is lack of a universal consensus on the cut-off value that will guide the clinician to determine the management of individual patients. Catalona and colleagues demonstrated that cancer risk in men with serum PSA levels between 4.0 and 10.0 ng/ml and a normal DRE, was 20.7%, which was equivalent to that found for a suspicious DRE alone (21%). As suspicious DRE is an indication for biopsy, the authors considered reasonable that TRUS-guided prostate biopsy should be recommended for all men with PSA level from 4.0 to 10 ng/ml as well (11).

Another complex issue is the selection of the optimal serum PSA cut-off value for the early detection of prostate cancer. The use of age-specific PSA ranges for men younger than 60 years may be acceptable for clinicians who consider it more important to identify more men with potentially curable cancers despite the increasing number of negative biopsies. Universal guidelines as to the proper management of individuals suspected to have prostate cancer do not exist due to the complexity and variability of the disease. Recommended detection strategies have their proponents and their critics, thus information about the potential risks and benefits of each intervention should be shared with the patients. Calculation of probabilities of having prostate cancer based on patient age, total PSA, and %-free PSA, which has recently begun to be used, may provide information on which urologists and patients could be base their decision-making as to the necessity for prostate cancer.

The diagnostic algorithm for the investigation of prostate cancer shown in Fig. 12.3 outlines our approach to this controversial issue. We rely on age-specific PSA reference ranges for men younger than 60 years and %-free PSA for men with total PSA between 2.5 and 10.0 ng/ml and normal DRE, to determine whether a prostate biopsy is required. PSA velocity is employed for the surveillance of men with normal PSA or a prior negative biopsy. In the future, modifications of this algorithm may prove necessary as more studies on the effectiveness of these parameters and the factors that affect %-free PSA are currently under evaluation. Furthermore, an algorithm may appear very effective in a patient population but the management of an individual patient could differ as it is influenced by personal factors including family history, life expectancy, and patient will.

References

1. Kim ED, Grayhack JT. Clinical symptoms and signs of prostate cancer. In: *Comprehensive textbook of genitourinary oncology* (ed. NJ Vogelzang, PT Scardino, WU Shipley *et al.*). Williams and Wilkins, Baltimore, 1996, 557–64.
2. Mc Neal JE, Redwine EA, Freiha FS *et al.* Zonal distribution of prostatic adenocarcinoma. *Am J Surg Pathol* 1988, **12**, 897–906.
3. Stamey TA. *Pathogenesis and treatment of urinary tract infections*. Williams and Wilkins, Baltimore, 1980.
4. Bostwick DG, Cooner WH, Dennis L *et al.* The association of benign prostatic hyperplasia and cancer of the prostate. *Cancer* 1992, **70** (Suppl), 291–301.
5. Stormont TJ, Farrow GM, Myers RP *et al.* Clinical stage B or T1c prostate cancer: nonpalpable disease identified by elevated serum prostate-specific antigen concentration. *Urology* 1993, **41**, 3–8.
6. Marshall VF, Fuller NF. Hemospermia. *J Urol* 1983, **129**, 377–8.
7. Venable DD, Hastings D, Misra RP. Unusual metastatic patterns of prostate adenocarcinoma. *J Urol* 1983, **130**, 980–5.
8. Campbell JR, Godsall JW, Bloch S. Neurologic complications in prostatic carcinoma. *Prostate* 1981, **2**, 417–23.
9. Crawford ED, Leewansangtong S, Goktas S *et al.* Efficiency of prostatic-specific antigen and digital rectal examination in screening, using 4.0 ng/ml and age-specific reference range as a cut-off for abnormal values. *Prostate* 1999, **38**, 296–302.
10. Faul P. Experience with the German annual preventive check-up examination. In: *Prostate cancer* (ed. GH Jacobi, R Hohenfeller). Williams and Wilkins, Baltimore, 1982, 57.
11. Catalona WJ, Richie JP, Ahmann FR *et al.* Comparison of DRE and serum PSA in the early detection of prostate cancer: results of a multicenter clinical trial of 6630 men. *J Urol* 1994, **151**, 1283–90.
12. Mueller EJ, Crain TW, Thompson IM *et al.* An evaluation of serial digital rectal examinations in screenimng for prostate cancer. *J Urol* 1992, **148**, 1445–7.
13. Cooner WH, Mosley RB, Rutherford CL Jr *et al.* Prostate cancer detection in a clinical urological practice by ultrasonography, digital rectal examination, prostate specific antigen. *J Urol* 1990, **143**, 1146–52.
14. Stamey TA, McNeal JE, Freiha FS *et al.* Morphometric and clinical studies on 68 consecutive radical prostatectomies. *J Urol* 1988, **139**, 1235–41.
15. Mettlin C, Lee F, Drago J *et al.* The American Cancer Society National Prostate Cancer Detection Project. Findings on the detection of early prostate cancer in 2425 men. *Cancer* 1991, **67**, 2949–57.
16. Lowe FC, Brendler CB. Evaluation of the urologic patient: History, physical examination, and urinalysis. In: *Campbell's Urology* (ed. PC Walsh, AB Retic, TA Stamey *et al.*). 1992, 307–31.
17. Byar DP, Mostofi FK and the Veterans Administration Cooperative Urological Research Group. Carcinoma of the prostate: prognostic evaluation of certain pathologic features in 208 radical prostatectomies. *J Urol* 1972, **10**, 5–13.
18. Spigelman SS, McNeal JE, Freiha FS *et al.* Rectal examination in volume determination of carcinoma of the prostate: clinical and anatomical correlations. *J Urol* 1986, **136**, 1228–30.
19. Huland H, Hübner D, Henke RP. Systematic biopsies and digital rectal examination to identify the nerve-sparing side for radical prostatectomy without risk of positive margin in patients with clinical stage T2,N0 prostatic carcinoma. *Urology* 1994, **44**, 211–4.
20. Obec C, Louis P, Civantos F *et al.* Comparison of digital rectal examination and biopsy results with the radical prostatectomy specimen. *J Urol* 1999, **161**, 494–9.
21. Schaller J, Akiyama K, Tsuda R *et al.* Isolation, characterization and amino-acid sequence of γ-seminoprotein, a glycoprotein from human seminal plasma. *Eur J Biochem* 1987, **170**, 111–20.
22. Belanger A, van Halbeek H, Graves HCB *et al.* Molecular mass and carbohydrate srtucture of prostate specific antigen. Studies for establishment of an international PSA standard. *Prostate* 1995, **27**, 187–97.
23. Pollen JJ, Dreilinger A. Immunohistochemical identification of prostatic acid phosphatase and prostate specific antigen in female peri-urethral glands. *Urology* 1984, **23**, 303–4.
24. Wang MC, Valenzuela LA, Murphy GP *et al.* Purification of a human prostate specific antigen. *Invest Urol* 1979, **17**, 159–63.
25. Stamey TA, Yang N, Hay AR *et al.* Prostate specific antigen as a serum marker for adenocarcinoma of the prostate. *N Eng J Med* 1987, **317**, 909–16.

26. Catalona WJ, Hudson MA, Scardino PT *et al.* Selection of optimal prostate specific antigen cut-offs of early detection of prostate cancer: receiver operating characteristic curves. *J Urol* 1994, **152**, 2037–42.

27. Catalona WJ, Smith DS, Ratliff TL *et al.* Measurement of prostate specific antigen in serum as a screening test for prostate cancer. *N Eng J Med* 1991, **324**, 1156–61.

28. Dalton DL. Elevated serum prostate-specific antigen due to acute bacterial prostatitis. *Urology* 1989, **33**, 465.

29. Hashui Y, Marutsuka K, Asada Y *et al.* Relationship between serum prostate-specific antigen and histological prostatitis in men with benign prostatic hyperplasia. *Prostate* 1994, **25**, 91–6.

30. Semjonow A, Roth S, Hamm M. RE: Nontraumatic elevation of prostate specific antigen following cardiac surgery and extracorporeal pulmonary bypass. *J Urol* 1995, **155**, 295–6.

31. Deliveliotis C, Alivizatos G, Stavropoulos NJ *et al.* Influence of digital examination, cystoscopy, transrectal ultrasonography and needle biopsy on the concentration of prostate specific antigen. *Urol Int* 1994, **53**, 186–90.

32. Oesterling JE, Rice DC, Glenski WJ *et al.* Effect of cystoscopy, prostate biopsy, and transurethral resection of prostate on serum prostate specific antigen. *Urology* 1993, **42**, 276–82.

33. Guess HA, Heyse JF, Gormley GJ. The effect of finasteride on prostate-specific antigen in men with benign prostatic hyperplasia. *Prostate* 1993, **22**, 31–7.

34. Gormley GJ, Ng J, Cook T *et al.* Effect of finasteride on prostate-specific antigen density. *Urology* 1994, **43**, 53–8.

35. Tchetgen MB, Song JT, Strawderman M *et al.* Ejaculation increases the serum prostate-specific antigen concentration. *Urology* 1996, **47**, 511–6.

36. Hagood PG, Parra RO, Rauscher JA. Nontraumatic elevation of prostate specific antigen following cardiac surgery and extracorporeal cardiopulmonary bypass. *J Urol* 1994, **152**, 2043–5.

37. Aus G, Skude G. Effect of ultrasound-guided core biopsy of prostate on serum concentration of prostate specific antigen and acid phosphatase activity. *Scand J Urol Nephrol* 1993, **26**, 21–3.

38. Leventhal EK, Rozanski TA, Morey AF *et al.* The effects of exercise and activity on serum PSA levels. *J Urol* 1993, **150**, 893–4.

39. Benson MC, Whang IS, Pantuck A *et al.* Prostate specific antigen density: a means of distinguishing benign prostatic hypertrophy and prostate cancer. *J Urol* 1992, **147**, 815–6.

40. Seaman E, Whang M, Olsson CA *et al.* PSA density (PSAD). Role in patient evaluation and management. *Urol Clin N Amer* 1993, **20**, 653–63.

41. Catalona WJ, Richie, deKernion JB *et al.* Comparison of prostate specific antigen concentration versus prostate specific antigen density in the early detection of prostate cancer: receiving operating characteristic curves. *J Urol* 1994, **152**, 2031–6.

42. Brawer MK, Aramburu EAG, Chen GL *et al.* The inability of prostate specific antigen density index to enhance the predictive value of PSA in the diagnosis of prostatic carcinoma. *J Urol* 1993, **150**, 369–73.

43. Bazinet M, Meshref AA, Trudel C *et al.* Prospective evaluation of prostate specific antigen density and systematic biopsies for early detection of prostatic carcinoma. *Urology* 1994, **43**, 44–51.

44. Epstein JI, Walsh PC, Carmichael M *et al.* Pathologic and clinical findings to predict tumor extent of non-palpable (stage) T1c prostate cancer. *JAMA* 1994, **278**, 368–74.

45. Beduschi MC, Oesterling JE. Prostate specific antigen density. *Urol Clin N Am* 1997, **24**, 323–32.

46. Oesterling JE, Jacobsen SJ, Chute CG *et al.* Serum prostate specific antigen in a community-based population of healthy men: Establishment of age-specific reference ranges. *JAMA* 1993, **270**, 860–4.

47. Morgan TO, Jacobsen SJ, McCarthy WF *et al.* Age-specific reference ranges for prostate specific antigen in African American men. *N Eng J Med* 1996, **335**, 304–10.

48. Oesterling JE, Kumamoto Y, Tsukamoto T *et al.* Serum prostate specific antigen in a community-based population of healthy Japanese men: Lower values than for similarly aged white men. *Br J Urol* 1995, **75**, 347–53.

49. Partin AW, Criley SR, Subong ENP *et al.* Standard versus age-specific antigen reference ranges among men with clinically localized prostate cancer: a pathological analysis. *J Urol* 1996, **155**, 1336–9.

50. Reissigl A, Bartch G. Prostate specific antigen as a screening test: the Austrian experience. *Urol Clin N Amer* 1997, **24** (2), 315–21.

51. Polascik TJ, Oesterling JE, Partin AW. Prostate specific antigen: A decade of discovery-what we have learned and where we are going. *J Urol* 1999, **162**, 293–306.

52. Carter HB, Pearson JD, Metter J *et al.* Longitudinal evaluation of prostate-specific antigen levels in men with and without prostate diseases. *JAMA* 1992, **267**, 2215–20.

53. Partin AW, Stutzman RE. Elevated prostate-specific antigen, abnormal prostate evaluation on digital rectal examination, and transrectal ultrasound and prostate biopsy. *Urol Clin North Amer* 1998, **25**, 581–9.

54. Christennsson A, Laurell C-B, Lilja H. Enzymatic activity of prostate-specific antigen and its reactions with extracellular serine proteinase inhibitors. *Eur J Biochem* 1990, **194**, 755–63.

55. Stenman UH, Leinonen J, Alfthan H *et al.* A complex between prostate specific antigen and alpha-1 antichymotrypsin is the major form of the prostate specific antigen in serum of patients with prostatic cancer: assay of the complex improves clinical sensitivity for cancer. *Cancer Res* 1991, **51**, 222–6.

56. Lilja H, Christensson A, Dahlen U *et al.* Prostate-specific antigen in serum occurs predominantly in complex with alpha 1-antichymotrypsin. *Clin Chem* 1991, **31**, 1618–25.

57. Vessella RL, Lange PH. Issues in the assessment of prostate-specific antigen immunoassays: Un update. *Urol Clin N Amer* 1997, **24** (2), 261–8.

58. Luderer AA, Chen YT, Soriano TF *et al.* Measurement of the proportion of free to total prostate specific antigen improves diagnostic performance of prostate specific antigen in the diagnostic gray zone of total prostate specific antigen. *Urology* 1995, **46**, 187–94.

59. Catalona WJ, Smith DS, Wolfert R *et al.* Evaluation of percentage of free serum prostate specific antigen to improve specificity of prostate cancer screening. *JAMA* 1995, **274**, 1214–20.

60. Prestigiacomo AF, Lilja H, Pettersson K *et al.* A comparison of the free fraction of serum prostate specific antigen in men with benign and cancerous prostates: the best case scenario. *J Urol* 1996, **156**, 350–4.

61. Partin AW, Catalona WJ, Southwick PC *et al.* Analysis of percent free prostate specific antigen (PSA) for prostate cancer detection: influence of total PSA, prostate volume, and age. *Urology* 1996, **48** (Suppl), 55–61.

62. Bangma CH, Kranse R, Blijengerg BG *et al.* The value of screening tests in the detection of prostate cancer. Results of a retrospective evaluation of 1726 men. *Urology* 1995, **46**, 773–8.

63. Catalona WJ, Smith DS, Ornestein DK. Prostate cancer detection in men with serum PSA concentrations of 2.6 to 4.0 ng/ml and benign prostate examination. Enhancement of specificity with free PSA measurements. *JAMA* 1997, **277**, 1452–5.

64. Vashi AR, Wojno KJ, Henricks W *et al.* Determination of the 'reflex-range' and appropriate cutpoints for percent free prostate-specific antigen in 413 men referred for prostatic evaluation using the AxSYM system. *Urology* 1997, **49**, 19–27.

65. Catalona WJ, Partin AW, Finlay JA *et al.* Use of percentage of free prostate-specific antigen to identify men at high risk of prostate cancer when PSA levels are 2.51 to 4 ng/ml and digital rectal examination is not suspicious for prostate cancer; an alternative model. *Urology* 1999, **54**, 220–4.

66. van Cangh PJ, de Nayer P, de Vischer L *et al.* Free to total prostate-specific antigen (PSA) improves the discrimination between prostate cancer and benign prostatic hyperplasia (BPH) in the diagnostic gray zone of 1.8 to 10 ng/ml total PSA. *Urology* 1996, **48**, 67–70.

67. Oesterling JE, Lilja H. Early detection and diagnosis. In: *Comprehensive textbook of genitourinary oncology* (ed. NJ Vogelzang , PT Scardino, WU Shipley *et al.*). Williams and Wilkins, Baltimore, 1996, 668–73.

68. Bjork T, Bjartell A, Abrahamsson PA *et al.* Alpha1-antichymotrypsin production in PSA-producing cells is common in prostate cancer but rare in benign prostatic hyperplasia. *Urology* 1994, **43**, 427–34.

69. Woodrum DL, Brawer MK, Partin AW *et al.* Interpretation of free prostate specific antigen clinical research studies for the detection of prostate cancer. *J Urol* 1998, **159**, 5–12.

70. Stenman UH, Hakama M, Knekt P *et al.* Serum concentrations of prostate specific antigen and its complex with alpha-1-antichymotrypsin before diagnosis of prostate cancer. *Lancet* 1994, **344**, 1594–8.

71. Gann PH, Hennekens CH and Stampfer MJ. A prospective evaluation of plasma prostate-specific antigen for detection of prostate cancer. *JAMA* 1995, **273**, 289–94.

72. Carter HB, Partin AW, Luderer AA *et al.* Percentage of free prostate specific antigen in sera predicts aggressiveness of prostate cancer a decade before diagnosis. *Urology* 1997, **49**, 379–84.

73. Kalish J, Cooner WH, Graham SD Jr. Serum PSA adjusted for volume of transitional zone (PSAT) is more accurate than PSA adjusted for total gland volume (PSAD) in detecting adenocarcinoma of the prostate. *Urology* 1994, **43**, 601–6.

74. Mc Neal JE. The prostate gland: morphology and pathobiology. *Monogr Urol* 1988, **9**, 36–54.

75. Djavan B, Marberger M, Zlotta A *et al.* PSA, f/tPSA, PSAD, PSA-TZ and PSA velocity for prostate cancer prediction: a multivariate analysis. *J Urol* 1998, **159** (253), A898.

76. Kurita Y, Terada H, Masuda K *et al.* Prostate specific antigen (PSA) value adjusted for transition zone volume and free PSA (γ-seminoprotein)/PSA ratio in the diagnosis of prostate cancer in patients with intermediate PSA levels. *Br J Urol* 1998, **82**, 224–30.

77. Horninger W, Reissigl A, Klocker H *et al.* Improvement of specificity in PSA-based screening by using PSA-transition zone density and %-free PSA in addition to total PSA levels. *Prostate* 1998, **37**, 133–7.

78. Sokoll LJ, Bruzek DJ, Cox JL *et al.* Is complexed PSA alone clinically useful? *J Urol* 1998, **159** (234), 895A.

79. Meyer GE, Brawer MK, Letran JL *et al.* Alpa1-antichymotrypsin complexed PSA in men undergoing prostate biopsy offers significant advantage for the detection of carcinoma over total PSA and free-to-total PSA. *J Urol* 1998, **159** (273), 72A.

80. Stamey TA, Barnhill SD, Zhang Z *et al.* Effectiveness of PROSTASURE in detecting prostate cancer (PCa) and benign prostatic hyperplasia (BPH) in men age 50 and older. *J Urol* 1996, **155** (Abstract), 436A.

81. Babaian RJ, Fritchie HA, Zhang Z *et al.* Evaluation of ProstAsure Index in the detection of prostate cancer: a preliminary report. *Urology* 1998, **51**, 132–6.

82. Berg T, Bradshaw RA, Carretero OA *et al.* A common nomenclature for members of the tissue (glandular) kallikrein gene families. *Agents Actions* 1992, **38** (Suppl), 19–25.

83. Schedlich LJ, Bennetts BH, Morris BJ. Primary structure of a human glandular kallikreine gene. *DNA* 1987, **6**, 429–37.

84. Watt KW, Lee PJ. M'Timkulu Chan WP *et al.* Human prostate-specific antigen: structural and functional similarity with serine proteases. *Proc Natl Acad Sci USA* 1986, **83**, 3166–70.

85. Young CY, Seay T, Hogen K *et al.* Prostate specific human kallikrein (hk2) as a novel marker for prostate cancer. *Prostate* 1996, **7** (Suppl), 17–24.

86. Darson MF, Pacelli A, Roche P *et al.* Human glandular kallikrein 2 (hk2) expression in prostatic intra-epithelial neoplasia and adenocarcinoma: a novel prostate cancer marker. *Urology* 1997, **49**, 857–62.

87. Kawakami M, Okaneya T, Furihata K *et al.* Detection of prostate cancer cells circulating in peripheral blood by reverse transcription-PCR for hKLK2. *Cancer Res* 1997, **57**, 4167–70.

88. Saedi MS, Hill TM, Kuus-Reichel K *et al.* The precursor form of the human kallikrein 2, a kallikrein homologous to prostate specific antigen, is present in human sera and is increased in prostate cancer and benign prostatic hyperplasia. *Clin Chem* 1998, **44**, 2115–9.

89. Kwiatkowski MK, Recker F, Piironen T *et al.* In prostatism patients the ratio of human glandular kallikrein to free PSA improves the discrimination between prostate cancer and benign hyperplasia within the diagnostic 'gray-zone' of total PSA 4 to 10 ng/ml. *Urology* 1998, **52**, 360–5.

90. Gutman AB, Gutman EB. An 'acid' phosphatase occurring in the serum of patients with metastasizing carcinoma of the prostate gland. *J Clin Invest* 1938, **17**, 473.

91. Huggins C, Hodges CV. Studies on prostate cancer: Effect of castration, of estrogen and of androgen injection on serum phosphatases in metastatic carcinoma of the prostate. *Cancer Res* 1941, **1**, 293.

92. Wild JJ, Reid JM. Progress in techniques of soft tissue examination by 15MC pulsed ultrasonography. In: *Ultrasound in biology and medicine* (ed. E Kelly). American Institute of Biological Sciences, Washington DC, 1957, 30–45.

93. Mettlin C, Murphy GP, Lee F *et al.* Characteristics of prostate cancers detected in a multimodality early detection program. *Cancer* 1994, **72**, 1701–8.

94. Lee F, Littrup PJ, Torp-Pederson ST *et al.* Prostate cancer: comparison of transrectal ultrasound and DRE for screening. *Radiology* 1988, **168**, 389–94.

95. Ezz El Din KE, de la Rochette JJ. Transrectal ultrasonography of the prostate. *Br J Urol* 1996, **78**, 2–9.

96. Lee F, Gray JM, McLeary RD *et al.* Transrectal ultrasound in the diagnosis of prostate cancer: location, echogenicity, histopathology, and staging. *Prostate* 1985, **7**, 117–29.

97. Stamey TA. Diagnosis of prostate cancer: a personal view. *J Urol* 1992, **147**, 830–2.

98. Ellis WJ, Chetner MP, Preston SD *et al.* Diagnosis of prostatic carcinoma: the yield of serum prostate-specific antigen, digital rectal examination and transrectal ultrasonography. *J Urol* 1994, **152**, 1520–5.

99. Hammerer P, Huland H. Systematic sextant biopsies in 651 patients referred for prostate evaluation. *J Urol* 1994, **151**, 99–102.

100. Shinohara K, Wheeler TM, Scardino PT. The appearance of prostate cancer on transrectal ultrasonography: correlation of imaging and pathological examinations. *J Urol* 1989, **142**, 76–82.

101. Ellis WJ, Brawer MK. The significance of isoechoic prostatic carcinoma. *J Urol* 1994, **152**, 2304–7.

102. Melchior SW, Brawer MK. Role of transrectal ultrasound and prostate biopsy. *J Clin Ultrasound* 1996, **24**, 463–71.

103. Lee F, Gray JM, McLeary RD *et al.* Prostatic evaluation by transrectal sonography: criteria for diagnosis of early carcinoma. *Radiology* 1986, **158**, 91–5.

104. Aarnik RG, Beerlage HP, de la Rochette JJMCH *et al.* Transrectal ultrasound of the prostate: Innovations and future applications. *J Urol* 1998, **159**, 1568–79.

105. Garg S, Fortling B, Chadwick D *et al.* Staging of prostate cancer using 3-dimensional transrectal ultrasoundimages: a pilot study. *J Urol* 1999, **162**, 1318–21.

106. Alexander AA. To color Doppler image the prostate or not: this is the question. *Radiology* 1995, **195**, 11–3.

107. Ikonen S, Karkkainen P, Kivisaari L *et al.* Magnetic resonance imaging of clinically localized prostate cancer. *J Urol* 1998, **159**, 915–9.

108. Perrotti M, Han KR, Epstein RE *et al.* Prospective evaluation of endorectal magnetic resonance imaging to detect tumor foci in men with prior negative prostatic biopsy: a pilot study. *J Urol* 1999, **162**, 1314–7.

109. Scheidler J, Hricak H, Vigneron DB *et al.* 3D 1H-MR spectroscopic imaging in localizing prostate cancer: Clinicopathologic study. *Radiology* 1999, **213**, 481–8.

110. Rietbergen JBW, Hoedemaeker RF, Boeken Kruger AE *et al.* The changing pattern of prostate cancer at the time of diagnosis: characteristics of screen detected prostate cancer in a population based screening study. *J Urol* 1999, **161**, 1192–8.

111. Schröder FH, Dennis LJ, Kirkels W *et al.* European randomized study of screening for prostate cancer. Progress report of Antwerp and Rotterdam pilot studies. *Cancer* 1995, **76**, 129–34.

112. Petros JA, Cooner WH. Prostatic biopsy. In: *Comprehensive textbook of genitourinary oncology* (ed. NJ Vogelzang, PT Scardino, WU Shipley *et al.*). Williams and Wilkins, Baltimore, 1996, 699–711.

113. Hodge KK, McNeal JE, Terris MK *et al.* Random systematic versus directed ultrasound guided transrectal core biopsies of the prostate. *J Urol* 1989, **142**, 71–4.

114. Rifkin MD, Alexander AA, Pisarchick PJ *et al.* Palpable masses in the prostate: superior accuracy of US-guided biopsy compared with accuracy of digitally guided biopsy. *Radiology* 1991, **179**, 41–2.

115. Weaver RP, Noble MJ, Weigel JW. Correlation of ultrasound-guided and digitally directed transrectal biopsies of palpable prostatic abnormalities. *J Urol* 1991, **145**, 516–8.

116. Rodriguez Larissa, Terris MK. Risks and complications of transrectal ultrasound guided prostate needle biopsy: a prospective study and review of the literature. *J Urol* 1998, **160**, 2115–20.

117. Rietbergen JB, Kruger AE, Kranse R *et al.* Complications of transrectal ultrasound-guided systematic sextant biopsies of the prostate: evaluation of complication rates and risk factors within a population-based screening program. *Urology* 1997, **49**, 875–80.

118. Norberg M, Holberg L, Häaggman M *et al.* Determinants of complications after multiple transrectal core biopsies of the prostate. *Eur Rad* 1996, **6**, 457–61.

119. Zoumboulis PS, Theotokas ID, Kehayas P *et al.* Natural evolution of prostate cancer: Contribution of transrectal ultrasound, guided biopsies, and cytologic and histologic examination. *Radiology* 1996, **201**, 465, 212.

120. Flanigan RC, Catalona WJ, Richie JP *et al.* Accuracy of digital rectal examination and transrectal ultrasonography in localising prostate cancer. *J Urol* 1994, **152**, 1506–9.

121. Eskew LA, Bare RL, Mccullough DL. Systematic 5 region prostate biopsy is superior to sextant method for diagnosing carcinoma of the prostate. *J Urol* 1997, **157**, 199–202.

122. Norberg M, Egevad L, Holmberg L *et al.* The sextant protocol for ultrasound-guided core biopsies of the prostate underestimates the presence of cancer. *Urology* 1997, **50**, 562–6.

123. Uzzo RG, Wei JT, Waldbaum RS *et al.* The influence of prostate size on cancer detection. *Urology* 1995, **46**, 831–6.

124. Letran JM, Meyer GE, Loberiza *et al.* The effect of prostate volume on the yield of needle biopsy. *J Urol* 1998, **160**, 1718–21.

125. Vashi AR, Wojno KJ, Gillespie B *et al.* A model for the number of cores per prostate biopsy based on patient age and prostate gland volume. *J Urol* 1998, **159**, 920–4.

126. Brown M, True LD, Ellis WJ *et al.* Does increased number of ultrasound-guided prostate needle biopsies enhance the yield of the chance of finding carcinoma. *J Urol* 1997, **157** (144), A563.

127. Ravery V, Billebaud T, Toublanc M *et al.* Diagnostic value of ten systematic TRUS-guided prostate biopsies. *Eur Urol* 1999, **35**, 298–303.

128. Bazinet M, Karakiewicz PI, Aprikian AG *et al.* Value of systematic transition zone biopsies in the early detection of prostate cancer. *J Urol* 1996, **155**, 605–6.

129. Terris MK, Pham TQ, Issa MM *et al.* Routine transition zone and seminal vesicle biopsies in all patients undergoing transrectal ultrasound guided prostate biopsies are not indicated. *J Urol* 1997, **157**, 204–6.

130. Fleshner NE, Fair WR. Indications for transition zone biopsy in the detection of prostatic carcinoma. *J Urol* 1997, **157**, 556–8.

131. Chang JJ, Shinohara K, Hovey RM *et al.* Prospective evaluation of systematic sextant transition biopsies in large prostates for cancer detection. *Urology* 1998, **52**, 89–93.

132. Beerlage HP, de Reijke TM, de la Rochette JJMCH. Considerations regarding prostate biopsies. *Eur Urol* 1998, **34**, 303–12.

133. Karakiewicz PI, Hanley JA, Bazinet M. Three dimensional computer-assisted analysis of sector biopsy of the prostate. *Urology* 1998, **52**, 208–12.

134. Chen ME, Troncoso P, Tang K *et al.* Comparison of prostate biopsy schemes by computer simulation. *Urology* 1999, **53**, 951–60.

135. Fleshner NE, O'Sullivan M, Fair WR. Prevalence and predictors of a positive repeat transrectal ultrasoung guided needle biopsy of the prostate. *J Urol* 1997, **158**, 505–9.

136. Ukimura O, Durrani O, Babaian RJ. Role of PSA and its indices in determing the need for repeat prostate biopsies. *Urology* 1997, **50**, 66–72.

137. Ellis WJ, Brawer MK. Repeat prostate needle biopsy: Who needs it? *J Urol* 1995, **153**, 1496–8.

138. Morgan TO, McLeod DG, Leifer ES *et al.* Prospective use of free prostate specific antigen to avoid repeat prostate biopsies in men with elevated total prostate specific antigen. *Urology* 1996, **48**, 76–80.

139. Durkan GC, Greene DR. Elevated serum prostate specific antigen levels in conjuction with an initial prostatic biopsy negative for carcinoma: who should undergo a repeat biopsy. *BJU Int* 1999, **83**, 34–8.

140. Rietbergen JB, Boeken Kruger AE, Hoedemaeker RF *et al.* Repeat screening for prostate cancer after 1-year followup in 984 biopsied men: Clinical and pathological features of detected cancer. *J Urol* 1998, **160**, 2121–5.

141. Keetch DW, Catalona WJ, Smith DS. Serial prostatic biopsies in men with persistently elevated serum prostate specific antigen values. *J Urol* 1994, **151**, 1571–4.

142. Rovner ES, Schanne FJ, Malkowicz SB. Transuretral biopsy of the prostate for persistently elevated or increasing prostate specific antigen following multiple negative transrectal biopsies. *J Urol* 1997, **158**, 138–42.

143. Roehrborn CG, Pickens GJ, Sanders JS. Diagnostic yield of repeated ultrasound guided biopsies stratified by specific histopathologic diagnosis and prostate specific antigen. *Urology* 1996, **47**, 347–52.

144. Lui PD, Terris MK, McNeal JE *et al.* Indications for ultrasound guided transition zone biopsies in the detection of prostate cancer. *J Urol* 1995, **153**, 1000–3.

145. Bostwick DG, Brawer MK. Prostatic intra-epithelial neoplasia and early invasion in prostate cancer. *Cancer* 1987, **59**, 788–94.

146. McNeal JE, Bostwick DG. Intraductal dysplasia: a pemalignant lesion of the prostate. *Hum Pathol* 1986, **17**, 64–71.

147. Davidson D, Bostwick DG, Qian J *et al.* Prostatic intra-epithelial neoplasia is arisk factor for adenocarcinoma: predictive accuracy in needle biopsies. *J Urol* 1995, **154**, 1295–9.

148. Aboseif S, Shinohara K, Weidner N *et al.* The significance of prostate intra-epithelial neoplasia. *Br J Urol* 1995, **76**, 355–9.

149. Shepherd D, Keetch DW, Humphrey PA *et al.* Repeat biopsy strategy in men with isolated prostatic intra-epithclial neoplasia on prostate needle biopsy. *J Urol* 1996, **156**, 460–2.

150. Raviv G, Janssen T, Zlotta AR *et al.* Prostatic intra-epithelial neoplasia: influence of clinical and pathological data on the detection of prostate cancer. *J Urol* 1996, **156**, 1050–4.

151. Brawer MK, Bigler SA, Sohlberg OE *et al.* Significance of prostatic intra-epithelial neoplasia on prostate needle biopsy. *Urology* 1991, **38**, 103–7.

152. Hayek OR, Noble CB, de la Taille A *et al.* The necessity of a second prostate biopsy cannot be predicted by PSA or PSA derivatives (density or free: total ratio) in men with prior negative prostatic biopsies. *Curr Opin Urol* 1999, **9**, 371–5.

153. Catalona WJ, Beiser JA, Smith DS. Serum free prostate specific antigen and prostate specific antigen density measurements for predicting cancer in men with prior negative prostatic biopsies. *J Urol* 1997, **158**, 2162–7.

154. Ornstein DK, Rao GS, Smith DS *et al.* The impact of systematic prostate biopsy on prostate cancer incidence in men with symptomatic benign prostatic hyperplasia undergoing transurethral resection of the prostate. *J Urol* 1997, **157**, 880–4.

155. Stamey TA. Editorial comment on: Eskew LA, Bare RL, Mccullough DL, Systematic 5 region prostate biopsy is

superior to sextant method for diagnosing carcinoma of the prostate. *J Urol* 1997, **157**, 202–3.

156. von Eschenbach A, Ho R, Murphy GP *et al.* American Cancer Society guidelines for the early detection of prostate cancer. Update, June 10,1997. *Cancer* 1997, **80**, 1805–7.

157. Cooner WH. Prostate-specific antigen, digital rectal examination, and transrectal ultrasonic examination of the prostate in prostate cancer detection. *Monogr Urol* 1991, **12**, 3.

13 | Imaging in prostate cancer

Rene G. Aarnink, Gerrit J. Jager, and
Jean J. M. C. H. de la Rosette

Introduction

Similar to the detection of colon cancer, breast cancer, and soft tissue tumors, tools used to confirm prostate cancer, determine prostate cancer stage, and monitor treatment effect include:

- physical examinations
- laboratory tests
- imaging studies.

Indeed, physical examination or digital rectal examination (DRE) has been the mainstay for prostate cancer detection. As the prostate is located close to the rectal wall, digital examination when palpating the rectum can identify lesions in the prostate that might correspond to the presence of prostate cancer. However, DRE can only reveal hard lesions on the dorsal side, since lesions in the ventral side of the prostate are usually impalpable. Furthermore, false-positives might occur due to the presence of calcifications in the prostate. This means that the overall accuracy of DRE in detecting prostate cancer is limited. A sensitivity and specificity of 38.7% and 96.4% has been reported for prostate cancer detection in 2999 men participating in the American Cancer Society National Prostate Cancer Detection Program (1). In another study, a sensitivity of 87% and a specificity of 60% for prostate cancer detection were reported in a selected group of 232 patients who underwent biopsies because of an elevated PSA or a suspicious DRE (2).

Prostatic acid phosphatase was in use as a prostate cancer marker since the early 1980s, but a more sensitive marker, prostate-specific antigen (PSA), has gradually replaced it. This prostate-specific antigen marker has the possibility to detect abnormal conditions, as increased levels above the normal value indicate the possible presence of prostate cancer. However, an elevated serum level can also occur in case of a benign disease of the prostate or prostatitis (inflammation). On the other hand, PSA levels might be in the normal range although prostate cancer is found at histopathologic inspection of biopsy cores or whole mount specimen. This means that PSA is neither an ideal marker for sensitivity and specificity to detect prostate cancer, but it is currently the only tumor marker available for the serum. PSA alone resulted in a sensitivity and specificity of 69.2% and 89.5%, respectively, (1) in a screening population, and 96% and 14%. in a selected population (2).

Imaging studies in prostate cancer detection showed significant changes in the past decades. Ultrasound was first introduced to detect prostate cancer in the 1970s. It received initial enthusiasm, it was even included in a triad together with PSA testing and rectal examination to make the diagnosis, but interest in ultrasound was lost because of a lack of diagnostic power. Recently, it has been reported that conventional gray-scale ultrasound has little advantages in detecting prostate cancer in a screening population. Currently, imaging modalities including MR scanning, CT scanning, PET scanning, and advanced ultrasound imaging receive renewed and increased interest because of significant improvement of the technology and addition of new information for diagnostic differentiation.

Due to the not optimal detection program, research on improvement of prostate cancer detection has focused on the identification of new tumor markers, as well as on the improvement of imaging modalities. To evaluate the efforts and progress in that field, we have monitored the number of papers appearing on each subject over the past 15 years (1984–98). We used the National Library of Medicine (3) (found on the Internet at URL: http://www.ncbi.nlm.nih.gov/PubMed/) to identify the number of papers per year. In Table 13.1, the subjects are listed, together with the maximum number of papers, the year of the maximum number of papers, and the growth assuming an exponential

Table 13.1 Query used in Medline: subject, prostate cancer and year

Subject	Max papers	Year of max. no. papers	Growth
Prostate cancer	2741	98	0.095
Digital rectal examination	106	98	0.206
Prostate specific antigen	837	98	0.259
Transrectal ultrasound	185	97	0.171
Tumor markers	779	98	0.311
Prostatic acid phosphatase	59	88	−0.036

increase in the number of papers. Figure 13.1 illustrates the number of papers that appeared on prostate cancer, and PSA, DRE and TRUS in combination with prostate cancer during the past 15 years, including trend lines assuming exponential growth. In Fig. 13.2 the estimated factor describing yearly growth is presented for all subjects mentioned in Table 13.1. From this figure, we can conclude that prostatic acid phosphatase is 'out' in prostate cancer, while tumor markers are the hottest topic in prostate cancer. Interesting is that PSA and DRE show a larger increase compared to TRUS, which might indicate that the first are less controversial in prostate cancer detection. The fact, however, that the absolute number of papers appearing on TRUS is higher than on DRE indicates that there still is a role for ultrasound in prostate cancer.

In this paper, we aimed to present an overview of the role of imaging modalities in the detection of prostate cancer. First, we present the rationale to improve the imaging of prostate cancer. Second, we focus on different imaging modalities used in prostate cancer detection, including ultrasound, magnetic resonance (imaging and spectroscopy), computed tomography, X-ray, nuclear imaging, and radioactive labeling. Finally, we present the role of imaging in prostate cancer detection and staging as advocated by the World Health Organization. The role of imaging in monitoring treatment effect, a rather new and unexplored area, has been left out of the discussion in this paper.

Prostate cancer prevalence and incidence, and the role for imaging

Prostate cancer is the most common cancer among American men, and the second leading cause of cancer-related deaths. In Europe, similar trends are observed. As treatment options increase and outcome improves with earlier stage cancers, detection of cancer should be attempted at an early stage. The established early-detection program of prostate cancer currently includes a digital rectal examination and a serum PSA level determination. If one or both indicate a suspicion for malignancy, ultrasound guided biopsies are indicated to make the final diagnosis.

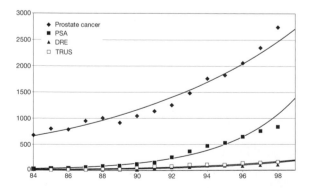

Fig. 13.1 The number of papers that appeared on prostate cancer as whole, and PSA, DRE and TRUS in combination with prostate cancer. Assuming an exponential growth, trend lines indicate the average increase in the past decade.

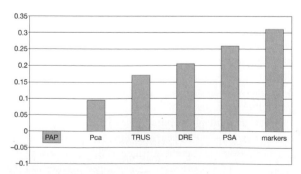

Fig. 13.2 The average increase in number of papers of the past 15 years for each subject. It is assumed that the number of papers increase exponentially, and an exponential fit was performed on the data.

Once the diagnosis of prostate cancer has been made, the grade and stage of the tumor should be established prior to initiating therapy. Initial discrimination between low-risk and high-risk patients for extra-prostatic tumor involvement, seminal vesicle invasion, and/or lymph node involvement is based on clinical stage, PSA, and biopsy Gleason score, combined in the Partin tables (4). High-risk patients are defined as those who have a PSA greater than 10 ng/ml and/or a Gleason score greater than 6. Low-risk patients with histologically proven prostate cancer are considered suitable for retropubic radical prostatectomy, the curative treatment of choice for organ-confined disease. In high-risk patients, additional tests are required to evaluate whether curative therapy is still possible for these patients. These additional tests include radionuclide bone scan to reveal bone metastases, computerized tomography (CT), and MRI to evaluate extra-prostatic extension, seminal vesicle invasion, and lymph node involvement. Depending on the findings, appropriate treatment will be selected, consisting of radical prostatectomy, radiotherapy (external or interstitial), or hormonal therapy. Also, alternative localized treatments can be considered, such as radiofrequency interstitial-tumor ablation, high-intensity focused ultrasound, and cryosurgery, but none of these treatments should be considered as established therapy for prostate cancer.

It is concluded that imaging plays a role in the diagnosis of prostate cancer, as well as in the staging of histologically proven prostate cancer. However, the role of imaging has not yet been fully employed, and in many aspects of imaging, research projects are performed to improve the detection, localization, and staging of prostate cancer. Also for treatment guidance and follow-up, imaging has found increasing interest, e.g. in the guidance of interstitial radiation therapy. We present the current status of ultrasound, magnetic resonance, computerized tomography, and nuclear imaging in displaying the prostate and prostate cancer.

Medical imaging modalities

Several imaging modalities have found their way in current clinical practice, and these modalities are either based on X-rays (CT imaging), sound (ultrasound imaging), magnetic fields, and radiofrequency waves (MR imaging), or the detection of radionuclides (nuclear imaging). The target of each imaging modality is to replace invasive procedures as a means to obtain the desired information, to add important information not available from other tests, assist during intervention, or to replace otherwise costly procedures. Sometimes its target is to provide detailed information of the anatomy of the object, but also physiological function might be of interest during the imaging session.

Ultrasound

Ultrasound scanners use reflections of pulsed sound waves emitted into the medium at high frequencies to display internal structures. The transducer is capable of producing sound waves that can be emitted into the surrounding medium for a given period of time, and reflected parts in periods not used for emission are used to construct a display of the examined tissue. Usually this is done along a number of lines covering the medium of interest, and reflections along each line are recorded. Reflections occur in regions with different acoustic properties, and the larger the difference in acoustic impedance the stronger the reflection. As the sound wave is attenuated by absorption and scattering, time-gain compensation is used to enhance and display regions that are further away from the transducer. The reflected and amplified signals are processed and converted to a 2D-grid displaying the amplitude of the reflected signals as intensity at locations corresponding to the anatomic origin of the examined tissue. Although many operations are needed to convert reflected sound waves to images, current machines are capable of displaying 20–30 images per second resulting in a real-time image.

Transrectal ultrasound of the prostate was introduced in the early 1970s in Japan (5) and the ultrasound chair developed for the purpose of screening at large has become famous in the urology world. Nowadays, transrectal ultrasound is applied in the left decubitus or lithotomy position using a high-frequency rectal probe. Due to the close approximation to the prostate, less penetration of ultrasound is required and higher frequencies can be applied ranging between 5 and 8 MHz. Transverse and longitudinal scans can be made allowing complete scanning of the prostate. Currently, transrectal imaging has become a routine procedure for assessing prostate diseases. Assessment of prostate size with ultrasound is well established in the urology clinic. Also, the use of ultrasound for biopsy guidance to obtain final diagnosis of prostate cancer has become widespread.

TRUS can also be used to reveal malignant areas in the prostate as prostate cancer might appear as a hypoechoic lesion in the image. A hypoechoic lesion observed in the peripheral zone, where the majority of cancers develop, is especially an indication of a malignant process. In Fig. 13.3, an example of a hypoechoic lesion in the prostate is presented showing a series of transverse sections in gray-scale ultrasound. However, not all prostate cancers appear hypoechoic, and not all hypoechoic lesions are malignant. Therefore, the detection of malignant tumors with ultrasound is a combination of findings, including echogenicity, prostate asymmetry, and bulging or disruption of the prostate capsule. However, the interpretation of the images is dependant on the expertise of the sonographer. Furthermore, the appearance of malignant lesions may vary in the image depending on lesion size and location, and transducer specifications. Due to these limitations, the detection of prostate cancer with ultrasound is limited, and the presence of malignancy should always be confirmed by histopathological analysis of removed tissue prior to initiating therapy.

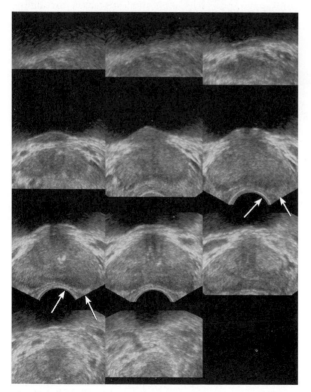

Fig. 13.3 Transverse images from base to apex at 4-mm intersection distances showing a hypoechoic lesion corresponding to a T2 malignancy in the prostate, proven by radical prostatectomy.

In the literature, a number of papers have been reported that studied the value of ultrasound in detecting malignancy in the prostate. Early studies reported high diagnostic accuracy in evaluating prostate diseases, in the range of 80% (6–9). Also, the results reported in the large study of Watanabe in 1980 were impressive. However, in the 1980s, reports indicated that TRUS was not an ideal technique to screen for prostate cancer due to a limited positive predictive value, although it is more sensitive in detecting cancer compared to rectal examination. The introduction of PSA in the clinical decision-making in the early 1990s further reduced the importance of TRUS in screening for prostate cancer, as PSA and DRE became the first-line parameters in the early detection of prostate cancer. The role of ultrasound shifted towards the guidance of biopsies in case of suspicion for malignancy indicated by these parameters and the evaluation of clinical stage of detected tumors. Curative therapy can be considered only an option in case of organ-confined disease, and extracapsular involvement is a contra-indication to perform, for example, radical prostatectomy. Identification of extra-prostatic extension or seminal vesicle involvement prior to surgery has been attempted with ultrasound, and clinical staging improved when adding ultrasound to the decision process (18–20). In Fig. 13.4, an extra-prostatic tumor is shown on gray-scale ultrasound in transverse and longitudinal recording, displaying a tumor with seminal vesicle invasion proven by staging biopsies. Others, however, concluded that the value of transrectal ultrasound as a pretreatment staging tool is limited, especially because of a low specificity in detecting extra-prostatic involvement Also, Hamper *et al.* concluded that transrectal ultrasound suffers from lack of sufficient spatial resolution to detect accurately invasion of the neurovascular bundle. However, ultrasound equipment has improved tremendously over the past decade leading to improvements in bandwidth and transducer sensitivity. Also software modifications resulted in improved ultrasound scanners, especially in filtering algorithms and beam forming. Despite these improvements, it is unexpected for ultrasound or any imaging modality to be able to detect microscopic extra-prostatic involvement with great accuracy.

In summary, ultrasound has developed from a detection technique in the 1970s to a staging technique in the 1980s and a biopsy guidance technique in the 1990s. Currently, transrectal ultrasound is advocated for assessment of prostate volume and to guide prostate sampling with biopsies (25). TRUS lacks

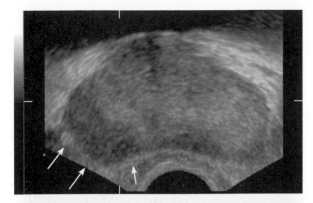

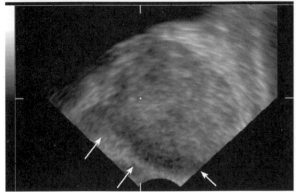

Fig. 13.4 A transverse and longitudinal image showing a hypoechoic lesion corresponding to a T3 malignancy in the prostate: invasion of the seminal vesicles, proven by staging biopsies.

sufficient sensitivity and specificity to be useful in a screening setting, and therefore the use of ultrasound to identify prostate cancer should be limited to a pre-screened group based on rectal examination and PSA. Identification of suspicious lesions should always be confirmed with histopathological examination of harvested tissue.

Prostate biopsies

Biopsies not only provide the confirmation of the presence of prostate cancer, they also provide prognostic information, and therefore an appropriate procedure to perform biopsies is essential. A first approach to standardize the procedure was suggested by Hodge *et al.* who advocated the sextant biopsy sessions for prostate tissue sampling (26). The sextant biopsy approach, with additional directed biopsies, provides an accurate method to detect prostate cancer in prostates pre-screened with DRE and PSA. Some reports mentioned

that sextant biopsy is not an optimal technique, e.g. the prostate volume is not taken into account. The five-region biopsy approach was reported to be superior to the sextant approach in identifying prostate cancer in an early but significant stage (27). By assuring that sufficient tissue is collected with each biopsy (a core of 1.5 cm), valuable additional information on cancer volume, Gleason grade, and staging information can be obtained. Also, the number of positive biopsies can be used to predict the pathological stage of prostate cancer. In case of increased risk for extra-prostatic extension, staging biopsies can be performed additionally by sampling the prostate capsule or the seminal vesicles (28).

The current biopsy procedure has limitations regarding the detection of all malignancies inside the prostate. Repeat biopsies are indicated in case of a negative first set of biopsies but prolonged elevation of PSA and/or suspicious DRE. Also, prescreening by DRE and PSA is not optimal and results in a large number of unnecessary biopsies in patients who show no cancer in removed tissue. We have estimated that in only one out of three patients with a clinical suspicion for malignancy, cancer is found in the removed biopsy cores (2). Next, in many cases the cancer that is found in the biopsy core represents only a limited reflection of the actual pathological stage of the tumor (29). Improvement of the indications to perform biopsies in combination with improved biopsy guidance is therefore an important requisite to improve the clinical workup of prostate diseases and especially prostate cancer.

Advanced transrectal ultrasound

The detection of prostate cancer with ultrasound imaging is mainly based on the identification of hypo-echoic lesions in the prostate that might correspond to malignancy. These lesions might result from, for example, a changed metabolism; however, such changes might also result in a more subtle change of gray-tone characteristics. Realizing that the perception of the human eye is limited, meaning not all information might be received from the images, computerized interpretation might add information to the differentiation process. One approach to adding computer interpretation to the differential diagnosis is to quantify spatial characteristics in the image and correlate quantitative measures to pathology. These spatial characteristics or texture can be described by the so-called co-occurrence analyses, which has been proposed for evaluation of prostate images as well (30). High diagnostic accuracy in the range of 80% has been reported in discriminating benign from malignant tissue based on texture descriptions of ultrasound data (30, 31). We performed a study to classify ultrasound data based on quantitative descriptions of texture obtained in biopsy study (32) and a radical prostatectomy study (33). Initial results (diagnostic accuracy of 75%) encouraged us to evaluate the technology in a larger group of radical prostatectomy patients. In a group of 62 consecutive radical prostatectomy patients, the identification of prostate cancer with quantitative texture descriptions was disappointing, resulting a diagnostic accuracy of less than 60% (unpublished data). Although texture analyses did provide diagnostic information, there is room for improvement. An alternative approach could be the application of artificial neural networks as recently reported by Loch (34). The network was even capable to detect iso-echoic tumors, which is a great improvement of conventional ultrasound. Overall, a diagnostic accuracy of 85% was claimed. An alternative to the processing of ultrasound images, inherently a result of scanner-specific processing of reflected RF data, could be the analyses of the reflected signals themselves. This would offer a scanner-independent analysis technique. Furthermore, due to processing of the signal prior to image display, some information is lost in the image. Spectral analyses of the unprocessed reflected signals might add important differential diagnosis, but this technology, by one author indicated as ultrasound spectroscopy (35), has a long way to go before it can be applied clinically.

Doppler ultrasound

Next to conventional gray-scale imaging, most ultrasound machines are equipped with Doppler techniques allowing the detection of moving reflectors in relation to the transducer position. The Doppler techniques allow the visualization of blood flow by detecting the shifts in frequency observed in reflected signals. In frequency Doppler imaging mode, a lower frequency is coded in a blue signal, and a higher frequency is coded red, meaning that the coded map provides information on velocity and direction of flow. In power Doppler imaging mode, not the frequency shift itself is used for color coding, but the power of the signal is presented to visualize blood flow, thus no longer providing directional information.

The rationale to display prostatic blood flow is that a relation is assumed between the local blood flow and the development of pathology. It is assumed that development of tumors is associated with a changed hemodynamic behavior of the tissue: to allow autonomous growth, the tumor develops the capability to grow new blood vessels, indicated as neovascularization. This neovascularization will result in a changed hemodynamic behavior in order to supply the tumor with nutrients and oxygen needed for proliferation. Accurate display of changed metabolism could therefore reveal important diagnostic information for differential diagnosis but this was only partially possible due to the spatial and temporal resolution of Doppler ultrasound techniques. Not only the spatial resolution improved due to technological improvements in the scanner, also the availability to enhance the signal intensities of the blood flow with contrast enhancers provided new possibilities.

The assumption that tumor growth relies on the development of additional and new blood vessels has been the ubject of a number of papers, and Bigler *et al.* demonstrated that prostate cancer is associated with an increased microvessel density (MVD) compared to benign tissue (36). Currently, most research to obtain MVD information is performed in pathology laboratories by counting microvessels with immunohistochemical assays using an antibody to human von Willebrand factor for assessing intra-tumor microvessel density. Quantification of tumor angiogenesis may allow stratification of patients to type of treatment and selection of expectant management for men with low tumor microvessel density. MVD is considered an independent predictor of pathologic stage and may thus provide prognostic information (37, 38). Using microvessel density in combination with PSA and Gleason score, the prediction of extra-prostatic extension significantly improved (39). Topographic analysis of neovascularity in human prostate cancer indicated a high vascularity of the cancer center, suggesting a high activity of angiogenic promoters in the center of the neoplasm (40). The orientation of microvessels was regular along the basement membrane in normal prostates, while abnormalities in shape, size, and structure of the vessels, as well as an increased proliferation, were found in malignant tissue (37). Recent reports confirm the finding of increased microvessel density in tumor tissue compared to surrounding normal tissue and increased microvessel density in higher Gleason score tumors (41). Borre *et al.* showed that microvessel density was a significant predictor of disease-specific survival in prostate cancer patients (42). Recently, Gettman *et al.* reported that microvessel density could not predict prostate cancer recurrence in patients with T2N0M0 prostate cancer treated with radical prostatectomy (43). Rubin *et al.* reported that microvessel density is not associated with Gleason sum, tumor stage, surgical margin status, or seminal vesicle invasion, based on data of 87 patients who underwent radical prostatectomy. (44).

From the reports presented above, it can be concluded that microvessel density does provide additional information, but does not paint the entire picture. One of the reasons may be that the proliferation of (new) vessels is not a goal as such, but a way for the tumor to increase the supply of nutrients and oxygen and removal of waste in order to continue its autonomous growth. In other words, the microvessel density count does not reflect the actual hemodynamics of tissue. This was the subject of study presented by Louvar *et al.* who reported that no significant differences in microvasculature parameters were noted between high and normal Doppler flow. Biopsies from regions with high flow had an average Gleason score of 6.7 compared with only 5.9 for biopsies from regions with normal Doppler flow (45). If local hemodynamics in an organ can be displayed accurately, the request for increased blood supply by tumors might become visible, and may be useful to detect tumor sites. The possibility of Doppler ultrasound to display flow patterns to detect malignancy in the prostate has been the subject of a number of publications (46–49). The Doppler studies mentioned on prostate cancer detection showed an improved positive predictive value when abnormal findings were shown in Doppler images. All reports, however, indicate limitations of Doppler velocity imaging of the prostate for cancer detection.

The ultrasound equipment, however, showed tremendous increase in computer power and most machines were transformed from analog to completely digital machines. This has greatly affected the technological possibilities of Doppler examination in the recent years. Recent studies indicated that Doppler imaging could be used to improve guidance to higher Gleason grade areas within the prostate (50, 51). Ismail concluded that coded-coded Doppler flow within the tumor and overlying capsule appeared to correlate with both tumor grade and stage, respectively (51). Based on

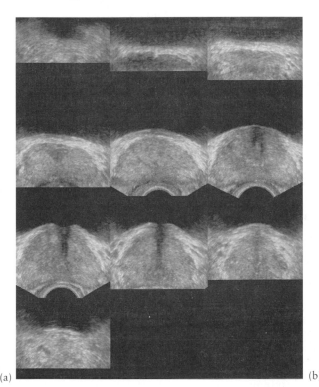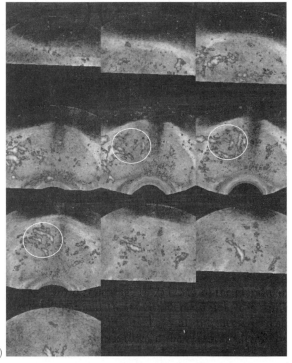

(a) (b)

Fig. 13.5 (a) Transverse images from base to apex at 4-mm intersection distances with no visible lesion. (b) Enhanced Doppler indicated an area with increased blood flow at the right ventral side of the gland. A ventral tumor was found at radical prostatectomy on the right side.

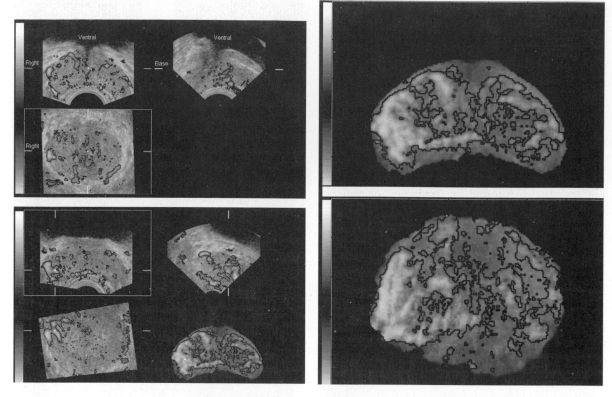

Fig. 13.6 Examples of enhanced Doppler studies of the prostate in combination with 3D-ultrasound: an instruction data-set is presented of a proven malignancy. 3D-reconstruction of Doppler signal intensities from dorsal to ventral view, and from base to apex view are presented indicating a malignancy on the right side at the base of the prostate.

data of 250 patients, Lavoipierre *et al.* advocated that Doppler sonography should become a routine part of transrectal sonography of the prostate gland to improve detection and targeting of lesions (52). Cho *et al.* (53) studied the role of color Doppler and power Doppler ultrasound in the identification of diffuse prostatic lesions and they presented that the majority of detected cancer showed increased blood flow in contrast to the majority of benign prostates.

A next step in Doppler imaging was the introduction of ultrasound contrast agent to enhance the Doppler signals obtained in the prostate (54). In theory, the addition of contrast media has the potential to improve both anatomical and hemodynamic information that could provide additional information for differential diagnosis (55, 56). In Fig. 13.5(a), a series of transverse gray-scale images is presented without visible lesions. Enhanced Doppler studies show increased blood flow activity in the right ventral zone (Fig. 13.5(b)), which was confirmed to be malig-

nant by histopathology of the whole-mount sections after radical prostatectomy. In combination with 3D-reconstruction algorithms, it is possible to display regions with increased activity as shown in Fig. 13.6. 3D-data is collected and presented in transverse, longitudinal, and sagittal sections and 3D-reconstruction can be displayed. The reconstructions shown indicate increased blood flow activity at the right base of the prostate, which was confirmed to be malignant after prostatectomy. Although no hard evidence is available at this moment, the increased Doppler signal intensity might be useful for additional guidance of the biopsy needle and for identification of malignant lesions. In combination with 3D-ultrasound, the vascular anatomy can be judged on symmetrical and focal changes in hemodynamics of the prostate that might correspond to development of tumor (55). However, data of a large patient population is required to define the exact role of enhanced Doppler imaging in identifying and judging prostate cancer.

Magnetic resonance

Magnetic resonance (MR) uses magnetic fields and radiofrequency waves to construct a display of the examined medium. The technique is based on a quantum mechanical phenomenon that is exhibited by atoms having an odd number of protons or neutrons that result in a non-zero nuclear magnetic moment, e.g. ^{1}H present in water and fatty tissue. These nuclei align their spins parallel or antiparallel to an applied external magnetic field. In equilibrium, a small population difference exists between the two states and this equilibrium can be distorted by irradiation of radiofrequency waves. The return to equilibrium is detected and the recorded data-set can be reconstructed to display anatomical images either in 2D or 3D.

Because of its ability to provide anatomical imaging with excellent display of details, MR has a great potential in displaying the anatomy of the prostate as well. The internal structures of the prostate can be clearly demonstrated on T2-weighted images, showing the peripheral zone of the prostate as an area with high-intensity signals. The presence of prostate cancer in the peripheral zone usually results in areas with relatively low-signal intensity (Fig. 13.7). Other reasons for low-intensity areas include the low-intensity signals returned from the transition zone, the presence of prostatitis, calculi, or post-biopsy hemorrhage. Detection of tumors in the central and transition zone based on low-intensity signal is thus not possible, whereas prostatitis and calcified tissue might result in false-negatives.

Due to the detailed anatomical display, MR could play an important role in detecting extra-prostatic involvement of proven prostate cancer. Capsular perforation is most often visible as a disruption of the prostate capsule and infiltration of the periprostatic fat. Involvement of the seminal vesicles is usually visible as abnormally low signal intensity within the lumen. Disappointingly, MRI has not proven to be superior to TRUS in staging of prostate cancer with the body coil technique (57). Initially, it was reported that endorectal coils resulted in more accurate staging (58), but more recent data showed similar results as for the body coil technique (59). Jager *et al.* demonstrated the ability to discriminate pT2 tumor from pT3 tumors with 68% accuracy (60). The criteria for detecting extra-prostatic extension included asymmetry of the neurovascular bundle, obliteration of the rectoprostatic angle, and bulging (61). Recently, it was reported that endorectal MR imaging can be used to improve the identification

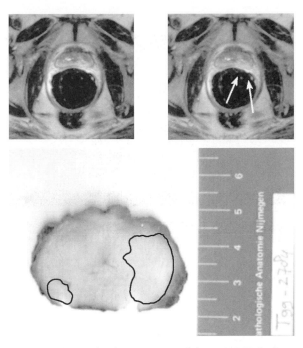

Fig. 13.7 T2-weighted MR image and dynamic MR findings of the prostate indicating a malignant tumor on the left side of the prostate. Whole-mount specimen were used a reference standard.

of established EPE and SVI in selected patients with prostate cancer (62). Further studies to identify the value in an unselected group of patients are needed to reveal the real clinical value of MR in detecting those patients with local extension of the disease.

Enhanced MR imaging

The assumed relation between local blood supply and development of malignant tumors has also found interest in MR imaging. As described for Doppler ultrasound studies, the local blood supply can be studied with a specific MR contrast agent as well. Gadopentetate dimeglumine (gadolinium-DTPA) has been introduced as a contrast medium to increase the diagnostic accuracy of MR imaging. MR contrast agents differ from ultrasound contrast agent in the fact that MR agents mainly display the blood perfusion/diffusion, while Doppler ultrasound reveals blood-flow velocities. While ultrasound contrast agents limited themselves to the circulation (blood-pool enhancer), MR contrast media have the possibility to highlight the permeability and diffusion behavior of the vessel wall and the interstitial space (56). Indeed, for bladder and breast cancer imaging, it was shown that malignant lesions demonstrate an earlier and faster enhancement compared to benign lesions, offering an additional possibility for differential diagnosis (63, 64). Time-enhancement features are related to the specific transient accumulation of contrast media in tumor tissue related to neovascular characteristics. Early data demonstrate the applicability of time-enhancement profiles to improve prostate cancer detection, as illustrated in Fig. 13.7 (65, 66). Furthermore, it is stated that fast dynamic MR imaging is useful in detecting extra-prostatic extension and seminal vesicle involvement (Fig. 13.8). Due to fast developments in the MR field, the application of Gd-enhanced MR imaging is far from established, and future research is needed to define its exact role in prostate cancer detection and staging, the optimal clinical setting and the appropriate patient group for additional imaging.

MR imaging of lymph nodes

Next to local staging of prostate cancer, MR imaging has also been proposed as a technique to evaluate the presence of lymph node involvement prior to treatment selection. By measuring the diameter of the lymph nodes, nodal metastasis can be detected (56). An example of lymph node evaluation by MR imaging is presented in Fig. 13.9, showing an enlarged lymph node. Detection of enlarged nodes should be followed by histological examination of the suspected nodes and a positive result is a contra-indication to perform curative radical prostatectomy.

An important limitation of imaging modalities in the evaluation of nodal metastasis is that outcome mainly relies on the enlargement of lymph nodes as a criterion for metastasis (see CT paragraph). However, most nodal metastases are microscopic and do not enlarge or distort the shape of the lymph node, meaning that metastasis might be present in normal-sized nodes reducing the sensitivity of shape-based imaging modalities. Currently, lymph node-specific MR contrast agents are under development, based on ultra-small superparamagnetic iron oxide particles. Whereas in normal lymph nodes, with functioning macrophages, the iron oxide particles are phagocytosed resulting in a decreased MRI signal intensity, in metastatic nodes lacking macrophages, the signal intensity remains unchanged (67). Application of such lymph node-specific contrast agents might improve the accuracy of MR imaging to detect lymph node involvement (68).

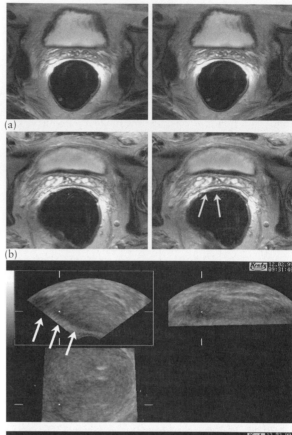

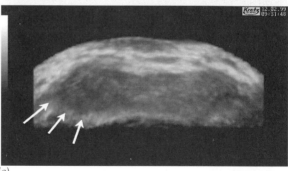

Fig. 13.8 (a) MR imaging of the seminal vesicle showing a normal image. Also the dynamic MR imaging did not show areas with early enhancement. (b) A second example of MR imaging of the seminal vesicles showing an enhancement of the seminal vesicle that corresponded to seminal vesicle invasion (SVI). (c) The 3D-ultrasound findings also indicated a suspicion for SVI, which was confirmed by the pathology.

MR spectroscopy

Next to visualization of dynamic behavior of local blood supply by enhanced MR, MR can be used to obtain metabolic information of the examined tissue.

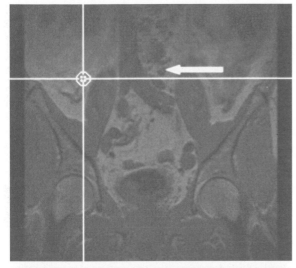

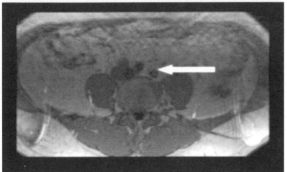

Fig. 13.9 Lymph node examination using MR imaging, showing an enlarged lymph node as indicated by the arrow.

imaging also improved the ability to determine the presence of prostate cancer and spatial extent when post-biopsy changes hinder interpretation with MR imaging alone (73). In a later study, it was concluded that metabolite spectra detected by MR could be used as *in vivo* markers for discriminating prostate cancer from BPH and healthy tissue in the central gland (74). An example of 2D-MR spectroscopic imaging of the human prostate is presented in Fig. 13.10, showing the difference in choline/citrate ratio between healthy and tumor tissue. Using these parametric images in a 3D-setting, the spatial extent of prostate tumor can be assessed, and the volume estimate of tumor with MR imaging might improve (72). With improvements in the robustness of the method, and somewhat better spatial and temporal resolution, MR spectroscopy might find its way to improve tumor visualization and cancer characterization. Recent developments have been reported including the combination of dynamic contrast-enhanced MR imaging and the MR spectroscopy imaging (75). It has been shown that T2-weighted MRI, ^{1}H MRS, and dynamic-enhanced MRI can be combined in a single patient examination, and by pooling the information of all examinations, the characterization of prostate cancer with MR techniques might be improved.

Such information related to metabolites can be an important addition to the anatomical display by standard MR techniques (69). Citrate is the most prominent metabolite signal in spectra obtained from human prostates with proton magnetic resonance spectroscopy (^{1}H MRS). Using localized ^{1}H MRS, local spectral content revealing metabolite levels can be used for quantitative examination of the tissue composition. It has been shown that prostate cancer can be made visible by displaying the ratio of choline and citrate signal as prostate cancer is characterized by a decreased level of citrate and an increased level of choline (69, 70). In the peripheral zone, tumor tissue can be distinguished from healthy tissue based on the choline/citrate ratio, also in the post-treatment evaluation (71, 72). The addition of MR spectroscopic imaging to MR

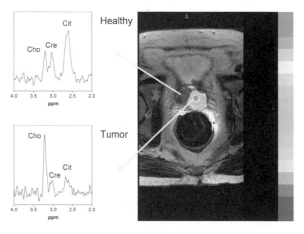

Fig. 13.10 An example of MR spectroscopy to visualize prostate cancer using a colored overlay of a choline/citrate ratio map on top of a T2-weighted MR image showing an increased choline/citrate ratio at the tumor region. The proton spectra displayed were selected from a 16 × 16 spectroscopic imaging plane (spatial resolution 0.8 cm³) and show patterns typical for healthy and tumor tissue.

Computerized tomography imaging

Computer tomography uses conventional X-ray technology and computer technology to create cross-sectional images of objects. Usually, the X-ray tube and the detectors rotate around the object of interest, and X-rays passing through a specific plane of the object can be recorded. By recording this illumination for various angles at various timing during rotation, a 2D-illumination map of the object can be reconstructed using the image reconstruction theorem stating that a 2D-distribution may be constructed from the projection data if one measures a sufficient number of projections of the object. This 2D-scanning can be extended to 3D by sequentially scanning many 2D-images. The 3D data-set can be reconstructed and slices of any particular plane can be constructed. Currently CT scanning is fast enough to even record different phases of the cardiac motion, providing at least 15 scans per second.

The value of CT in detecting and local staging prostate cancer has been limited: it is in general not possible to distinguish prostate cancer from benign tissue in the prostate. It was concluded that CT scanning fails to demonstrate the required precision needed to evaluate local tumor spread (76). Its ability to detect extra-prostatic extension or seminal vesicle involvement in a reliable manner has been considered limited (77).

The ability of CT to detect pelvic lymph node involvement, an exclusion criterion of curative radical prostatectomy, has been studied but results have also been disappointing. The detection of lymph node metastasis with CT was reported to be of limited value (78), although van Poppel *et al.* reported a very high diagnostic accuracy and optimal specificity of CT scanning in combination with fine-needle aspiration biopsies (79). The mean reported sensitivity is approximately 35% (80). Reasons for poor performance might be that the detection of positive lymph nodes with CT is based on distorted shape or enlarged size, and microscopic nodal metastases might not influence the actual size and shape. The most appropriate threshold in nodal size to identify nodal metastasis is still a point of discussion, and reported upper limits vary between 1.6 and 0.6 cm, but the clinical threshold should be below 1.0 cm (81).

In general, it was concluded that the use of routine imaging of lymph nodes, including CT, in all patients with proven malignancy should not be recommended (82), and that imaging of lymph nodes is of value in a selected group of patients at high risk for nodal metastases to prevent them from an unnecessary surgery. High-risk patients are those patients with a Gleason score greater than 6, and/or a PSA exceeding 10 ng/ml, who are candidates for curative therapy. If suspicion of lymph node involvement is indicated by imaging, adequate action should be performed either by taking image-guided biopsy (fine-needle aspiration biopsy FNAB) (80) or image-guided laparoscopic pelvic lymph node dissection (83). FNAB can be performed with CT or MR imaging, both having their specific advantages and disadvantages.

In addition to lymph node imaging, CT scanning is currently applied in the planning of radiation therapies, such as conformal radiation and brachytherapy. CT is used to detect seeds post-implantation and to calculate the dosimetry based on the seed distribution (84). Furthermore, accurate determination of the planning target volume, prior to conformal radiotherapy of prostate cancer, is a prerequisite for successful therapy, and CT is often used to determine the target volume assuming certain margins to encompass prostate movement and position variation (85).

Nuclear imaging

Nuclear imaging techniques use radiopharmaceuticals administered to the object of interest, e.g. the blood circulation, to obtain knowledge of physiological function. Once administered, an external detector is used to obtain the spatial distribution of the tracer or to record the temporal changes in concentration in the organ or tissue of interest. For accurate representation of the actual situation, the tracer should not perturb the function of the organ. Usually, a scintillation camera is used to obtain radionuclide images, reflecting the distribution of the radiopharmaceuticals. By comparing the actual behavior to the predicted behavior of the radionuclides, one can make a diagnosis based on local distribution.

Since hematogeneous metastases of prostate cancer are most common in the axial skeleton, identification of bone metastases is recommended using radionuclide imaging. Technetium is often used as a tracer to mark osteoblastic activity in areas of cortical bone with increased bone turnover. Radionuclide imaging has proven to be a sensitive technique for detection of bone metastasis (86) but it might result in a false-positive outcome due to previous trauma, degenerative disease, or metabolic abnormalities. In low PSA ranges, the number of patients with positive bone scans was very low, with metastases discovered in less than 1% of patients with a PSA below 20 ng/ml (87). It was therefore recommended that PSA should dictate whether a bone scan should be performed.

Next to the tracer Technetium to detect bone metastasis, alternative tracers have been reported to be useful in imaging of prostate cancer. For instance, areas with increased indium concentration in the prostate have been reported to correlate with the presence of prostate cancer (88). Using single-photon emission tomography (SPECT) and a murine monoclonal antibody targeting prostate-specific membrane antigen, increased photon emission correlated to the presence of prostate cancer (89). Such an increased activity at cancer sites can be used to evaluate whether the cancer shows local extension and whether lymph nodes are involved, both findings having impact on therapeutic approach.

Positron emission tomography also uses tracers but these tracers are labeled with positron emitting isotopes (90). In PET scanning, the disintegration of the labeled atom is associated with the release of two photons. As these photons take off at an angle of 180 degrees, no collimators are needed, but the timing between the detection of the photons can be used to estimate whether the photons originate from a single event. ^{18}fluorine (^{18}F)-labeled deoxyglucose has been proposed as a helpful tracer to identify prostate cancer (91). First results indicated that current settings are insufficient for accurate identification of the presence of prostate cancers, but variations in tracer might provide new insights in the application of PET scanning in the evaluation of prostatic diseases (92).

Conclusions and recommendations

Conventional techniques such as gray-scale ultrasound, CT scanning, and MR scanning all showed limited value in screening for prostate cancer. As a result, screening with imaging modalities is currently not advocated, but the application of imaging should be restricted to specific areas. In general, imaging modalities should only be applied when the outcome of the imaging studies can actually change the path of prostate cancer therapy and follow up.

The recommendations for the use of imaging modalities in the identification and evaluation of prostate cancer include:

- Ultrasound should be used for a first evaluation in a patient population with a suspicion of prostate cancer identified by a positive DRE and/or an elevated PSA. To exclude or confirm prostate cancer, ultrasound-guided biopsies should be taken, using a systematic sextant biopsy procedure and if applicable additional targeted biopsies of hypoechoic lesions.

- Once the presence of prostate cancer has been confirmed by histopathology, staging biopsies of the seminal vesicles or the prostatic capsule can be performed under ultrasound guidance. In addition, MR scans can be performed in patients with

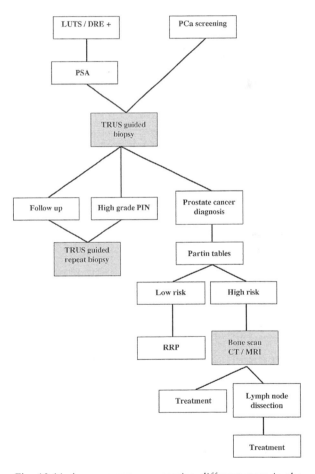

Fig. 13.11 A nomogram representing different steps in the evaluation of the presence of prostate cancer and the selection of appropriate therapy. Applications of imaging modalities are shaded.

increased risk for extra-prostatic involvement to display a detailed view of the prostate anatomy and lymph nodes. It should be borne in mind that MR, and probably all imaging modalities, are not capable of revealing microscopic extra-prostatic extension. The selection of increased-risk patients should be based on a PSA > 10 ng/ml, and/or or a biopsy Gleason score greater than 6 (meaning that a Gleason component of 4 or 5 is present in the biopsy core).

● Bone metastasis should be evaluated only in newly diagnosed patients with a PSA value greater than 10 ng/ml, as the probability of a positive bone scan is extremely low in the low PSA range. In the nomogram presented in Fig. 13.11, the recommendations of the WHO committee on Detection and Staging of Prostate Cancer are presented with the imaging aspects presented as highlighted boxes.

Despite great developments and promising early results, no image modality has been identified that offered the diagnostic accuracy needed for screening of prostate cancer. Alterations in techniques and addition of dynamic studies hold great promises, but these techniques are currently only available in a research setting. Prove of diagnostic power and cost effectiveness is needed before such modified techniques can be advocated for routine use. It is therefore the task of researchers to provide the data needed to establish the future role of these techniques, and just as important to advocate the current setting of diagnostic work up as it should be applied routinely for prostate cancer detection.

Acknowledgement

The authors acknowledge the assistance of Marc Engelbrecht and Professor Dr Jelle Barentsz (MR imaging), and Dr Marinette van der Graaf, Dr Ferdi van Dorsten, and Professor Dr Arend Heerschap (MR spectroscopy) of the Department of Radiology for their assistance in preparing this paper.

References

1. Mettlin CJ, Murphy GP, Babaian RJ *et al*. Observations on the early detection of prostate cancer from the American Cancer Society National Prostate Cancer Detection Project. *Cancer* 1997, **80**, 1814–7.

2. Aarnink RG, Beerlage HP, De la Rosette JJMCH *et al*. Transrectal ultrasound of the prostate: innovations and future applications. *J Urol* 1998, **159**, 1568–79.
3. National Library of Medicine. Medline library. *http://www.ncbi.nlm.nih.gov/PubMed*, 1999. Ref Type: Internet Communication
4. Partin AW, Yoo J, Carter HB *et al*. The use of prostate specific antigen, clinical stage and Gleason score to predict pathological stage in men with localized prostate cancer. *J Urol* 1993, **150**, 110–4.
5. Watanabe H, Igari D, Tanahasi Y *et al*. Development and application of new equipment for transrectal ultrasonography. *JCU J Clin Ultrasound* 1974, **2**, 91–8.
6. Brooman PJ, Griffiths GJ, Roberts E *et al*. Per rectal ultrasound in the investigation of prostatic disease. *Clin Radiol* 1981, **32**, 669–76.
7. Harada K, Igari D, Tanahashi Y. Gray scale transrectal ultransonography of the prostate. *JCU J Clin Ultrasound* 1979, **7**, 45–9.
8. Peeling WB, Griffiths GJ, Evans KT *et al*. Diagnosis and staging of prostatic cancer by transrectal ultrasonography. A preliminary study. *Br J Urol* 1979, **51**, 565–9.
9. Watanabe H, Igari D, Tanahashi Y *et al*. Transrectal ultrasonotomography of the prostate. *J Urol* 1975, **114**, 734–9.
10. Watanabe H, Date S, Ohe H *et al*. A survey of 3,000 examinations by transrectal ultrasonotomography. *Prostate* 1980, **1**, 271–8.
11. Chodak GW, Wald V, Parmer E *et al*. Comparison of digital examination and transrectal ultrasonography for the diagnosis of prostatic cancer. *J Urol* 1986, **135**, 951–4.
12. Lee F, Torp-Pedersen ST, McLeary RD. Diagnosis of prostate cancer by transrectal ultrasound. *Urol Clin North Am* 1989, **16**, 663–73.
13. Lee F, Littrup PJ, Torp-Pedersen ST *et al*. Prostate cancer: comparison of transrectal US and digital rectal examination for screening. *Radiology* 1988, **168**, 389–94.
14. Lee F, Torp-Pedersen ST, Siders DB *et al*. Transrectal ultrasound in the diagnosis and staging of prostatic carcinoma. *Radiology* 1989, **170**, 609–15.
15. Watanabe H. History and applications of transrectal sonography of the prostate. *Urol Clin North Am* 1989, **16**, 617–22.
16. Torp-Pedersen S, Juul N, Jakobsen H. Transrectal prostatic ultrasonography. Equipment, normal findings, benign hyperplasia and cancer. *Scand J Urol Nephrol* 1988, **107** (Suppl), 19–25.
17. Pontes JE, Ohe H, Watanabe H *et al*. Transrectal ultrasonography of the prostate. *Cancer* 1984, **53**, 1369–72.
18. Vijverberg PL, Giessen MC, Kurth KH *et al*. Is preoperative transrectal ultrasonography of value in localized prostatic carcinoma? A blind comparative study between preoperative transrectal ultrasonography and the histopathological radical prostatectomy specimen. *Eur J Surg Oncol* 1992, **18**, 449–55.
19. Salo JO, Kivisaari L, Rannikko S *et al*. Computerized tomography and transrectal ultrasound in the assessment of local extension of prostatic cancer before radical retropubic prostatectomy. *J Urol* 1987, **137**, 435–8.

20. Hamper UM, Sheth S, Walsh PC *et al.* Carcinoma of the prostate: value of transrectal sonography in detecting extension into the neurovascular bundle. *AJR Am J Roentgenol* 1990, **155**, 1015–9.

21. Rorvik J, Halvorsen OJ, Servoll E *et al.* Transrectal ultrasonography to assess local extent of prostatic cancer before radical prostatectomy. *Br J Urol* 1994, **73**, 65–9.

22. Jansen H, Gallee MP, Schroder FH. Analysis of sonographic pattern in prostatic cancer: comparison of longitudinal and transversal transrectal ultrasound with subsequent radical prostatectomy specimens. *Eur Urol* 1990, **18**, 174–8.

23. Whittingham TA. New and future developments in ultrasonic imaging. *Br J Radiol* 1997, **70** (Spec No), S119-S132.

24. Smith JAJ, Scardino PT, Resnick MI *et al.* Transrectal ultrasound versus digital rectal examination for the staging of carcinoma of the prostate: results of a prospective, multi- institutional trial. *J Urol* 1997, **157**, 902–6.

25. Smith JAJ. Transrectal ultrasonography for the detection and staging of carcinoma of the prostate. *J Clin Ultrasound* 1996, **24**, 455–61.

26. Hodge KK, McNeal JE, Terris MK *et al.* Random systematic versus directed ultrasound guided transrectal core biopsies of the prostate. *J Urol* 1989, **142**, 71–4.

27. Eskew LA, Bare RL, McCullough DL. Systematic 5 region prostate biopsy is superior to sextant method for diagnosing carcinoma of the prostate. *J Urol* 1997, **157**, 199–202.

28. Lee F, Bahn DK, Siders DB *et al.* The role of TRUS-guided biopsies for determination of internal and external spread of prostate cancer. *Semin Urol Oncol* 1998, **16**, 129–36.

29. Ruijter ET, van de Kaa C, Schalken JA *et al.* Histological grade heterogeneity in multifocal prostate cancer. Biological and clinical implications. *J Pathol* 1996, **180**, 295–9.

30. Kratzik C, Schuster E, Hainz A *et al.* Texture analysis–a new method of differentiating prostatic carcinoma from prostatic hypertrophy. *Urol Res* 1988, **16**, 395–7.

31. Basset O, Sun Z, Mestas JL *et al.* Texture analysis of ultrasonic images of the prostate by means of co- occurrence matrices. *Ultrason Imaging* 1993, **15**, 218–15737.

32. de la Rosette JJMCH, Giesen RJ, Huynen AL *et al.* Computerized analysis of transrectal ultrasonography images in the detection of prostate carcinoma. *Br J Urol* 1995, **75**, 485–91.

33. Giesen RJ, Huynen AL, Aarnink RG *et al.* Computer analysis of transrectal ultrasound images of the prostate for the detection of carcinoma: a prospective study in radical prostatectomy specimens. *J Urol* 1995, **154**, 1397–400.

34. Loch T, Leuschner I, Genberg C *et al.* Artificial neural network analysis (ANNA) of prostatic transrectal ultrasound. *Prostate* 1999, **39**, 198–204.

35. Gartner T, Zacharias M, Jenderka KV *et al.* [Equipment-independent ultrasound tissue characterization of testis and prostate]. Gerateunabhangige Ultraschall-Gewebecharakterisierung von Hoden und Prostata. *Radiologe* 1998, **38**, 424–33.

36. Bigler SA, Deering RE, Brawer MK. Comparison of microscopic vascularity in benign and malignant prostate tissue. *Hum Pathol* 1993, **24**, 220–6.

37. Brawer MK. Quantitative microvessel density. A staging and prognostic marker for human prostatic carcinoma. *Cancer* 1996, **78**, 345–9.

38. Weidner N, Folkman J. Tumoral vascularity as a prognostic factor in cancer. *Important Adv Oncol* 1996, **1** 167–90.

39. Bostwick DG, Wheeler TM, Blute M *et al.* Optimized microvessel density analysis improves prediction of cancer stage from prostate needle biopsies. *Urology* 1996, **48**, 47–57.

40. Siegal JA, Yu E, Brawer MK. Topography of neovascularity in human prostate carcinoma. *Cancer* 1995, **75**, 2545–51.

41. Mydlo JH, Kral JG, Volpe M *et al.* An analysis of microvessel density, androgen receptor, p53 and HER-2/neu expression and Gleason score in prostate cancer: preliminary results and therapeutic implications. *Eur Urol* 1998, **34**, 426–32.

42. Borre M, Offersen BV, Nerstrom B *et al.* Microvessel density predicts survival in prostate cancer patients subjected to watchful waiting. *Br J Cancer* 1998, **78**, 940–4.

43. Gettman MT, Bergstralh EJ, Blute M *et al.* Prediction of patient outcome in pathologic stage T2 adenocarcinoma of the prostate: lack of significance for microvessel density analysis. *Urology* 1998, **51**, 79–85.

44. Rubin MA, Buyyounouski M, Bagiella E *et al.* Microvessel density in prostate cancer: lack of correlation with tumor grade, pathologic stage, and clinical outcome. *Urology* 1999, **53**, 542–7.

45. Louvar E, Littrup PJ, Goldstein A *et al.* Correlation of color Doppler flow in the prostate with tissue microvascularity. *Cancer* 1998, **83**, 135–40.

46. Kelly IM, Lees WR, Rickards D. Prostate cancer and the role of color Doppler US. *Radiology* 1993, **189**, 153–6.

47. Newman JS, Bree RL, Rubin JM. Prostate cancer: diagnosis with color Doppler sonography with histologic correlation of each biopsy site. *Radiology* 1995, **195**, 86–90.

48. Patel U, Rickards D. The diagnostic value of color Doppler flow in the peripheral zone of the prostate, with histological correlation. *Br J Urol* 1994, **74**, 590–5.

49. Rifkin MD, Sudakoff GS, Alexander AA. Prostate: techniques, results, and potential applications of color Doppler US scanning. *Radiology* 1993, **186**, 509–13.

50. Cornud F, Belin X, Piron D *et al.* Color Doppler-guided prostate biopsies in 591 patients with an elevated serum PSA level: impact on Gleason score for nonpalpable lesions. *Urology* 1997, **49**, 709–15.

51. Ismail M, Petersen RO, Alexander AA *et al.* Color Doppler imaging in predicting the biologic behavior of prostate cancer: correlation with disease-free survival. *Urology* 1997, **50**, 906–12.

52. Lavoipierre AM, Snow RM, Frydenberg M *et al.* Prostatic cancer: role of color Doppler imaging in transrectal sonography. *Am J Roentgenol* 1998, **171**, 205–10.

53. Cho JY, Kim SH, Lee SE. Diffuse prostatic lesions: role of color Doppler and power Doppler ultrasonography. *J Ultrasound Med* 1998, **17**, 283–7.

54. Ragde H, Kenny GM, Murphy GP *et al.* Transrectal ultrasound microbubble contrast angiography of the prostate. *Prostate* 1997, **32**, 279–83.

55. Bogers JA, Sedelaar JPM, Beerlage HP *et al.* Contrast-enhanced 3D power Doppler angiography of the human prostate: correlation with biopsy outcome. *Urology* 1999, **54**, 97–104.

56. Aarnink RG, Beerlage HP, de la Rosette JJMCH *et al.* Contrast angiosonography: a technology to improve Doppler ultrasound examinations of the prostate. *Eur Urol* 1999, **35**, 9–20.

57. Rifkin MD, Zerhouni EA, Gatsonis CA *et al.* Comparison of magnetic resonance imaging and ultrasonography in staging early prostate cancer. Results of a multi-institutional cooperative trial. *N Engl J Med* 1990, **323**, 621–6.

58. Schnall MD, Imai Y, Tomaszewski J *et al.* Prostate cancer: local staging with endorectal surface coil MR imaging. *Radiology* 1991, **178**, 797–802.

59. Tempany CM, Zhou X, Zerhouni EA *et al.* Staging of prostate cancer: results of Radiology Diagnostic Oncology Group project comparison of three MR imaging techniques. *Radiology* 1994, **192**, 47–54.

60. Jager GJ, Ruijter ET, van de Kaa C *et al.* Local staging of prostate cancer with endorectal MR imaging: correlation with histopathology. *Am J Roentgenol* 1996, **166**, 845–52.

61. Yu KK, Hricak H, Alagappan R *et al.* Detection of extracapsular extension of prostate carcinoma with endorectal and phased-array coil MR imaging: multivariate feature analysis. *Radiology* 1997, **202**, 697–702.

62. D'Amico AV, Schnall M, Whittington R *et al.* Endorectal coil magnetic resonance imaging identifies locally advanced prostate cancer in select patients with clinically localized disease. *Urology* 1998, **51**, 449–54.

63. Boetes C, Barentsz JO, Mus RD *et al.* MR characterization of suspicious breast lesions with a gadolinium-enhanced TurboFLASH subtraction technique. *Radiology* 1994, **193**, 777–81.

64. Barentsz JO, Jager GJ, van Vierzen PB *et al.* Staging urinary bladder cancer after transurethral biopsy: value of fast dynamic contrast-enhanced MR imaging. *Radiology* 1996, **201**, 185–93.

65. Turnbull LW, Buckley DL, Turnbull LS *et al.* Differentiation of prostatic carcinoma and benign prostatic hyperplasia: correlation between dynamic Gd-DTPA-enhanced MR imaging and histopathology. *J Magn Reson Imaging* 1999, **9**, 311–6.

66. Jager GJ, Barentsz JO, Oosterhof GO *et al.* Pelvic adenopathy in prostatic and urinary bladder carcinoma: MR imaging with a three-dimensional TI-weighted magnetization-prepared- rapid gradient-echo sequence. *Am J Roentgenol* 1996, 1503–7.

67. Weissleder R, Elizondo G, Wittenberg J *et al.* Ultrasmall superparamagnetic iron oxide: characterization of a new class of contrast agents for MR imaging. *Radiology* 1990, **175**, 489–93.

68. Harisinghani MG, Saini S, Weissleder R *et al.* MR lymphangiography using ultrasmall superparamagnetic iron oxide in patients with primary abdominal and pelvic malignancies: radiographic- pathologic correlation. *Am J Roentgenol* 1999, **172**, 1347–51.

69. Heerschap A, Jager GJ, van der Graaf M *et al.* Proton MR spectroscopy of the normal human prostate with an endorectal coil and a double spin-echo pulse sequence. *Magn Reson Med* 1997, **37**, 204–13.

70. Heerschap A, Jager GJ, van der Graaf M *et al.* In vivo proton MR spectroscopy reveals altered metabolite content in malignant prostate tissue. *Anticancer Res* 1997, **17**, 1455–60.

71. Kurhanewicz J, Vigneron DB, Hricak H *et al.* Three-dimensional H-1 MR spectroscopic imaging of the in situ human prostate with high (0.24–0.7-cm3) spatial resolution. *Radiology* 1996, **198**, 795–805.

72. Kurhanewicz J, Vigneron DB, Hricak H *et al.* Prostate cancer: metabolic response to cryosurgery as detected with 3D H-1 MR spectroscopic imaging. *Radiology* 1996, **200**, 489–96.

73. Kaji Y, Kurhanewicz J, Hricak H *et al.* Localizing prostate cancer in the presence of postbiopsy changes on MR images: role of proton MR spectroscopic imaging. *Radiology* 1998, **206**, 785–90.

74. Kim JK, Kim DY, Lee YH *et al.* In vivo differential diagnosis of prostate cancer and benign prostatic hyperplasia: localized proton magnetic resonance spectroscopy using external-body surface coil. *Magn Reson Imaging* 1998, **16**, 1281–8.

75. Liney GP, Turnbull LW, Knowles AJ. In vivo magnetic resonance spectroscopy and dynamic contrast enhanced imaging of the prostate gland. *NMR Biomed* 1999, **12**, 39–44.

76. Engeler CE, Wasserman NF, Zhang G. Preoperative assessment of prostatic carcinoma by computerized tomography. Weaknesses and new perspectives. *Urology* 1992, **40**, 346–50.

77. Rorvik J, Halvorsen, OJ, Espeland A *et al.* Inability of refined CT to assess local extent of prostatic cancer. *Acta Radiol* 1993, **34**, 39–42.

78. Tiguert R, Gheiler EL, Tefilli MV *et al.* Lymph node size does not correlate with the presence of prostate cancer metastasis. *Urology* 1999, **53**, 367–71.

79. Poppel Hv, Ameye F, Oyen R *et al.* Accuracy of combined computerized tomography and fine needle aspiration cytology in lymph node staging of localized prostatic carcinoma [see comments]. *J Urol* 1994, **151**, 1310–4.

80. Wolf JSJ, Cher M, Dall *et al.* The use and accuracy of cross-sectional imaging and fine needle aspiration cytology for detection of pelvic lymph node metastases before radical prostatectomy. *J Urol* 1995, **153**, 993–9.

81. Jager GJ. Sensitivity of frozen section examination of pelvic lymph nodes for metastatic prostate carcinoma [letter]. *Cancer* 1996, **77**, 1003–5.

82. Flanigan RC, McKay TC, Olson M *et al.* Limited efficacy of preoperative computed tomographic scanning for the evaluation of lymph node metastasis in patients before radical prostatectomy. *Urology* 1996, **48**, 428–32.

83. Hoenig DM, Chi S, Porter C *et al.* Risk of nodal metastases at laparoscopic pelvic lymphadenectomy using PSA, Gleason score, and clinical stage in men with localized prostate cancer. *J Endourol* 1997, **11**, 263–5.

84. Prestidge BR, Bice WS, Kiefer EJ *et al.* Timing of computed tomography-based postimplant assessment following permanent transperineal prostate brachytherapy. *Int J Radiat Oncol Biol Phys* 1998, **40**, 1111–5.

85. Tinger A, Michalski JM, Cheng A *et al.* A critical evaluation of the planning target volume for 3-D conformal radiotherapy of prostate cancer. *Int J Radiat Oncol Biol Phys* 1998, **42**, 213–21.

86. Haukaas S, Roervik J, Halvorsen OJ *et al.* When is bone scintigraphy necessary in the assessment of newly diagnosed, untreated prostate cancer? *Br J Urol* 1997, **79**, 770–6.

87. Chybowski FM, Keller JJ, Bergstralh EJ *et al.* Predicting radionuclide bone scan findings in patients with newly diagnosed, untreated prostate cancer: prostate specific antigen is superior to all other clinical parameters. *J Urol* 1991, **145**, 313–8.

88. Lamb HM, Faulds D. Capromab pendetide: a review of its use as an imaging agent in prostate cancer. *Drugs Aging* 1998, **12**, 293–304.

89. Sodee DB, Ellis RJ, Samuels MA *et al.* Prostate cancer and prostate bed SPECT imaging with ProstaScint: semiquantitative correlation with prostatic biopsy results. *Prostate* 1998, **37**, 140–8.

90. Hoh CK, Schiepers C, Seltzer MA *et al.* PET in oncology: will it replace the other modalities? *Semin Nucl Med* 1997, **27**, 94–106.

91. Effert PJ, Bares R, Handt S *et al.* Metabolic imaging of untreated prostate cancer by positron emission tomography with 18fluorine-labeled deoxyglucose. *J Urol* 1996, **155**, 994–8.

92. Hoh CK, Seltzer MA, Franklin J *et al.* Positron emission tomography in urological oncology. *J Urol* 1998, **159**, 347–56.

14 | Prognostic and predictive markers in prostate cancer

Bhaskar V. S. Kallakury and Jeffrey S. Ross

Introduction

Prostate cancer has surpassed lung cancer in becoming the most commonly diagnosed cancer in American men. It is second to lung cancer in causing cancer deaths in this group (1) and is responsible for 3% of all deaths in men over the age of 55 years (2). The incidence of prostate cancer increases more rapidly with age than any other cancer. The clinical patterns of prostate cancer development and progression have changed markedly in recent years (3–4) and it is estimated that during the years 1985–2000 there will have been a 37% increase in prostate cancer deaths per year and a 90% increase in prostate cancer cases diagnosed (5). Prostate cancer is rare in men under 30 years of age and rarely occurs in men less than 50 years old (6–7). The peak incidence of the disease is between ages 65 and 75 years, and 75% of newly diagnosed patients are 65–80 years of age (6). The frequency of the disease increases steadily with age and although rates of 100% after 80 years of age have been reported, the overall frequency of prostate cancer in elderly males is closer to 50% (6–7). Prostate cancer is more common in African-Americans and much less common among Asians than among whites (8). The highest mortality rate for prostate cancer in the world is found in African-American men in the US; the rate being 2- to 3-fold higher in this group than among whites, even after adjusting for socioeconomic factors (8). Currently, the search for epidemiologic factors has produced no compelling evidence to implicate any particular agent as a cause of prostate cancer (9). However, although loosely related, the documented observations can be grouped into four categories: genetic influences; endogenous hormonal changes; exposure to environmental agents; and exposure to infectious organisms (10). The potential role of genetic factors is based on the observation of an increased frequency of the disease among relatives of prostate cancer patients. It has been reported that human prostate cancer can be inherited in a Mendelian fashion, best fitting an autosomal dominant model (11). Much effort is underway to identify the specific genetic markers of predisposition for prostate cancer (12). Although cytogenetic analyses of prostate cancer have not indicated any consistent chromosomal deletions, limited studies indicate that some late stage prostatic carcinomas have a high incidence of a deletion in chromosome 10q or 7q (13).

Androgens appear to function as permissive factors required for the development of both prostate cancer and benign glandular hyperplasia (BPH). Cancers of the prostate typically regress after androgen stimulation is ablated. Males castrated prior to puberty never develop prostate cancer, and prostate cancer can be induced in certain breeds of rats by exogenous estrogens and androgens. In addition, prostatic carcinomas are often encountered immediately adjacent to histologic foci of glandular atrophy (10). However, the exact mechanisms by which sex hormone levels influence the development of prostate cancer remain to be determined. Environmental factors have been implicated, not only by differences in the geographic incidence but by an increased frequency of prostate cancer among those exposed to cadmium oxide dust, substances in exhaust fumes, fertilizers, and certain industrial settings (14). It has also been observed that the first generation to emigrate from low-incidence to high-incidence areas retain their low incidence of prostate cancer but their children, born and raised in the high-incidence environment, develop an intermediate frequency of disease (10). Viral particles have been reported in prostate cancers but the evidence for their etiologic role has not been clearly established (15).

General pathology of prostate cancer

Malignant tumors of the prostate

Of the malignant neoplasms of the prostate gland, 96% are acinar adenocarcinomas (Table 14.1). Although rare, sarcomas of the prostate comprise a small but significant group of tumors. Prostatic carcinomas can be divided into two major categories based on their site of origin:

(1) carcinomas of the central or transition zone of the gland;

(2) carcinomas arising in the peripheral lobes.

Approximately 90% of prostate cancers arise from the peripheral lobes and these cancers are the most well-characterized.

Gross features of prostatic carcinoma

Most clinical carcinomas of the prostate arise in the posterior lobe but may also originate in any of the other lobes. Grossly, prostatic carcinoma may be difficult to see but may be identified as a firm gray or yellowish, poorly delineated area. Sometimes, multiple tumor foci are seen and have been documented in up to 75–85% of radical prostatectomy specimens that were studied by step-wise sectioning (16). Foci of necrosis

are usually not apparent unless the tumor reaches large proportions.

Microscopic features of prostate cancer

Adenocarcinomas are heterogeneous tumors characterized by back to back prostatic acini in which the cells lining the acinus form a single layer. The basal cell layer is usually absent. Prominent large eosinophilic nucleoli are commonly present in the tumor cells. Adenocarcinomas are infiltrating tumors growing in sheets, cords, or isolated compressed glands. Perineural invasion is common and may be helpful in both the diagnosis and prediction of outcome for well-differentiated tumors. Well-differentiated adenocarcinomas are often confined to a single prostate lobe and are usually small in volume. High-grade tumors are often larger, more infiltrating, multi-focal, and typically involve more than one prostate lobe.

Epithelial neoplasms

Large-duct carcinomas are characterized by the presence of malignant cells originating from the lining of the large dilated central ducts of the gland. These tumors often display papillary foci (17–19) and occasionally by clear cell changes (20). Tumor cells typically immunostain positively for prostate-specific antigen (PSA) and prostatic acid phosphatase (PAP). Although usually of low to intermediate aggressiveness, these tumors may, on occasion, spread rapidly.

Mucinous carcinomas are tumors that produce prominent lakes of extracellular mucin thus resembling colloid carcinomas of the colon and breast. They are associated with a cribiform pattern in the mucinous areas and invariably stain for both PAP and PSA (21). These tumors do not respond well to hormonal therapy and have an aggressive biological behavior with the propensity to develop bone metastases.

Adenoid cystic carcinomas are extremely uncommon variants of adenocarcinomas and closely resemble their counterpart in the salivary glands. The origin of these tumors is unclear but is thought to arise from peri-uretheral seromucinous glands rather than the prostatic glandular epithelium and are negative for both PAP and PSA (22).

Adenosquamous carcinomas are another rare variant of prostatic adenocarcinoma. The most common situation in which an adenosquamous carcinoma is encountered is when an adenocarcinoma undergoes partial squamous metaplasia after exposure to radiation

Table 14.1 Tumors of the prostate

Epithelial neoplasms	Non-epithelial neoplasms

1. Adenocarcinoma
    Pure ductal
    Mucinous
    Adenoid cystic
    Adenosquamous
    Papillary
    Signet-ring cell
    Endometrioid
	1. Mesenchymal tumors

2. Small cell carcinoma	2. Leiomyosarcoma
3. Transitional cell a carcinom	3. Embryonal rhabdomyosarcoma
4. Carcinosarcoma	4. Granulocytic sarcoma
5. Sarcomatoid carcinoma	5. Other sarcoma types
6. Pure squamous cell carcinoma	6. Lymphoma/leukemia
7. Basal cell carcinoma	7. Germ-cell tumors
8. Carcinoid tumors	8. Metastatic neoplasms

therapy (23). Squamous cell carcinoma differentiation has also been reported in conventional adenocarcinoma following estrogen therapy (24). It is likely that this tumor arises from pleuripotent undifferentiated stem cells.

Papillary adenocarcinomas arise in the large peri-uretheral prostatic ducts and may represent either a variant of prostatic adenocarcinoma or a form of non-prostatic carcinoma of peri-uretheral glands or meta-plastic urethral mucosa. These tumors are PAP-positive (19) and pursue a clinical course similar to that of the usual acinar type prostatic adenocarcinoma.

Signet-ring carcinomas are another rare histologic pattern of prostatic carcinoma and are considered to be high-grade poorly differentiated carcinomas (25). The signet-ring cells are negative for neutral and acid mucins, but are immunoreactive for PAP and PSA (26).

Endometrioid adenocarcinomas commonly present with obstructive symptoms due to their protrusion into the prostatic urethra and the verumontanum (27). These tumors probably arise from prostatic ducts and are not of Mullerian origin (28). Although these tumors closely resemble adenocarcinomas arising from the endometrium, they immunoreact with PSA and PAP, and are associated with an aggressive clinical behavior (28).

Small-cell carcinomas are thought to arise from mul-tipotential undifferentiated prostatic epithelium and are associated with uniformly poor prognosis with a median survival of 7.7 months (29). This group includes both neuroendocrine carcinomas and poorly differentiated adenocarcinomas. Neuroendocrine dif-ferentiation is associated with the presence of specific biomarkers and is an aggressive tumor in most cases.

Prostatic transitional cell carcinomas are thought to arise from the reserve cells that lie between the luminal epithelium and the basement membrane in the peri-urethral ducts of the prostatic urethral glandular epithe-lium (30). These lesions are PSA and PAP negative. Advanced cases do not respond to hormonal therapy.

Lymphoepithelioma-like carcinomas are extremely rare poorly differentiated carcinomas with a syncitial growth pattern and prominent lymphocytic stroma (17). Carcinosarcomas of the prostate are biphasic tumors that contain an adenocarcinoma and a recog-nizable sarcomatous component such as chondrosar-coma, osteosarcoma, liposarcoma, or angiosarcoma (31). Some authorities consider these tumors to be sar-comatoid carcinomas (32). Theories as to their histo-genesis include: sarcomatous transformation of an existing adenocarcinoma or apparent biphasic differen-tiation from a single precursor stem cell. The prognosis is uniformly poor with a mean survival of less than two years. Other uncommon malignant epithelial neo-plasms include pure squamous cell carcinomas (33), basal cell carcinomas and carcinoid tumors.

Non-epithelial neoplasms

Mesenchymal tumors of the prostate include the embryonal rhabdomyosarcoma (34) and leiomyosar-coma (35). Both types have occurred at all ages, but mesenchymal tumors in the young tend to differentiate towards rhabdomyosarcoma, while those in the older patients differentiate towards leiomyosarcoma. These lesions are typically at an advanced stage at diagnosis and feature a poor survival rate. Other rarely diag-nosed sarcomas include granulocytic sarcoma, osteosarcoma, malignant fibrous histiocytoma, malig-nant schwannoma, myxosarcoma, fibrosarcoma, and angiosarcoma.

Primary malignant lymphomas may involve the prostate and typically occur in elderly men (mean age of 60) and clinically present with prostate enlargement and urinary obstruction (36). All subtypes of lym-phoma, including Hodgkin's disease, have been observed. They are associated with poor prognosis with mean survival of 14 months (range 2–44 months).

Germ-cell tumors may rarely involve the prostate gland with reports of both endodermal sinus tumor (37) and malignant mixed germ-cell tumor (38) in the literature. These tumors are associated with a grave prognosis.

The most frequent metastatic tumors involving the prostate are lymphomas and leukemias (36). Other metastatic neoplasms include adenocarcinomas from the gastro-intestinal tract and lung; malignant melanomas; seminomas; and malignant rhabdoid tumor.

Prostatic intra-epithelial neoplasia

In-situ carcinoma or prostatic intra-epithelial neoplasia (PIN) is an intraluminal proliferation of the secretory cells of the prostatic duct-acinar system that displays a spectrum of dysplastic cytologic features ranging from minimal atypia to those that are ultimately indistin-guishable from adenocarcinoma (39). This intraglandu-lar proliferation is consistently enveloped by a basal cell layer that may be focally disrupted in high grade

PIN. The classification of PIN into low-grade and high-grade PIN is chiefly based on the cytologic characteristics of the cells (40–41). The presence of a basal cell layer enveloping the atypical acinar glandular cells is a prerequisite for the diagnosis of PIN. The four common morphologic patterns of PIN (of no apparent clinico-pathologic significance) are: micropapillary, tufting, flat, and cribiform patterns (40). For patients with a similar age range, there is an increased incidence of PIN in the prostates with carcinoma (82%), compared to benign prostate tissue samples (43%) (42). Patients with PIN in biopsy specimens have been noted to have intermediate elevations of their serum PSA levels (43). High-grade PIN appears to share many molecular genetic features that are also identified in the adjacent adenocarcinomas that have developed in the same patients (44). The genetic, histochemical, and immunochemical similarities between PIN and prostatic carcinoma strongly favors that PIN is the pre-invasive phase of at least a subset of cases of prostate cancer.

The diagnosis of prostate cancer

The predominant method by with prostate cancer is diagnosed in the US today is by ultrasound-guided transrectal biopsy (Table 14.2) (45). The sextant biopsy approach remains the most popular (46). National screening programs using serum measurements of prostate-specific antigen (PSA) (47) yield approximately three negative needle biopsy sets for each case positive for malignancy. Various new approaches to serum-based screening have utilized free versus total PSA, prostate-specific membrane antigen, and molecular techniques designed to detect cancer-specific genetic abnormalities in circulation (48). Although the diagnosis of carcinoma is readily made in most cases, a variety of atypical, psedocarcinomatous, and pre-malignant lesions can be encountered in needle biopsies and lead to an 'equivocal' pathology report (49–51).

Table 14.2 The diagnosis of prostate cancer

1. Serum PSA screening
2. Digital rectal exam
3. Transrectal ultrasound
4. Guided or unguided needle biopsy
5. Transurethral resection for BPH
6. Metastasis biopsy (lymph node, liver, bone marrow)

Spread and metastasis of prostatic carcinoma

Capsular involvement is reported to be very common in prostatic adenocarcinoma with incidence as high as 90% in one series (52). The existence of a distinct prostatic capsule has been questioned and it is now concluded that the prostate is devoid of a true capsule but has an outer fibromuscular band that is referred to as its capsule. Patients with focal intra-capsular penetration by the tumor are reported to have an intermediate prognostic risk between those with organ-onfined disease and those with diffuse trans-capsular penetration (53). Peri-neural invasion with migration of the tumor along the peri-neural sheath is recognized as a low-resistant pathway of tumor penetration across the prostatic capsule. The presence of peri-neural invasion on needle biopsy has been reported to be a specific marker for capsular penetration of the tumor in a prostatectomy specimen (54).

Seminal vesicle involvement by adenocarcinoma is associated with poorly differentiated tumors with large volume; a high incidence of extracapsular invasion and lymph node metastasis; and a poor prognosis (55). Three patterns of seminal vesicle involvement have been reported:

(1) direct spread along the ejaculatory duct into seminal vesicle;

(2) spread outside the prostate, through the capsule and into the seminal vesicle;

(3) isolated deposits of tumor in seminal vesicle with no contiguous primary cancer in prostate.

Type 2 seminal vesicle involvement is associated with a significantly higher risk of lymph node metastasis (55).

Regarding the capsular margins of resection, there is a significant difference in tumor prognosis between patients with negative margins and either focally positive or extensively positive margins (53). When patients with positive lymph nodes and/or seminal vesicle involvement were included, there was a significant difference in tumor progression between focally involved and extensively involved margins, although this difference lacked significance when these patients were excluded from the analysis (53). Resection margin positivity is also linked to higher levels of serum PSA at the time of disease diagnosis (56–57).

The presence of nodal metastases is almost invariably associated with significant tumor progression. The first station of nodal involvement is in the pelvic chains from which the tumor spreads to the retroperitoneal lymph nodes. The overall incidence of nodal metastases averages 40% (58). Metastases also can occur in the supradiaphragmatic lymph node groups. On occasion, involvement of the left supraclavicular or mediastinal nodes may be the presenting sign of the disease. Bone metastases are typically osteoblastic, but can also be entirely osteolytic or mixed. When extensive, they can be accompanied by hypocalcemia, hypophosphatemia, and elevated serum alkaline phosphatase levels. The lumber spine, sacrum, and the pelvis are the most common locations, but any bone can be involved (59). Rarely, parenchymal metastases involving visceral organs such as the liver can be the presenting symptoms of prostatic carcinoma.

Traditional morphologic predictors of prognosis

Grading of prostate cancer

The microscopic grade of a prostate cancer correlates significantly with the local extent of the disease, incidence of lymph node, and bone metastasis, and the response to various therapies and overall disease outcome. To date, 12 different methods of grading have been proposed, although only a select group of grading systems have achieved significant use in clinical practice (Table 14.3). The most commonly used grading system in North America today is that developed by Gleason (60). The Gleason system uses two numerical scores, one for the predominant pattern and the second for the next most common pattern in a given tumor, the final grade being the summation of the two scores. A summary of other grading systems is given in Table 14.3.

Correlation of grading with other parameters

In a large series, McNeal *et al.* (61) reported a strong correlation between cancer volume, percentage of poorly differentiated carcinoma (Gleason pattern 4 and/or 5), and nodal metastases. They found that when the tumor volume was less than 1 cm^3, the predominant Gleason histologic patterns were those of 1 and 2 and the cancer was found mainly in the transition zone of the prostate. Tumor grade has often correlated with non-morphologic markers of disease aggressiveness, including increased cell proliferation, aneuploid DNA content, oncogene activation, and tumor-suppressor gene mutation (see following section). Although the Gleason histologic grade of prostatic adenocarcinoma is one of the strongest predictors of biologic behavior and metastatic potential, it does not appear to be sufficiently reliable when used alone for the prediction of the pathological stage (62).

Comparison of specimen source for diagnosis and grading

The tumor grade of the needle core biopsy has been successfully correlated with the grade obtained from fine-needle aspiration biopsies (63–64). The correlation of needle biopsy grade with the final grade at radical prostatectomy has achieved the best result for moderately and poorly differentiated adenocarcinomas (65). Discrepancies between the Gleason's score on the biopsies and the corresponding radical prostatectomy specimens are greatest when the Gleason scores were low and the quantity of tumor in the biopsy specimens was limited (66). In addition, it has been documented that needle biopsy accuracy may be higher when the grading pathologists are experienced sub-specialists in urologic pathology, compared to the more frequent grade changes at radical prostatectomy seen when community hospital pathologists performed the original biopsy grading (67).

Tumor volume

Tumor volume is a significant predictor of pathologic stage, lymph node, and distant metastasis and overall disease outcome (68–69). Accurate measurement of tumor volume requires careful processing of radical prostatectomy specimens. Pre-operative estimates of tumor volume have been marginally successful given the limited accuracy of ultrasound, computer tomography, and magnetic resonance imaging in measuring prostate cancer tumor size. The number and length of involvement of multiple (sextant or octant) needle biopsy cores has been successful at predicting overall tumor volume, pathologic stage, and disease outcome.

Table 14.3 Comparison of grading systems for prostate cancer

Gleason	Mostofi	M. D. Anderson	Bocking	Gaeta	Broders
1. Uniform small glands in lobules.	1. Well differentiated glands with mild nuclear anaplasia.	1. 75–100% of tumor forms glands	1. Uniform glands with no nuclear anaplasia.	1. Well-defined glands with small nucleii and inconspicuous nucleoli.	1. 75–100% of tumor is gland forming.
2. Similar to pattern 1 with glands being irregular.	2. Tumor–forming glands with moderate nuclear anaplasia.	2. 50–75% of tumor forms glands	2. Pleomorphic irregular glands with variable-sized nucleoli.	2. Glands with pleomorphic nucleii and prominent nucleoli.	2. 50–75% of tumor is gland forming.
3. Infiltrative irregular glands, cribiform or papillary pattern.	3. Tumor–forming glands with marked nuclear anaplasia or no glands are found.	3. 25–50% of tumor forms glands.	3. No glands, large nucleii with nucleoli.	3. Infiltrative, cribiform or sebaceous pattern ± glands with pleomorphic nucleii and prominent nucleoli.	3. 25–50% of tumor is gland forming.
4. Infiltrative markedly irregular glands, hyper-nephroma like large cells.		4. 0–25% of tumor forms glands.		4. No glands. Cells with pleomorphic nucleii and prominent nucleoli, mitosis > 3/hpf	4. 0–25% of tumor is gland forming.
5. Infiltrative anaplastic cells, very poorly differentiated.					

Staging of prostatic cancer

Recently, the American Joint Committee and International Union Against Cancer published a new TNM system for pathologic staging (70–71). A comparison of staging systems is summarized in Table 14.4. Although these systems differ slightly in detail, they all recognize that:

(1) early stage prostate cancer can be non-palpable;

(2) palpable tumors can be of different sizes and of various histologic grades;

(3) tumors may extend beyond the prostate without metastatic disease;

(4) tumors with regional metastasis may be biologically different than those with distant metastases.

Table 14.4 Comparison of staging systems for prostate cancer

Whitmore/Jewett	AJCC (American Joint Cancer Committee)	American Urological System	Prout
A No clinical neoplasm.	**T1** No clinical neoplasm.	**A** Incidental finding.	**A** No clinical neoplasm.
A1 Tumor < 3 foci.	**T1a** Tumor ≤ 3 foci.	**A1** Focal.	**A1** Well-differentiated carcinoma, < 3 microscopic foci.
A2 Tumor > 3 foci.	**T1b** Tumor > 3 foci.	**A2** Diffuse.	**A2** Multi-focal/diffuse carcinoma.
B Palpable neoplasm.	**T2** Palpable neoplasm.	**B** Confined to prostate.	**B** Palpable tumor.
B1 Focal, ≤ 1.5 cm, 1 lobe.	**T2a** Focal, ≤ 1.5 cm, 1 lobe.	**B1** Small, discrete nodule.	**B1** ≤ 2 cm, no capsular involvement, normal acid phosphatase.
B2 Diffuse, > 1.5 cm, > 1 lobe.	**T2b** Diffuse, > 1.5 cm, > 1 lobe.	**B2** Large, multiple nodules or areas.	**B2** Diffuse carcinoma involves > 35% of gland. No capsular penetration. Normal acid phosphatase.
C Local invasion.	**T3** Local invasion, bladder, seminal vesicles, prostatic capsule, not fixed.	**C** Localized to peri prostatic area.	**C** Extensive local tumor, capsular penetration. Involves any combination of seminal vesicle, bladder neck, pelvic side wall involvement. Negative bone scan and acid phosphatase.
C1 Bladder, seminal vesicles, prostate capsule, not fixed.	**T4** Other sites, fixed.	**C1** No involvement of seminal vesicles < 70 g.	**D1** Metastasis to pelvic nodes.
C2 Other sites, fixed.	**N1–3** Regional node involvement.	**C2** Seminal vesicle involvement, > 70 g.	**D2** Bone or nodal metastases above aortic bifurcation or visceral involvement.
D Metastases.	**M1** Distant metastasis	**D** Metastatic disease.	
D1 Regional nodes involved.		**D1** Pelvic nodes involved.	
D2 Distant sites.		**D2** Bone, distant nodes, organs, soft tissues.	

Low-stage cancers (stages A and B) in the young may behave no more aggressively than similar tumors in the elderly (72). In younger patients, when tumors recur after primary treatments, aggressive hormone-independent clones may develop increasing the cancer stage with time and elevating the risk of cancer related death in that individual (72).

Ancillary and molecular prognostic factors

A variety of molecular-based assays of genes and proteins (Table 14.5) have been studied for their ability to predict outcome and target therapy in prostate cancer (73–74).

Hormone receptors

Biochemical and immunohistochemical measurements of estrogen and progesterone hormone receptors have played a significant role in the prognosis assessment and planning of therapy in breast carcinoma (75). Assays of estrogen and progesterone receptors have not been shown to have a statistically significant predictive value in prostate cancer. Androgen-receptor assays, however, have received significant attention as potential markers of disease outcome (76). Although androgen receptor loss and clinical lack of anti-androgen therapy benefit have been associated with high-grade and high-stage prostate cancer, androgen-receptor activity has not independently predicted disease outcome. Androgen-receptor expression can be heterogeneous in prostate cancer, which may reflect receptor-genetic instability and the future development of androgen-independent tumor growth (77). The major use of androgen-receptor assays in prostate cancer has been in the selection of therapy for patients with symptomatic metastatic disease and in older men in whom radical surgery is contra-indicated. Assays of androgen-receptor activity have not been used to select patients for pre-operative neo-adjuvant androgen-ablation therapy prior to prostatectomy. Research interest in androgen-receptor activity has focused recently on the relationship between expression of various genes associated with prostate cancer progression and the androgen-receptor status (78). Further characterization of androgen-receptor activity in prostate cancer appears warranted both to better understand the events that produce the capability of androgen-independent growth for some aggressive tumors and the interaction of the androgen receptor with other prognosis markers.

Cell-proliferation markers

A variety of techniques have been developed to measure the rate of cell proliferation in prostate cancer. The two main methods have been the direct immunohistochemical staining using cell-proliferation markers and the calculation of the S-phase from flow cytometry or image analysis derived quantitative DNA histograms. Both proliferating cell nuclear antigen immunostaining (PCNA) and Ki-67 antibodies have been used to study prostate cancer. Both of these markers measure cells in the S- or synthesis-phase as well as portions of the G1 compartment and G2 compartment. The recently developed MIB-1 Ki-67 clone is effective in fixed-processed tissues and has become the technique of choice (79–80). Although clinically defined proliferation ranges remain under study for prostate cancer, it is generally accepted that greater than 16–20% MIB-1 staining is associated with a high proliferation rate and an adverse prognosis.

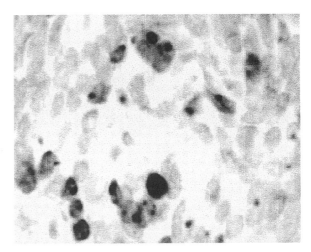

Fig. 14.1 Prostate cancer cell proliferation index determined by immunostaining for the MIB 1 clone of the Ki-67 proliferation marker. The labeling index for this case was 23%. This is a high rate of proliferation for prostate cancer and is associated with high-grade, high-stage disease with a propensity for recurrence after surgical or radiation therapy.

Table 14.5 Ancillary factors in predicting prognosis in prostate cancer

1. Hormone receptors
2. Cell-proliferation markers and cell-cycle proteins
3. DNA ploidy
4. Morphometric analysis
5. Tumor vascularity and micro-vessel density
6. Nuclear matrix proteins
7. Growth factors
8. Cell-adhesion molecules
9. Invasion-associated proteases
10. Dominant oncogenes
11. HER-2*neu* oncogene
12. p53 tumor-suppressor gene
13. Other tumor-suppressor genes
14. Apoptosis and Bcl-2

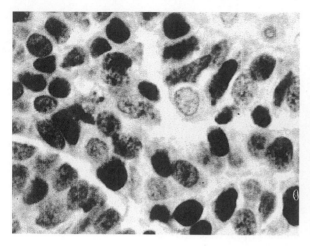

Fig. 14.2 Immunostaining for the p34^{cdc2} cyclin-dependent kinase. This protein has been associated with the transition of cells from the S- into the G$_2$-phase of the cell cycle. Over-expression of p34^{cdc2} has been linked to high-grade aggressive prostate cancer with high recurrence rates.

MIB-1 over-expression (Fig.14.1) has also been associated with primary therapy failure (80). S-phase calculations by flow cytometry or image analysis have been less clinically useful in prostate cancer. Cell-cycle regulatory proteins have also been linked to adverse outcome in prostate cancer including over-expression of p34^{cdc2} cyclin dependent kinase (81) (Fig. 14.2) and loss of expression of p27^{Kip1} cyclin-dependent kinase inhibitor (82).

DNA ploidy determination

The majority of retrospective studies have shown that aneuploid DNA content in prostate cancer independently predicts poor prognosis for the disease (83–88). Recently, DNA ploidy measurements have been successfully performed on needle biopsy specimens using the tissue section image analysis technique (Fig. 14.3) (89). An aneuploid DNA ploidy status determined on needle biopsies has successfully correlated with the ploidy status of corresponding radical prostatectomy specimens and independently predicted disease outcome with a 3-fold increase in post-surgical disease recurrence rates and a 20-fold increase in metastatic disease (89).

Morphometrics

A variety of morphometric techniques have been applied on prostate cancer specimens with the nuclear-

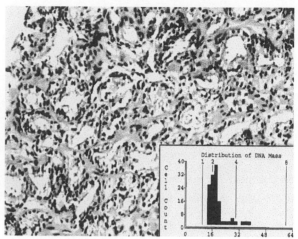

Fig. 14.3 DNA ploidy in prostate cancer. In this prostate cancer needle-biopsy specimen, the DNA ploidy histogram determined by the tissue section image analysis technique revealed a hypertetraploid aneuploid pattern. Ploidy patterns of needle-biopsy specimens have been correlated with post-prostatectomy disease relapse and can also be used to confirm the accuracy of tumor grading. Needle-biopsy specimens featuring a low histologic grade and an aneuploid histogram are significantly more likely to be upgraded on the radical prostatectomy specimen.

roundness factor measurement achieving the most significant potential clinical utility. Prostate cancers featuring near-perfect round nuclei are typically well-differentiated and slow growing. Tumors with irregular nuclear contours and correspondingly low nuclear roundness have been associated with high tumor-grade and a propensity for the development of distant metastasis and shortened survival (90).

Tumor vascularity and microvessel density

Tumor angiogenesis has also correlated with metastasis in prostate cancer as measured by microvessel-counting studies (91). Angiogenesis is an essential component of solid tumor growth and disease progression. Accordingly, neovascularity has been found to be an important feature of prostate cancer, as measured by microvessel density. Significantly higher microvessel counts have been obtained in areas of adenocarcinoma than in the benign tissues of radical prostatectomy specimens (92). Interestingly, prostate cancers appear to have the greatest concentration of microvessels in the centers of the tumoral areas, which may account for the infrequency of necrosis in prostate cancer (93).

In addition to its biologic importance, neovascularity has been found in several studies to be a powerful predictor of prognosis in prostate cancer. Increased microvascularity has been found to correlate with the pathologic stage of the disease (94–95). Microvessel density has been associated with the presence of metastasis (91) and with a significant risk for disease progression after radical prostatectomy (94). The application of microvessel counts to needle biopsies of prostate cancer, where it could be used prospectively to plan therapy, has not received significant study.

Color Doppler flow has been shown to be an important aid to gray-scale sonography in the detection of prostatic carcinoma, and has recently been correlated with tumor grade and stage (96–99). However, little evidence has been presented to date linking the sonographic findings to microvessel counts in the respective tissue samples. In fact, in one study, microvessel density and tumor size was no different in specimens with normal or increased color Doppler flow (99).

Nuclear matrix proteins

Nuclear matrix proteins function to maintain the structure, shape, and higher order of DNA organization within a cell (100). Nuclear matrix proteins have been characterized in prostate cancer and may define subsets of the disease with differing biology and clinical behavior (100).

Growth factors

A variety of growth factors have been studied in prostate cancer including the epidermal growth factor (EGF) and its receptor. The results have been conflicting, i.e. although epidermal growth factor assays of prostate cancer specimens show higher levels than seen in the normal prostate, high-grade tumors appear to have lower EGF content than do well-differentiated lesions (101). Increased expression of basic fibroblast growth factor (bFGF) has been linked to adverse outcome (74). Growth factors appear to operate in networks in the prostate and further studies are necessary to elucidate the various interactions of these trophic proteins on disease outcome.

Cell-adhesion molecules

E-cadherin, a cell-adhesion molecule associated with cell–cell and cell–matrix interaction, leukocyte function, and tumor invasion, and metastasis in a variety of neoplasms, has been associated with disease outcome in prostate cancer (102–104). Decreased expression of E-cadherin has been shown to associate with high tumor-grade and aneuploidy (105). Recent evidence suggests that a major chromosomal deletion on chromosome 16 may be a major event in the development of prostate cancer (106). It has been further suggested that this deletion may involve the E-cadherin gene and that E-cadherin protein, in addition to its cell-adhesion role, may be functioning as a tumor-suppressor protein. Alternatively, the loss of E-cadherin expression in prostate cancer may be related to gene methylation (Fig. 14.4). Further immunohistochemical and molecular genetic studies appear warranted to pursue this potential important association.

The CD44 cell-adhesion molecule has also been linked to outcome in prostate cancer. Loss of expression of the CD44 protein standard form has also been associated with other adverse prognostic factors such as high tumor-grade and aneuploid DNA content (107–108) (Fig. 14.5). Integrins have also been widely studied in prostate cancer and implicated as potential indicators of aggressive disease (98). Decreased expres-

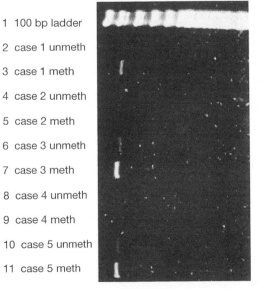

Fig. 14.4 Hypermethylation of the E-cadherin promoter gene in prostate cancer. E-cadherin promoter gene hypermethylation is detected by sodium bisulfite treatment and PCR with methylation specific primers. In lanes 3, 7, and 11, the positive bands at the bottom of the lanes indicate the presence of bisulfite-resistant DNA characteristic of gene methylation.

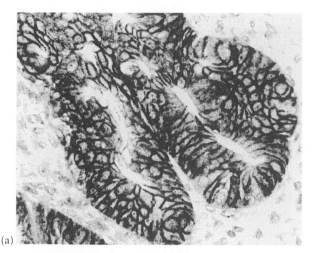

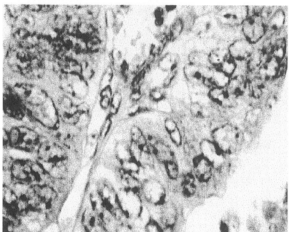

(a)

(b)

Fig. 14.5 CD44s immunostaining in prostate cancer. (a) Continuous membranous staining for CD44s is seen in a low-grade tumor. (b) There is complete loss of the cytoplasmic membraneous CD44s immunoreactivity. CD44s expression loss has been associated with high-grade, aneuploid prostate cancer with high recurrence rates.

sion of β_4 integrin subunit and γ-2 laminin 5 subunit have linked to adverse disease outcome (74).

Tumor proteases

Cathepsin D, a lysosomal protease and autocrine mitogen, has been associated with prognosis in breast cancer (109). In prostate cancer, increased tumor cathepsin D immunoreactivity has been correlated with pathologic stage (110), as well as with tumor grade and DNA content (111). Increased expression of tumor

collagenases has also been linked to adverse disease outcome (74).

Dominant oncogenes

In comparison with their significance in adenocarcinomas of the respiratory and gastro-intestinal tract, the roles of dominant oncogenes in the development and progression of prostate cancer appear to be limited (74, 112–113). The ras gene, commonly mutated in epithelial adenocarcinomas in the gastro-intestinal, hepatobiliary, and respiratory tracts, is not frequently altered in human prostate cancers, cell lines, or experimental models (114). Amplification of the myc gene has been studied in prostate cancer, but could not be linked to disease progression (114).

The HER-2/neu gene in prostate cancer

The HER-2/neu (c-erb-B2) gene has been associated with adverse outcome in breast cancer (115) and testing for HER-2/neu status has achieved near standard of practice for selecting therapy for breast cancer (115). For prostate cancer, immunohistochemistry based studies have conflicted, but tend to favor that overexpression of HER-2/neu protein is associated with an adverse outcome (114). Recently, HER-2/neu gene

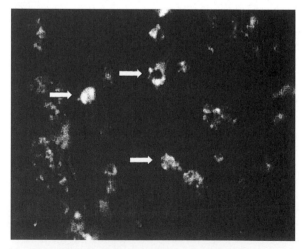

Fig. 14.6 HER-2/neu gene amplification detected by fluorescence in situ hybridization (FISH) in a high-grade invasive prostate cancer. *Arrows* indicate multiple nuclei with bright fluorescent signals indicating amplification of the HER-2/neu gene. HER-2/neu amplification in prostate cancer has been associated with high-grade, aneuploid disease with high rates of disease relapse, and a tendency to develop androgen-independent disease metastatic disease.

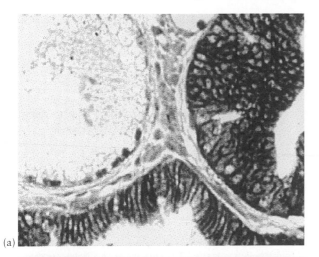

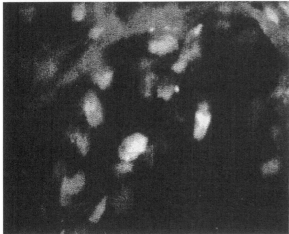

Fig. 14.7 HER-2/neu gene amplification and protein over-expression in prostatic intra-epithelial neoplasia (PIN). (a) A membranous staining pattern indicating over-expression of the HER-2/neu protein. (b) Multiple nuclei with amplified copies of the HER-2/neu gene. Abnormalities of the HER-2/neu gene and protein have generally been similar in both invasive and PIN foci when measured simultaneously on the same prostatectomy specimen.

amplification has been measured in prostate cancer by a fluorescence *in situ* hybridization technique (Figs 14.6 and 14.7) and associated with other adverse prognostic factors (116), recurrence after surgery (117–118), and recurrence after radiation therapy (80). In that advanced breast cancer has been shown to respond to anti-HER-2/neu treatments (Herceptin™) (115), clinical trials using both vaccination and systemic humanized anti-HER2/neu antibodies (Herceptin™) in prostate cancer have now been started.

The p53 tumor-suppressor gene

Tumor-suppressor genes encode protein products that normally suppress cell proliferation in a regulated fashion. The p53 gene, arguably the most frequently mutated gene in human cancer, appears to function as a 'guardian of the genome' protecting somatic cells against the accumulation of genomic mutations. p53 Protein over-accumulation has been reported frequently in prostate cancer with immunoreactivity ranging from 13% to 23% on average (119). A positive association between nuclear p53 immunoreactivity and aggressive biologic behavior of prostate cancer has been confirmed in four independent studies (120–123). p53 Mutations appear to be very frequent in metastatic prostate cancer (122). Although immunohistochemistry can be an inaccurate predictor of p53 gene status, when molecular biologic techniques are utilized, it has been reported that 42% of prostate cancers can harbor mutant p53 sequences (124) (Fig. 14.8). Mutations of the p53 locus in benign prostate tissue have been reported, suggesting that p53 mutations may occur early in the pathogenesis of prostate cancer (125–126). New studies of p53 status, including functional assays, must be performed on needle-biopsy specimens to achieve prognostic value for prospective treatment planning in prostate cancer.

Other tumor suppressors

The retinoblastoma gene on chromosome 13 may also function as a tumor suppressor in prostate cancer, but probably is altered in only a very small subset of cases (119). Other known tumor-suppressor genes that may play a role include the DCC gene on chromosome 18q and the APC gene on chromosome 5q (127). The glutathione S-transferase-π gene is (GSTP1) involved in the intracellular detoxification of certain carcinogens and is deactivated in the vast majority of prostatic carcinomas, due to hypermethylation of regulatory sequences, resulting in loss of expression of the gene (128). The GSTP1 methylation status may also have potential for the development of a blood-based assay to improve on the specificity of prostate cancer screening. The KAI-1 gene may function as a metastasis-suppressor gene in prostate cancer (74).

Apoptosis and bcl-2

The oncoprotein encoded by the bcl-2 gene functions to suppress apoptosis (programmed cell death) and has

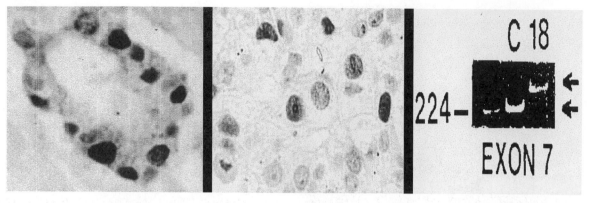

Fig. 14.8 p53 Status in prostate cancer. At the *left* and *center*, multiple immunoreactive nuclei are consistent with p53 protein over-expression generally, but not exclusively associated with p53 gene mutation. The single-strand conformation polymorphism analysis shown at the right indicates the presence of p53 gene mutation. Although original reports found a relatively low rate of p53 gene mutations in prostate cancer, recent studies have found higher rates and have associated p53 abnormalities with adverse prognosis for the disease.

been associated with human B-cell lymphoma. Bcl-2 expression has been studied in prostate cancer, initially by immunohistochemical techniques, and found to react with primary and metastatic prostate cancer specimens obtained from patients refractory to hormonal therapy (73) (Fig. 14.9). Bcl-2 immunoreactivity is most intense in basal cells rather than secretory cells (129) and may be limited to normal prostatic and seminal vesicle epithelium, as well as rare cases of poorly differentiated but not well-differentiated prostatic carcinomas (130). In prostate cancer, over-expression of bcl-2 protein was not associated with

Table 14.6 Potential molecular-based therapies for advanced prostate cancer

1. Anti-HER-2/*neu* antibody therapy (HERCEPTIN™)
2. Anti-HER2/*neu* vaccination
3. Gene therapy to restore cell-cycle regulation
4. Deme thylation (gene therapy) to restore adhesion
5. Gene therapy to restore androgen dependence

rearrangements in the 2.8 kb major breakpoint region or with accumulation of p53 protein (131).

New markers and new therapies

The development of new molecular markers of prostate cancer progression has led to the early stages of testing for novel therapies. Potential new therapies directed at prostate cancer are summarized in Table 14.6.

References

1. Boring CC, Squires TS, Tong T. Cancer Statistics 1991. *CA* 1991, **41**, 19–36.
2. Seidman H, Mushinski MH, Geib SK *et al*. Probabilities of eventually developing or dying of cancer—United States, 1985. *CA* 1985, **35**, 36–56.
3. Mettlin CJ, Murphy GP, Ho R *et al*. The national cancer database report on longitudinal observations on prostate cancer. *Cancer* 1996, **77**, 2162–6.
4. Lu-Yao GL, Greenberg R. Changes in prostate cancer incidence and treatment in USA. *Lancet* 1994, **343**, 251–4.

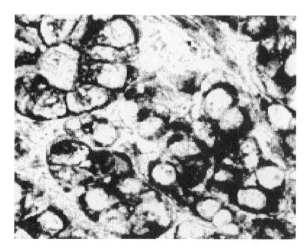

Fig. 14.9 Bcl-2 staining in prostate cancer. The immunoreactivitiy for bcl-2 shown in the photomicrograph has been associated with androgen-independent and anti-androgen resistant prostate cancer.

5. Carter HB, Coffey D. The prostate: an increasing medical problem. *Prostate* 1990, **16**, 39–48.

6. Wynder EL, Mabuchi K, Whitmore WF Jr. Epidemiology of cancer of the prostate *Cancer* 1971, **28**, 344–60.

7. Shimada H, Misugi K, Sasaki Y *et al.* Carcinoma of the prostate in childhood and adolescence. Report of a case and review of the literature. *Cancer* 1980, **46**, 2534–42.

8. Levine RL, Wilchinsky M. Adenocarcinoma of the prostate: a comparison of the disease in blacks versus whites. *J Urol* 1979, **121**, 761–2.

9. Carter BS, Carter HB, Isaacs JT. Epidemiologic evidence regarding predisposing factors to prostate cancer. *Prostate* 1990, **16**, 187–97.

10. Catalona WJ, Scott WW. Carcinoma of the prostate. In: *Campbell's urology* (5th edn) (ed. PC Walsh, RF Gittes, AD Perlmutter *et al.*). WB Saunders, Philadelphia, 1986, Ch.32.

11. Carter BS, Beaty TH, Steinberg GD *et al.* Mendelian inheritance of familial prostate cancer. *Proc Natl Acad Sci USA* 1992, **89**, 3367–71.

12. Coffey DS. Prostate cancer. An overview of an increasing dilemma. *Cancer* 1993, **71**, 880–6.

13. Atkin NB, Baker MC. Chromosomal study of five cases of the prostate. *Hum Genet* 1985, **70**, 359–64.

14. Winkelstein W Jr, Ernster VL. Epidemiology and etiology. In: *Prostatic cancer* (ed. GP Murphy). Littleton, MA, PSG Publishing Co, 1979, 1–17.

15. Dmochowski L, Ohtsuki Y, Seman G *et al.* Search for oncogenic viruses in human prostate cancer. *Cancer Treatment Reports* 1977, **61**, 119–27.

16. Byar DP, Mostofi FK. The Veterans Administration Cooperative Urological Research Group: Carcinoma of the Prostate, prognostic evaluation of certain pathologic features in 208 radical prostatectomies. Examined by the step-section technique. *Cancer* 1972, **29**, 5–13.

17. Randolph TL, Amin MB, Ro JY *et al.* Histologic variants of adenocarcinoma and other carcinomas of prostate: pathologic criteria and clinical significance. *Mod Pathol* 1997, **10**, 612–29.

18. Mostofi FK, Davis CJ, Sesterhenn IA. Pathology of carcinomaof the prostate. *Cancer* 1992, **70**, 235–53.

19. Kuhajda FP, Gipson T, Mendelsohn G. Papillary adenocarcinomas of the prostate. An immunohistochemical study. *Cancer* 1984, **54**, 1328–32.

20. Cantrell BB, Leifer G, DeKlerk DP *et al.* Papillary adenocarcinoma of the prostatic urethera with clear cell appearance. *Cancer* 1981, **48**, 2661–7.

21. Epstein JI, Lieberman PH. Mucinous adenocarcinoma of the prostate gland. *Am J Surg Pathol* 1985, **9**, 299–308.

22. Kuhajda FP, Mann RB. Adenoid cystic carcinoma of the prostate. A case report with immunoperoxidase staining for prostate-specific acid phosphatase and prostate-specific antigen. *Am J Clin Path* 1984, **81**, 257–60.

23. Saito R, Davis BK, Ollapally EP. Adenosquamous carcinoma of the prostate. *Hum Pathol* 1984, **15**, 87–9.

24. Devaney DM, Dorman A, Leader M. Adenosquamous carcinoma of the prostate, a case report. *Hum Pathol* 1991, **22**, 1046–50.

25. Alline KM, Cohen MB. Signet-ring carcinoma of the prostate. *Arch Pathol Lab Med* 1992, **116**, 99–102.

26. Ro JY, El-Naggar A, Ayala AG *et al.* Signet-ring-cell carcinoma of the prostate. Electron-microscopic and immunohistochemical studies of 8 cases. *Am J Surg Path* 1988, **12**, 453–60.

27. Bostwick DG, Kindrachuk RW, Rouse RV. Prostatic adenocarcinoma with endometrioid features. Clinical pathologic and ultrastructural findings. *Am J Surg Path* 1985, **9**, 595–609.

28. Ro JY, Ayala AG, Wishnow KI *et al.* Prostatic duct adenocarcinoma with endometrioid features: immunohistochemical and electron microscopic study. *Sem Diagn Pathol* 1988, **5**, 301–11.

29. Ro JY, Tetu B, Ayala AG *et al.* Small cell carcinoma of the prostate. Immunohistochemical and electron microscopic studies of 18 cases. *Cancer* 1987, **59**, 977–82.

30. Johnson DE, Hogan JM, Ayala AG. Transitional cell carcinoma of the prostate. A clinical morphological study. *Cancer* 1972, **29**, 287–93.

31. Lauwers GY, Schevechuk M, Armenekas N *et al.* Carcinosarcoma of the prostate. *Am J Surg Path* 1993, **17**, 342–9.

32. Shannon RL, Ro JY, Grignon DJ *et al.* Sarcomatoid carcinoma of the prostate, a clinical pathologic study of 12 patients. *Cancer* 1992, **69**, 2676–82.

33. Uchibayashi T, Hisazumi H, Hasegawa M *et al.* Squamous cell carcinoma of the prostate. *Scand J Urol Nephrol* 1997, **31**, 224–228.

34. King DG, Finney RP. Embryonal rhabdomyosarcoma of the prostate. *J Urol* 1977, **117**, 88–90.

35. Smith BH, Dehner LP. Sarcoma of the prostate gland. *Am J Clin Pathol* 1972, **58**, 43–50.

36. Bostwick DG, Mann RB. Malignant lymphomas involving the prostate. A study of 13 cases. *Cancer* 1985, **56**, 2932–8.

37. Benson RC Jr, Segura JW and Carney JA. Primary yolk-sac (endodermal sinus) tumor of the prostate. *Cancer* 1978, **41**, 1395–8.

38. Michel F, Gattegno B, Roland J *et al.* Primary non-seminomatous germ cell tumor of the prostate. *J Urol* 1986, **135**, 597–9.

39. Brawer MK. Prostatic intra-epithelial neoplasia: a premalignant lesion. *Hum Pathol* 1992, **23**, 242–8.

40. Bostwick DG, Amin MB, Dundore B *et al.* Architectural patterns of high grade prostatic intra-epithelial neoplasia. *Hum Pathol* 1993, **24**, 298–310.

41. Bostwick DG. Premalignant lesions of the prostate. *Sem Diagn Pathol* 1988, **5**, 240–53.

42. Quinn BD, Cho KR, Epstein JI. Relationship of severe dysplasia to stage B adenocarcinoma of prostate. *Cancer* 1990, **65**, 2328–37.

43. Brawer MK, Lange PH. Prostate-specific antigen and pre-malignant change: implications for early detection. *CA-A* 1989, **39**, 361–75.

44. Bostwick DG. Clinical utility of prostatic intra-epithelial neoplasia. *Mayo Clin Proc* 1995, **70**, 395–6.

45. Brawer MK. The diagnosis of prostatic carcinoma. *Cancer* 1993, **71**, 899–905.

46. Peller PA, Young DC, Marmaduke DP *et al.* Sextant prostate biopsies. *Cancer* 1995, **75**, 530–8.

47. Oesterling JE. Prostate specific antigen. *Cancer* 1995, **75**, 1795–804.

48. Katz AE, de VriesGM, Begg MD *et al.* Enhanced reverse transcriptase-polymerase chain reaction for prostate specific antigen as an indicator of true pathologic stage in patients with prostate cancer. *Cancer* 1995, **75**, 1642–8.

49. Jones EC, Young RH. The differential diagnosis of prostatic carcinoma. *Am J Clin Pathol* 1994, **101**, 48–64.

50. Humphrey PA, Walther PJ. Adenocarcinoma of the prostate. *Am J Clin Pathol* 1993, **99**, 746–59.

51. Algaba F, Epstein JI, Aldape HC *et al.* Assessment of prostate carcinoma in core needle biopsy- definition of minimal criteria for the diagnosis of cancer in biopsy material. *Cancer* 1996, **78**, 376–81.

52. Robinette MA, Robson CJ, Farrow GA *et al.* Giant serial step sections of the prostate in assessment of the accuracy of clinical staging in patients with localized prostatic carcinoma. *J Urol* 1984, **133** (Suppl) (Abstract), 242A.

53. Epstein JI, Bizo VG, Walsh PC. Correlation of pathologic findings with progression after radical retropubic prostatectomy. *Cancer* 1993, **71**, 3582–93.

54. Bastacky SI, Walsh PC, Epstein JI. Relationship between peri-neural tumor invasion on needle biopsy and radical prostatectomy capsular penetration in clinical stage B carcinoma of the prostate. *Am J Surg Path* 1993, **17**, 336–41.

55. Ohori AM, Scardino PT, Lapin SL *et al.* The mechanisms and prognostic significance of seminal vesicle involvement by prostate cancer. *Am J Surg Pathol* 1993, **17**, 1252–61.

56. Humphrey PA, Frazier HA, Vollmer RT *et al.* Stratification of pathologic features in radical prostatectomy specimens that are predictive of elevated initial postoperative serum prostate-specific antigen levels. *Cancer* 1993, **71**, 1821–7.

57. Epstein JI, Partin AW, Sauvageot J *et al.* Prediction of progression following radical prostatectomy. *Am J Surg Pathol* 1996, **20**, 286–92.

58. Fowler J Jr, Whitmore WF. The incidence and extent of pelvic lymph node metastasis in apparently localized prostatic cancer. *Cancer* 1981, **47**, 2941–5.

59. Dodds PR, Karid EVJ, Lytton B. The role of vertibal veins in the dissemination of prostatic carcinoma. *J Urol* 1981, **126**, 753–5.

60. Gleason DF. Histologic grading and clinical staging of prostatic carcinoma. P.171. In: *Urologic pathology: the prostate* (ed. M Tannenbaum). Lea and Febiger, Philadelphia, 1977.

61. McNeal JE, Villers AA, Redwine EA *et al.* Histologic differentiation, cancer volume, and pelvic lymph node metastasis in adenocarcinoma of the prostate. *Cancer* 1990, **66**, 1225–33.

62. Oesterling JE, Brendler CB, Epstein JI *et al.* Correlation of clinical stage, serum prostatic acid phosphatase and preoperative Gleason grade with final pathologic stage in 275 patients with clinically localized adenocarcinoma of the prostate. *J Urol* 1987, **138**, 92–8.

63. Epstein JA. Prostatic biopsy. A morphologic correlation of aspiration cytology with needle biopsy histology. *Cancer* 1976, **38**, 2078–87.

64. Eble JN, Angermeier PA. The roles of fine needle aspiration and needle core biopsies in the diagnosis of primary prostatic cancer. *Hum Pathol* 1992, **23**, 249–57.

65. Bostwick DG. Gleason grading of prostatic needle biopsies. Correlation with grade in 316 matched prostatectomies. *Am J Surg Path* 1994, **18**, 796–803.

66. Mills SE, Fowler JE. Gleason histologic grading of prostatic carcinoma. Correlations between biopsy and prostatectomy specimens. *Cancer* 1986, **57**, 346–9.

67. Steinberg DM, Sauvageot J, Piantadosi S *et al.* Correlation of prostate needle biopsy and radical prostatectomy Gleason grade in academic and community settings. *Am J Surg Pathol* 1997, **21**, 566–76.

68. McNeal JE. Cancer volume and site of origin of adenocarcinoma of the prostate: relationship to local and distant spread. *Hum Pathol* 1992, **23**, 258–66.

69. Stamey TA, Freiha FS, McNeal JE *et al.* Localized prostate cancer. *Cancer* 1993, **71**, 933–8.

70. Montie JE. Staging of prostate cancer. *Cancer* 1995, **75**, 1814–8.

71. Ohori M, Wheeler TM, Scardino PT. The new American Joint Committee on Cancer and International Union against Cancer TNM classification of prostate cancer. *Cancer* 1994, **73**, 104–14.

72. Blute ML, Zinche H, Farrow GM. Long-term follow-up of young patients with stage A adenocarcinoma of the prostate. *J Urol* 1986, **136**, 840–3.

73. Foster CS, Abel PD. Clinical and molecular techniques for diagnosis and monitoring of prostate cancer. *Hum Pathol* 1992, **23**, 395–401.

74. Isaacs JT. Molecular markers for prostate cancer metastasis. *Am J Pathol* 1997, **150**, 1511–21.

75. Sadi MV, Walsh PC, Barrack ER. Immunohistochemical study of androgen receptors in metastatic prostate cancer. *Cancer* 1991, **67**, 3057–64.

76. Newmark JR, Hardy DO, Tonb DC *et al.* Androgen receptor gene mutations in human prostate cancer. *Proc Natl Acad Sci* 1992, **89**, 6319–23.

77. Sadi MV, Barrack ER. Image analysis of androgen receptor immunostaining in metastatic prostate cancer. *Cancer* 1993, **71**, 2574–80.

78. Collembell M, Symmans F, Gil S *et al.* Detection of the apoptosis suppressing oncoprotein bcl-2 in hormone-refractory human prostate cancers. *Am J Pathol* 1993, **143**, 390–400.

79. Goel A, Abou-Ellela A, DeRose PB *et al.* The prognostic significance of proliferation in prostate cancer. *J Urol Pathol* 1996, **4**, 213–23.

80. Scalzo DA, Kallakury BVS, Gaddipati RV *et al.* Cell proliferation rate by MIB-1 immunohistochemistry predicts post radiation recurrence of prostatic adenocarcinomas. *Am J Clin Pathol* 1998, **109**, 163–8.

81. Kallakury BVS, Sheehan CE, Ambros RA *et al.* Prognostic significance of $p34^{cdc2}$ and cyclin D1 protein expression in prostatic adenocarcinomas. *Cancer* 1997, **80**, 753–63.

82. Yang RM, Naitoh J, Murphy M *et al.* Low p27 expression predicts poor disease-free survival in patients with prostate cancer. *J Urol* 1998, **59**, 941–5.

83. Ross JS, Nazeer T, Church K *et al.* Contribution of her-2/neu oncogene expression to tumor grade and DNA content analysis in the prediction of prostatic carcinoma metastasis. *Cancer* 1993, **72**, 3020–8.

84. Winkler HC, Rainwater LM, Myers RP *et al.* Stage D1 prostatic carcinoma: Significance of DNA ploidy patterns studied by flow cytometry. *Mayo Clin Proc* 1988, **63**, 103–12.

85. Peters AJM, Miles BJ, Kubus JJ *et al.* The prognostic significance of the nuclear DNA content in localized prostatic adenocarcinoma. *Anal Quant Cytol Histol* 1990, **12**, 359–65.

86. Peters-Gee JM, Miles BJ, Cerny JC *et al.* Prognostic significance of DNA quantification in stage D1 prostatic carcinoma with the use of image analysis. *Cancer* 1992, **70**, 1159–65.

87. Foster CH, McLoughlin J, Bashir I *et al.* Markers of the metastatic phenotype in prostate cancer. *Hum Pathol* 1992, **23**, 381–94.

88. Montgomery BT, Nativ O, Blute M *et al.* Stage B prostate adenocarcinoma: Flow cytometric nuclear DNA ploidy analysis. *Arch Surg* 1990, **125**, 327–31.

89. Ross JS, Figge H, Bui HX *et al.* Prediction of pathologic stage and post prostatectomy disease recurrence by DNA ploidy analysis of initial needle biopsy specimens of prostate cancer. *Cancer* 1994, **74**, 2811–8.

90. Mohler JL, Metts JC, Zhang X-Z *et al.* Nuclear morphometry in automatic biopsy and radical prostatectomy specimens of prostatic carcinoma. *Analyt Quant Cytol Histol* 1994, **16**, 415–20.

91. Weidner N, Carroll PR, Flax J *et al.* Tumor angiogenesis correlates with metastasis in invasive prostate carcinoma. *Am J Pathol* 1993, **143**, 401–9.

92. Bigler SA, Deering RE, Brawer MK. Comparison of microscopic vascularity in benign and malignant prostate tissue. *Hum Pathol* 1993, **24**, 220–6.

93. Siegal JA, Enyou YU, Brawer MK. Topography of neovascularity in human prostate carcinoma. *Cancer* 1995, **75**, 2545–51.

94. Silberman MA, Partin AW, Veltri RW *et al.* Tumor angiogensis correlates with progression after radical prostatectomy but not with pathologic stage in Gleason 5 to 7 adenocarcinomaof the prostate. *Cancer* 1997, **79**, 772–9.

95. Brawer MK, Deering RE, Brown M *et al.* Predictors of pathologic stage in prostatic carcinoma. *Cancer* 1994, **73**, 678–87.

96. Rifkin MD, Sudakoff GS, Alexander AA. Prostate: techniques, results, and potential applications of color Doppler US scanning. *Radiology* 1993, **186**, 509–13.

97. Newman JS, Bree RL, Rubin JM. Prostate cancer: diagnosis with color doppler sonography with histologic correlation of each biopsy site. *Radiology* 1995, **195**, 86–90.

98. Mohamed I, Peterson RO, Alexander AA *et al.* Color doppler imaging in predicting the biologic behavior of prostate cancer: correlation with disease-free survival. *Urology* 1997, **50**, 906–12.

99. Louvar E, Littrup PJ, Goldstein A *et al.* Correlation of color doppler flow in the prostate with tissue microvascularity. *Cancer* 1998, **83**, 135–40.

100. Partin AW, Getzenberg RH, CarMichael MJ *et al.* Nuclear matrix protein patterns in human benign prostatic hyperplasia and prostate cancer. *Cancer Res* 1993, **53**, 744–6.

101. Ware JL. Prostate cancer progression. Implications of histopathology. *Am J Pathol* 1994, **145**, 983–93.

102. Bussemakers MJ, van-Moorselaar RJ, Giroldi LA *et al.* Decreased expression of e-cadherin in the progression of rat prostatic cancer. *Cancer Res* 1992, **52**, 2916–22.

103. Giroldi LA, Schalken JA. Decreased expression of the intercellular adhesion molecule e-cadherin in prostate cancer: Biological significance and clinical implications. *Cancer Metastasis Rev* 1993, **12**, 29–37.

104. Umbas R, Schalken JA, Aalders TW. Expression of the cellular adhesion molecule e-cadherin is reduced or absent in high grade prostate cancer. *Cancer Res* 1992, **52**, 5104–9.

105. Ross JS, Figge HL, Bui HX *et al.* E-cadherin expression in prostatic carcinoma biopsies: Correlation with tumor grade, DNA content, pathologic stage and clinical outcome. *Modern Pathol* 1994, **7**, 835–41.

106. Sandberg AA. Chromosomal abnormalities and related events in prostate cancer. *Hum Pathol* 1992, **23**, 368–80.

107. Kallakury BVS, Yang F, Figge J *et al.* Decreased levels of CD44 protein and mRNA in prostate carcinoma: Correlation with tumor grade and ploidy. *Cancer* 1996, **78**, 1461–9.

108. Cohen MB, Griebling TL, Ahaghotu CA *et al.* Cellular adhesion molecules in urologic malignancies. *Am J Clin Pathol* 1997, **107**, 56–63.

109. Pujol P, Maudelond T, Daures JP *et al.* A prospective study of the prognostic value of cathepsin D levels in breast cancer cytosol. *Cancer* 1993, 71, 2006–2012.

110. Makar R, Mason A, Kittleson JM *et al.* Immunohistochemical analysis of cathepsin D in prostate carcinoma. *Mod Pathol* 1994, 7, 747–51.

111. Ross JS, Nazeer T, Figge HL *et al.* Quantitative immunohistochemical determination of cathepsin D levels in prostatic carcinoma biopsies. *Am J Clin Pathol* 1995, **104**, 36–41.

112. Peehl DM. Oncogenes in prostate cancer. *Cancer* 1993, 71, 1159–64.

113. Wang YZ, Wong YC. Oncogenes and tumor-suppressor genes in prostate cancer: a review. *Urol Oncol* 1997, **3**, 41–6.

114. Netlo GJ, Humphrey PA. Molecular biologic aspects of human prostatic carcinoma. *Am J Clin Pathol* 1994, **102**, S57–S64.

115. Ross JS, Fletcher JA. The HER-2/neu Oncogene: prognostic factor, predictive factor and target of therapy. *Semin Cancer Biol* 1999, **9**, 125–38.

116. Ross JS, Sheehan C, Hayner-Buchan A *et al.* HER-2/neu gene amplification status in prostate cancer by fluorescence in-situ hybridization. *Hum Pathol* 1997, **28**, 827–33.

117. Ross JS, Sheehan CE, Hayner-Buchan AM *et al.* Prognostic significance of HER-2/neu gene amplification status by fluorescence in-situ hybridization in prostatic cancer. *Cancer* 1997, **79**, 2162–70.

118. Kallakury BVS, Sheehan CE and Ambros. Correlation of p34^{cdc2} cyclin dependent kinase over-expression, CD44s downregulation and HER-2/neu oncogene amplification with recurrence in prostatic adenocarcinomas. *J Clin Oncol* 1998, **16**, 1302–9.

119. Ross JS, Kallakury BVS, Figge J. Pathology and molecular biology of prostate cancer. In: *Imaging of the prostate* (ed. MD Rifkin). Lippincott Raven Press, New York, 1997.

120. Kallakury BVS, Figge J, Ross JS *et al.* Association of p53 immunoreactivity with high Gleason grade in prostatic adenocarcinoma. *Hum Pathol* 1994, **25**, 92–7.

121. Bookstein R, MacGrogan D, Hilsenbeck SG *et al.* p53 is mutated in a subset of advanced-stage prostate cancers. *Cancer Research* 1993, **53**, 3369–73.

122. Visakorpi T, Kallioniemi O-P, Heikkinen A *et al.* Small subgroup of aggressive, highly proliferative prostatic carcinomas defined by p53 accumulation. *J Natl Cancer Inst* 1992, **84**, 883–7.

123. Navone N, Troncoso P, Pisters L *et al.* p53 Protein accumulation and gene mutation in the progression of human prostate carcinoma. *J Natl Cancer Inst* 1993, **85**, 1657–69.

124. Chi S-G, White RWd, Meyers FJ *et al.* p53 in prostate cancer: frequent expressed transition mutations. *J Natl Cancer Inst* 1994, **86**, 926–33.

125. Kallakury BVS, Jennings TA, Ross JS *et al.* Alteration of the p53 gene locus in benign hyperplastic prostatic epithelium associated with high grade prostatic adeno-carcinoma. *Diagn Molec Pathol* 1994, **3**, 227–32.

126. Meyers FJ, Chi S-G, Fishman JR *et al.* p53 mutations in benign prostatic hyperplasia. *J Natl Cancer Inst* 1993, **85**, 1856–8.

127. Brewster SF, Browne S, Brown KW. Somatic allelic loss at the DCC, APC, nm23 H1 and p53 tumor-suppressor gene loci in human prostatic carcinoma. *J Urol* 1994, **151**, 1073–7.

128. Lee W-H, Morton RA, Epstein JI *et al.* Cytidine methylation of regulatory sequences near the ?-class glutathione-S-transferase gene accompanies human prostatic carcinogenesis. *Proc Natl Acad Sci* 1994, **91**, 1733–7.

129. Krajewski S, Bodrug S, Krajewska M *et al.* Immunohistochemical analysis of Mcl-1 protein in human tissues. Differential regulation of Mcl-1 and bcl-2 protein production suggests a unique role for Mcl-1 in control of programmed cell death *in vivo. Am J Pathol* 1995, **146**, 1309–19.

130. Shabaik AS, Krajewski S, Burgan A *et al.* bcl-2 protooncogene expression in normal, hyperplastic, and neoplastic prostate tissue. *J Urol Pathol* 1995, **3**, 17–27.

131. Kallakury BVS, Figge J Leibovich B *et al.* Increased bcl-2 protein levels in prostatic adenocarcinomas are not associated with rearrangements in the 2.8 kb major breakpoint region or with p53 protein accumulation. *Mod Pathol* 1996, **9**, 41–7.

15 | Clinical use of prostate-specific antigen changes

R. Clements

Introduction

Prostate cancer is now the second-commonest male cancer in both the United States and the United Kingdom, with the second-highest death rate. Curative treatment is available for organ-confined prostate cancer, but the prognosis for metastatic prostate cancer remains poor. The disease is uniformly fatal once it has spread outside the prostate, as there is no effective curative systemic treatment available. In these circumstances it is logical to seek to identify early prostate cancer, and an accurate specific test of early disease is needed. Prostate-specific antigen (PSA) is currently the best single test for prostate cancer diagnosis and monitoring. The use of PSA has transformed the diagnosis of prostate cancer in the last 15 years. It is one of the most important tumor markers in oncology, but it cannot identify whether the detected cancer will be of clinical significance in an individual patient. PSA is an organ-specific and not a tumor-specific marker, and is produced by abnormal and normal prostatic tissue; a change in its value is not specific for prostate cancer. Serum measurements of PSA can be used in the diagnosis, staging, and prognosis of patients with prostate cancer and there is a linear relationship between serum PSA levels and the extent of the primary prostate tumor. However, despite markedly improving the detection of organ-confined prostate cancer in North America and Europe in recent years, PSA remains an imperfect diagnostic marker and a variety of approaches are being investigated to improve its specificity in the diagnosis of prostate cancer. Unfortunately, the sensitivity and specificity of a diagnostic test are inversely proportional, and mechanisms that increase the specificity tend to decrease the sensitivity. Even the newer PSA-based indices, such as PSA density and PSA velocity, remain imperfect for prostate cancer diagnosis. PSA measurements also have now an

established role in the surveillance of patients with proven cancer for monitoring response to treatment and disease progression. Most recently, gene therapy for prostate cancer, based on a PSA promoter, may be possible and may offer a novel theoretical therapeutic approach for prostate cancer (1).

Biological and physiological features of PSA

When PSA was introduced, it was the first serum test that could be used in the diagnosis of organ-confined prostate cancer. Prostatic acid phosphatase (PAP), the original serum marker used for prostate cancer assessment, had been available for about 50 years. That marker was used as an indicator of metastatic prostate cancer but has no role in the diagnosis of organ-confined prostate cancer. Its clinical value was additionally limited because an elevated PAP level was not always associated with metastatic prostate cancer.

The PSA protein is present within the prostate in young men with no prostatic disease, in patients with prostatitis, and in benign and malignant prostate tissue, and is present in ejaculate and serum. Despite its name, there is a growing body of evidence that PSA is not a prostate-specific protein. In males, it may be present in peri-anal and peri-urethral glands and in salivary glands. In females, it may be detected in normal and abnormal breast tissue and in human breast milk, nipple aspirate, and breast cyst fluid (2); it can also be present in female peri-urethral glands, ovary, endometrium, amniotic fluid, and salivary glands. However the serum PSA level is unlikely to be affected by PSA produced at any of these sites. The clinical use of serum PSA in females is outside the scope of this chapter. It should be noted however that recent studies suggest that women with PSA-positive breast cancer have better disease-free survival and overall survival compared to those females with PSA-negative breast cancer and additionally PSA levels in fluid aspirated from the nipple may be associated with the risk of development of breast cancer (2).

The PSA molecule is a single chain glyco-protein with a peptide length of 237 amino acids and has a molecular weight of about 34 kDa. It is encoded by a gene sequence (hK3) located on the long arm of chromosome 19, as part of the human kallikrein gene locus. The hK1 gene for tissue kallikrein and the hK2 gene for human prostate glandular kallikrein are found at the same locus. PSA is a member of the kallikrein gene family and is a protease, with a proteolytic action that is similar to chymotrypsin. PSA is produced in prostatic epithelial cells from which it is secreted into the prostatic ducts. It then becomes concentrated in the seminal plasma where its level in semen is approximately a million times higher than in serum. PSA is believed to reach the serum by diffusion from the prostate epithelial cells through the basement membrane and into the stroma of the prostate; from there it passes into prostatic capillaries and lymphatics to reach the systemic circulation. The considerably increased concentrations of PSA in patients with prostate cancer are believed to be due to derangement of prostatic architecture caused by the cancer. There may be increased diffusion of PSA due to breakdown of the basement membrane by the tumor cells and loss of tissue polarization, and also PSA secretion directly into the extracellular fluid and thence in to the blood.

The action of PSA is on the gel proteins in fresh ejaculate to liquefy the seminal coagulum, and thus promote the activation and release of spermatozoa from the ejaculate. PSA does not exist as an enzymatically active molecule in the serum. The enzyme activity is regulated by being bound as stable complexes to serine protease inhibitors. A small amount of PSA in serum is unbound or 'free' PSA (molecular weight 34 kDa). PSA binds to α_1 antichymotrypsin (ACT) (molecular weight approximately 100 kDa) and α-2-macroglobulin (AMG) (molecular weight approximately 800 kDa) to form inactive complexes. The protease inhibitors ACT and AMG form covalent complexes with the enzymatically active PSA molecule. The PSA–ACT complex is the major PSA form found in serum. 'Free' non-complexed PSA accounts for about 15% of the measurable PSA in serum. PSA immunoassays only measure free PSA and the PSA–ACT complex; in serum the ratio free PSA: PSA–ACT is approximately 1:4. Current PSA assays do not measure the PSA–AMG complex.

There are over 20 different PSA assay techniques in use. The Tandem-R PSA assay produced by Hybritech Laboratories is one of the most frequently used assays. This is a radioimmunometric assay and uses a murine monoclonal antibody to identify the PSA molecule. The radioisotope-labeled second antibody then binds to the complex of the PSA antigen and the murine antibody. The Tandem E assay (Hybritech Laboratories) works similarly but uses an enzyme-labeled rather than a radioisotope-labeled second antibody. The IMx assay (Abbott Laboratories) and the Pros-Check assay (Yang Laboratories) are radioimmunometric assays. The IMx assay also uses a murine monoclonal antibody, and a radioisotope-labeled goat anti-mouse polyclonal antibody to bind with the PSA antigen–antibody complex; the Pros-Check assay uses polyclonal rabbit anti-PSA antibodies. Other assay techniques are also in use. It can be difficult for a clinician to assess patients if unfamiliar assays have been used, or if multiple assays have been used in the same patient on different occasions, as they use alternative techniques and have differing reference ranges. A PSA reference standard was introduced in 1995, and this should simplify the use of different assays and reduce variability within and between assays. It has been found that if assays are calibrated against PSA–ACT rather than against minor forms of free PSA in serum, the difference between monoclonal and polyclonal assays virtually disappears (3). The currently used 'normal' reference ranges for PSA were historically based on normal healthy men but did not take into account the findings of the Digital Rectal Examination (DRE). A threshold of 4 ng/ml has been usually taken as the upper limit of normal, but a level of 3 ng/ml may be a more appropriate threshold. There has been considerable recent research interest on measurements of the proportions of 'free PSA' and PSA bound to ACT. This follows the discovery that prostate cancer cells commonly produce ACT, and that such production is rare in benign prostatic hyperplasia (4). The role of %-free PSA measurements will be discussed later in this chapter. New ultrasensitive PSA assays are now available, which are able to measure picogram levels of PSA in serum. They are unlikely to be useful for diagnosis, but may have a future role in giving earlier biochemical warning of relapse after radical prostatectomy (5).

Clinical use of PSA measurements in diagnosis

PSA currently plays a crucial role in the diagnosis of prostate cancer, but the diagnostic performance of the PSA test is reduced by significant false-positive test results. As great emphasis may be placed on individual PSA readings, the effect of other situations on the serum PSA level should be considered, and it is helpful to have a repeat second PSA reading to provide confirmation of any PSA elevation, and to assess the significance of an individual elevated level before making potentially important decisions about performing a systematic sextant prostate biopsy. It is important to ensure that other factors, which might elevate PSA and thus suggest potential cancer, have been eliminated. There can be marked short-term variability between repeat PSA measurements within men both with and without prostate cancer. It has been quoted that physiological variation combined with inter-assay variation could be as much as 30% for 95% of men and $\geq$ 30% for 5% of men (6).

Variations in serum PSA levels

The half-life of total PSA in the serum is between two and three days (7), although 'free PSA' has a half-life of less than two hours. In consequence of this half-life of total PSA, large temporary elevations in total serum PSA levels may take over a week to return to baseline levels.

Sample handling

PSA is stable for 24 h at room temperature. Concentrations of PSA in serum may decrease during storage (8). With storage at room temperature the loss is usually 5–10%. Both total and free PSA are lost during storage and this may affect the ratio of free to total PSA. For long-term storage, it is recommended that samples should be frozen, and stored at –70°C.

Diurnal variation

No significant diurnal variation in serum PSA levels has been demonstrated, and a blood sample can be drawn for PSA analysis at any time during the day.

Ejaculation

Ejaculation appears to have a slight effect on PSA. In young men aged under 40, there was a slight decrease in serum PSA on the 1st and 7th day after ejaculation (9). PSA is however rarely used in clinical practice as a test in young men, but in a group of older men aged between 40 and 79 years investigated by Tchetgen *et al.* (10), serum PSA increased after ejaculation in 87% of men by a mean of 0.8 ng/ml at 1 h and 0.2 ng/ml at 24 h; this returned to the normal level in 97% of the men in 48 h. This study advocated that men should abstain from ejaculation for 48 h prior to blood samples being drawn for PSA measurement.

Effect of digital rectal examination (DRE)

It was initially considered that DRE might affect serum PSA levels, but subsequent studies have shown that any increase in PSA after DRE is not clinically significant and does not alter treatment decisions. The free PSA fraction appears to increase to a greater extent than total PSA after DRE, and this could lead to an overestimation of benign prostatic hyperplasia (11).

Effect of prostatic massage

Stamey reported that prostatic massage may adversely affect PSA levels (7), and that such an increase in PSA may last over one week. This observation has not been confirmed to be clinically significant by subsequent studies.

Prostatitis

Urinary tract infection can cause serum PSA elevation. Acute prostatitic inflammation can lead to a considerable increase in the serum PSA concentration, probably due to increased vascular permeability within the inflamed prostate causing increased leakage of PSA into the circulation. A normal serum PSA level is usually restored after treatment of prostatitis with appropriate antibiotics, but this may take a period of 6–8 weeks. Some authorities consider sub-clinical acute prostatitis to be the cause of PSA elevation in asymptomatic men with no evidence of cancer on prostatic biopsies (12). They believe that treatment of men with subclinical prostatitis with antibiotics could lead to normalization of the serum PSA concentration. This hypothesis was investigated by Tchetgen *et al.* (13) in a study of 60 men with minor elevation of the serum PSA level and no clinical evidence of prostatitis. Each man received a 3-week course of Ciprofloxacin. No significant difference in serum PSA was noted between the control group and those receiving Ciprofloxacin, and in this study a short course of Ciprofloxacin did not lower the serum PSA concentration sufficiently to avoid a prostatic biopsy.

Retention of urine

Acute urinary retention may cause an acute rise in serum PSA levels. Semjonov and colleagues (14) reported a group of seven patients with acute retention whose retention was relieved by suprapubic cystostomy. There was a 2.4-fold increase in PSA in these patients. Histological examination of the prostate after acute urinary retention may show microscopic prostatic infarcts and it may be postulated that such events can lead to the release of PSA from the prostate into the circulation.

Urological procedures

Cystoscopy and transrectal ultrasound (TRUS) do not appear to alter serum PSA levels. TRUS-guided prostate biopsy and transurethral prostatectomy (TURP) does however markedly increase serum levels. All diagnostic serum PSA samples should be drawn before prostatic biopsy. After prostatic biopsy or TURP, serum PSA measurement should be deferred for a period of at least 6 weeks.

Testosterone

Androgen deprivation causes a rapid decrease in serum PSA levels, but exogenous testosterone does not appear to increase PSA levels in healthy males. Ultrasound-determined prostate volume, semen PSA, and serum PSA levels did not change significantly following the administration of exogenous testosterone to 31 healthy volunteers aged under 40 (15).

Finasteride

Finasteride is a type II 5α-reductase inhibitor used for the medical treatment of men with benign prostatic hyperplasia. By preventing the conversion of testosterone to its tissue active form, finasteride reduces dihydrotestosterone in plasma and prostate tissue. Its effects are predominantly on the prostate, and were reported in a large study involving 1645 men (16). A dose of 5 mg daily for 12 months reduced prostate size by about 20%, increased urine flow rate by about 20%, and improved symptom scores by about 20%. Serum PSA levels decreased by 46% compared to no change with placebo treatment (16). Data from finasteride clinical trials have shown that when PSA levels in finasteride-treated patients are doubled, the distribution of PSA in such patients parallels the range of values in placebo treated patients. This has led to a recommendation that to interpret PSA levels for prostate cancer diagnosis in finasteride treated men, one should double the measured PSA in serum. Because BPH and prostate cancer may co-exist, it is important to consider the effect of finasteride on PSA levels used for prostate cancer diagnosis. Oesterling and colleagues recently (17) reported a study that provided evidence of the effect of finasteride on PSA levels in 72 men with BPH, and 77 men with both BPH and untreated prostate cancer. The latter group of men can serve as a model for latent prostate cancer. This study found a median decrease of PSA of approximately 50% with finasteride treatment, although there was a range of PSA suppression in individual patients. The study confirmed the value of doubling the PSA levels for the interpretation of PSA in finasteride-treated men, and finasteride did not mask the elevations of PSA due to cancer in the men in this study. This study concluded that PSA remains an effective screening tool for prostate cancer in finasteride-treated patients. Current attention has been focused on the proportions of PSA components in serum. It appears that the percentage of free PSA does not change significantly with finasteride (18). In a double-blind study of 40 men given placebo or 5 mg finasteride daily for 9 months, there was a 50% decrease in total PSA with finasteride, but the mean %-free PSA did not change significantly with finasteride.

α1-Adrenoreceptor blockers

There is relatively little data about the effect on serum PSA levels of α-adrenergic antagonists used in the treatment of BPH. Terazosin does not appear to affect the free or total PSA levels in men with BPH and therefore administration of this medication will not interfere with PSA measurements used for prostate cancer diagnosis (19).

Cardiac catheterization

Cardiac surgery and extra-corporeal cardio-pulmonary bypass can increase PSA (20). This was reported by Hagood and colleagues who studied 68 patients with acute retention after cardiac surgery and noted a PSA increase in 56%. The mean PSA level was 9.1 ng/ml. This was not due to urethral catheterization as in a control group of 23 patients, the PSA only increased in one patient with urethral catheterization.

Dialysis

A prospective study of the impact of haemodialysis on total and free PSA levels in 149 men was reported in 1999 (21). Free PSA molecules passed through high-flux membranes, but complexed PSA molecules failed to pass through high- or low-flux membranes. Thus total PSA measurements can be used for prostate cancer diagnosis and monitoring in patients on dialysis, but free PSA and free:total PSA ratios should only be used in patients treated by haemodialysis with low flux membranes.

Exercise

Physical exercise does not appear to raise PSA. Bicycle riding does not increase the serum PSA level (22), and a graded exercise stress test in hospitalized patients did not significantly increase PSA levels (23). Nonetheless, it has been recommended that PSA levels used for serial measurements should be performed in similar situations, e.g. in ambulant patients.

Contemporary transrectal ultrasound-guided prostate biopsy

The most common indications for prostate biopsy are a palpable abnormality of the prostate on DRE, or an alteration in the serum PSA level. Serum PSA levels are used in diagnosis to identify those men who need further investigation by a transrectal biopsy of the prostate under ultrasound guidance to confirm or exclude the presence of prostate cancer. Such a screening investigation for an otherwise healthy patient should be without serious complications and it is thus important to ensure that an appropriate indication for performing a biopsy exists. PSA is the commonest primary test used in the detection of prostate cancer

but it is not foolproof, as not all prostate cancers cause a detectable elevation in PSA. PSA is produced by normal prostate cells and prostatic adenocarcinoma cells, and the expression of PSA determined immuno-histochemically decreases with increasing tumor grade (24). The power of PSA as a screening test for prostate cancer is based on the observation that with the Yang polyclonal assay, normal prostate tissue contributes 0.1 ng/ml/g tissue to the serum PSA level. PSA is elevated by 0.3 ng/ml/g of BPH tissue, whilst the elevation is 3 ng/ml/g of cancer tissue (25). Using PSA as the primary modality for prostate cancer detection can be problematic. The manufacturers' upper limit of normal with the monoclonal 'Hybritech' PSA assay is 4 ng/ml. This threshold level is unsatisfactory because the histological status of the 'normal' prostate in early studies was not accurately confirmed and it is known that up to 20% of patients with newly diagnosed organ-confined prostate cancer may have PSA levels below 4 ng/ml. The detection rates in recent North American PSA-based prostate cancer detection programs have varied from 1.5% to 4.1% (26). Many biopsies demonstrate no malignancy if the PSA level has been used as the sole determinant of the need for prostate biopsy, and considerable effort has been spent in the last decade in trying to decrease the number of unnecessary biopsies. A false-negative rate of up to 23% may be found with an initial sextant biopsy of the prostate. When the PSA level remains elevated or increases further with time, further biopsy must be considered, either repeating the sextant biopsy or sampling other areas of the prostate.

Although TRUS-guided transrectal biopsy has a low morbidity, complications may occur, but are rarely serious. Minor complications of biopsy are very common, the most common being persistent hematuria; other minor complications are those of rectal bleeding, and pelvic and perineal discomfort (27, 28, 29). A cause for concern following prostate biopsy would be heavy and prolonged hematuria resulting in urinary retention requiring urethral catheterization. In a series of patients investigated by sextant biopsy, the minor bleeding complications appeared to be unrelated to the total number of biopsy cores, or to previous aspirin or non-steroid anti-inflammatory drug use (30). Much attention has been given to the infectious complications of prostate biopsy. When biopsy is performed under antibiotic cover, infections are rare but can result in fever, urinary tract infection, and rigors occasionally necessitating hospitalization. Death from anaerobic infection following prostate biopsy has been reported (31), further reminding us of the importance of ensuring that an appropriate indication for biopsy is present in each individual patient. Various prophylactic antibiotic regimens are used but there is currently little consensus on the optimum prophylactic antibiotic or the timing and duration of its administration. The most common regimen is currently to use a quinalone, e.g. ciprofloxacin or ofloxacin, plus metronidazole.

Part of the problem in understanding the multitude of studies related to PSA is the variation in biopsy techniques used in different centers. Biopsy protocols need to be considered in detail as an understanding of the potential variation of the different biopsy approaches used (and their associated thoroughness of prostate sampling) is related to an understanding of the interpretation of studies on the value of PSA, PSA density, age-related PSA, and PSA velocity in prostate cancer diagnosis.

A combination of DRE and PSA is the best technique for identifying patients with prostate cancer. Palpable abnormalities of the prostate must be biopsied irrespective of the PSA level. If the prostate is palpably normal, biopsy is performed on the basis of the PSA level and a threshold level of 3 or 4 ng/ml is usually used. In cancer diagnosis, there is now little role for prostate ultrasound without biopsy. In a patient in whom the prostate is palpably benign, current diagnostic algorithms would recommend that a prostate biopsy should be performed if the PSA level is above 10 ng/ml. It is usual to avoid biopsy in the palpably normal gland if the PSA level is below 4 ng/ml, although about 20% of cancers in some studies have a PSA below 4 ng/ml. In a screening study in my own institution, three patients with cancer were detected with PSA below 1 ng/ml; the sole indication for biopsy was abnormality of the DRE. The serum PSA range between 4 and 10 ng/ml is difficult to assess, as 80% of such biopsies with a palpably normal prostate and this PSA range are benign. It is currently usual practice to perform a sextant biopsy if the serum PSA is in this PSA range, but it is for this PSA range that the refinements of PSA levels such as PSA density, PSA velocity, and age–specific PSA ranges are targeted.

TRUS-guided biopsies may be directed at specific areas, e.g. either palpable abnormalities, or at focal sonographic abnormalities (peripheral or transition zone hypoechoic areas on gray-scale sonography, or areas of hypervascularity on power or color Doppler sonography). The optimum biopsy protocol is still not established. Previous practice in the past 15 years has concentrated on peripheral zone hypoechoic areas and has relatively ignored alterations of echo-texture in the transition zone, as most cancers occur in the peripheral zone (32). Recent studies have confirmed the value of color and power Doppler in highlighting areas for biopsy (33), but most urologists and many radiologists do not use color or power Doppler for TRUS scanning and biopsy. Systematic biopsies are usually taken in addition to focal ultrasound-guided biopsies in an attempt to detect isoechoic cancer, as approximately 25% of prostate cancers are isoechoic and may be missed without systematic biopsy (34). Systematic biopsy protocols originally used four core (quadrant) or six core (sextant) procedures, but the sextant biopsy procedure is now the standard and some institutions biopsy additional further sites systematically, as part of their standard systematic biopsy procedure. The original sextant procedure advocated by Hodge and colleagues (35) involved taking three cores from each lobe in parallel lines at the base, mid-gland, and apex of each lobe. A recent study from Vienna (36) has suggested that there may be advantages in taking the six cores at mid-gland level, as a fan of six cores in the peripheral zone, rather than using the traditional parallel line approach. In this study comparing the conventional double-line approach with the fan approach, cancer was found in 20 out of 54 patients (37%) with the fan approach, whilst it was only found in 16 out of 53 patients (30.1%) with the double-line approach. My personal unpublished experience with a fan approach in two similar groups of 50 patients has not confirmed the value of this approach.

Other authors have proposed different variations to the sextant biopsy procedure. Some have advocated taking more lateral cores at mid-gland level (37). In the latter paper, cancer was found in 121 of 273 patients; routine sextant biopsies found 88% of these tumors, but 17 of the 22 missed cancers were detected by the lateral biopsy cores. Combining these lateral cores with mid-line cores gives the five-region (13-core) approach (38). Some patients with a persistent elevated PSA and negative previous biopsy have cancer in the anterior part of the transition zone and to diagnose such cancers, transition zone cores taken anteriorly may be needed (39, 40, 41). These are often taken on a subsequent occasion rather than at the initial biopsy procedure, but may be taken at the original procedure in some institutions. Many patients with an elevated PSA level have negative systematic sextant biopsies at the original sextant biopsy, and yet are found to have prostate cancer at a repeat systematic biopsy (42, 43). It may be argued that the cores from a repeat systematic biopsy should be taken at sites away from those sampled at the original biopsy procedure. It could also be argued that the additional areas should be sampled at the primary biopsy procedure, i.e. taking a more extensive sample of the gland, and an 18-core biopsy protocol was recently described (44). There is concern about the number of cores needed to adequately sample the prostate of different overall gland volumes, as from a mathematical model it would appear that the standard sextant biopsy only optimally samples a minority of prostate glands (45). Several papers have subsequently investigated this aspect, and Letran and colleagues demonstrated that sextant biopsy was adequate for smaller glands, but the yield of sextant biopsy decreased significantly when the total prostate volume exceeded 55 cm^3 (46).

A new diagnostic tool to aid prostate biopsy is the use of sonographic contrast agents. Various such agents are in the development stage by commercial pharmaceutical companies; two agents—Levovist, (Schering) and Sonovue, (Sonus Pharmaceuticals)—are now commercially available. Studies describing the use of these agents in the diagnosis of prostate cancer have been recently reported. Rickards and colleagues (47) reported a study of 22 men given Sonovue in whom 132 biopsies had been undertaken. Areas of biopsy before and after contrast administration were correlated with histological results; Sonovue increased the sensitivity to cancer detection from 46% to 64 % but decreased the specificity from 75% to 56%. Another recently reported study from Innsbruck, Austria (48) using Levovist gave a sensitivity of 53%, specificity of 72%, and a positive predictive value of 70% in a study of 44 patients with prostate cancer. The newest potential sonographic technique that may be valuable in identifying areas for prostate biopsy is the use of second harmonic imaging with contrast; this technique is still under development and there are currently no reports on its use in the selection of sites for prostate biopsy in the literature.

The current optimum protocol for transrectal ultrasound-guided biopsy appears to be either a combination of targeted biopsies with color or power Doppler plus a sextant biopsy, or an extended systematic biopsy involving more than six areas. Lavoipierre and colleagues (33) reported a study involving 256 patients scanned by both conventional gray-scale and color Doppler imaging. Targeted biopsies of focal abnormalities on gray-scale and color Doppler were taken, and in addition a sextant biopsy was performed on all patients. Altogether 100 cancers were detected (39% of patients studied); 16 of these cancers were only demon-

strated by color Doppler. Nine cancers were found by sextant biopsies, yet gray-scale and color Doppler failed to reveal any abnormality in these nine patients. Many studies evaluating the use of PSA, and PSA-derived indices, such as PSAD and PSAV, have used less thorough sampling procedures than the above, and this raises problems in assessing the value of these different indices in cancer detection.

PSA *in the diagnosis of prostate cancer*

PSA density and PSA transition zone density

Many patients with a palpably normal prostate have a PSA level above 4 ng/ml and systematic sextant biopsy yields benign prostate hyperplasia or prostatic inflammation but not prostate cancer. Frequent attempts have been made in the past decade to improve the specificity of PSA measurements by relating the serum PSA to the overall prostate gland volume. More recent work has attempted to correlate the PSA to the transition zone volume in addition, to correct more accurately for the proportion of serum PSA due to benign transition zone glandular hyperplasia. The volume-corrected PSA approach stems from the work of Stamey and Kabalin (25) who found that in BPH, serum PSA levels were elevated by approximately 0.3 ng/ml/g BPH tissue, whereas in prostatic cancer the levels were elevated 3.5 ng/ml/g of prostate.

One of the first methods of relating the PSA to the prostate volume measured sonographically or by magnetic resonance was the PSA density (PSAD). This concept was introduced by Benson (49); the PSAD quotient is obtained by dividing the serum PSA by the overall prostate gland volume. In Benson's study, 20 patients with cancer had a higher mean PSAD (0.58 ng/ml/ml) compared to 41 patients with BPH who had a mean PSAD of 0.04 ng/ml/ml. Subsequently Seaman (50) reported the value of PSAD in a retrospective series of 3494 men. PSAD was found useful in devising a biopsy protocol for men with a serum PSA between 4 and 10 ng/ml. In 773 men with PSA measurements in this range, the mean PSAD of men with cancer was higher than those with benign prostate disease. It was recommended that a systematic sextant biopsy should be performed if the PSAD was greater than 0.15 ng/ml/ml, but might be avoided if below this level.

The PSAD calculation assumes that one can make an adjustment for the proportion of PSA resulting from the prostate epithelial cells in BPH, and this gives an indication of the excess PSA due to cancer. Some authors have revised the PSAD threshold of 0.15 ng/ml/ml, and would advocate a threshold of 0.10 or 0.12. Littrup and co-workers from the American Cancer Society National Prostate cancer detection project (51) investigated a cohort of 2999 men and found by decision analysis that the use of PSAD with a threshold of ≥ 0.12 could reduce biopsies by 16–55% with a 4–25% loss of cancer detection. They analyzed various strategies for biopsy reduction and found that the greatest biopsy reduction relative to cancer yield and lowest cost per cancer detected occurred with PSAD-driven biopsy protocols.

Some authors have found the PSAD concept unhelpful and claim it offers little benefit over PSA alone. This may be because of inaccuracy in measurement of the prostate volume (as this is usually measured using the formula for an ellipse, and the prostate shape does change with increasing size), or differing epithelial: stromal ratios in the prostate in different sample populations. A disappointing impression of PSAD may also be due to the effect of overall prostate size, and the efficiency of prostate sampling by sextant biopsy in large prostates, reinforcing the points considered earlier about differences in sampling protocols in different reported series.

The PSAD approach has been developed further as the 'PSA transition zone density' (PSATZD) (52), which recognizes that the density of PSA in the two parts of the prostate is different. The transition zone expressed about 2.5 times more PSA than the peripheral zone in this study giving different zonal densities of 0.14 ng/ml/g in the transition zone, and 0.052 ng/ml/g in the peripheral zone. Both the total prostate volume and transition zone volumes can be determined sonographically, and the peripheral zone volume calculated by subtraction. It was hoped this newest approach might help to improve the PSA density concept, but early reports of PSA transition zone density have been discouraging. Lin and colleagues in Seattle (53) assessed 917 men with total PSA measurements prior to ultrasound-guided biopsy, in a protocol where the overall prostate volume and the transition zone volume was measured in each patient. Cancer was found in 276 patients. In the overall series of patients, total PSA was as useful as any other PSA index for cancer detection, but in men with a PSA between 4.0 and 10 ng/ml, PSAD and PSATZD were more predictive than PSA alone. In this series of men, PSA transition zone density did not give additional information to that obtained

from the PSA density. The disadvantage with the use of both the PSAD and PSATZD is the need to obtain a prostate volume measurement. Whilst avoiding prostate biopsy in some patients, the volume determination necessitates TRUS; this is costly and causes patient discomfort and adds to patient anxiety. These considerations tend to limit the overall value of the PSA density approach.

Age-specific reference ranges

PSA levels increase with age. This has generally been considered to be due to an increase in prostatic mass with age due to benign prostatic hyperplasia, but other processes, which may be age-related, such as prostatic infarction, inflammation, and 'leakage' of the prostatic epithelium, may be involved. These pathological processes can affect the PSA released into the serum. Age-related PSA ranges could be used as an alternative approach to increase the specificity of individual PSA levels in cancer diagnosis, as the standard serum PSA reference range does not account for age differences. Oesterling *et al.* (54) first proposed age-related reference normal ranges for serum PSA measurements on the basis of a study of PSA, DRE, and prostate biopsy in men in whom no evidence of cancer had been found. In these men, PSA levels and prostate volume were determined as a function of age and it was found that the median serum PSA concentration increased with each decade of age. In the age decade between 40 and 49 years, no man had a serum PSA level above 4 ng/ml. In the age decade between 70 and 79 years, 19% men had a serum PSA of more than 4 ng/ml. Subsequent reports have shown that age related ranges make PSA a more sensitive marker for prostate cancer, with increased detection, in men under 60 years of age and a more specific marker, decreasing the number of negative biopsies, for men over 60. The aim of these age-specific reference ranges is 2-fold. First they aim to make PSA a more discriminating marker for early stage prostate cancer in younger men aged below 60. Second they aim to decrease the number of negative biopsies in older men, in whom surgical treatment of early-stage disease may be less likely and where it might be argued that establishing a diagnosis of cancer may be considered less important. It is impossible for any individual physician to quantify these aims and gauge whether the increased number of biopsies in younger men justify the costs, and similarly it is difficult to qualify the balance between decreased sensitivity and increased specificity in older men. Health economists and the public must make these difficult judgments. The critical question perhaps is whether these undetected cancers in older men would have been clinically significant disease.

From a large study (55), involving review of almost 80 000 of men from the Prostate Cancer Awareness Week in 1993, the following age specific reference ranges were recommended:

- age 40 to 49 = 0–2.4 ng/ml
- age 50 to 59 = 0–3.8 ng/ml
- age 60 to 69 = 0–5.6 ng/ml
- age 70 to 79 = 0–6.9 ng/ml.

Some reports have disputed the value of age-specific PSA reference ranges. Borer and colleagues (56) reviewed 1280 prostate biopsies in 1046 men aged 60–80. By the use of age-specific reference ranges, 73 of the 1280 (5.7%) biopsies in this study would have been avoided; 15 of those 73 biopsies had cancer, while 9 of those 15 cancers were considered unfavorable because of a Gleason score of 5 or more, and 2 of these 9 were in patients aged 63 and 65 years of age. The authors felt that age-specific PSA reference ranges could not be used to assess the need for prostate biopsy, as in their study 60% of the potentially missed cancers had unfavorable histology. Another report observed that the conventional PSA threshold of 4 ng/ml resulted in 1091 life-years saved compared with 757 life-years saved with age-specific thresholds (57). Catalona and colleagues (58) have criticized age-specific PSA reference ranges as they felt that the decrease in cancer detection in older men was inappropriate. They concluded that a threshold of 4 ng/ml should be used in men of all ages. In their series, 6630 men aged over 50 were assessed by serum PSA and DRE; men underwent biopsy on the basis of an abnormal DRE or serum PSA over 4 ng/ml, and 264 cancers were detected. They found that in men aged 50–59 years, a decrease in the PSA cut-off from 4 to 4.5 ng/ml would have produced a 45% increase in the number of biopsies. They noted that an increase in the PSA cut-off point for men aged 60–69 from 4 ng/ml to 4.5 ng/ml would have decreased the number of biopsies in this age band by 15% but missed 8% of all confined cancers. In men aged over 70 years, an increase in the cut-off point to 6.5 ng/ml would have caused 44% fewer biopsies but would have missed 47% of all confined cancers. This is a very controversial subject, particularly with the decreased sensitivity of cancer-detection in older men. There are now further studies

available and whilst the use of age-specific reference ranges in older men remains controversial, the approach does appear more acceptable approach for men under 50.

PSA velocity

PSA velocity (PSAV) is the rate of change in PSA levels with time, and the use of PSAV to identify men requiring prostate biopsy was introduced by Carter (59). Based on the database from the Baltimore longitudinal study of aging, Carter investigated PSA levels over a minimum 7-year period and noted a linear increase in PSA with time in patients with BPH, but a transition to an exponential rise in PSA in patients with cancer. An increase of 0.04 ± 0.02 ng/ml/year was suggested as normal. From this it was deduced that a change of 0.75 ng/ml/year would act as an index alerting to the presence of cancer. PSAV has a high specificity; less than 5% of men without prostate cancer have a PSAV suggestive of cancer (60). It has been considered that a percentage change of PSA may be useful, but Littrup and co-workers (51) found that a 20% annual change in PSA was less useful than the absolute change in PSA with time. In their study, a PSA velocity of 0.6 ng/ml/year was the optimum threshold PSA change, but a threshold of 1.0 ng/ml/year was better for patients with PSA levels ≥ 4 ng/ml. Other groups (61) have not found the PSA velocity concept useful. These contradictory results may be related to the substantial individual variation in the PSA levels that may be observed in individual patients—a short-term variation in PSA of ≥ 0.75 ng/ml may occur. Alternatively it may represent the variations in biopsy protocols in different centers referred to earlier, when different equipment and different criteria for identifying areas for biopsy sampling have been used.

PSA velocity has been incorporated into some longitudinal studies for the detection of early prostate cancer, as with the increasing use of routine PSA measurements many men now have a cumulative PSA record that spans at least 2 years. To facilitate the use of these PSA changes with time, it is helpful for doctors making clinical decisions about prostate cancer diagnosis or disease progression, if biochemical laboratories print an individual man's PSA results as a cumulative PSA record. There is sufficient individual short-term variability between PSA measurements that it is rarely practical to decide whether to biopsy or not from a single short-term PSA change. The optimum number of PSA measurements and the time interval between measurements has not been fully assessed, although a study (62) has suggested a minimum of three consecutive PSA measurements in a 2-year period. As well as their use in initial diagnosis of cancer, PSAV measurements may also be used to monitor patients with cancer managed by 'watchful waiting' to identify those with a rapidly rising PSA. These patients may warrant closer surveillance, but it is not proven whether this subset of patients does have a more aggressive biological behavior (63).

%-Free PSA

The percentage of free PSA has been the subject of much current urological research, which has been reviewed recently (64). The presence of multiple forms of PSA was first discovered in 1991 (65). α-1-Chymotrypsin (ACT) and α-2-macroglobulin (AMG) bind with PSA to form inactive complexes, whilst a small amount of PSA in serum is unbound or 'free' PSA. The potential of these molecular forms of PSA to be used in cancer diagnosis became apparent when it was found that the %-free PSA is lower in men with prostate cancer than in men with normal prostate glands or benign prostatic hyperplasia. In recent years, many research programs have tried to increase the specificity of serum tests in the diagnosis of prostate cancer in the palpably normal iso-echoic prostate by measuring the %-free PSA; these studies have again tried to limit the number of benign systematic sextant biopsies of the prostate, particularly in patients with a PSA level in the 4–10 ng/ml range. A low percentage of free PSA is an indicator suggestive of prostate cancer (66, 67), but the ideal threshold for clinical practice remains to be determined.

A study by Oesterling and colleagues (68) investigated 422 men and attempted to establish reference ranges of free, complexed, and total PSA in healthy men aged 40–75 years. The individual reference ranges were established but it was found that the ratios between these individual ranges did not correlate well with patient age. It was suggested that %-free PSA might increase the performance of the PSA test in the 3–10 ng/ml range by 20–25% (69). Results of trials to evaluate the value of this approach are currently somewhat contradictory (70), but appear to confirm the value of %-free PSA in improving the specificity of prostate cancer detection. Vashi and colleagues (71) used a study of sextant biopsy in 413 men with a PSA between 2–20 ng/ml to define the optimal total PSA range for use of %-free PSA. In this study, 225 men

(54%) had benign disease and 188 (46%) had prostate cancer. The authors found that %-free PSA was most advantageous in men with total PSA between 3 and 10 ng/ml, and termed this the 'reflex range' when they recommended that %-free PSA measurements should be used. When the total PSA value was in the 3.0–4.0 ng/ml range, the threshold value for %-free PSA was 0.19%. This gave a biopsy rate of 73% and a cancer detection rate of 44%, for a sensitivity of 90%. The corresponding threshold for %-free PSA was 0.24% for total PSA levels in the 4.1–10.0 ng/ml range; this gave an improvement in the biopsy rate to 60% with a sensitivity of 95%, but failed to detect 5% of cancers.

Various studies have suggested that measurement of %-free PSA would increase the specificity of prostate cancer screening but the suggested cut-offs have ranged from 15% to 25%. Studies by other workers have confirmed the report by Luderer and co-workers (67) that the use of free PSA measurements was unhelpful in cancer detection when the total PSA level exceeds 10 ng/ml, due to the higher specificity and positive predictive value of total PSA levels above 10 ng/ml.

It is clear that the use of %-free PSA measurements can improve the specificity of cancer detection when the total PSA is *mildly* elevated. The value of %-free PSA in prostate cancer diagnosis has been reported in a recent study (72) of 1709 men investigated in five North American centers. The mean %-free PSA in 229 men with cancer was 9.1%, whereas it was 18.9% in men without cancer. In the 4–9.9 ng/ml total PSA range, use of a 15% free PSA cut-off gave a sensitivity of 85%, specificity 32%, and positive predictive value of 39%. A 20% free PSA cut-off gave sensitivity of 97%, 12% specificity, and positive predictive value 36% in the same men.

If 15% free PSA had been used as a criterion for TRUS-guided sextant prostate biopsy in those men with serum PSA levels in the range 4.0–9.9 ng/ml, the number of biopsies would have been decreased by 21% with a concomitant decrease in cancer detection of 14.6%. Use of 20% free PSA would have decreased the biopsies by 13.7% with only a 3% decrease in cancer detection. Age variations of free PSA were noted.

A recent study from Sweden (73) retrospectively assessed the role of free PSA as a predictor of prostate cancer. The %-free PSA level was measured in the frozen serum samples of 1748 men who had been previously screened in 1988 and 1989. Five-year follow up details on new cancers in this group of men were obtained from the Swedish cancer registry. The combination of a total PSA below 3 ng/ml and %-free PSA

> 18% defined a population with a very low risk of prostate cancer during the screening study and subsequent 5 years. The report advocated that men in this group could have avoided DRE as part of the screening study.

Prostate-specific membrane antigen (PSMA)

One of the newest serum tests that might be used in prostate cancer management is prostate-specific membrane antigen (PSMA) (74). The PSM antigen is a marker for prostatic epithelial cells, but has also been identified in testis, epididymis, and seminal vesicle. It is a 750 amino acid membrane-bound glycoprotein and it has been identified by immuno-cytochemistry in both benign and malignant prostate tissue. PSMA levels were greater in patients with prostate cancer than men with benign prostatic hyperplasia or normal prostate glands (75); in this series, some men with prostate cancer were found to have increased PSMA levels and low levels of PSA. The expression of PSMA does appear to be increased with progressive prostate cancer and does not appear to be increased in patients with hormone refractory disease (76). Murphy and colleagues (77) compared PSMA with total PSA and found no advantage with PSMA compared with total PSA in the diagnosis of cancer in 226 men in a screening project. In this particular study, it was found that PSAD gave the best diagnostic information, but PSMA did offer the best correlation with tumor stage. Thus PSMA may have prognostic significance. Theoretically PSMA should be better than PSA as a marker in patients receiving androgen-eprivation treatment because its expression is increased in the absence of hormone. Expression of the PSM antigen forms the basis of the recently developed immunoscintigraphic Prostascint scan. This technique uses a [111] In-labeled murine monoclonal antibody that identifies PSMA expression in soft tissues such as lymph nodes, and is being investigated as a test for identifying metastatic prostate cancer (78, 79). FDA protocol studies have revealed correlation between areas of increased isotope concentration and biopsy proven tumors.

PSA and staging of prostate cancer

Through using serum PSA measurements, urologists and radiologists now usually detect prostate cancer at an earlier stage than in previous decades, and a direct correlation between serum PSA levels and the stage of the primary prostate cancer has been found (7). In another PSA-based screening program using a threshold of 4 ng/ml, 70% of cancers are T1 or T2; if the PSA level is over 10 ng/ml, only 45% of patients have T1 or T2 cancers (80). However, by themselves PSA levels cannot be used to predict the stage of the primary tumor in an individual patient.

Metastatic prostate cancer

Fifteen years ago, about one-third of patients with prostate cancer had skeletal metastases at the time of diagnosis. Currently only about 5% of men with newly diagnosed prostate cancer have skeletal metastases when their cancer is detected (81). Radio-isotope skeletal scintigraphy is a highly sensitive but relatively expensive method for assessing potential metastases in the axial skeleton. The urological practice of assessing all patients with newly diagnosed prostate cancer by skeletal scintigraphy was developed before the advent of PSA, when isotope bone scans were more accurate than plain radiography or acid phosphatase in detecting metastases in bone. As bone metastases are now less frequent at the time of diagnosis, an appropriate imaging strategy for the use of scintigraphy is needed, as there appears to be scope to eliminate the isotope scan in many patients with newly diagnosed prostate cancer. This approach was first considered by Chybowski and workers from the Mayo Clinic (82) who evaluated prostate cancer stage, serum acid phosphatase, and serum PSA in 521 patients with untreated prostate cancer, and compared these findings with the bone scan appearances. Serum PSA levels had the best correlation with bone scan findings. It was found that in 306 men with a serum PSA below 20 ng/ml, only one patient—a man with a PSA of 18.2 ng/ml—had a positive bone scan, giving a negative predictive value of 99.7%. This study was important as it allowed health planners to question whether a staging bone scan was an essential test in newly diagnosed asymptomatic untreated patients with prostate cancer with a low serum PSA. From the Mayo Clinic series, it was recommended that men with no symptoms of bone pain and a PSA of 10 ng/ml or less did not require an isotope bone scan. A subsequent study from the same institution (83) reported a study of 852 patients with newly diagnosed untreated prostate cancer and a PSA level below 20 ng/ml. Seven of these 852 patients had a positive bone scan. Five of these seven had significant musculo-skeletal symptoms related to their metastases and only one patient with a PSA below 10 ng/ml was asymptomatic yet had a positive bone scan. My own experience and that of other authors (84) has also confirmed that the bone scan can be eliminated in patients with no skeletal symptoms and a PSA below 10 ng/ml, and urological practice has now changed in many centers to reflect this approach.

A selective approach could also be used for the other radiological investigations that are used for staging soft tissue metastatic prostate cancer—computed tomography (CT) and magnetic resonance (MR). Threshold PSA levels for the use of these modalities have not been clearly identified (85). An initial study (86) of 300 newly diagnosed patients with prostate cancer examined with CT and MR scanning demonstrated a low likelihood of lymph node metastases if the PSA was below 20 ng/ml. Spencer and colleagues (87) reported a selected series of 102 men with newly diagnosed prostate cancer investigated with skeletal scintigraphy and contrast enhanced CT scans (for nodal staging) as pre-operative investigations. There was no statistical difference between the mean PSA values of the 13 men with lymph node metastases (106 ng/ml) and the 89 men without lymphadenopathy (101 ng/ml). Ten men had positive pelvic lymph nodes alone; three further men had retro-peritoneal and pelvic lymph nodes. One man had CT evidence of pelvic lymphadenopathy and a PSA level below 20 ng/ml, namely 18.6 ng/ml; 18% of men had positive skeletal scintigraphy, and one man (who had symptomatic bone pain) had a skeletal metastasis with a PSA level below 20 ng/ml. Patients in this study had not been diagnosed through a prostate cancer screening program, and thus many of the patients had more advanced disease than may be seen in other centers' series. Most of these men were symptomatic with outflow tract obstruction or acute urinary retention, and the proportion of abnormalities was thus higher than would be expected in other series where cancer was detected through PSA screening. If staging imaging had been restricted to those men with a PSA value above 20 ng/ml, 30 of the 102 patients would have avoided imaging tests. The use of these imaging tests had a sensitivity of 92% and a specificity of 67%. If a Gleason score above 5 or a PSA level over 20 ng/ml had qualified imaging the sensitivity of imaging would have been 96% but 12 further men would have required these imaging tests. Further work is needed to clarify a PSA-based policy for the selective use of CT and MR in these patients.

Measurement of free to total PSA does not appear to help with staging the primary tumor within the prostate. This was shown from a review of 307 patients with prostate cancer (88), 170 of whom underwent radical prostatectomy. There was no statistically significant difference between patients with T2 and T3 tumors, and the ratio of free to total PSA did not help in the pre- operative prediction of tumor stage and volume.

PSA in follow-up

The main biochemical criteria used for predicting the prognosis and likely outcome of definitive treatment, whether surgical or radiation therapy, are the pretreatment PSA and the subsequent monitoring of the serum PSA level following definitive treatment. A rising PSA level following a course of radical therapy implies residual or recurrent or progressive disease and raises issues about future management. The PSA doubling time (PSADT) can be measured in untreated patients with prostate cancer, and may provide information about the biological potential of the tumor to supplement the absolute pretreatment level. Other workers are exploring the possibility of measuring intracellular PSA levels in material obtained from the prostate as a fine-needle aspirate, as a prognostic factor for prostate cancer (89). Accelerated PSA doubling times may be identified in some patients with progressive disease after radiation therapy (90) or surgery. PSA doubling times have also been suggested as a surrogate end-point in clinical trials for hormone-refractory prostate cancer (91). This approach was outlined in a study of 30 patients receiving oral idarubicin; 26 patients were assessable and in 23 the PSA increased exponentially with time, with a median PSADT of 2.1 months, similar to the PSADT of patients receiving anti-androgen treatment alone.

The radio-isotope bone scan is a sensitive test and can be used to monitor symptomatic prostate cancer patients after treatment, but in asymptomatic prostate cancer patients the role of scintigraphy is not established. Serial PSA monitoring is a logical theoretical approach for monitoring asymptomatic patients, but currently no level has been found to identify a threshold to perform a bone scan when PSA levels rise in asymptomatic patients after treatment. A retrospective study of our own patients who had been in therapeutic trials (84) identified 59 patients with serial bone scans and serial PSA measurements. In three men, new bone metastases were observed by bone scintigraphy without a corresponding rise in PSA. In 13 men, the PSA levels rose in advance of new metastases on the scintigram. In the remaining 41 cases any change of the serum PSA level and scintigram appearance occurred in parallel. We felt that serial PSA levels were able to monitor disease progression in metastatic prostate cancer better than skeletal scintigraphy but that neither technique in isolation gave complete accuracy.

Radical prostatectomy

Following successful radical prostatectomy, the serum PSA level should be undetectable. The serum total PSA half-life after surgery has been measured at 3 days (7). Frequent sampling of PSA after prostatectomy enables two components to be identified. One has a half-life of 1–2 h and represents free PSA; the other has a half-life of 3 days and represents PSA complexed to α-chymotrypsin (92). Unfortunately about 35% of men will develop a rise in serum PSA in the 10 years after surgery. Pound and colleagues (93) found that they were able to predict the probability of long-term cure after radical prostatectomy by using pathological stage as a surrogate end point. The factors indicating a patient's likelihood of having an undetectable PSA at 10 years after surgery are pretreatment PSA, Gleason score, and pathological stage. An analysis of post-operative PSA levels in a series of 1977 men treated by radical prostatectomy at the Johns Hopkins Hospital, Baltimore, Maryland between 1982 and 1997 was reported by Pound and colleagues (93); 315 men (15%) showed recurrent disease, and a detectable PSA greater than 0.2 ng/ml was the only evidence of recurrent disease in 201 men. In these men, serum PSA level increases demonstrated an exponential growth curve and PSA doubling times were correlated. A PSA doubling time cut-off of 10 months provided the most statistically significant prediction of time to distant disease progression after PSA elevation. The median time to development of metastases after PSA elevation was 5 years (mean 8 years). In this group's experience, no patient had local recurrence or distant metastases with an undetectable PSA level at the time of progression; 23% of men with biochemical progression had an undetectable PSA for at least 5 years after surgery, and 4% had an undetectable PSA for 10 years before there was biochemical evidence of progression. The overall 10- and 15-year metastases-free survival rates were 87% and 82%, respectively. Men with a pre-operative PSA level between 10 and 20 ng/ml demonstrated a lower rate of recurrent disease than men with a preoperative PSA level greater than 20 ng/ml. A report from

another center (94), however, has noted recurrent disease in 3 of 394 men (2.3%) after radical prostatectomy where clinical evidence of disease progression occurred despite undetectable serum PSA levels

PSA assays with significant improved sensitivity are being developed and can be used to detect the presence of minimal prostate cancer. In theory, such ultrasensitive PSA assays might help to identify more aggressive tumors and facilitate administration of early adjuvant therapy after failed primary treatment. The Immulite ® third-generation PSA assay (Diagnostic Products Corporation, Los Angeles, California, USA) claims a working range of 0.01–20 ng/ml. Experience with this assay after radical prostatectomy has allowed PSA to be detected in some patients in whom PSA could not be detected with conventional detection ranges (5). Patients with minimal risk of early cancer recurrence were correctly identified with the Immulite assay. Two-thirds of those not cured by prostatectomy were identified post-operatively with this assay, and all patients with biochemical or clinical recurrence of prostate cancer were correctly identified by 2 years after prostatectomy.

Radical radiotherapy

The last decade has seen increasing numbers of patients with early prostate cancer treated by radical prostatectomy, and a relative decrease in those treated by radiation therapy. Following radical prostatectomy, the serum PSA should become undetectable and any increase in the serum PSA is indicative of recurrent disease. The situation is less clear following radiation therapy. Serum PSA levels may initially increase following radiation therapy due to cell damage, inflammation, and tissue necrosis, but should subsequently fall. The levels usually start to decrease from the third and fourth week after the start of radiotherapy, with a half-life of 2–3 months. However, they seldom reach the undetectable levels seen following surgery. There may be a continued fall for 12 months after radiation therapy (95). Kavadi and colleagues (96) showed that patients whose PSA did not fall to at least 4 ng/ml by 6 months after treatment were likely to demonstrate a high rate of recurrent disease. There is controversy about the PSA levels that indicate successful treatment with no clear absolute PSA nadir level identified to indicate successful treatment. In a study reported from the Massachusetts General Hospital (97), the ability of a PSA nadir to act as an early surrogate for subsequent freedom from biochemical progression was investigated in 314 men with T1–2 prostate

cancer treated by conventional external beam radiotherapy. 123 patients with a PSA nadir below 0.5 ng/ml had
a 90% freedom from PSA failure; those 103 patients
with a PSA nadir of 0.6–1 ng/ml had a 55% association,
and those 88 men with a PSA nadir above 1 ng/ml had a
34% association. A good correlation was identified
between the pretreatment PSA level and the likelihood of
obtaining an undetectable PSA nadir. This was 74% if
the pretreatment PSA was below 4 ng/ml, 42% in those
men with a PSA level between 4 ng/ml and 10 ng/ml,
and 32% in those men with a pretreatment serum PSA
level over 10 ng/ml. The time required to reach the PSA
nadir does not appear to be critical. A multi-institution
pooled analysis of 1765 patients treated at six North
American centers with external beam radiation therapy
alone was reported in 1999 (98). The institutions submitted details of patients with T1b, T1c, T2, Nx, M0
prostate cancer together with details of initial PSA levels
and follow up for at least 24 months with at least four
post-treatment PSA levels. The mean pretreatment level
was 18.9 ng/ml (range 0.2–2028 ng/ml); 14% of patients
had a PSA level of 4 ng/ml or less; 24% had a PSA level
over 20 ng/ml. Four separate prognostic groups were
identified:

- group 1: initial PSA below 9.2 ng/ml
- group 2: PSA between 9.2–19.7 ng/ml
- group 3: PSA over 19.7 ng/ml and Gleason score below 6
- group 4: PSA over 19.7 ng/ml and Gleason score between 7 and 10.

Estimates of the rate of survival free of biochemical
failure at five years were identified: group 1 81%,
group 2 69%, group 3 47%, group 4 29%. A rising
PSA may occur some years before there is evidence of
clinical failure, and patients with a rising PSA may
never have clinical metastases. Nonetheless, a rise in
PSA is indicative of disease activity, and may be used as
an indication for additional therapy. The American
Society of Therapeutic Radiology and Oncology issued
consensus guidelines of biochemical recurrence in 1997
(99): three consecutive rises in PSA values or any rise in
PSA great enough to provoke androgen suppression
with backdating of the failure time to the midpoint
between the last non-rising PSA and the first rising PSA
value. Studies using immuno-peroxidase stains for PSA
have shown that the PSA produced in patients following radiation therapy represents malignant cells and
not residual benign prostate epithelial cells (100).
TRUS-guided biopsy is required to fully assess local

recurrence after radical radiotherapy, but computed
tomography has a role in the assessment of symptomatic soft tissue relapse. Indications for CT scanning in
such circumstances will be largely determined by PSA
levels; upper-abdominal rather than pelvic retroperitoneal lymph node disease may predominate in such
patients and the CT scan should encompass the entire
abdomen and pelvis.

Some patients with erectile dysfunction after radiation therapy may now be treated with sildenafil
(Viagra). Recent reports have suggested a favorable
improvement in erectile function in 74% of patients
treated after external beam therapy (101) and in 81%
of patients after prostate brachytherapy (102). The
manufacturer (Pfizer Inc) (personal communication) is
not aware of any effect of sildenafil on PSA levels in
men, although specific investigation of this has not
been undertaken. Treatment with sildenafil would not
appear to have an effect on serum PSA levels used for
monitoring patients with prostate cancer after cancer
treatment. Erectile dysfunction and prostate cancer will
tend to occur in men at a similar age. In view of the
widespread use of PSA in all aspects of prostate cancer
diagnosis and treatment, and the potential extensive
use of sildenafil, it may be worth obtaining more
precise clarification that the PSA level is unaffected by
sildenafil therapy.

Intermittent endocrine therapy

The use of PSA to monitor treatment has led to
renewed interest in this therapeutic approach. This
treatment is based on the hypothesis that androgen
replacement at the end of a period of apoptotic regression may enable stem cells to differentiate and thus
become androgen-dependent. Akakura and colleagues
(103) reported the effects of intermittent androgen suppression therapy in four men with stage C and three
men with stage D prostate cancer. When the PSA level
was in the normal range after 6 months treatment,
treatment was interrupted for 2–11 months. Androgen
withdrawal was restarted when the PSA level increased
to about 20 ng/ml. This cycle was subsequently
repeated. Further studies are needed to assess whether
PSA can usefully monitor tumor progression in patients
with this intermittent therapeutic approach.

Hormone refractory prostate cancer

Metastatic prostate cancer usually shows regression
with androgen-ablation therapy but most patients with

metastatic prostate cancer will suffer a relapse because of androgen-independent tumor growth. The median period for this relapse is 12–18 months, with a median survival of about 3 years. Prostate tumors represent a heterogeneous group of cell patterns. The cell death induced by androgen treatment is incomplete and ultimately with treatment, cells with androgen-independent tumor growth become selected, i.e. the tumor becomes 'hormone refractory prostate cancer'. Various studies have explored the use of different aspects of PSA as a prognostic indicator of hormone refractory prostate cancer in an attempt to identify which patients with hormone refractory prostate cancer may benefit from further treatment, and to establish whether PSA response is a valid surrogate end-point. Pretreatment PSA, time to reach PSA nadir, percentage decrease in PSA with treatment, and PSA doubling times are some of the parameters currently under consideration. Absolute PSA levels have not been useful as PSA expression by the tumor may alter during treatment, and there may be alterations in protein binding rather than changes in tumor cell mass. Initial reports looked at pretreatment PSA levels as a threshold level for identifying patients with a poorer prognosis. An early study (104) identified that patients with hormone refractory prostate cancer with an initial pretreatment serum PSA level above 100 ng/ml had a significant decrease in survival. Some other studies have not confirmed this. Kelly and colleagues (105) looked at percentage change in PSA in hormone refractory prostate cancer and reported a significant improvement in survival in patients with a 50% decrease in PSA with treatment. Suramin directly modulates PSA release and another report PSA from phase I studies of suramin (106) demonstrated an increase in survival in patients with a greater than 50% decrease in PSA. The role of PSA levels is unclear in hormone refractory prostate cancer with no clear relation between serum PSA and clinical outcome, and no clear definition of response criteria. Further studies into the use of PSA in predicting outcome of hormone refractory prostate cancer are needed.

Conclusions

PSA has become the essential test in the investigation and management of patients with prostate cancer. New concepts, such as the use of PSAD, age-specific reference ranges, PSA velocity, free to total PSA ratios, coupled with technical developments in ultrasound

imaging, such as power Doppler, sonographic contrast agents, and second harmonic imaging, may improve the specificity of PSA as a diagnostic test in the next decade and decrease the number of benign biopsies performed, particularly for patients with intermediate PSA elevations in the 4–10 ng/ml range. The role of PSA in the follow-up of prostate cancer after treatment is well established and offers valuable prognostic information. A serum test that can be used for early diagnosis and will differentiate those prostate cancers that will progress clinically from those that are clinically indolent is however needed.

References

1. Dannull J, Belldegrun AS. Development of gene therapy for prostate cancer using a novel promoter of prostate-specific antigen. *Br J Urol* 1997, **79**, 97–103.
2. Yu H, Berkel H. Prostate-specific antigen (PSA) in women. *J La State Med Soc* 1999, **151**, 209–13.
3. Stamey TA. Some comments on progress in the standardization of immunoassays for prostate-specific antigen. *Br J Urol* 1997, **79**, 49–52.
4. Björk T, Bjartell A, Abrahamsson PA *et al*. Alpha-1-antichymotrypsin production in PSA-producing cells is common in prostate cancer but rare in benign prostatic hyperplasia. *Urology* 1994, **43**, 427–34.
5. Witherspoon LR. Early detection of cancer relapse after prostatectomy using very sensitive prostate-specific antigen measurements. *Br J Urol* 1997, **79**, 82–6.
6. Prestigiacomo AF, Stamey TA. Physiological variation of serum prostate specific antigen in the 4.0 to 10.0 ng/ml range in male volunteers. *J Urol* 1996, **155**, 1977–80.
7. Stamey TA, Yang N, Hay AR *et al*. Prostate-specific-antigen as a serum marker for adenocarcinoma of the prostate. *New Eng J Med* 1987, **317**, 909–16.
8. Leinonen J, Lovgren T, Vornanen T *et al*. Double label time resolved immunofluorometric assay of prostate-specific antigen and of its complex with alpha 1-antichymotrypsin. *Clinical Chemistry* 1993, **39**, 2098–103.
9. Simak R, Madersbacher S, Zhang ZF *et al*. The impact of ejaculation on serum prostate specific antigen. *J Urol* 1993, **150**, 895–7.
10. Tchetgen MB, Song JT, Strawderman M *et al*. Ejaculation increases the serum prostate-specific antigen concentration. *Urology* 1996, **478**, 511–6.
11. Collins GN, Martin PJ, Wynn-Davies A *et al*. The effect of digital rectal examination, flexible cystoscopy and prostatic biopsy on free and total prostate specific antigen and free-to-total prostate specific antigen ratio in clinical practice. *J Urol* 1997, **157**, 1744–7.
12. Nadler RB, Humphrey PA, Smith DS *et al*. Effect of inflammation and benign prostatic hyperplasia on elevated serum prostate-specific antigen levels. *J Urol* 1995, **154**, 407–13.

13. Tchetgen MB, Wojno KJ, Oesterling JE *et al.* The effect of a short course of antibiotics on the serum PSA concentration. *J Urol* 1996, **155**, 425A.

14. Semjonow A, Roth S, Hamm M *et al.* Re: Non traumatic elevation of prostate specific antigen following cardiac surgery and extracorporeal cardiopulmonary bypass. *J Urol* 1996, **155**, 295–6.

15. Cooper CS, Perry PJ, Sparks AET *et al.* Effect of exogenous testosterone on prostate volume, serum and semen prostate specific antigen levels in healthy young men. *J Urol* 1998, **159**, 441–3.

16. Finasteride (MK-906) in the treatment of benign prostatic hyperplasia. The finasteride study group. *Prostate* 1993, **22**, 291–9.

17. Oesterling JE, Roy J, Agha A, *et al.* Biologic variability of prostate-specific antigen and its usefulness as a marker for prostate cancer: effects of finasteride. Finasteride study group. *Urology* 1998, **51** (Suppl), 58–63.

18. Pannek J, Marks LS, Pearson JD *et al.* Influence of finasteride on free and total serum prostate specific antigen levels in men with benign prostatic hyperplasia. *J Urol* 1998, **159**, 449–53.

19. Roehrborn CG, Oesterling JE, Olson PJ *et al.* Serial prostate-specific antigen measurements in men with clinically benign prostatic hyperplasia during a 12-month placebo controlled study with terazosin. HYCAT Investigator Group. Hytrin community assessment trial. *Urology* 1997, **50**, 556–61.

20. Hagood PG, Parra RO, Rauscher JA. Non traumatic elevation of prostate specific antigen following cardiac surgery and extracorporeal cardiopulmonary bypass. *J Urol* 1994, **152**, 2043–5.

21. Djavan B, Shariat S, Ghawidel K *et al.* Impact of chronic dialysis on serum PSA, free PSA, and free/total PSA ratio: is prostate cancer detection compromised in patients receiving long term dialysis? *Urology* 1999, **53**, 1169–74.

22. Safford III HR, Crawford ED, Mackenzie SH *et al.* The effect of bicycle riding on serum prostate specific antigen levels. *J Urol* 1996, **156**, 103–5.

23. Leventhal EK, Rozanski TA, Morey AF *et al.* The effects of exercise and activity on serum PSA levels. *J Urol* 1993, **150**, 893–4.

24. Abrahamsson PA, Lilja H, Falkmer S *et al.* Immunohistochemical distribution of the three predominant secretory proteins in the parenchyma of hyperplastic and neoplastic prostate glands. *Prostate* 1988, **12**, 39–46.

25. Stamey TA, Kabalin JN. Prostate specific antigen in the diagnosis and treatment of adenocarcinoma of the prostate.I.Untreated patients. *J Urol* 1989, **141**, 1070–5.

26. Arcangeli CG, Ornstein DK, Keetch DW *et al.* Prostate-specific antigen as a screening test for prostate cancer. *Urol Clin N A* 1997, **24**, 299–306.

27. Clements R, Aideyan OU, Griffiths GJ *et al.* Side effects and patient acceptability of transrectal biopsy of the prostate. *Clin Rad* 1993, **47**, 125–6.

28. Norberg M, Holmberg L, Haggman M *et al.* Determinants of complications after multiple transrectal core biopsies of the prostate. *Eur Rad* 1996, **6**, 457–61.

29. Rodriguez LV, Terris MK. Risks and complications of transrectal ultrasound guided prostate needle biopsy; a prospective study and review of the literature. *J Urol* 1998, **160**, 2115–20.

30. Siegal JA, Yu E, Brawer MK. Topography of neovascularity in human prostate carcinoma. *Cancer* 1995, **75**, 2545–51.

31. Brewster SF, Rooney N, Kabala J *et al.* Fatal anaerobic infection following transrectal biopsy of a rare prostatic tumor. *Br J Urol* 1993, **77**, 977–8.

32. McNeal JE, Redwine EA, Freiha FS *et al.* Zonal distribution of prostatic adenocarcinoma. *Am J Surg Path* 1988, **12**, 897–906.

33. Lavoipierre AM, Snow RM, Frydenberg M *et al.* Prostatic cancer: role of color Doppler imaging in transrectal sonography. *Am J Radiol* 1998, **171**, 205–10.

34. Ellis WJ, Brawer MK. The significance of isoechoic prostate cancer. *J Urol* 1994, **152**, 2304–7.

35. Hodge KK, McNeal JE, Terris MK *et al.* Random systematic versus directed ultrasound guided transrectal core biopsies of the prostate. *J Urol* 1989, **142**, 71–5.

36. Brossner C, Madersbacher S, Klinger HC *et al.* A comparative study of a double-line versus a fan-shaped technique for obtaining transrectal ultrasound-guided biopsies of the prostate. *Eur Urol* 1998, **33**, 556–61.

37. Chang JJ, Shinohara K, Bhargava V *et al.* Prospective evaluation of lateral biopsies of the peripheral zone for prostate cancer detection. *J Urol* 1998, **160**, 2111–4.

38. Eskew LA, Bare RL, McCullogh DL. Systematic 5 region prostate biopsy is superior to sextant method for diagnosing carcinoma of the prostate. *J Urol* 1997, **157**, 199–203.

39. Stamey TA, Dietrick DD, Issa MM. Large, organ confined, impalpable transition zone prostate cancer: association with metastatic levels of prostate specific antigen. *J Urol* 1993, **149**, 510–25.

40. Keetch DW, Catalona WJ. Prostatic transition zone biopsies in men with previous negative biopsies and persistently elevated serum prostate specific antigen values. *J Urol* 1995, **154**, 1795–7.

41. Onder AU, Yalcin V, Arar O *et al.* Impact of transition zone biopsies in detection and evaluation of prostate cancer. *Eur Urol* 1998, **33**, 542–8.

42. Ellis WJ, Brawer MK. Repeat prostate needle biopsy: who needs it? *J Urol* 1995, **153**, 1496–8.

43. Rabbani F, Stroumbakis N, Kava BR *et al.* Incidence and clinical significance of false-negative sextant prostate biopsies. *J Urol* 1998, **159**, 1247–50.

44. Nava L, Montorsi F, Consonni P *et al.* Results of a prospective randomised study comparing 6, 12, and 18 transrectal ultrasound guided sextant biopsies in patients with elevated PSA, normal DRE, and normal prostatic ultrasound. *J Urol* 1997, **157**, 59.

45. Vashi AR, Wojno KJ, Gillespie B *et al.* A model for the number of cores per prostate biopsy based on the patient age and prostate gland volume. *J Urol* 1998, **159**, 920–4.

46. Letran JL, Meyer GE, Loberiza FR *et al.* The effect of prostate volume on the yield of needle biopsy. *J Urol* 1998, **160**, 1718–21.

47. Rickards D, Gillams AR, Deng J *et al.* Do intravascular ultrasound Doppler contrast agents improve transrectal

ultrasound diagnosis of prostate cancer? *Radiology* 1998, **200**, 259.

48. Frauscher F, Helweg G, Strasser H *et al.* Contrast enhanced color Doppler ultrasound in the diagnostic evaluation of prostate cancer. *Eur Rad* 1999, **19** (Suppl 1), S18.

49. Benson MC, Whang IS, Pantuck A *et al.* Prostate specific antigen density: a means of distinguishing benign prostatic hyperplasia and prostate cancer. *J Urol* 1992, **147**, 815–6.

50. Seaman E, Whang M, Olsson CA *et al.* PSA density (PSAD): Role in patient evaluation and management. *Urol Clin N Am* 1993, **20**, 653–63.

51. Littrup PJ, Kane RA, Mettlin CJ *et al.* Cost-effective prostate cancer detection. Reduction of low-yield biopsies. Investigators of the American Cancer Society National Prostate Cancer Detection Project. *Cancer* 1994, **74**, 3146–58.

52. Recker F, Kwiatkowski MK, Pettersson K *et al.* Enhanced expression of prostate-specific antigen in the transition zone of the prostate. *Eur Urol* 1998, **33**, 549–55.

53. Lin DW, Gold MH, Ransom S *et al.* Transition zone prostate specific antigen density: lack of use in prediction of prostatic carcinoma. *J Urol* 1998, **160**, 77–82.

54. Oesterling JE, Jacobsen SJ, Chute CG *et al.* The establishment of age-specific reference ranges for prostate-specific antigen. *J Urol* 1993, **149**, 510A.

55. De Antonio EP, Crawford ED, Oesterling JE *et al.* Age and race specific reference ranges for prostate-specific antigen from a large community-based study. *Urology* 1996, **48**, 234–9.

56. Borer JG, Sherman J, Solomon MC *et al.* Age specific prostate specific antigen reference ranges: population specific. *J Urol* 1998, **159**, 444–8.

57. Pettaway J, Brawer MK. Age specific vs 4.0 ng/ml as PSA cutoff in the screening population. *J Urol* 1995, **153** (Suppl), 946A.

58. Catalona WJ, Hudson MA, Scardino PT *et al.* Selection of optimal prostate specific antigen cutoffs for early detection of prostate cancer: receiver operating characteristic curves. *J Urol* 1994, **152**, 2037–42.

59. Carter HB, Pearson JD, Metter J *et al.* Longitudinal evaluation of prostate-specific antigen levels in men with and without prostate disease. *JAMA* 1992, **267**, 2215–20.

60. Carter HB, Pearson JD. Prostate-specific antigen velocity and repeated measures of prostate-specific antigen. *Urol Clin N Am* 1997, **24**, 333–8.

61. Brawer MK, Beatie J, Wener MH *et al.* Screening for prostatic carcinoma with prostate specific antigen: results of the second year. *J Urol* 1993, **150**, 106–9.

62. Carter HB, Pearson JD, Waclawin Z *et al.* Prostate-specific antigen variability in men without prostate cancer: effect of sampling interval on prostate-specific antigen velocity. *Urology* 1995, **45**, 591–6.

63. Nam RK, Klotz LH, Jewett MA *et al.* Prostate specific antigen velocity as a measure of the natural history of prostate cancer: defining a 'rapid riser' subset. *Br J Urol* 1998, **81**, 100–4.

64. Woodrum DL, Brawer MK, Partin AW *et al.* Interpretation of free prostate specific antigen clinical research studies for the detection of prostate cancer. *J Urol* 1998, **159**, 5–12.

65. Lilja H, Christensson A, Dahlén U *et al.* Prostate-specific antigen in serum occurs predominantly in complex with α1-antichymotrypsin. *Clinical Chemistry* 1991, **37**, 1618–25.

66. Catalona WJ, Smith DS, Wolfert RL *et al.* Evaluation of percentage of free serum prostate-specific antigen to improve specificity of prostate cancer screening. *JAMA* 1995, **274**, 1214–20.

67. Luderer AA, Chen Y, Soriano TF *et al.* Measurement of the proportion of free to total prostate-specific antigen improves diagnostic performance of prostate-specific antigen in the diagnostic gray zone of total prostate-specific antigen. *Urology* 1995, **46**, 187–94.

68. Oesterling JE, Jacobsen SJ, Klee GG *et al.* Free, complexed and total serum prostate specific antigen: The establishment of appropriate reference ranges for their concentrations and ratios. *J Urol* 1995, **154**, 1090–5.

69. Beduschi MC, Oesterling JE. Percent free prostate-specific antigen: the next frontier in prostate-specific antigen testing. *Urology* 1998, **51**, 98–109.

70. Catalona WJ, Partin AW, Slawin KM *et al.* Use of the percentage of free prostate-specific antigen to enhance differentiation of prostate cancer from benign prostatic disease. *JAMA* 1998, **279**, 1542–7.

71. Vashi AR, Wojno KJ, Henricks WH *et al.* Determination of the 'reflex range' and appropriate cutpoints for percent free PSA in 413 men referred for prostatic evaluation using the AxSYM system. *Urology* 1997, **49**, 19–27.

72. Mettlin C, Chesley AE, Murphy GP *et al.* Association of free PSA percent, total PSA, age, and gland volume in the detection of prostate cancer. *Prostate* 1999, **39**, 153–8.

73. Tornblom M, Norming U, Adolfsson J *et al.* Diagnostic value of percent free prostate-specific antigen: retrospective analysis of a population-based screening study with emphasis on men with PSA levels less than 3.0 ng/ml. *Urology* 1999, **53**, 945–50.

74. Israeli RS, Grob M, Fair WR. Prostate-specific membrane antigen and other prostatic tumor markers on the horizon. *Urol Clin N Am* 1997, **24**, 439–50.

75. Murphy GP, Holmes EH, Boynton AL *et al.* Comparison of prostate-specific antigen, prostate-specific membrane antigen and LNCaP-based enzyme linked immunosorbent assays in prostatic cancer patients and patients with benign prostatic enlargement. *Prostate* 1995, **26**, 164–8.

76. Murphy GP, Elgamamal A-AA, Su SL *et al.* Current evaluation of the tissue localization and diagnostic utility of prostate specific membrane antigen. *Cancer* 1998, **83**, 2259–69.

77. Murphy GP, Barren RJ, Erikson SJ *et al.* Evaluation and comparison of two new prostate carcinoma markers. *Cancer* 1996, **78**, 809–18.

78. Murphy GP, Maguire RT, Rogers B *et al.* Comparison of serum PSMA, PSA levels with results of Cytogen-356 ProstatScint scanning in prostatic cancer patients. *Prostate* 1997, **33**, 281–5.

79. Sodee DB, Ellis RJ, Samuels MA *et al.* Prostate cancer and prostate bed SPECT imaging with ProstaScint:

semiquantitative correlation with prostatic biopsy results. *Prostate* 1998, **37**, 140–8.

80. Smith DS, Catalona WJ. The nature of prostate cancer detected through prostate specific antigen based screening. *J Urol* 1994, **152**, 1732–6.

81. Lee CT, Oesterling JE. Using prostate-specific antigen to eliminate the staging radionuclide bone scan. *Urol Clin N Am* 1997, **24**, 389–94.

82. Chybowski FM, Larson-Keller JJ, Bergstrahl EJ *et al.* Predicting radionuclide bone scan findings in patients with newly diagnosed, untreated prostate cancer: Prostate specific antigen is superior to all other parameters. *J Urol* 1991, **145**, 313–8.

83. Oesterling JE, Martin SK, Bergstrahl EJ *et al.* The use of prostate-specific antigen in staging patients with newly diagnosed prostate cancer. *JAMA* 1993, **269**, 57–60.

84. Sissons GRJ, Clements R, Peeling WB *et al.* Can serum prostate -specific antigen replace bone scintigraphy in the follow-up of metatstatic prostate cancer? *Br J Radiol* 1992, **65**, 861–4.

85. Levran Z, Gonzalez JA, Diokno AC *et al.* Are pelvic computed tomography, bone scan and pelvic lymphadenectomy necessary in the staging of prostatic cancer? *Br J Urol* 1995, **75**, 778–81.

86. Miller PD, Eardley I, Kirby RS. Prostate specific antigen and bone scan correlation in the staging and monitoring of patients with prostate cancer. *Br J Urol* 1992, **70**, 295–8.

87. Spencer JA, Chng WJ, Hudson E *et al.* Prostate specific antigen level and Gleason score in predicting the stage of newly diagnosed prostate cancer. *Br J Radiol* 1998, **71**, 1130–5.

88. Noldus J, Graefen M, Huland E *et al.* The value of the ratio of free-to-total prostate specific antigen for staging purposes in previously untreated prostate cancer. *J Urol* 1998, **159**, 2004–8.

89. Pousette A, Carlstrom K, Tribukait B *et al.* Prostate-specific antigen in tissue from fine-needle aspiration biopsies. *Br J Urol* 1997, **79** (Suppl), 104–6.

90. Stamey TA, Ferrari MK, Schmid HP. The value of serial prostate-specific antigen determinations 5 years after radiotherapy. *J Urol* 1994, **152**, 492–5.

91. Schmid HP, Semjonow A, Maibach R. Prostate-specific antigen doubling time: a potential surrogate end point in hormone-refractory prostate cancer. *J Clin Oncol* 1999, **17**, 1645–6.

92. van Strahlen J, Bossens M, de Reijke T *et al.* Biological half-life of prostate specific antigen after radical prostatectomy. *Eur J Clin Chem Clin Biochem* 1994, **32**, 53–5.

93. Pound CR, Partin AW, Eisenberger MA *et al.* Natural history of progression after PSA elevation following radical prostatectomy. *JAMA* 1999, **281**, 1591–7.

94. Oefelein MG, Smith N, Carter M *et al.* The incidence of prostate cancer progression with undetectable serum prostate specific antigen in a series of 394 radical prostatectomies. *J Urol* 1995, **154**, 2128–31.

95. Zagars G, Pollack A. The fall and rise of prostate-specific antigen: kinetics of serum prostate-specific antigen levels after radiation therapy for prostate cancer. *Cancer* 1993, **72**, 832–42.

96. Kavadi V, Zagars G, Pollack A. Serum prostate-specific antigen after radiation therapy for clinically localized prostate cancer: Prognostic implications. *International Journal of Radiation Oncology Biology and Physics* 1994, 30, 279–281.

97. Zeitman AL, Tibbs M, Dallow KC *et al.* Use of PSA nadir to predict subsequent biochemical outcome following external beam radiation therapy for T1–2 adenocarcinoma of the prostate. *Radiother Oncol* 1996, **40**, 159–62.

98. Shipley WU, Thames HD, Sandler HM *et al.* Radiation therapy for clinically localised prostate cancer: a multi-institutional pooled analysis. *JAMA* 1999, **281**, 1598–604.

99. ASTRO Consensus Statement. Guidelines for PSA following radiation therapy. *Int J Rad Oncol Biol Physics* 1997, **37**, 1035–41.

100. Grob BM, Schellhammer PF, Brassil D *et al.* Changes in the immunohistochemical staining of PSA, PAP, and TURP-27 following irradiation therapy for clinically localized prostate cancer. *Urology* 1994, **44**, 525–29.

101. Zelefsky MJ, McKee AB, Lee H *et al.* Efficacy of oral sildenafil in patients with erectile dysfunction after radiotherapy for carcinoma of the prostate. *Urology* 1999, **53**, 775–8.

102. Merrick GS, Butler WM, Lief JH *et al.* Efficacy of sildenafil citrate in prostate brachytherapy patients with erectile dysfunction. *Urology* 1999, **53**, 1112–6.

103. Akakura K, Bruchovsky N, Goldenberg SL *et al.* Effects of intermittent androgen suppression on androgen-dependent tumors. *Cancer* 1993, **71**, 2782–90.

104. Fossa SD, Paus E, Lindegaard M *et al.* Prostate-specific antigen and other prognostic factors in patients with hormone-resistant prostate cancer undergoing experimental treatment. *Br J Urol* 1992, **69**, 175–9.

105. Kelly WK, Scher HI, Mazumdar M *et al.* Prostate-specific antigen as a measure of disease outcome in metastatic hormone-refractory prostate cancer. *J Clin Oncol* 1993, **11**, 607–15.

106. Sridhara R, Eisenberger MA, Sinibaldi VJ *et al.* Evaluation of prostate-specific antigen as a surrogate marker for response of hormone refractory prostate cancer to suramin therapy. *J Clin Oncol* 1995, **13**, 2944–53.

Section IV

16 | Radical prostatectomy in the management of localized prostate cancer

David L. Shepherd, Michael Harris, and Ian Thompson

Introduction

With carcinoma of the prostate having achieved the status of the most common cancer in US men, and with the majority of currently diagnosed prostate cancers being clinically localized, the importance of surgical extirpation of the disease has grown. Evidence is growing that a substantial number of men diagnosed at this time derive substantial benefit from treatment and that, of all treatments available, radical prostatectomy offers the highest likelihood of long-term, disease-free survival. In this chapter, we will provide the background for the efficacy of prostate cancer early detection, for treatment with radical prostatectomy, and thereafter, technical details regarding both radical retropubic and perineal prostatectomy.

Evidence of the efficacy of early diagnosis and treatment

With the advent of PSA screening, a phenomenon that increased substantially between 1987 and 1990, the US witnessed a major increase in disease incidence. In the SEER tumor registry system, disease incidence increased from 84.4/100 000 population to 163/100 000 population between the years 1984 and 1991. The incidence rate in Utah reached a high in 1992 of 236.2/100 000 population (1). Several interesting observations have resulted from this natural experiment. First was that the tumors detected were not the so-called 'autopsy tumors', tumors that were noted incidentally at the time of death in a majority of men. These autopsy tumors were generally of microscopic dimensions and well-differentiated. A number of authors have found that the volume of tumors detected through PSA screening is dramatically larger than these autopsy tumors (almost certainly as needle biopsies

only sample a fraction of the gland) and that the vast majority (> 90%) of tumors are moderately or poorly differentiated (1, 2).

Shortly after the recognition of a major increase in the detection of clinically-significant prostate cancer with PSA screening, the observation was made that a shift was occurring in tumor stage. While previous reports had noted that many patients were found with pathologically-advanced prostate cancer, the rate of pT3 (pathologically-advanced) disease was falling. From the Washington University screening series, Smith reported the results of annual PSA screening in 10 248 healthy, community-dwelling men (1). Over a period of 4 years, the rate of pathologically advanced disease fell from 33% to 27%. A similar result was noted at Stanford University where, between 1988 and 1996 with PSA screening, the rate of patients with seminal vesicle invasion fell from 18% to 5%, the rate of positive margins from 30% to 14%, and the rate of organ confined disease rose from 40% to 75% (1).

The next step witnessed in the natural experiment of PSA screening was a dramatic fall in prostate cancer incidence. Such was not unexpected as a sensitive screening test had not been available prior to 1987. Once men with the disease in the general population were diagnosed, the total numbers of men diagnosed annually fell precipitously. In Utah, where a dramatic increase in incidence was initially seen, the incidence rate fell from 236.2/100 000 in 1992 to 195 and 164/100 000 population during the subsequent two years (1).

Probably the best evidence of the efficacy of PSA screening has been demonstrated by a fall in prostate cancer mortality. This fall in mortality has been realized in several geographic regions—only those where PSA screening has been operational—and includes Olmsted County, Minnesota, Canada, and the SEER regions of the United States (1–4). While in the absence of a randomized, prospective controlled study (currently being conducted, PLCO: the Prostate, Lung, Colorectal, and Ovarian Cancer Screening Study of the National Cancer Institute), definite evidence of the effectiveness of prostate cancer screening is not conclusively demonstrated, these data presented above provide a compelling rationale for the early detection and treatment of this disease.

Who is the optimal patient for therapy?

Whitmore first coined the paradigm that the patient for whom therapy is indicated has a tumor that both *requires treatment* and *can be cured*. Regarding the first half of the paradigm, if the tumor is destined to do well over the patients life-expectancy, treatment would be unnecessary. Regarding the second, if the disease is so advanced as to make treatment only an academic exercise, treatment is also unnecessary as it will be ineffective. Factors that should be considered when selecting a patient for radical prostatectomy are described below.

Age

The optimal patient for treatment of prostate cancer is a man who is at risk of disease progression and death over the course of his lifetime. Albertsen, in a study of patients with prostate cancer who were followed without treatment, found that in most patients, death from disease occurred after 10–15 years following diagnosis. Thus, with the exception of men who may have very aggressive tumors (for whom treatment may be unsuccessful and therefore unnecessary), it is only a man with a 10-year or more life-expectancy for whom screening and treatment will be beneficial (5). For a man in his 50s, screening and treatment is therefore very reasonable. For the average man in his late 70s, treatment may be unnecessary. However, the physician should carefully examine the older man. We have been disappointed on many an occasion after witnessing disease recurrence and progression in men over age 70, in whom non-aggressive initial therapy was elected merely because of the patient's age.

PSA

One of the most powerful predictors of outcome of treatment is PSA. PSA relates to a number of factors regarding

the tumor. It is an excellent surrogate for tumor volume and therefore also relates directly to the likelihood of positive margins, seminal vesicle invasion, nodal disease, and metastatic disease. Assuming that metastatic disease has been ruled out by a normal radioisotopic bone scan, PSA can be used successfully to predict which man will require pelvic lymph node dissection. At both Washington University and Johns Hopkins University, institutions with very large series of patients treated with radical prostatectomy, PSA predicted the likelihood of disease progression. At Washington University, 7-year progression-free survivals were 93% (PSA < 2.5 ng/ml), 80% (PSA 2.5–4.0 ng/ml), 76% (PSA 4.0–10.0 ng/ml), and 40% for PSA values > 10.0 ng/ml (1). Results at 10 years at Hopkins were 87% (0–4 ng/ml), 75% (4–10 ng/ml), 30% (10–20 ng/ml), and 28% (> 20 ng/ml). Thus, the optimal candidate for radical prostatectomy has a PSA < 10 ng/ml. Patients with higher PSA values should be counseled regarding the high likelihood of the need for adjuvant therapy (6–9).

Tumor grade

Differentiation of prostate cancer is a powerful predictor of the outcome of radical prostatectomy in every series that has been reported. While results with well-differentiated tumors are excellent, high failure rates have been observed with patients who have poorly differentiated tumors. It must be realized, however, that many patients with such poorly differentiated disease have overt metastases identified prior to radical prostatectomy—either positive bone scans, positive pelvic lymph node dissections, or palpable evidence (e.g. seminal vesicles) of extraprostatic extension. Nevertheless, several large series have presented durable, excellent long-term, disease-free survivals—even in men with high-grade disease. One such example is the Washington University series that has reported a 48% progression-free survival at 7 years of follow-up (10–12). The question of how to manage the patient with well-differentiated disease is difficult to answer. Certainly, the older patient with low-volume, well-differentiated disease (e.g. T1a disease) is probably best managed expectantly. However, the young man with low-grade disease has a substantial risk of disease progression—both in stage and in grade—and may be best managed early and definitively with surgical extirpation.

Clinical stage

In general, digital rectal examination is a poor predictor of ultimate clinical stage. We have found, for example, that in the years prior to PSA, tumors that were felt to be organ-confined by DRE, were more likely to have extra-prostatic spread than to be organ-confined (13). However, it is generally the case that if extra-prostatic disease is appreciated on DRE, in excess of 75% of the time, pathologic staging will confirm that the disease is not organ-confined. Thus, the optimal candidate for radical prostatectomy should have no evidence of palpable seminal vesicle or extra-prostatic tumor extension.

What is the best method of radical prostatectomy?

At our institutions, we have found that the results of radical prostatectomy are quite similar, whether performed retropubically or perineally. Unfortunately, most urologic surgeons are facile with one or the other procedure and this technical detail generally determines the approach. However, for some surgeons who are equally comfortable and skilled in both approaches, there are some features that may make one or the other a better choice for an individual patient.

Patient *habitus*

In general, an obese patient has better access to the perineum than via the retropubic approach. Pre-operatively, the patient should be examined closely as, on occasion, an obese patient has a high-riding prostate that is not amenable to perineal prostatectomy.

Gland size

A prostate larger than 60–80 g can be difficult to remove intact via a perineal approach. While not an absolute contra-indication, we prefer to perform a retropubic prostatectomy on such patients.

Risk of positive nodes

In general, we recommend perineal prostatectomy for men with a < 3–5% risk of positive lymph nodes. We and others have developed nomograms for this purpose and we use these to assist in patient counseling to determine whether node dissection is necessary or appropriate (14). For patients with a greater risk of nodal disease, we generally recommend a retropubic approach with simultaneous lymphadenectomy. On

occasion, however, an educated patient with a higher risk of nodal disease may opt for a perineal approach to reduce the post-operative recovery time. We have been concerned in such patients, however, about decision-making related to the management of PSA recurrences and the risk of radiating a prostatic fossa when nodal involvement is present. In general, using our approach, about half of patients undergo a perineal prostatectomy and half a retropubic approach.

Other considerations

In general, a perineal prostatectomy results in a more rapid patient recovery. A majority of patients are discharged within 24 h and it is a rare patient who cannot return to work within a few days. Most require minimal to no post-operative analgesia. We have been impressed that urinary continence seems to return more quickly with this approach and that potency is no different than with the retropubic approach. On the other hand, rectal injury has traditionally been higher with the perineal approach and, through a series of investigations, we have found that a small subset of patients will complain of some degree of fecal incontinence following perineal prostatectomy (3).

Nerve-sparing radical retropubic prostatectomy

Patient selection

The ideal candidate for a nerve-sparing radical retropubic candidate is determined by pre-operative and intra-operative criteria. The patient must be potent pre-operatively and wish to be potent post-operatively (10). Ideally, the patient should be younger than 60 years of age. Post-operative potency is best in this age group; up to a 75% potency rate can be achieved by sparing both nerves in these men (11). This is in contrast to a 48% potency rate in older men undergoing unilateral nerve-sparring procedure (11). Pre-operative clinical staging should indicate localized prostate cancer and a life expectancy of ten years or greater.

The anatomical margin for technical error between the cavernosal nerves and prostate cancer is, at best, 3–4 mm (10). In addition, the earliest signs of extra-prostatic cancer extension appear along these nerves where they penetrate the prostate capsule (12). Surgeons must therefore incorporate all available clinical staging tools to thoughtfully select candidates with localized cancer and exercise precise technical skill in order to avoid a positive margin of resection and preserve potency.

The most basic clinical staging criterion are the patient's total serum PSA, biopsy Gleason score, and findings of the digital rectal examination. Partin combined these criterion to construct his nomogram that is widely used to estimate the probability of extra-prostatic cancer. Based on this nomogram, the ideal candidate for a nerve-sparing radical prostatectomy would have a serum PSA less than 10 ng/dl, a Gleason score less than 8, and a benign digital rectal examination (13).

While a low PSA and Gleason score are preferred, each of these criteria considered individually, however, are only guidelines to select the appropriate candidate for a nerve-sparing procedure. Serum PSA elevations are not cancer-specific and partially represent benign prostate processes such as hypertrophy and inflammation. A biopsy Gleason score greater than 7, however, is a reasonably specific indicator of a high-grade cancer in the prostate. Steinberg found an 87% correlation between a high-grade cancer on biopsy and the radical prostatectomy specimen. These high-grade tumors are significantly associated with a higher incidence of a positive margin (14–16).

A prostate nodule should lead the surgeon to intra-operatively consider a wide excision of the ipsilateral neurovascular bundle (NVB). This finding in itself, however, does not pre-operatively mandate excision of the NVB, as it is an unreliable indicator of the location of cancer in the prostate. Eggleston and Walsh reported that over 80% of patients with a unilateral prostate nodule had cancer in both lobes of the resected prostate. By routinely excising the NVB ipsilateral to a prostate nodule, Smith *et al.* demonstrated a 10% reduction of positive margins. We recommend particular caution in sparing a NVB on the side of an apical prostate nodule because positive margins are most common at the prostate apex and the NVB is most intimately associated with the prostate at this location (8, 9). If the NVB appears fixed during the apical dissection and does not easily separate from the prostate capsule, suspect peri-neural invasion and widely excise that bundle (17–19).

Particular caution is also recommended when sparing the NVB on the prostate side where peri-neural invasion was identified on the prostate biopsy. When present, peri-neural invasion is a strong indicator of extra-prostatic disease and a independent predictor of eventual biochemical failure (4, 5, 6). When the NVB

ipsilateral to biopsy demonstrated peri-neural invasion is resected, Epstein reported a 17% reduction in the incidence of positive margins (7).

Through careful pre-operative patient selection and precise operative technique, a nerve-sparing prostatectomy can achieve complete excision of prostate cancer in 64% of patients (20). Bilateral nerve-sparing procedures can preserve potency rate of 68% of men without increasing the incidence of positive margins (16, 17, 18, 20). Patients with partial or complete impotence following a bilateral nerve-sparing prostatectomy can expect an excellent response to sildenafil. Zippe demonstrated an 80% potency and partner satisfaction rate in these patients (21).

Technique

The nerve-sparing radical prostatectomy as initially described by Walsh is now widely employed and has been modified by several leading experts (22). The below description of the operation is such a modification.

Patient preparation

Blood transfusions

Advances in technique and improved understanding of the peri-prostatic venous anatomy have limited the average blood loss to approximately 600 cm^3. The frequency of blood transfusions at most centers have accordingly declined. A blood transfusion can generally be avoided if the blood loss is < 1000 cm^3. The experience of the surgeon is a key factor determining the average blood loss. If a surgeon's average loss is > 1000 cm^3, alternatives to heterogeneic blood transfusions such as pre-operative autologous blood banking and acute normovolemic hemodilution should be considered.

Bowel preparation

A rectal injury is encountered during a retropubic prostatectomy in < 3% of cases (23, 24). One prefers an operative field that is clear of gross contamination in the event of such an injury. We therefore typically ask our patients to adhere to a clear liquid diet 24 h before surgery and administer an enema the evening before and morning of surgery. A formal antibiotic and mechanical bowel prep is not employed. In the rare event of a rectal injury, it is closed primarily in two layers with 2.0 absorbable suture. We separate this repair from the vesico-urethral anastamosis by an interposing pad of fat. Such management has resulted in no fistula or post-operative wound infections.

Peri-operative antibiotics

An oral fluoroquinalone is started the morning of surgery and continued post-operatively until the pelvic drain is removed. This regimen is clinically effective and more economical than parental antibiotics. After drain removal, the patient is kept off antibiotics until the day before the catheter is removed. We then start an 8-day course of a broad spectrum antibiotic.

Patient position

The patient is flexed at the lumbar region to expose the retropubic space. Abducting the patient's legs in stirrups allows the assistant to apply perineal pressure with a sponge stick and expose the urethral stump during the placement of anastomotic sutures or areas of venous bleeding for hemostasis. We experienced a less than 1% incidence of deep venous thrombosis and no cases of nerve palsies with this positioning. Many surgeons, however, find perineal pressure can be satisfactorily applied with the patient in a supine position without leg abduction.

Prostate apex and urethra exposure

The endo-pelvic fascia

The endopelvic fascia is exposed through a midline infra-umbilical extra-peritoneal incision and the aid of a Balfor retractor with a malleable center blade. Use a sponge-stick to retract the prostate medially and place this fascia on tension. Enter the peri-prostatic space by popping through the fascia approximately 4 mm lateral to the prostate surface with the Metz scissor tips. An incision that is more medial risks opening the peri-prostatic venous plexus. An incision that is too lateral will damage the musculature of the lateral pelvic sidewall and result in hemorrhage that is very difficult to control. Expose the base of the prostate by extending this incision posteriorly to the rectum and anteriorly to the insertion of the pubo-prostatic ligament. Exercise caution to avoid the veins behind this fascial plane. If such a vein is encountered, carefully ligate it. Next,

buff the prostate by sweeping all strands of pelvic sidewall muscles off with a clean Kippner. Insert your finger to palpate the urethra. Pack a #10 sponge in this space and dissect the contra-lateral peri-prostatic space in an identical fashion.

The pubo-prostatic ligaments

Preservation of the pubo-prostatic ligaments is felt to promote a more rapid return of post-operative continence. The ultimate continence achieved through the preservation of these ligaments is not, however, superior to the rates published for patient that have had these ligaments divided. Sacrificing these ligaments affords a more secure tie on the dorsal venous complex (DVC). We therefore routinely divide these ligaments by pressing the prostate posteriorly with a sponge-stick and cutting them as close to their pubic bone insertion as possible. If these ligaments are short and intimately associated with the DVC, however, it is far better to preserve them and proceed directly to securing the DVC than prematurely injuring the complex and suffering excess blood loss.

Securing the dorsal venous complex

Control of the DVC begins by placing several 2.0 monofilament sutures on a UR-5 needle to secure the veins that aphorize over the anterior and lateral aspects of the prostate in a manner originally described by Meyers (25). Next, face the anesthesiologist and pinch the complex with your left hand to develop the groove between it and the urethra. Pass the right-angle clamp through this groove to pass a #1 vicryl suture around the DVC. Establish proximal control by securing this suture as close to the urogenital diaphragm as possible (Fig. 16.1).

Dividing the dorsal venous complex

Replace the right-angle clamp anterior to the urethra and stretch the DVC over the opened tips of this clamp by pressing prostate base down with a sponge-stick. Divide the DVC with electrocautery to expose the urethra. A pair of forceps and a 0-chromic suture on a UR-5 needle should be readily available to compress and over-sew the cut edges of the DVC if the proximal tie is lost at this time.

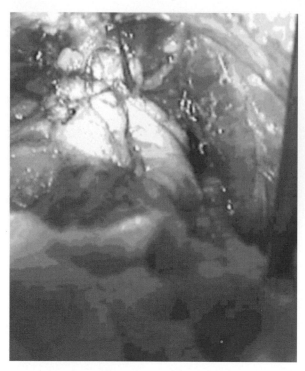

Fig. 16.1 View into the pelvis of the dorsal venous complex tie from the head of the table.

The apical dissection

Urethral dissection and division

Apply cephalad traction to the prostate to expose the apex. Sharply dissect away peri-urethral muscle fibers inserting onto the anterior prostate apex. Place a right-angle clamp between the urethra and recto-urethralis muscle and elevate the urethra. Incise the anterior and lateral aspects of the urethra without injuring the catheter. A balance between leaving the longest possible urethral stump to preserve continence and ensuring an adequate surgical margin can be met by planning this incision approximately 4 mm distal from the prostate apex. Next, expose the posterior urethra by lifting the catheter away with a second right-angle clamp to complete the urethral division.

Urethral anastomotic sutures

Many surgeons feel that the urethra is maximally exposed before it is completely divided and prefer to place their proximal anastomotic sutures at that time.

We find it equally easy to expose the urethra by applying perineal pressure after the prostate is completely removed. This keeps the urethral safe from injury by inadvertent traction on the anastomotic sutures during the remainder of the operation.

Division of the catheter

We routinely preserve the majority of the catheter length and use it to apply gentle traction to the prostate apex while sparing the cavernosal nerves. To do this, occlude the balloon port by clamping the intra-pelvic portion of the catheter with a right-angle clamp. Divide the catheter as it exits the penis and pull the cut catheter end into the pelvis. Apply a Kelly clamp to this end and remove the right-angle clamp.

Division of the recto-urethralis muscle

Apply gentle cephalad and posterior pressure to the anterior prostate. The recto-urethalis muscle should be obvious as it extends from the rhabdosphincter and inserts onto the apex of the prostate. Two methods of dividing this muscle are equally effective and should be specifically tailored to each patient's unique anatomy. For a thick recto-urethralis muscle, we prefer to insert the tips of a delicate right-angle clamp under the lateral borders of this muscle band and elevate it from the underlying cavernosal nerves and pre-rectal fat. For a patient with a thin recto-urethralis muscle, this maneuver is not as necessary and we directly divide this muscle with Metz scissors in the midline until the lemon-yellow pre-rectal fat is encountered. The cavernosal nerves abut the lateral borders of this muscle.

Sparing the cavernosal nerves

The anterior lateral pelvic fascia

The cavernosal nerves course along the posterio-lateral aspects of the prostate and are confined to this space by the anterior and posterior divisions of the lateral pelvic fascia. To liberate these bundles, most surgeon start by sharply dissecting the anterior pelvic fascia off of the prostate. It is often easiest to divide this fascia after elevating the proximal edge where it folds over the prostate base with a right-angle clamp. Continue the dissection sharply to the prostate apex. The cavernosal nerves should fall away laterally.

The posterior lateral pelvic fascia

Next, identify the point where the neurovascular bundle courses from the prostate apex to the urogenital diaphragm. At this point separate each bundle from the prostate by dividing the posterior fascia. This will release the bundles laterally and keep both layers of Denovier's fascia on the posterior aspect of the prostate as an additional margin.

Liberating the cavernosal neurovascular bundle

Use the urethral catheter to apply gentle counter traction anterolaterally to the prostate and continue liberating the bundle in a retrograde fashion. Apply small clips in parallel with the bundle to control obvious veins draining into the prostate as described by Walsh during this dissection (22). It is essential to keep tension on each bundle to a minimum during this dissection. For this reason, begin liberating the contralateral bundle before completing liberating the nerve from one side. Continue the dissection by alternating the dissection between the right and left sides until the level of the seminal vesicals are reached. Pack the pelvis at this point to tamponade venous bleeding during the remainder of the operation.

Securing the vascular pedicles and the seminal vesical dissection

Retract the prostate upward to expose Denovier's fascia covering the seminal vesicals. We divide Denovier's fascia approximately 10 mm below the prostate base to expose the seminal vesicals. The prostate vascular pedicles are at the lateral ends of this incision. These are controlled with #1 Vicryl ties and divided until the plane between the seminal vesicals and the bladder is encountered. We next expose the medial aspects of the seminal vesicals by isolation and division of the ampullae of the vas deferens. Dissection of each seminal vesical thereafter centers on identifying, clipping, and dividing the seminal vesical arteries as they enter the tips and mid-lateral aspects (Fig. 16.2).

Sparing the bladder neck

We routinely favor preservation of the circular bladder neck musculature in patients that have not had a previous transurethral resection of the prostate. Preservation

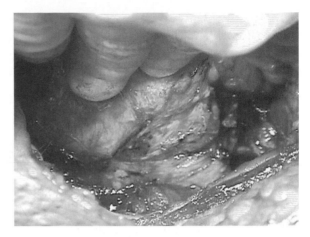

Fig. 16.2 View of prostate retracted. Denovier's fascia is open, exposing the seminal vesicals prior to securing the lateral vascular pedicle.

of this 'internal sphincter' has been demonstrated to promote a more rapid return of post-operative continence (24). The ultimate continence rates achieved with or without bladder neck sparing are ultimately the same.

To spare the bladder neck, retract the prostate upward and away from the bladder. It is easiest to initially identify the proper plane posteriorly behind the seminal vesicals. Continue this plane laterally and progressively spiral around the prostate sharply or with the electrocautery until the funnel of the bladder neck is obvious. At this point, remove the catheter and sharply separate the prostate from the bladder.

Pelvic hemostasis

Expose the pelvis by placing the bladder neck behind the malleable center blade. Systematically remove the pelvic packs and inspect the seminal vesical fossae, lateral pelvic vascular pedicles, cavernosal bundles, genito-urinary diaphragm, and DVC for bleeding. Use the least number of 4-0 chromic sutures and strictly avoid electrocautery to control bleeding from the cavernosal bundles.

The anastomosis

Place a 16 french Robnel urethral catheter and apply perineal pressure with a sponge stick to expose the urethral stump. We use a 2-0 absorbable monofilament suture on a UR-6 to place four quadrant sutures at the 2, 5, 7, and 10 o'clock position. For easy placement of

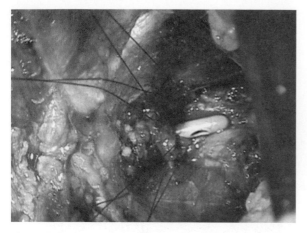

Fig. 16.3 Surgeon's view of the urethra with the anastamotic sutures in place.

these sutures, position yourself so that you face the anesthesiology screen and orient the needle driver perpendicular to the floor. We prefer to pass the needle from within the urethral to ensure that mucosa and an adequate amount of urethral wall is anchored in these stitches. Replace the Robnel with an 18 french silastic 30 cm^3 balloon catheter after placing all four sutures (Fig. 16.3).

Thread a free SH needle on the end of each proximal anastamotic sutures to secure the corresponding bladder neck sutures. Simultaneously anchor this stitch in the circular bladder neck fibers and avert the bladder mucosa. This reliably results in strong and expeditious mucosa–mucosa re-anastomosis. Insert the catheter into the bladder neck and inflate the balloon to hold it in the bladder. Securely tie the anastamotic sutures and place a closed-suction pelvic drain (Fig. 16.4).

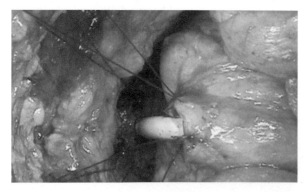

Fig. 16.4 Surgeon's view of the catheter stenting the urethrovesical anastamosis prior to securing the sutures.

Post-operative management

Pain control

The replacement of narcotic-based patient-controlled analgesia and epidurals with ketorolac has resulted in a dramatic decrease in post-radical prostatectomy patient discomfort, length of hospitalization, and cost of care (27). We use ketorolac in all patients without renal compromise, a history of peptic ulcer disease, or sensitivity to this agent. We recommend 30 mg intravenously at the time of wound closure followed by 15 mg intravenously every 6 h for the first 48 h. Thereafter, we prefer 15 mg of intravenous ketorolac or 1000 mg of acetaminophen for incisional pain over oral narcotics.

Drain management

Keep the pelvic drain in place until the output decreases to < 50 cm^3 per hour for 16 consecutive hours. The urethral catheter is removed on POD #14.

Radical perineal prostatectomy

Surgical technique

Following appropriate evaluation and counseling for radical prostatectomy, the decisions regarding erectile nerve preservation and use of neo-adjuvant hormone therapy are discussed. The following description of radical perineal prostatectomy should be adapted to the specific needs of the individual patient. On the day prior to surgery, a mechanical bowel prep is accomplished. On the morning of surgery, a 1% neomycin enema is administered. A pre-operative dose of a second-generation cephalosporin is infused intravenously. Thigh-high anti-thrombotic stockings and pneumatic compression devices are utilized to prevent deep venous thrombosis.

A spinal or general anesthetic is utilized. Epidural anesthesia is not necessary, as the length of surgery is predictable and post-operative pain is minimal. Following induction of anesthesia, the patient is placed in the lithotomy position using Allen stirrups (Allen Medical Systems, Bedford Heights, Ohio). A 6-inch roll is placed under the sacrum and the hips are further flexed, exposing the perineum (Fig. 16.5).

An O'Conor–Sullivan drape (American V. Mueller, Chicago, Illinois) is placed such that the rectal sheath is in the rectum. A curved Lowsley prostatic tractor is

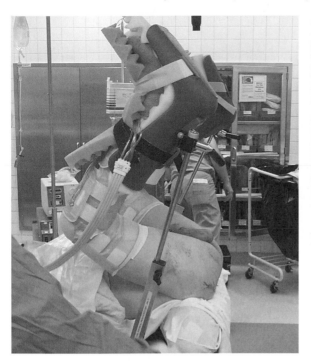

Fig. 16.5 The Allen Stirrups support the legs and a 6-inch jell roll elevates the sacrum to provide exposure to the perineum. Adequate exposure does not require that the perineum is parallel to the floor.

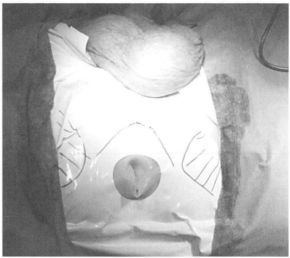

Fig. 16.6 The incision apex is in the mid-perineum and the lateral ends are medial to the ischial tuberosities. The incision remains anterior to the mid-anal line to avoid compromise of anal function.

placed per urethra and the wings opened in the bladder. A curved incision is placed with the apex in the mid-perineum and the ends just anterior to the mid-anal line, 1-cm medial to the ischial tuberosities (Fig. 16.6). Allis clamps are used to secure the edge of the drape to the incision. The incision is carried through the central tendon and Scarpa's fascia to develop the ischio-rectal space. Generous tissue is left over the intact external anal sphincter in developing the ischio-rectal space. Dissection will proceed through the fibrous condensation in the midline of the pelvic floor, anterior to the rectum, and associated with the fibrous raphe of the bulbous spongiosum. The midline raphe of the bulbous spongiosum muscles is elevated with a forceps and the attachments of the fibrous raphe are divided with electrocautery until the recto-urethralis muscle is visualized. The levator ani muscles are evident just lateral to the recto-urethralis muscle where they converge on their rectal attachments (Fig. 16.7). Using the scissors, slightly opened, like a comb, the rectum is easily swept posteriorly away from the apex of the prostate. Remaining vertically oriented recto-urethralis fibers are cauterized. The scissors are spread with the tips on the prostatic apex (Fig. 16.8). The

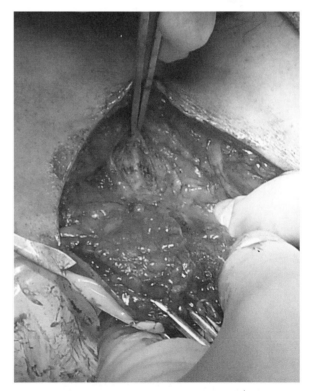

Fig. 16.7 Elevation of the midline fibrous raphe of the bulbo-spongiosum muscles helps identify the 'safe-entry' to the recto-urethralis muscles.

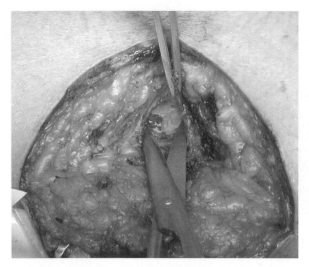

Fig. 16.8 The levator ani muscles attach to the rectum with the recto-urethralis muscles in the midline. The recto-urethralis muscles are vertical at the prostatic apex, but run parallel to the rectum at the level of the prostate base. Care must be taken to dissect anterior to all recto-urethralis fibers on the posterior aspect of Denonvillier's fascia to avoid rectal injury.

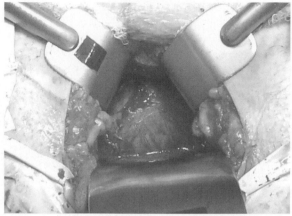

Fig. 16.9 The Thompson–Farley retractor is flush with the skin yet provides optimal exposure through the anterior triangle of the pelvic outlet. In non-nerve sparing cases, all periprostatic tissues are swept medial from the levator ani muscles to maximize margin control.

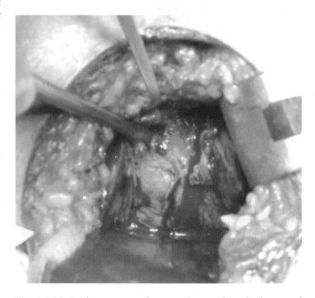

Fig. 16.10 Right cavernosal nerves invested in the layers of Denonvillier's fascia are dissected carefully off of the prostate. Tissue lateral to the nerve bundles is not dissected. The right retractor is to be placed gently over the padded nerve bundle.

white Denonvillier's fascia is visualized once the recto urethralis muscles are divided. The dissecting finger is used to develop this plane and mobilize the rectum posteriorly off of Denonvillier's fascia. The rectum is also swept posteriorly off of the inside of the levator ani muscles and the levator ani are divided to provide improved exposure. A sponge stick is used to sweep the rectum off of Denonvillier's fascia overlying the seminal vesicles. A fixed retraction system, such as the Thompson Retractor (Thompson Surgical, Inc., Traverse City, Michigan) or the Bookwalter Retractor Set (Codman and Shurleff, Inc., Randolph, Massachusetts) greatly facilitates exposure and frees up the surgical assistant's hands. A 2-inch malleable blade is used to retract the rectum posteriorly and two double-angled blades are placed antero-laterally, inside of the levators (Fig. 16.9).

For fully potent men with unilateral, non-apical tumors, who desire nerve preservation, unilateral cavernosal nerve preservation is considered. In such cases, Denonvillier's fascia is incised from lateral of the midline, over the medial aspect of the ipsilateral seminal vesical to the contra-lateral aspect at the apex near the urethra. With careful, sharp dissection, the fascia and associated cavernosal nerves are mobilized laterally off of the lateral aspect of the prostate (Fig. 16.10). A clear plane can be developed between the prostate and the layers of Denonvillier's fascia investing the cavernosal nerves. This plane is developed around the lateral aspect of the prostate from apex to the seminal vesicles. Branches of the nerves that penetrate the prostate at the apex and base should be divided sharply to avoid injury to the nerve bundles being spared. The vascular pedicle at the prostate base should be ligated adjacent to the prostate with care to avoid a traction injury to the nerve bundles. Once the dissection is completed, a damp sponge is used to pad a gentle double angled retractor to hold the nerve bundles out of the way of the operating field. In non-nerve sparing procedures, all peri-prostatic tissue is swept from the levators medially and left on the prostate to enhance tumor-free margins of resection. Denonvillier's fascia and the endopelvic fascia are left intact overlying the posterior and lateral aspects of the prostate, respectively.

Denonvillier's fascia overlying the seminal vesicles is incised transversely exposing the vas and seminal vesicles. The vas is isolated, divided, and then dissected away from the prostate for 5–6 cm. The vas is then hemoclipped and divided (Fig. 16.10). This dissection essentially accomplishes the dissection of the medial aspect of the seminal vesical and the posterior bladder neck. The seminal vesical is grasped with a Russian forceps and tracted medially. Metzenbaum scissors are used to sweep remaining Denonvillier's fascia laterally, then the scissors are spread along the lateral aspect of the seminal vesical. The prostate pedicles are thus identified, ligated, and divided (Fig. 16.11). The

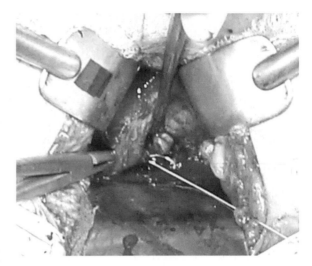

Fig. 16.12 The proximal prostate pedicles are ligated and divided.

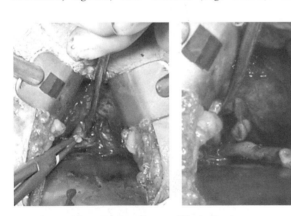

Fig. 16.11 After opening Denonvillier's fascia transversely cephalad to the prostate base, the vas is dissected for 5 cm and clipped. The posterior bladder neck and medial seminal vesicle dissection is then complete.

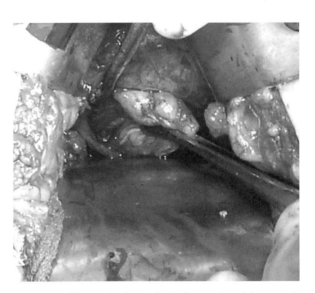

Fig. 16.13 The seminal vesicle is dissected and its vessels clipped.

seminal vesical is then dissected to the blood vessels at its tip, which are hemoclipped and divided (Fig. 16.12). The bladder neck is swept downward with a 'push' to identify the circular smooth muscles. This plane is developed laterally and anteriorly revealing any remaining pedicle vessels, which are ligated and divided. The endopelvic fascia is scored with cautery along the bladder neck, laterally to the anterior aspect of the prostate to aid in separation of the bladder neck

from the prostate (Fig. 16.13). Attention is then turned to the prostatic apex.

The skeletal muscles near the prostatic apex are separated to expose the urethra distal to the apex. One to two millimeters thick of pelvic floor muscle is separated from the pelvic floor and left overlying the apex of the prostate to ensure adequate margin around the apex. Care is taken to avoid violating the prostate anterior to the urethra at the apex. The urethra is separated from the prostate circumferentially by rolling a 'push' dissector between the urethra and the apex of the prostate. The apical pedicles are divided with cautery (Fig.

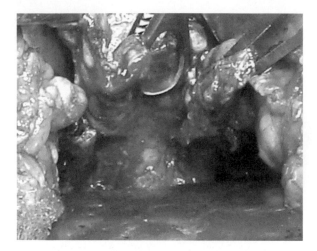

Fig. 16.14 The posterior bladder-neck fibers are pushed off of the prostate base, initiating the anatomic bladder-neck dissection.

16.14). The Lowsley tractor is removed and additional length of urethra is dissected out of the apex up to the veru montanum. The urethra is then divided sharply.

Tissue anterior to the prostate is swept away from the pubis and the pubo-prostatic ligaments are divided with cautery. A ring clamp is placed on the anterior tissue with one ring inside the urethra to provide downward traction on the prostate, to expose anterior attachments to the bladder neck. These attachments are divided with cautery. Occasionally venous bleeding from the dorsal venous complex necessitates ligation with an absorbable suture. With traction on the prostate, the plane of dissection between the bladder neck and the prostate base is developed exposing the urethra as it enters the prostate base. The urethra is dissected out of the prostatic base and divided leaving a 1-cm stump of urethra protruding from an intact bladder neck (Fig. 16.15).

The operative field is irrigated and any remaining bleeding points controlled prior to starting the anastomosis. The urethral ends are anatomized with 3–0 chromic suture, by placing the anterior sutures first and working around to the posterior aspect (Fig. 16.16). Once the anastomosis is complete (about 8 sutures), the urethra is injected with sterile saline retrograde from the meatus and the anastomosis is distended to identify any leaks needing an additional suture. An 18F catheter is then passed into the bladder and the bladder irrigated free of any clots.

In men with prior transurethral prostatectomy, very large glands, or cancer near the bladder neck, bladder neck preservation is not intended. In this situation, the bladder is entered anteriorly after dividing the pubo-

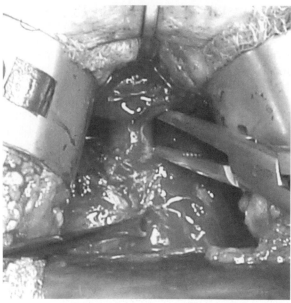

Fig. 16.15 The urethra is dissected from the peri-apical tissues. Using a 'peanut' dissector, the urethra is dissected out of the apex of the prostate up to the veru montanum.

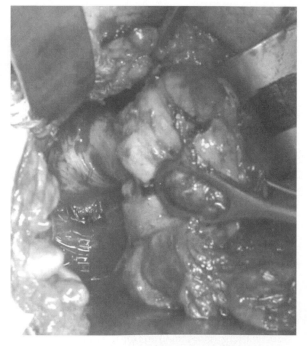

Fig. 16.16 With downward traction, the bladder is anatomically dissected off from the prostate. The proximal prostatic urethra is dissected out of the base of the prostate. The 'end-to-end' urethro-urethrostomy is accomplished. Note that the bladder neck is intact and the anastomotic sutures do not incorporate bladder-neck fibers. In cases where the urethra is thin and delicate, the anastomotic sutures incorporate some bladder-neck muscle fibers.

prostatic ligaments. The bladder neck is excised off from the prostate taking care to keep safe distance from the ureteral orifices. The bladder neck is then tailored to a snug 18F opening without necessarily averting the urothelium. The anastomosis is then accomplished in a similar manner being sure to include urothelium in each anastomotic suture. The 'tennis racquet' closure of the bladder neck is reinforced with another layer.

The retractors are removed. The rectum is inspected for injury or thin areas and, if present, are repaired or reinforced, respectively. The levator ani muscles are re-approximated in the midline with a penrose drain overlying the rectum. The central tendon is re-approximated. The subcutaneous tissues are closed and the skin is closed with a subcuticular stitch on the right side and one on the left (Fig. 16.17).

A Belladonna and opiate suppository is placed per rectum. The catheter is taped without tension to the lower abdomen and the patient taken to recovery. Ambulation and diet are advanced on the day of surgery. The penrose drain is removed prior to discharge on the morning post-operative day one. The catheter is removed 10 days later for intact bladder-neck cases and 17 days later for 'tennis racquet' bladder-neck closure cases. Activities, except bicycle riding, are unrestricted when the catheter is removed.

Using the above description, over the past 6 years a single surgeon's (MJH) experience in 340 cases is reviewed. Transfusions are utilized 1% of the time and all in the first 140 cases. No transfusions have been administered in the recent 200 cases. Surgery time is typically 90 min for non-nerve sparing cases and 120 min for nerve sparing cases (range 54–165 min). Patients are home on post-operative day one, nearly every case. While 40% of cases have extra-capsular disease, positive margins are seen 19% of cases without seminal vesicle invasion. The majority of margin-positive cases have focal (< 2 mm^2) margin positivity. After the catheter is removed, 32% of patients are free of pad-use within the first week. By the first month, second month, fourth month, and one year, 55%, 74%, 87%, and 94% of patients, respectively, are free of pad-usage. Most remaining men use one pad daily for minimal stress incontinence. Two men have been treated with artificial sphincter implantation and eight men have been treated with 1–5 collagen implants. Distal urethral strictures and anastomotic strictures have occurred in 2% each. One patient developed a recurrent urethro-cutaneous fistula, which required excision and Gracilis muscle interposition flap. He is continent and cancer-free 5 years post-operation. One man has experienced anal incompetence, while 4% note fecal urgency or poor control of flatus.

In conclusion, radical prostatectomy (either retropubic or perineal) provide an efficient therapeutic modality for the management of localized prostate cancer.

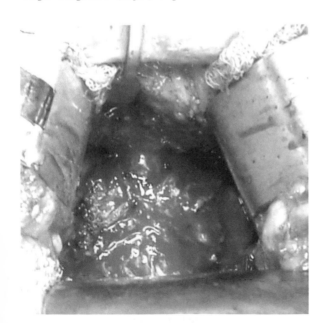

Fig. 16.17 A subcuticular suture completes the closure. Each side is closed separately to prevent contraction across the midline of the perineum.

References

1. Albertsen PD, Aaranson NK, Muller MJ *et al.* Health-related quality of life among patients with metastatic porstate cancer. *Urology* 1997, **49**, 207–16.
2. Villers AA, McNeal JE, Redwine EA *et al.* The role of peri-neural space invasion in the local spread of prostatic adenocarcinoma. *J Urol* 1989, **142**, 763–8.
3. Partin AW, Yoo J, Carter HB *et al.* The use of prostate specific antigen, clinical stage and Gleason score to predict pathologic stage in men with localized prostate cancer. *J Urol* 1993, **150**, 110–4.
4. Ravery V, Boccon LA, Dauge MC *et al.* Systematic biopsies accurately predict extracapsular extension of prostate cancer and persistent/recurrent detectable PSA after radical prostatectomy. *Urology* 1994, **44**, 371–6.
5. Ukimura O, Troncoso P, Romirez EI *et al.* Prostate cancer staging: correlation between ultrasound determined tumor contact length and pathologically confirmed extra-prostatic extension. *J Urol* 1998, **159**, 1251–9.
6. de la Taille A, Rubin MA, Bagiella E *et al.* Can peri-neural invasion predict prostate specific antigen recurrence? *J Urol* 1999, **162**, 103–6.
7. Epstein JI. The role of peri-neural invasion and other biopsy characteristics as prognostic markers for localized prostate cancer. *Semin Urol Oncol* 1998, **16**, 124–8.

8. Stamey TA, Villers AA, McNeal JE *et al*. Positive surgical margins at radical prostatectomy: importance of the apical dissection. *J Urol* 1990, **143**, 1166–72.

9. Watson RB, Grantos F *et al*. Postive surgical margins with radical prostatectomy: detailed pathological analysis and prognosis. *J Urol* 1996, **48**, 80.

10. Lepor H, Gregerman M, Crosby R, *et al*. Precise localization of the autonomic nerves from the pelvic plexus to the corpora cavernosa: a detailed anatomical study of the adult male pelvis. *J Urol* 1985, **133**, 207–12.

11. Eggleston JI, Walsh PC. Radical prostatectomy with preservation of sexual function: pathologyical findings in the first 100 cases. *J Urol* 1985, **134**, 1146–8.

12. Catalona WJ. Patient selection for, results of, and impact on tumor resection of potency-sparing radical prostatectomy. *Urol Clin North Am* 1990, **17**, 819–26.

13. Thompson IM, Ernst JJ, Gangai MP, Spence CR. Adenocarcinoma of the prostate: Results of routine urological screening. *J Urol*, 1984, **132**, 690.

14. Bishoff JT, Reyes A., Thompson IM *et al*. Pelvic lymphadenectomy can be omitted in selected patients with prostate cancer: Development of a system of patient selection. *Urology* 1995, **45**, 270.

15. Watson RB *et al*. Positive surgical margins with radical prostatectomy: detailed pathological analysis and prognosis. *Urology* 1996, **48**, 80–90.

16. Wahle S, Reznicek M, Falloy B. *et al*. Incidence of surgical margin involvement in various forms of radical prostatectomy. *Urology* 1990, **36**, 23–26.

17. Catalona WJ, Dresner SM. Nerve-sparing radical prostatectomy: estraprostatic tumor estension and preservation of erectile function. *J Urol* 1985, **134**, 1149–51.

18. Jones EC. Resection margin status in radical retropubic prostatectomy specimens: relationship tootype of operation, tumor size, tumor grade and local tumor extension. *J Urol* 1990, **144**, 89–93.

19. Smith RC, Partin AW, Epstein JL *et al*. Extended followup of the influence of wide excision of the neurovascular bundle(s) on prognosis in men with clinically localized prostate cancer and extensive capsular perforation. *J Urol* 1996, **156**, 454–7.

20. Catalona WJ. Potency, continence, complication rates in 1,870 consecutive radical retropubic prostatectomies. *J Urol* 1999, **162**, 433–8.

21. Zippe CD, Kedia AW, Kediol K *et al*. Treatment of erectile dysfunction after radical prostataectomy with sildenafil citrate. *Urology* 1998, **52** (6), 963–6.

22. Walsh PC. Anatomic radical retropubic prostatectomy. In: *Campbell's urology* (7th edn) 1998.

23. Heinzer H, Graefen M, Noldus J *et al*. Early complications of anatomical redical retropubic prostatectomy: lessons from a single-center experience. *Urologia Internationalis* 1997, **59** (1), 30–3.

24. Hautmann RE, Sauter TW, Wenderoth UK *et al*. Radical retropubic prostatectomy: morbidity and urinary continence in 418 consecutive cases. *Urology* 1994, **43** (Suppl 2), 47–51.

25. Meyers RP. Improving the exposure of the prostate in radical retropubic prostatectomy: longitudinal bunching of the deep venous plexus. *J Urol* 1989, **142**, 1282–4.

26. Klein EA. Early Continence after Radical Prostatectomy. *J Urol* 1992, **148**, 92–5.

27. See WA and Fuller JR. An outcome study of patient-controlled morphine analgeisa, with or without ketorolac, following radical retropubic prostatectomy. *J Urol* 1995, **154**, 1429–32.

17 | External-beam radiotherapy in the management of localized prostate cancer

Christopher M. Nutting and D. P. Dearnaley

Introduction

Prostate cancer detection has increased by an estimated 30 000–50 000 cases per year in the USA as a result of biochemical testing using prostate-specific antigen (PSA) (1), so that prostate cancer (CAP) is now the most commonly diagnosed male malignancy in North America. In Europe and the UK, the uptake of PSA testing has been slower, Schroder suggesting that 20% of European men undergo regular PSA testing compared to 70% in the USA (2). The figure in the UK is probably much lower and is reflected in the ratio of prostate cancer incidence to mortality in the UK (12 496 cases diagnosed in 1988; 9629 deaths in 1992) compared with the USA (projected incidence in 1994, 200 000 cases; 35 000 deaths in 1990) (3, 4). The considerable majority of the 'newly' diagnosed cancers are of early stage and potentially curable. In the UK, a rapidly increasing rate of CAP diagnosis over the next 5–10 years, and a corresponding demand for potentially curative treatment options, should be anticipated. In both the UK and North America, radical radiotherapy has been the most commonly used curative modality (5), although the proportion of men in the USA (particularly those aged 70 years or less) undergoing radical prostatectomy has risen rapidly (6). The increase in diagnosis of CAP has substantial implications for the provision of services to deliver radiotherapy or perform prostatectomy; for example, the demand for radiation treatment has increased by 3- to 4-fold in some centers (7, 8) and there is, therefore, an increasing urgency to determine the optimal selection of patients for radical local treatment and to decide on the most effective and appropriate radiation therapy techniques.

The seminal paper by Chodak and colleagues (9) reporting the results of 'watch and wait' management of T1/2 CAP has shown that tumor grade is of overriding importance in determining outcome. Cause-specific mortality was only 13% at 10 years for grades 1 or 2 tumors compared to 66% in men with grade 3 cancers. Metastases occurred in 19%, 42%, and 74% of patients with grade 1, 2, or 3 cancers, respectively, 10 years after diagnosis, clearly demonstrating the progressive nature of the disease in men with a reasonable life-expectancy. A retrospective analysis by Schroder and Chodak (data presented at British Prostate Group Symposium 1996), studied 2558 men treated with total prostatectomy compared with 815 men managed with a 'watch and wait' policy. For those patients with high-grade, localized tumors, surgical treatment gave a 78%, 10-year survival compared to 34% for men treated by watch and wait policy (*P* = 0.004). On multivariate analysis, expectant management predicted for poor survival. Such data needs confirmation from prospective randomized studies. Patient recruitment continues in Sweden and North America, although unfortunately in the UK the Medical Research Council study comparing radiotherapy with prostatectomy or expectant management has failed because of poor recruitment.

Results of external-beam radiotherapy treatment for localized prostate cancer

The long-term results of external-beam radiotherapy for CAP derived from reports from the Patterns of Care Surveys, RTOG studies, and large single-institute series (5, 10–14) are shown in Table 17.1. Results from the Royal Marsden NHS Trust in 388 clinically staged patients treated between 1970 and 1989 showed broadly similar results with 5–10-year actuarial local control rates of 88(77%) for T1, 80(65%) for T2, and 74(68%) for T3 cancers. It should be noted that these series do not contain patients who have had pathologi-

Table 17.1   External-beam radiotherapy for carcinoma of the prostate: long-term results from Patterns of Care Surveys, RTOG studies, and large single-institute series

		Local recurrence			Evidence of disease survivial (%)			Overall survival (%)		
	No.	5 years	10 years	15 years	5 years	10 years	15 years	5 years	10 years	15 years
T1Nx	583	3–6	4–8	17	84–85	52–68	39	83–95	52–76	41–46
T2Nx	1117	12–14	17–29	32–35	66–90	27–85	15–42	74–78	43–70	22–36
T3Nx	2292	12–26	19–31	25–56	32–60	14–46	17–40	56–72	32–42	23–27

Ref. nos: 17, 11, 12, 14.

cal lymph node staging and, as might be expected, the 11-year cause-specific mortality in 104 patients with T1B-T2 N0 surgically staged disease treated in RTOG trial 7706 was 90%, and 87% of patients were clinically free of local recurrence (15). The survival in this group of patients exceeded that of an aged-matched control population, and in general, for patients with T1 and T2A disease, overall results are generally similar to those reported after radical prostatectomy (16).

It is clear from these studies that results for more advanced T2C, T3–4 tumors have been less favorable. Survival of these patients is affected by the presence of undiagnosed metastatic disease, and understaging of pelvic lymph nodes at the time of initial treatment. Additionally, however, a general finding is that large tumors have poorer local control, failure rates rising from 25% for tumors palpably less than 25 cm^3 to more than 50% for tumors with a product of their diameter with greater than 25 cm^3 (17). Most local recurrences are detected by digital rectal examination (DRE) and the true rate determined by post-radiation biopsy is probably higher. There is general agreement that a positive biopsy 24 months after radiotherapy indicates persisting disease (18). The reported rates of positive biopsy specimens vary considerably and the true incidence of positive biopsy results in patients with normal DRE is uncertain (19). Reported incidence of positive biopsy vary from 18% to 45% post-treatment and increases with disease bulk from 15% for men with B1 disease (< 1.5 cm nodule) to 68–79% for men with bulky stage B or C cancer (20, 21).

Prostate-specific antigen (PSA) and external-beam radiotherapy

It is becoming clear that PSA estimation both before and after irradiation can give useful information to guide prognosis and selection of patients for treatment, as well as being a very sensitive indicator of disease recurrence. Hanks and colleagues (22) studied 110 patients with T1–3 CAP with a mean follow-up of 12.6 years and found long-term biochemical control of 72% for T1 cancers, 54% for T2A cancers falling to 22% and 28% for bulkier T2 and T3 cancers, respectively. A favorable outcome was also seen in patients with cancers that had a low Gleason score, who had a 75% rate of biochemical control compared to only 18% for Gleason sum 7, and 0% for Gleason sum 8 or 9. It has also been shown that pretreatment PSA levels are of critical importance (23–25). For example, Hanks and colleagues (25) found that of 120 patients with PSA more than 20 ng/ml at presentation, only 28% remained biochemically free of progressive disease at 4 years, although 81% still had no evidence of distant metastases. The nadir level of PSA following radiotherapy also appears to be a powerful predictor of outcome, although it remains uncertain as to whether 1.0 ng/ml or 0.5 ng/ml gives optimal discrimination (26, 27). Groups from Harvard and DeKalb have suggested that it is important to achieve nadir values of 0.5 ng/ml. Zietman and colleagues (23) showed that 63% of 314 men with T1–2 NxM0 carcinomas were free of biochemical progression after radical radiotherapy at 5 years. If the PSA nadir was 0.5 ng/ml or less, then biochemical recurrence free rate was 90% compared to 46% if the PSA nadir was higher. The likelihood of reaching a PSA nadir was clearly related to initial PSA but not to Gleason score. Critz and colleagues (28), using a combination of external-beam radiotherapy and interstitial treatment, described a group of 536 patients with T1, T2 N0 cancers; 80% achieved a nadir of 0.5 ng/ml or less, and 5- and 10-year biochemical disease-free survival rates were 95 and 84%, respectively, compared with 29% at 5 years for those with a higher nadir level; all patients with a nadir of more than 1.0 ng/ml ultimately failed. Presenting levels of PSA may be useful in determining which patients are most suitable for treatment using dose-escalation techniques. For example, Hanks and colleagues (25) analyzed 375 consecutive patients treated with conformal radiotherapy techniques. Dividing patients into those who received above or below 71 Gy showed an advantage in biochemical disease-free recurrence for those patients presenting with PSA levels more than 10 and 20 ng/ml, but not for those with PSA levels below 10 ng/ml at the time of presentation. In the future, PSA levels in combination with clinical staging and Gleason score will be used to stratify patients for appropriate treatment and PSA will be valuable as a proxy endpoint in studies looking at different treatment combinations and radiotherapy techniques.

The importance of local tumor control

Long-term clinically judged local tumor control is good for patients with stage T1 cancers (83% at 15 years) but becomes increasingly less secure with increasing T stage, falling to 65–68% for T2 and 44–75% for T3 cancers (Table 17.1). As above, prostate biopsy may show higher rates of recurrence than can be detected clinically and biochemical (PSA) failure rates are certainly significantly higher (24). Review of Royal Marsden Hospital patients showed 57% metastasis-free survival at 5 years in patients with clinically assessed locally controlled disease, compared to 26% of patients with local recurrence (*P* < 0.01), and local control remained highly significant (*P* < 0.001), when included as a time-dependent variable in a multivariate analysis of outcome (survival and development of metastases). These findings are in accordance with other series, which have documented distant metastases developing in 19–41% of patients with stages A–C disease and local control of disease compared with 57–83% for patients who have developed local failure (16). Local failure has been reported to be the most important determinant on multivariate analysis in predicting the development of metastatic disease for all stages of disease (29). Additionally, this study demonstrated that distant metastases developed, on average, later in patients with local failure than in those patients who had local control of disease, strongly suggesting that local failure itself was an important determinant of outcome. Using Monte Carlo simulation techniques, Yorke and colleagues (30) estimated that 50% of the

metastases in patients with local recurrence were due to local treatment failure.

Complications after radiotherapy

Radiation-induced complications are-dose limiting and current 'standard' radiotherapy doses and fractionation schedules have been derived from years of clinical experience to give acceptable morbidity. Acute side-effects from radiotherapy to the pelvis include proctitis causing rectal discomfort and diarrhea, cystitis producing dysuria and frequency of micturition, and occasional skin reactions. Reported incidence ranges from 70% to 90% for mild, 20–45% for moderate, and 1–4% for severe or prolonged reactions (31–33). Such side-effects depend upon the volume of tissue treated (pelvis or prostate only) (34) and also relate to treatment technique. Acute side-effects are expected to settle within 4–6 weeks of completing radiotherapy treatment. Late complications may develop months or years after treatment and are potentially of more concern. Late gastro-intestinal side-effects include persistent rectal discharge, tenesmus, rectal bleeding, and rectal stricture. Major late genito-urinary complications include chronic cystitis, bladder ulcers, urinary incontinence, urethral stricture, and impotence.

Results from over 1000 patients treated in recent single-institute series suggest an overall moderate complication rate of 16–19%, with severe complications requiring surgical correction in 1–3% of patients (12, 35, 36). The Patterns of Care study group has defined major complications as those requiring hospital admission for investigation or management. Of 619 patients treated, 4.5% had such complications (gastro-intestinal 2.6%, urological 1.8%) and complications were related to treatment technique, being higher in patients treated with only anterior/posterior radiation fields or in whom only one radiation field was treated each day. Doses above 70 Gy were also associated with increased complications (37). These series were updated with a 10-year follow-up (38); at that time, 2% of patients had needed surgical correction of complications, a further 2% had had a major complication not requiring surgery, and two patients had died from treatment-related side-effects. The actuarial 5- and 10-year complication-free rates were 93% and 86%, respectively. A further series of 313 with stage T1 tumors had a similar complication rate, with less than 2% requiring surgical correction. An increase in the overall complication rate from 6% to 11% was noted for patients treated with doses below and above 65 Gy, respectively (39). The remaining complication is of importance, which has been estimated to occur in 30–40% of treated patients, usually developing during the 6 months after treatment (40). In a recent randomized study by the RTOG (41), 76% of men who were sexually potent before treatment reported return of sexual function. In a report of conformal radiotherapy (42), 62% of men reported return of sexual function. 'Quality-of-Life' questionnaires may lead to a higher estimate of sexual dysfunction (43), although this may be little different from an aged matched control population (44).

Methods to improve the results of radiotherapy

As described above, the local control of CAP becomes increasingly uncertain with increasing tumor stage and tumor bulk. Potential methods to improve results are shown in Table 17.2. The development of late radia-tion side-effects (most notably radiation induced proc-titis) has limited the total dose of irradiation that can be given using standard techniques to approximately 70 Gy. A retrospective review of 1348 men with stage B or C prostate cancer showed an actuarial 5-year local recurrence rate for stage B disease of 29% for doses under 60 Gy, decreasing to 18% and 12% for doses up to 64 Gy and 70 Gy, respectively (45). Conformal radiotherapy techniques are now available, which closely confine the high-dose irradiation volume to the prostate (± seminal vesicles) and these techniques have allowed exploration of high-dose therapy. Preliminary results showed that late radiation-induced side-effects can be relatively modest. Two series from the Memorial Sloan Kettering Cancer Center and Fox Chase Cancer Center have strongly suggested that bio-chemical control rates are significantly improved for patients with presenting PSA levels over 10 ng/ml or other unfavorable features (Table 17.3) (46, 47). Dose escalation, therefore, seems justified. However, as dis-cussed above, radiotherapy-induced side-effects restrict attempts to increase the delivered radiation dose above 70 Gy using conventional photon irradiation, rectal bleeding increasing from 12% to 20% (48). There is little clinical data concerning volume/complication rela-tionships for either rectum or bladder, but there is an expectation of decreased side-effects using either conformal-radiotherapy or interstitial-treatment approaches. The calculation of dose–volume histogram (DVH) and normal tissue complication probability (NTCP) (49, 50) will eventually permit refinement of mathematical models of radiation toxicity, and it is essential that clinical and physics data are collected prospectively. One such study (51), including 41 patients, has suggested that there is a dose–volume relationship for rectal bleeding. A high probability of complications ranged contiguously between 60 CGE

Table 17.2 Methods to improve local control with radiotherapy in carcinoma of the prostate

Increased radiation dose	Conformal radiotherapy
	Interstitial irradiation
Particle-beam radiotherapy	Protons
	Neutrons
Combined modality treatment with androgen deprivation	Neoadjuvant
	Adjuvant
Combined modality treatment with total prostatectomy	

Table 17.3 Effect of radiation dose on biochemical (PSA) control (5-year actuarial results)

	Memorial Sloan Kettering Cancer Center Dose (Gy)				Fox Chase Cancer Center Dose (Gy)			
	64.8/70.2	75.6/81				70	76	
No.					No.			
167	85%*	95%*	P = 0.5	PSA < 10	96	82%	84%	P = 0.9
269	54%*	79%*	P = 0.04	PSA 10–19	70	35%	75%	P = 0.02
307	20%*	53%*	P = 0.03	PSA > 20	66	10%	32%	P = 0.02

* Unfavorable factors PSA > 10, Stage ≥ T3, Gleason ≥ 7. *Figures extrapolated from graphical data.
Zelefsky *et al.* and Hanks *et al.* (46, 47).

(Cobalt Grey Equivalent) to 70% of the anterior rectal wall and 75 CGE to 30%. A further complicating factor is that inherent radiosensitivity may vary between patients (52–54) and tests to detect sensitive patient populations would be most helpful in deselecting patients from radical radiotherapy treatments particularly using dose escalation techniques.

Conformal radiotherapy

Prostate cancer has become the focus of attention for conformal radiotherapy, particularly in the USA. Accurate patient positioning, computed tomography (CT) planning with 3-dimensional reconstruction of volumes of interest, clear definition of treatment margins, and meticulous verification procedures of the shaped fields produced by customized shaped blocks or multi-leaf collimation (MLC), are necessary components of this approach (5, 55). Multiple planar and complex non-coplanar beam operations have been designed (56, 57), although any clear advantages over more simple arrangements, particularly with more moderate degrees of dose escalation, are not overwhelming (58–61). The amount of normal tissue treated to the 90% isodose may be reduced by 42%, with 46% and 41% reductions in the volumes of bowel and bladder, respectively (62). In the UK, the Institute of Cancer Research and the Royal Marsden NHS Trust (ICR/RMNHST) recruited men with prostate cancer for treatment with a standard dose of 64 Gy in daily 2-Gy fractions (63). The men were randomly assigned conformal or conventional radiotherapy treatment. The primary endpoint was the development of late radiation complications (> 3 months after treatment) measured with the Radiation Therapy and Oncology Group (RTOG) score. Indicators of disease (cancer) control were also recorded.

In the 225 men treated, significantly fewer men developed radiation-induced proctitis and bleeding in the conformal group than in the conventional group (37% vs. 56% > RTOG grade 1, $P = 0.004$; 5% vs. 15% > RTOG grade 2, $P = 0.01$). There were no differences between groups in bladder function after treatment (53% vs. 59% >grade 1, $P = 0.34$; 20% vs. 23% > grade 2, $P = 0.61$). After median follow-up of 3–6 years, there was no significant difference between groups in local tumor control (conformal 78% (95% CI 66–86), conventional 83% (64–90)).

Dose-escalation studies have been reported by three North American groups (57, 64, 65). Using meticulous planning and immobilization techniques, does of 75 Gy have been well tolerated (albeit with a relatively short follow-up) and, currently, doses in excess of 80 Gy are being delivered. Further National Cancer Institute sponsored dose-escalation trials are under way, comparing doses of 68.4 Gy, 73.8 Gy, and 79.8 Gy, in a multicenter Phase II study. The ICR/RMNHST commenced a randomized study comparing 74 Gy with 64 Gy in conjunction with the use of neoadjuvant androgen deprivation (8) and recently the Medical Research Council Radiotherapy Working Party has adopted this study nationally.

Combined modality treatment using androgen deprivation and radiotherapy

Neoadjuvant androgen deprivation offers potential advantages in two ways (Fig. 17.1). First, combined modality treatment may lead to increased tumor-cell kill. This mechanism may depend on synergistic enhancement in cell death by apoptosis induced by both treatment modalities (66), and hence to the

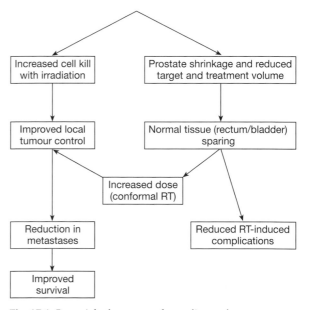

Fig. 17.1 Potential advantages of neoadjuvant hormone treatment in combination with radiotherapy (RT).

improvements in local control. Second, initial shrinkage of the prostate and prostate cancer can lead to a beneficial modification of radiation treatment volume. Reducing the radiation target volume may favorably affect the therapeutic ratio, either by reducing radiation sequeal for a standard radiation dose or by permitting dose escalation (using conformal radiation techniques), which should increase tumor control probability whilst maintaining acceptable level of radiation complications.

Reduction of prostate and radiation volumes

A series of 22 patients at the Royal Marsden NHS Trust were intensively studied during the course of a 3–6-month period of androgen deprivation using a LHRH agonist prior to the commencement of radiotherapy. Monthly ultrasound examinations were made (67) during androgen deprivation and prostate volume reduced by approximately 50%. The median volume pretreatment of 66 ml (range 40–130 ml) reduced to 30 ml (range 30–47 ml) after a median of 17 weeks therapy. The majority of patients had stabilized prostate volumes (within 10% of previous estimate) by week 13, although patients with large prostates took up to 6 months to obtain maximum response defined in this way. It was notable how the majority of patients had significant improvement in symptoms of urinary

outflow obstruction prior to radiotherapy. Planning CT scans were taken before and after the hormonal treatment. Results were correlated with ultrasound findings (68). Radiotherapy planning was performed using both conventional and conformal techniques to treat the target volume (prostate ± seminal vesicles) with a 1-cm margin. Results of this analysis are shown in Table 17.4, which demonstrates how androgen deprivation has a complimentary effect to conformal techniques in reducing the volumes of normal tissues treated by radiotherapy. Using both initial androgen deprivation and conformal irradiation techniques, decreased the volume of rectum treated to the 90% isodose by 59%, with a similar 58% reduction in volume of bladder irradiated with an overall 71% reduction in radiation target volume. Similar findings have been reported by other centers. In a study from the Memorial Sloan Kettering Cancer Center on 22 patients with bulky prostate cancers, neoadjuvant hormone therapy reduced the target volume by a mean of 25% with a reduction of 25% in volume of rectum and 50% in volumes of bladder treated (69). Similarly, Forman and colleagues reported an average of 37% reduction in prostate volume after 3 months of hormonal therapy with 23% reduction of the volume of rectum and 21% reduction of the volume of bladder receiving 64 Gy (70). Recently, work in our hospital has looked at changes in MRI characteristics of localized prostate cancer before and after neoadjuvant androgen depravation. In 55 patients with visible tumors, 14 completely disappeared after hormonal

Table 17.4 Modification of radiation treatment volume by neoadjuvant androgen deprivation and conformal radiotherapy

	Prostate volume (cm^3)		Radiotherapy target volume (cm^3) (90% isodose)		Rectal volume (cm^3) (90% isodose)		Bladder volume (cm^3) (90% isodose)	
	TRUS	CT	CONV*	CONF†	CONV*	CONF†	CONV*	CONF†
Pre-androgen deprivation	70 (40–131)	84 (29–200)	616	280	68	36	114	73
Post-androgen deprivation	33 (11–100)	47 (14–107)	363	176	53	28	65	48
% Reduction in volume by:								
Androgen deprivation	53%	44%	41%		22%		43%	
Conformal RT	–	–	54%		47%		36%	
Both	–	–	71%		59%		58%	

* Coventional and †conformal radiation planning methods. A 1-cm margin was given around the target tissues – prostate ± seminal vesicles.

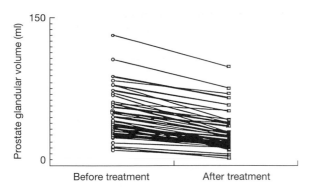

Fig. 17.2 Prostate glandular volume change with neoadjuvant hormone deprivation treatment in 55 patients.

treatment and overall tumor volume decreased by 65% (95% CI 55–76) (Fig. 17.2). Dynamic-contrast enhanced image acquisition after bolus injection of God-EDTA showed significant reduction in capillary permeability in all patients. These reductions in tumor volume, vascular permeability suggest an alternative means of monitoring tumor response to NAAD (71).

Clinical trials of neoadjuvant hormonal treatment and radiotherapy

Three phase III trials have now reported the results of comparisons of radiotherapy with or without neoadjuvant androgen deprivation. The first and largest undertaken by the Radiotherapy and Oncology Group (RTOG) randomized 471 patients with large primary tumors (T2 to T4) and no evidence of distant metastases to receive goserelin 3.6 mg every 4 weeks and flutamide 250 mg, three times daily for 2 months before radiation therapy and during irradiation treatment (Group I) or radiation therapy alone (Group II). Median follow-up for patients who were treated between 1987 and 1991 is now 6 years, and the most recent reported results have continued to show highly significant benefits in 5-year rates of local disease control (Group I 75%, Group II 64% P = 0.002), freedom from distance metastases (Group I 71%, Group II 61% P = 0.3), and no evidence of disease including PSA failure (Group I 39%, Group II 20% P < 0.0001). Improvements in these endpoints has been maintained after 8-years follow-up and for the first time survival in Groups I (51%) may be showing some

indication of improvement compared to Group II (42%), although this result does not yet reach statistical significance (P = 0.2) (72). A similar small study by the Canadian Urologic Oncology Group has recently reported preliminary results. A total of 208 patients with stage B2 to C prostate cancer were randomly allocated to a 12-weeks neoadjuvant course of cyproterone acetate followed by radiotherapy (Group I) or radiotherapy alone (Group II). Time to reach PSA nadir was shorter in the combined modality group (P = 0.007) and the average nadir was lower (P = 0.003). Over the study period, more patients in the combined group remained free of clinical (71% vs. 49% P = 0.02) or biochemical (47% vs. 22% P=0.001) recurrence. Additionally, at 18 months there was a significant improvement in the number of patients who had negative biopsies (73). Finally, a small three-arm randomized study has been reported by a Quebec Group (74). Between 1991 and 1994, 120 patients were randomized to receive radiotherapy alone, radiotherapy with an initial 3-month course of neoadjuvant maximum androgen blockade, or additionally to continue maximum androgen blockade for a total of 11 months. Two-year biopsy results have been reported showing residual cancer in 65%, 28%, and 5% of these three groups, respectively. Testosterone levels were not reported at time of biopsies and the results in the third group may have been confounded by continued androgen suppression. Nevertheless, these clinical studies taken together offer strong support for the contention that initial androgen deprivation improves the local control that can be achieved with external-beam irradiation alone. Non-randomized studies of experimental radiotherapy approaches have also produced similar results. For example, in a trial of dose-escalation and conformal radiotherapy 10% (3 out of 31) of patients had positive biopsies, if initial hormone therapy was given compared to 46% (48 out of 105), if radiation alone was used (46), and in a protocol using hyperfractionated radiotherapy, the incidence of positive biopsies was 50% (9 out of 18) without hormone treatment compared to 0% (0 out of 23) when initial androgen deprivation was use (75). Our own results in over 450 patients treated with combined modality therapy have given comparable results to the randomized studies and, in particular, in a sequential series of 45 patients in 2 years, biopsies have been negative in 80–90% of patients, depending upon initial presenting features. A potential disadvantage of even short-course androgen deprivation is that impotence is produced, at least during the time of androgen deprivation, in the major-

Table 17.5 Testosterone levels before and after neoadjuvant androgen deprivation using LHRHa

	No.	Testosterone (nmol/l)			LH (IU/L)**	
		Median	Range	No. < 10 nmol/l	Median	Range
Pre–LHRHa treatment*	115	16	5–39	3	5	(1–27)
≥ 6 months after last LHRHa treatment	115	16	1–45	13	10	(1–41)
		$P = 0.18$			$P < 0.0001$	

* 3–6 Months treatment with monthly depot preparations of goserelin or leuprorelin.
** Luteinizing Hormone (IU/L)

ity of patients. We have studied a group of 115 patients and demonstrated that testosterone levels recover to pretreatment levels in the considerable majority of men within 6–9 months, although luteinising hormone (LH) levels remain elevated in the majority. A small proportion of men (under 10%) with initially normal testosterone levels remain with subnormal values (< 10 ng/l) post-treatment (Table 17.5). Despite recovery of hormone levels, the rate of impotence may be higher after combined modality treatment, and among 159 patients who received initial androgen suppression, the 2-year actuarial incidence of impotence was 43% compared with 27%, for 385 patients treated with radiation alone ($P < 0.001$) (46). Recovery of sexual ability after a period of androgen suppression may be more difficult than maintenance of potency when treatment is given using radiotherapy alone (Fig. 17.3).

Animal models in neoadjuvant androgen deprivation and radiotherapy

Laboratory research on combined modality treatment has been hampered by a lack of readily available experimental models. Two groups, however, have made interesting contributions. Zietman and colleagues at the Massachusetts General Hospital have explored the combination of androgen deprivation and radiotherapy using a transplantable androgen-depended Shionogi adenocarcinoma in athymic nude mice (76). When orchiectomy was performed 12 days prior to radiation (neoadjuvant therapy), there was a significant decline in the TCD50 (dose that controls 50% of tumors). TCD50 reduced from 86 Gy to 43 Gy comparing radiotherapy alone, and neoadjuvant orchiectomy and radiotherapy. Interestingly, however, orchiectomy performed 1–12 days after irradiation (adjuvant therapy) had a much smaller effect (TCD50 of 69 Gy and 75 Gy, respectively). Experiments by researchers at the

MD Anderson (77), using the Dunning R3327-G rat prostate tumor, have also demonstrated a supra-additive interaction between androgen ablation and radiotherapy. This occurred when androgen ablation preceded radiotherapy by 3 days, when the apoptotic index increased 5- to 10-fold compared to controls, but no supra-additive effect was seen when androgen ablation was commenced at the same time as irradiation. These studies suggest that the timing and sequencing of combined hormonal and radiotherapy treatments may be critical to obtain optimal results.

The role of radiotherapy in pathological T3 disease

Pathological analysis of total prostatectomy specimens in stage T2 cancer shows pT3 disease in 30–50% of cases (78–80). Retrospective review of the literature has suggested that local recurrence occurred in 23% of patients treated without post-operative radiotherapy compared to 3% with irradiation (81). Subsequent reports have supported the idea that immediate adjuvant radiotherapy reduces the instant of local recurrence (82–84) and following post-operative radiotherapy recurrence rates have been shown to be 5% or less (83, 85–87). If radiotherapy is delayed until after evidence of local recurrence, higher radiation doses are required and treatment morbidity may be greater for less certain local control (70%) (87). A recent report on 46 patients with PSA relapse alone showed biochemical disease control (PSA < 0.3 ng/ml) in 59% of patients, with actuarial freedom from recurrence of 50% at 5 years (88). It has been suggested that radiation therapy improves long-term outcome by controlling loco-regional disease (84, 89–91). A recent report (92, 93) of 288 patients managed the Mayo Clinic showed a significant improvement in biochemical disease control (PSA < 0.3 ng/ml) in those patients given post-operative radiotherapy, but (as yet) no dif-

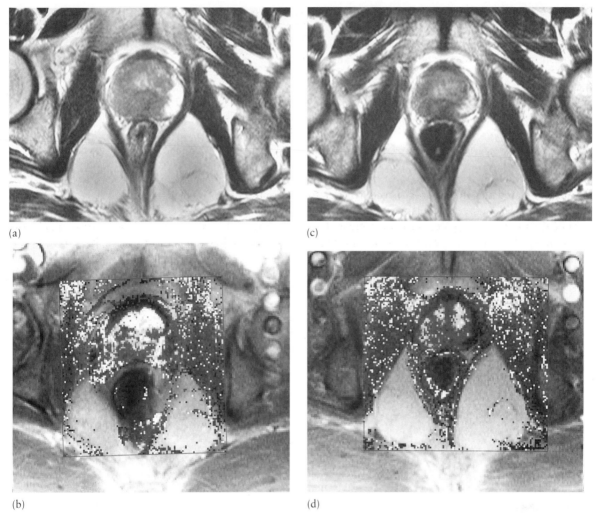

(a)

(c)

(b)

(d)

Fig. 17.3 T2-weighted MR image of a 51-year-old man with prostate cancer (T3B N1 M0, presenting PSA = 22 ng/ml, Gleason score 5) before treatment: (a) a large tumor is visible in the *right* peripheral zone. (b) Permeability map in the same patient before treatment: high capillary permeability is seen in the *left* side of the tumor and in the central gland compared to the peripheral zone (maximum permeability depicted 1/min). (c) T2-weighted image of the same patient after 3 months of hormone deprivation (PSA = 1 ng/ml): the gland and the tumor are smaller. (d) Permeability map after treatment: there is a marked reduction in the capillary permeability of all tissues, particularly the tumor.

ference in the distant failure rate at 5 years, of 8% vs. 10% ($P = 0.09$). It cannot, therefore, be assumed that improved local disease control will necessarily translate into therapeutic gain, and post-operative radiotherapy runs the risk of producing an increase in side-effects from the combined-modality approach. It is, therefore, appropriate that randomized studies are undertaken to define clearly the role of post-operative radiotherapy in pT3 disease. Recently there have been two such studies. In RTOG Protocol 91–19, patients with pT3 disease (capsular invasion, positive margins, positive seminal vesicles) were randomized to immediate radiotherapy (60–64 Gy) or observation. The EORTC Protocol

No.22911, which is still in progress, randomizes similar patients between radiotherapy (60 Gy) and observation, and aims to recruit a total of 700 patients. Results from these comprehensive studies should guide selection of patients for such treatment.

Conclusion

In prostate cancer, as for cancer arising at other sites, radiotherapy alone is capable of sterilizing the primary tumor, and can improve loco-regional control in conjunction with radical surgery. However, assessment of the real value of radical treatment to the patient is made difficult because of the long natural history of disease in many patients and the competing causes of death. The rapid increase in diagnosis of localized carcinoma of the prostate, due to increased public awareness and PSA testing, highlights the requirement for improving patient selection and minimizing treatment related side-effects.

Local control may be improved by increasing tumor dose by a variety of methods including 'conformal' radiotherapy, or interstitial treatment. Late damage to rectum and bladder/urethra limits dose escalation, and high degrees of technical skill are required if these approaches are to be safely implemented.

Neoadjuvant androgen deprivation has been shown to be complementary to radiotherapy and improves local control without significant excess (and probably with reduced) toxicity. As in breast cancer, adjuvant treatment may improve recurrence-free and overall survival at the cost of long-term hormone side-effects. Alternative hormonal strategies to LHRH and maximal androgen-blockade would be of interest. Ongoing clinical studies will address some of these issues but enthusiasm for 'high tech' therapies should not obscure the overall aims of treatment, which can only be accurately assessed in prospective randomized studies, with end-points including overall survival and quality-of-life assessments, as well as biochemical data on disease control.

For the future, improved understanding of the biology of prostate cancer may lead to more optimal patient selection for treatment. Optimization of dose and radiotherapy techniques using DVH and TCP/NTCP considerations should improve uncomplicated tumor control probabilities. The role of normal tissue sensitivity testing deserves further study and the indications for and duration of neoadjuvant and adjuvant hormone therapy must be clarified. Finally, new modalities should to be tested and integrated as they become available.

References

1. Mettlin C. The status of prostate cancer early detection. *Cancer* 1993, **72** (Suppl 3), 1050–5.
2. Schroder FH. Screening for prostate cancer (letter). *Lancet* 1994, **343**, 1438–9.
3. Cancer Research Campaign. Cancer of the prostate. *Factsheet* 1994, **20** (1).
4. Boring CC, Squires TS, Tong T. Cancer statistics. *Cancer* 1993, **43** (1), 7–26.
5. Hanks GE. Treatment of early stage prostate cancer: Radiotherapy. In: *Important advances in oncology* (ed. VT De Vita, S Hellman, SA Rosenberg). JB Lippincott, Philadelphia, 1994, 225–39.
6. Lu-Yao GL, McLeuan D, Wasson J *et al.* An assessment of radical prostatectomy. Time trends, geographic variation, and outcomes. The Prostate Patient Outcomes Research Team. *JAMA* 1993, **269**, 2633–6.
7. De Jong B, Crommelin M, van der Heijden LH *et al.* Patterns of radiotherapy for cancer patients in southeastern Netherlands, 1975–1989. *Radiother Oncol* 1994, **31**, 213–21.
8. Deamaley DP. Radiotherapy for prostate cancer: the changing scene. *Clin Oncol* 1995, 7(2), 147–50.
9. Chodak GW, Thisted RA, Gerber GS *et al.* Results of conservative management of clinically localized prostate cancer. *NEJM* 1994, **330** (4), 242–8.
10. Hanks GE, Hanlon A, Owen JB *et al.* Patterns of radiation treatment of elderly patients with prostate cancer. *Cancer* 1994, **74** (Suppl 7), 2174–7.
11. Goffinet DR, Bagshaw MA. Radiation therapy of prostate carcinoma: thirty year experience at Stanford University. In: *EORTC genitourinary group monograph 8. Treatment of prostatic cancer—facts and controversies* (ed. PH Schroder). Wiley-Liss Inc, New York, Chichester, Brisbane, Toronto, Singapore, 1990, 209–22.
12. Zagars GK, von Eschenbach AC, Johnson DE *et al.* Adenocarcinoma of the prostate: an analysis of 551 patients treated with external-beam radiation. *Cancer* 1987, **60** (7), 1489–99.
13. Zagars GK, von Eschenbach AC, Johnson DE *et al.* The role of radiation therapy in stages A2 and B adenocarcinoma of the prostate. *Int J Radiat Oncol Biol Phys* 1988, **14**, 701–9.
14. Perez CA, Pilepich MV, Garcia D *et al.* Definitive radiation therapy in carcinoma of the prostate localized to the pelvis: experience at the Mallinckrodt Institute of Radiology. *Natl Cancer Int Monogr* 1988, 7, 85–94.
15. Hanks GE, Asbell S, Krall JM *et al.* Outcome for lymph node dissection negative T-lb, T-2 (A-2, B) prostate cancer treated with external-beam radiation therapy in RTOG 77–06. *Int J Radiat Oncol Biol Phys* 1991, **21** (4), 1099–103.
16. Leibel SA, Zelefsky MJ, Kutcher OJ *et al.* The biological basis and clinical application of 3-dimensional conformal external-beam radiation therapy in carcinoma of the prostate. *Semin Oncol* 1994, **21** (5), 580–97.
17. Pilepich MV, Krall JM, Sause WT *et al.* Prognostic factors in carcinoma of the prostate-analysis of RTOG study 7506. *Int J Radiat Oncol Biol Phys* 1987, **13** (3), 339–49.
18. Crook J, Robertson S, Collin G *et al.* Clinical relevance of trans-rectal ultrasound, biopsy and serum prostate-specific antigen following extemal beam radiotherapy for carcinoma of the prostate. *Int J Radiat Oncol Biol Phys* 1993, **27** (1), 31–7.
19. Zietman AL, Shipley WU. Willett GC. Residual disease after radical surgery or radiation therapy for prostate cancer. Clinical significance and therapeutic implications. *Cancer* 1993, **71**, 859–69.

20. Scardino PT, Bretas F. Interstitial radiotherapy. In: *Adenocarcinoma of the prostate* (ed. AW Bruce, J Trachtenberg). Springer Verlag, London, 1987, 145–58.

21. Freiha FS, Bagshaw MA. Carcinoma of the prostate: results of post- irradiation biopsy. *Prostate* 1984, 5 (1), 19–25.

22. Hanks OE, Hanlon AL, Hudes G *et al.* Patterns-of-failure analysis of patients with high pretreatment prostate-specific antigen levels treated by radiation therapy: the need for improved systemic and locoregional treatment. *J Clin Oncol* 1996, 14 (4), 1093–97.

23. Zietman AL, Tibbs MK, Dallow KC *et al.* Use of PSA nadir to predict subsequent biochemical outcome following external beam radiation therapy for T1–2 adenocarcinoma of the prostate. *Radiother Oncol* 1996, 40 (2), 159–162.

24. Horwitz EM, Vicini PA, Ziaja EL *et al.* Assessing the variability of outcome for patients treated with localised prostate irradiation using different definitions of biochemical control. *Radiat Oncol Biol Phys* 1996, 36 (3), 565–71.

25. Hanks GE, Lee WR, Hanlon AL *et al.* Conformal technique dose escalation for prostate cancer: biochemical evidence of improved cancer control with higher doses in patients with pretreatment prostate specific antigen > or = 10 ng/ml. *Int J Radiat Oncol Biol Phys* 1996, 35 (5), 861–8.

26. McLaughlin PW, Sandler HM, Jiroutek MR. Prostate specific antigen following prostate radiotherapy: how low can you go? *J Clin Oncol* 1996, 14 (II), 2889–92.

27. McNeil C. PSA levels after radiotherapy: how low must they go? *J Natl Cancer Inst* 1996, 88 (12), 791–2.

28. Critz PA, Levinson AK, Williams WH *et al.* Prostate specific antigen nadir: the optimum level after irradiation for prostate cancer. *J Clin Oncol* 1996, 14 (11), 2893–900.

29. Fuks Z, Leibel SA, Wallner KE *et al.* The effect of local control on metastatic dissemination in carcinoma of the prostate: long-term results in patients treated with 125I implantation. *Int J Radiat Biol Oncol Phys* 1991, 21, 537–47.

30. Yorke ED, Fuks Z, Norton L *et al.* Modeling the development of metastasis from primary and locally recurrent tumors: comparison with a clinical data base for prostatic cancer. *Cancer Res* 1993, 53, 2987–93.

31. Duncan W, Warde P, Catton CN. Carcinoma of the prostate: results of radical radiotherapy (1970–1985). *Int J Radiat Oncol Biol Phys* 1993, 26 (2), 203–10.

32. Amdur RJ, Parsons JT, Fitzgerald LT *et al.* Adenocarcinoma of the prostate treated with external-beam radiation therapy: 5-year minimum follow-up. *Radiotherapy and Oncology* 1990, 18 (3), 235–46.

33. Mithal NP, Hoskin PJ. External beam radiotherapy for carcinoma of the prostate: a retrospective study. *Clin Oncol* 1993, 5 (5), 297–301.

34. Sagerman RH, Chun HC, King GA *et al.* External beam radiotherapy for carcinoma of the prostate. *Cancer* 1989, 63 (12), 2468–74.

35. Aristizabal SA, Steinbronn D, Heusinkveld RS. External beam radiotherapy in cancer of the prostate. *Radiother Oncol* 1984, 1, 309–15.

36. Forman JD, Zinreich E, Lee Ding-J *et al.* Improving the therapeutic ratio of external beam irradiation for carcinoma of the prostate. *Int J Radiat Oncol Biol Phys* 1985, 11, 2073–80.

37. Leibel SA, Hanks OE, Kramer S. Patterns of care outcome studies: Results of the national practice in adenocarcinoma of the prostate. *Int J Radiat Oncol Biol Phys* 1984, 10 (3), 401–9.

38. Hanks OE, Diamond JJ, Krall JM *et al.* A ten year follow-up of 682 patients treated for prostate cancer with radiation therapy in the United States. *Int J Radiat Oncol Biol Phys* 1987, 13 (4), 499–505.

39. Hanks OE, Krall JM, Martz KL *et al.* The outcome of treatment of 313 patients with T-1 (UICC) prostate cancer treated with external beam irradiation. *Int J Radiat Oncol Biol Phys* 1988, 14 (2), 243–8.

40. De Wit L, Ang KK, van der Schueren E. Acute side-effects and late complications after radiotherapy of localized carcinoma of the prostate. *Cancer Treat Rev* 1983, 10, 79–89.

41. Pilepich MV, Krall JM, al Sarraf M *et al.* Androgen deprivation with radiation therapy compared with radiation therapy alone for locally advanced prostatic carcinoma: a randomized comparative trial of the Radiation Therapy Oncology Group. *Urology* 1995, 45 (4), 616–23.

42. Roach MI, Chinn DM, Holland J *et al.* A pilot survey of sexual function and quality of life following 3D conformal radiotherapy for clinically localized prostate cancer. *Int J Radiat Oncol Biol Phys* 1996, 35 (5), 869–74.

43. Helgason AR, Fredrikson M, Adolfsson J *et al.* Decreased sexual capacity after external radiation therapy for prostate cancer impairs quality of life. *Int J Radiat Oncol Biol Phys* 1995, (1), 33–9.

44. Fransson P, Widmark A. Self assessed sexual function after pelvic irradiation for prostate carcinoma. Comparison with an age-matched control group. *Cancer* 1996, 78 (5), 1066–78.

45. Hanks GE, Martz KL, Diamond JJ. The effect of dose on local control of prostate cancer. *Int J Radiat Oncol Biol Phys* 1988, 15, 1299–305.

46. Zelefsky MJ, Leibel SA, Gaudin PB *et al.* Dose escalation with three–dimensional conformal radiation therapy affects the outcome in prostate cancer. *Int J Radiat Oncol Biol Phys* 1998, 41 (3), 491–500.

47. Hanks GE, Hanlon AL, Schultheiss TE. Dose escalation with 3D conformal treatment: five-year outcomes, treatment optimization, and future directions. *Int J Radiat Oncol Biol Phys* 1998, 41 (3), 501–10.

48. Pilepich MV, Asbell SO, Krall JM *et al.* Correlation of radiotherapeutic parameters and treatment related morbidity-analysis of RTOG study 77-06. *Int J Radiat Oncol Biol Phys* 1987, 13 (7), 1007–12.

49. Emami B, Lyman J, Brown A *et al.* Tolerance of normal tissue to therapeutic irradiation. *Int J Radiat Oncol Biol Phys* 1991, 21, 109–22.

50. Kutcher GJ, Burman C, Brewster L. Histogram reduction method for calculating complication probabilities for 3-dimensional treatment planning evaluations. *Int J Radiat Oncol Biol Phys* 1991, 21, 137–46.

51. Hartford AC, Niemierko A, Adams JA. Conformal irradiation of the prostate: estimating long term rectal

bleeding risk using dose-volume histograms. *Int J Radiat Oncol Biol Phys* 1996, **36** (3), 721–30.

52. Johansen J, Bentzen SM, Overgaard J *et al.* Relationship between the in vitro radiosensitivity of skin fibroblasts and the expression of subcutaneous fibrosis, telangiectasia, and skin erythema after radiotherapy. *Radiother Oncol* 1996, **40** (2), 101–9.

53. Burnet NG, Nyman JIT. The relationship between cellular radiation sensitivity and tissue response may provide the basis for individualising radiotherapy schedules. *Radiother Oncol* 1994, **33**, 228–38.

54. Brock W A, Tucker SL, Geara FB. Fibroblast radiosensitivity versus acute and late normal skin responses in patients treated for breast cancer. *Int J Radiat Oncol Biol Phys* 1995, **32**, 1371–9.

55. Rosenthal SA, Roach MD, Goldsmith BJ *et al.* Immobilization improves the reproducibility of patient positioning during six-field confoffilal radiation therapy for prostate carcinoma. *Int J Radiat Oncol Biol Phys* 1993, **27** (4), 921–926.

56. Ten Haken RK, Perez-Tamayo C, Tesser RJ *et al.* Boost treatment of the prostate using shaped, fixed fields. *Int J Radiat Oncol Biol Phys* 1989, **16**, 193–200.

57. Leibel SA, Heimann R, Kutcher JG *et al.* Three-dimensional conformal radiation therapy in locally advanced carcinoma of the prostate: preliminary results of a phase I dose-escalation study. *Int J Radiat Oncol Biol Phys* 1994, **28** (1), 55–65.

58. Mesina CF, Sharman R, Rissman LS *et al.* Comparison of a standard four-field boost technique with a customized non-axial external beam technique for the treatment of adenocarcinoma of the prostate (Abstract). *Int J Radiat Oncol Biol Phys* 1993, **27** (Suppl), 193.

59. Sailer SL, Rosenman JG, Symon JR. The tetrad and hexad: maximum beam separation as a starting point for noncoplanar 3-D treatment planning: prostate cancer as a test case. *Int J Radiat Oncol Biol Phys* 1994, **30** (2), 439–46.

60. Sandler H, McLaughlin PW, Ten Haken R. 3-D conformal radiotherapy for the treatment of prostate cancer: low risk of chronic rectal morbidity observed in a large series of patients. *Int J Radiat Oncol Biol Phys* 1993, **27** (Suppl 1), 135.

61. Neal AJ, Oldham M, Dearnaley DP. Comparison of treatment techniques for conformal radiotherapy of the prostate using dose-volume histograms and normal tissue complication probabilities. *Radiother Oncol* 1995, **37** (1), 29–34.

62. Dearnaley DP, Nahum A, Lee M *et al.* Radiotherapy of prostate cancer: reducing the treated volume. Conformal therapy, hormone cytoreduction and protons (Meeting abstract). *Br J Cancer* 1994, **70** (Suppl 22), 187.

63. Deamaley DP, Khoo VS, Norman A *et al.* Comparison of radiation side–effects of conformal and conventional radiotherapy in prostate cancer: a randomized trial. *Lancet* 1999, **353** (9149), 267–72.

64. Sandler HM, Perez-Tamayo C, Ten Haken RK *et al.* Dose escalation for stage C (T3) prostate cancer: minimal rectal toxicity observed using conformal therapy. *Radiother Oncol* 1992, **23**, 53–4.

65. Epstein BE, Hanks GE. Radiation therapy techniques and dose selection in the treatment of prostate cancer. *Semin Radiat Oncol* 1993, **3** (3), 179–86.

66. Meyn RE, Stephens LC, Ang KK. Heterogeneity in the development of apoptosis in irradiated murine tumors of different histologies. *Int J Radiat Biol Phys* 1993, **64** (5), 583–91.

67. Shearer RJ, Davies JH, Gelister JSK *et al.* Hormonal cytoreduction and radiotherapy for carcinoma of the prostate. *Br J Urol* 1992, **69** (5), 521–4.

68. Deamaley DP, Shearer RJ, Ellingham L *et al.* Rationale and initial results of adjuvant hormone therapy and irradiation for prostate cancer. In: *Sex hormones and antihormones in endocrine dependent pathology: basic and clinical aspects* (ed. M Motta, M Serio). Elsevier Science, Amsterdam, Lausanne, New York, Oxford, Shannon, Tokyo, 1994, 197–208.

69. Zelefsky MJ, Leibel SA, Burman CM *et al.* Neoadjuvant hormonal therapy improves the therapeutic ratio in patients with bulky prostatic cancer treated with three-dimensional conformal radiation therapy. *Int J Radiat Oncol Biol Phys* 1994, **42** 755–61.

70. Forman JD, Kumar R, Haas G *et al.* Neoadjuvant hormonal downsizing of localized carcinoma of the prostate: effects on the volume of normal tissue irradiation. *Cancer Invest* 1995, **13** (1), 8–15.

71. Padhani AR, Husband JE, Revell P *et al.* Prostate cancer morphology and vascular permeability after androgen deprivation treatment. *Radiology* 1998, **209**, 182.

72. Pilepich MV, Winter K, Roach M. Phase III Radiation Oncology Group (RTOG) 86–10 of androgen deprivation before and during radiotherapy in locally advanced carcinoma of the prostate. *Proc Am Soc Clin Oncol* 1998, **1185** (17), 308a.

73. Porter A, Ethliali M, Manji M. A phase III randomized trial to evaluate the efficacy of neoadjuvant therapy prior to curative radiotherapy in locally advanced prostate cancer patients. A Canadian Urologic Oncology Group Study. *Proc Am Clin Oncol* 1998, **17** (315a), 1123.

74. Laverdiere J, Gomez JL, Cusan L. Beneficial effect of combination hormonal therapy administered prior and following extemal beam radiation therapy in localized prostate cancer. *Int J Radiat Oncol Biol Phys* 1997, **37** (2), 247–52.

75. Forman JD, Shamsa F, Maughan RL *et al.* Improving the therapeutic ratio of radiation in locally advanced prostate cancer: mixed neutron/photon vs. hyperfractionated photon irradiation. *Radiat Oncol Invest* 1996, **4**, 129–34.

76. Zietman AL, Prince EA, Nakfoor BM *et al.* Androgen deprivation and radiation therapy: sequencing studies using the Sionogi in NiNo tumor system. *Int J Radiat Oncol Biol Phys* 1997, **38** (5), 1067–70.

77. Joon DL, Hasegawa M, Sikes C. Supra-additive apoptotic response of R3327-G rat prostate tumors to androgen ablation and radiation. *Int J Radiat Oncol Biol Phys* 1997, **38** (5), 1071–7.

78. Lange PH, Narayan P. Understaging and undergrading of prostate cancer: argument for postoperative

radiation as adjuvant therapy. *Urology* 1983, **21**, 113–8.

79. Eggleston JC, Walsh PC. Radical prostatectomy with preservation of sexual function: pathological findings in the first 100 cases. *J Urol* 1985, **134** (6), 1146–8.

80. Feneley MR, Gillatt DA, Hehir M *et al*. A review of radical prostatectomy from 3 centers in the UK: clinical presentation and outcome. *Br J Urol* 1996, **78** (6), 911–20.

81. Hanks OE, Dawson AK. The role of external-beam radiation therapy after prostatectomy for prostate cancer. *Cancer* 1986, **58**, 2406–10.

82. Ray GR, Bagshaw MA, Freiha F. External-beam radiation salvage for residual or recurrent local tumor following radical prostatectomy. *J Urol* 1984, **132**, 926–30.

83. Bahnson RR, Gamett JE, Grayhack JT. Adjuvant radiation therapy in stage C and D, prostatic adenocarcinoma: preliminary results. *Urology* 1986, **27** (5), 403–6.

84. Eisbruch A, Perez CA, Roessler EH *et al*. Adjuvant irradiation after prostatectomy for carcinoma of the prostate with positive surgical margins. *Cancer* 1994, **73** (2), 384–7.

85. Lange PH, Lightner DJ, Medini E. The effect of radiation therapy after radical prostatectomy in patients with elevated prostate specific antigen levels. *J Urol* 1990, **144** (4), 927–33.

86. Lange PH, Moon DT, Narayan P *et al*. Radiation therapy as adjuvant treatment after radical prostatectomy: patient tolerance and preliminary results. *J Urol* 1986, **136**, 45–59.

87. Anscher MS, Prosnitz LR. Radiotherapy vs. hormonal therapy for the management of locally recurrent prostate cancer following radical prostatectomy. *Int J Radiat Oncol Biol Phys* 1989, **17** (5), 953–8.

88. Schild SE, Buskirk SJ, Wong WW. The use of radiotherapy for patients with isolated elevation of serum prostate specific antigen following radical prostatectomy. *J Urol* 1996, **156** (5), 1725–9.

89. Carter GE, Lieskovsky G, Skinner DG *et al*. Results of local and/or systemic adjuvant therapy in the management of pathological stage C or Dl prostate cancer following radical prostatectomy. *J Urol* 1989, **142**, 1266–70.

90. Cheng WS, Frydenberg M, Bergstralh EJ *et al*. Radical prostatectomy for pathologic Stage C prostate cancer: Influence of pathologic variables and adjuvant treatment on disease outcome. *Urology* 1993, **42**, 283–91.

91. Freeman JA, Leiskovsky G and Cook DW. Radical retropubic prostatectomy and post operative adjuvant radiation for pathological stage C (PcN0) prostate cancer from 1976 to 1989: intermediate findings. *J Urol* 1989, **149** (5), 1029–34.

92. Schild SE, Wong WW, Grado GL. The results of radical retropubic prostatectomy and adjuvant therapy for pathological stage C prostate cancer. *Int J Radiat Oncol Biol Phys* 1996, **34** (3), 535–41.

93. Schild SE. Regarding postoperative radiotherapy for pathologic stage C prostate cancer: in response to Dr Lawrence and Mr Collins. *Int J Radiat Oncol Biol Phys* 1996, **36** (3), 757–9.

18 | Cryosurgical ablation of the prostate in the management of localized prostate cancer

John P. Long

Introduction

The task of determining the most effective therapy for patients diagnosed with clinically localized prostate carcinoma (PCA) is a challenging one for both physicians and patients alike. PCA remains a major health concern in many industrialized countries, (1) and remains the most common malignancy and second most common cause of cancer-related deaths in American males (2). Despite a voluminous literature investigating this disease, defining a standard of treatment for individual patients who present with a new diagnosis of PCA remains problematic. Historically, the dominant treatment options for localized PCA have been radical prostatectomy (3, 4) and external-beam radiotherapy (5, 6). In fact these two therapies account for nearly 80% of initial treatments administered to patients with PCA in the US (7). More recently, particularly over the past 5 years, novel or modified treatments for localized PCA have been introduced including ultrasound-guided interstitial brachytherapy (8, 9) 3-dimensional conformal radiotherapy (10, 11), high-dose combination radiotherapy (12), HDR Iridium192 brachytherapy (13, 14), proton-beam radiotherapy, (15) high-intensity focused ultrasound (HIFU) thermotherapy (16), and cryo-ablation (17–21). Unfortunately, no randomized prospective comparison with adequate follow-up has ever been completed comparing any two of these approaches. Obviously without such information treatment recommendations must be made on the basis of the available literature, but this is problematic since often both patient selection and definitions of treatment success (regardless of the treatment) vary considerably among reports that document post-treatment outcomes (22, 23).

Over the past 5 years over 40 reports have been published pertaining to the use of transrectal ultrasound-guided cryo-ablation of the prostate for treating patients with PCA, with variable and inconsistent results. A number of authors have suggested very promising preliminary results with regard to cancer-related outcomes such as biochemical disease-free survivals or negative biopsy rates, (24) while others have raised concerns regarding the potential morbidities of this procedure and the feasibility of safely accomplishing whole-gland ablations (25). The purpose of this chapter is to review the evolution of this interesting technology and to summarize the current clinical experience with using cryo-ablation to treat patients with localized prostate cancer.

Cryo-ablation history

The first report of cryo-ablation of the human prostate was in 1966 when Gonder and Soanes published the results of using a transurethral single cryoprobe in ablating peri-urethral adenomatous tissue in patients with outlet obstructive symptoms (26). Subsequently, several reports appeared pertaining to its use as a possible treatment for patients with both metastatic and localized adenocarcinoma of the prostate. Later a transperineal approach, applying the cryoprobes directly to the surface of the prostate, was also described. Collectively over the next 15 years, these procedures were employed in several institutions as an alternative to more conventional means of managing patients with various stages of PCA, with a number of reports demonstrating mixed results (27–29). Fundamentally these applications of cryo-ablation to the prostate suffered from the inability to monitor the cryodestruction in real time; treatment endpoints were occasionally determined by direct palpation only.

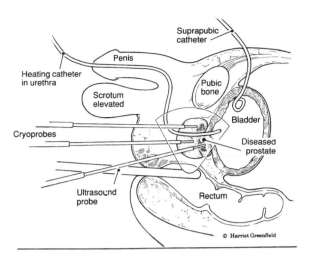

Fig. 18.1 Graphic illustration of transperineal cryo-ablation of the prostate. Post-treatment urinary drainage can be either with a suprapubic tube, as here, or with urethral catheters.

Ultimately these forms of cryo-ablation were generally abandoned due to modest rates of local recurrence along with frequent morbidities (30).

With the development of transrectal ultrasonographic imaging, interest in percutaneous cryo-ablation of the prostate was renewed in the late 1980s. Three critical modifications to the older techniques were made. The first was the use of real-time transrectal ultrasonographic monitoring of both the cryoprobe placement, as well as the propagation of the advancing ice. The second was the development of 3-mm cryoprobes, which could be placed transperineally into targeted areas of the prostate. Lastly, a urethral warming system was devised to maintain sufficient viability of the peri-urethral tissues to lower tissue-sloughing rates relative to the older approaches (Fig. 18.1).

Using these components, two small-animal studies were performed investigating cryo-ablation in a canine prostate model. The first indicated that the leading edge of the propagating ice ball could be safely followed in real time by TRUS imaging (31), and the second indicated that percutanous cryoprobes could be used to produce necrosis in canine prostate tissue (32). Using this somewhat limited testing, a first-generation cryo-ablation system (Accuprobe™, CMS) was developed that supported active freezing from no more than five cryoprobes simultaneously (28). This number was chosen somewhat arbitrarily and, not surprisingly, the probe pattern initially suggested for treating human prostates involved five probe sites. Prior to marketing

(i.e. prior to obtaining 510K designation) this device, no studies had been completed that were directed toward validating the actual five-probe technique itself in either animal or pre-prostatectomy models. Notably specific questions pertaining to the use of cryo-ablation to treat PCA in humans, such as (to list some) patient selection, probe distribution, mechanisms of urethral warming, number of freezes, ideal target volumes, ideal rates of freezing, or establishing correlations between histologic effects and specific temperature endpoints in prostate tissue, were not explored. As a result, although it was probably true that, as claimed at the time, there was little doubt that cryo-ablation could destroy PCA tissue, initial marketing was done amid the absence of data that defined an ideal technique of applying this technology to the human prostate.

The first clinical experience in humans with percutaneous transrectal ultrasound-guided cryo-ablation was published in 1993 when Onik reported early results after treatment of 63 patients with localized prostate carcinoma (33). Given that this was the first focal ablative therapy introduced for treating PCA, and that it may have been marketed prematurely, it is fair to say that since that time cryo-ablation has been a work in evolution. Perhaps not surprisingly, a number of technical variations have been proposed since the initial report, and the absence of a validated treatment protocol prior to marketing is probably the reason why the clinical results presented in over 40 peer-reviewed reports since then have been somewhat mixed.

Mechanisms of tissue injury

Cryo-ablation is the best developed of several forms of tissue ablation, which (when applied in the human prostate) attempt to eradicate all foci of prostate cancer in a given gland *in situ* without the use of surgical extirpation. Unlike radiation (mitotic arrest) or androgen deprivation (apoptosis), the mechanism whereby cryo-ablation produces cytotoxicity is the induction of targeted areas of coagulative necrosis in the prostate gland. There are two mechanisms whereby this is believed to occur (34). First involves 'direct' injury to the targeted cells, which is effected in one of two ways. The accumulation of extracellular ice in the interstitial compartment is very desiccating and results in a toxic accumulation of toxins within the cell; during thawing the osmotic shift reverses, resulting in lysis of both the intracellular organelles and the cell membrane itself. The second mechanism of 'direct' injury is through the accumulation of intracellular ice, which produces shear forces within the cell disruptive enough to destroy all organelles and the cell membrane itself. The accumulation of intracellular ice may be enhanced by rapid freezing rates, particularly at rates which exceed 25°C/min (35). The second mechanism of cryo- injury is the 'indirect' or ischaemic mechanism. Some believe that this may be the most important mechanism whereby cryo-ablation can produce large areas of necrosis in a targeted tissue field. (i.e. as opposed to cell monolayers *in vitro*) (34). Rapid freezing clearly induces thrombosis both in a microvascular level as well as for larger arterioles, producing large areas of field infarcts. Although the temperatures necessary to generate coagulative necrosis may vary amongst different tissues (34), recent evidence has clearly indicated that –40°C to –50°C is the critical threshold for achieving reliable areas of coagulative necrosis in human prostate tissue (36).

Cryo-ablation: features of effective treatment of prostate cancer

PCA poses a particular challenge to focal ablation techniques such as cryo-ablation, in that it is difficult to reliably define the location or extent of local tumor burden in the prostate. For example, it has been shown that prostate cancers are usually multi-focal, typically consisting of two to five tumors per gland (37). Unfortunately there is still no radiographic modality that can identify with satisfactory degrees of resolution the intraprostatic tumor volume distribution to a reliable degree. Thus, until such time that clinically significant foci (> 0.5 cm³) of prostate carcinoma can be accurately identified pre-operatively, the application of cryo-ablation in treating patients with PCA must be directed toward treating the *entire prostate gland* as the ideal means of eradicating the disease.

Because effective cryo-ablation relies on temperature changes in order to produce coagulative necrosis in the desired tissue target, the temperature thresholds necessary to produce a reliable correlation between treatment parameters and histopathology (i.e. coagulative necrosis in the target area) need to be well defined. As stated, for human prostate tissue, these targets currently appear to be less than –40°C to –50°C. At the present time, the only way to assess the extent of prostate tissue ablation is to use temperature monitoring in real time during freezing. While it is conceivable

that models could be constructed to predict reliably the 3-dimensional areas of coagulative necrosis that will be created in the prostate based on a given set of treatment variables (tissue composition, duration of freeze, etc.), such 'operator-independent' models are lacking. Currently the best means of providing real-time temperature monitoring during focal cryo-ablation involves the interstitial placement of multiple thermocouples in strategic locations in and around the targeted treatment area.

Finally, treating PCA with cryo-ablation is also challenging because of the need to avoid damage to a number of important structures that are within or adjacent to the freezing zone—most important of these being the rectum, urethra, voluntary urinary sphincter complex, and bladder neck. Histopathologic studies of cryolesions consistently indicate a fairly sharp demarcation between treatment effect and normal tissue. This feature of cryo-ablation can be exploited by using precise cryoprobe placement to maximize coagulative necrosis in the glandular prostate and minimize freezing effect in the surrounding structures. As will be seen, adequate urethral warming and probe distribution are critical elements of technique if these goals are going to be achieved.

Cryo-ablation: technical variations

Multiple freeze-thaw cycles

It has been demonstrated that cellular destruction occurs during both the freeze and the thaw (rapid freeze, slow thaw) portions of a cryo-ablation cycle (34). Two freeze-thaw cycles have been shown to produce more efficient cell kill when compared to single cycles, both in human prostate monolayers *in vitro* (35)—although this may not be as important as reaching –40°C in human prostate models *in vivo* (38). Further, two freeze-thaw cycles during prostate cryo-ablation in humans have been associated with lower positive biopsy rates, as well as improved PSA results, when compared to single-freeze cycles, without any apparent increase in developing cryo-related morbidities (18, 19, 39). Finally, in single-probe temperature mapping experiments performed on patients prior to radical prostatectomy, two consecutive 10-min freeze cycles produced a larger area of coagulative necrosis than a single 20-min freeze (36). Thus the available literature supports the use of a minimum of two freeze-thaw cycles, although whether there is any additional benefit to more than two cycles is not known.

Urethral warming

The primary objective of the use of urethral warming catheter systems during cryo-ablation is to minimize urethral sloughing. The first urethral warming system was marketed as a non-significant risk device until approximately July 1994. Initial experiences with this system were notable for fairly low rates of urethral sloughing ranging from 4% to 10% (33, 40, 41). Due apparently to concerns submitted to the FDA surrounding the safety of this particular device, it was taken off the market in mid-1994 for approximately 18 months, while it underwent regulatory review. During this time period numerous authors reported a sharp increase in post-cryo-ablation TURP and overall urethral sloughing rates due to the use of alternate urethral warmers or warming systems, which did not have many of the features of the original one (14–16, 20, 21). As expected, the safety of the original warmers was easily confirmed during this period and, since 1996, approved urethral warming catheters have been widely available. The precise mechanisms by which adequate urethral warming ensures the most protective heat transfer during cryo-ablation are still being evaluated; however, currently it is clear that the warming system as originally designed was effective in reducing slough-related morbidities. With current techniques, anticipated post-cryo-ablation sloughing rates lie between 3% and 9% (17, 42) provided that the appropriate warming catheters are used, and that patients have not been radiated. Studies directed toward improving catheter design and urethral warming efficiency are ongoing, with the hopeful result that slough rates will decline even further as new systems are marketed.

Thermocouple monitoring

Early in the experience with performing cryo-ablation of the prostate, several authors in particular noted that real-time interpretation of the leading edge of the ice ball on sonographic imaging underestimated the actual extent of cellular destruction (19, 43, 44). In addition, a number of reports in the cryobiological literature had documented in several human tissues fairly reliable coagulative necrosis when temperatures of $-40°C$ to $-50°C$ were achieved in the target areas (34). As a result some programs began to place thermocouples at the margins of the targeted treatment zones (e.g. neurovascular bundles, apex) to ensure that these cytotoxic temperatures were achieved during freezing. Wong and Bahn were among the first to relate improved PSA rates and post-cryobiopsy results with thermocouple monitoring when compared to patients in whom this had not been used (19, 20, 45). Currently it is evident that transrectal ultrasonography alone is inadequate for monitoring and planning a successful cryo-ablation. Although the precise number of thermocouples that constitute a satisfactory number of data points to ensure an adequate freeze is still being evaluated, a minimum of four to perhaps five thermocouple positions around the periphery of the prostate as well as at the apex of the prostate is recommended.

Probe number/probe distribution

The device first used to perform percutaneous cryo-ablation in patients with PCA was manufactured with exit ports for fve cryoprobes (46). Not surprisingly, the initial report on this procedure described a technique involving the placement of five cryoprobes radically around the urethra. To what degree this probe distribution effectively produced reliably confluent areas of coagulative necrosis around the urethra had not been confirmed in human prostate settings, and was based to some extent on patterns of ice propagation using five cryoprobes in agar phantoms.

Recently temperature mapping studies done in patients with localized prostate cancer, who agreed to undergo focal cryo-ablation of the prostate prior to undergoing a radical prostatectomy, have begun to define the mechanics of freezing in human prostate tissue more clearly (36). These studies found that for single probes engaged in two consecutive 10-min freeze-thaw cycles, a radius of approximately 7–8 mm from the cryoprobe correlated consistently with a $-40°$ to $-50°C$ degree isotherm. Subsequent histopathological evaluation of the surgical specimens after 3-mm step-sectioning indicated that this isotherm also consistently correlated with zones of complete coagulative necrosis. Temperatures ranging from $-20°$ to $-40°C$ (i.e. 8–10 mm radii) correlated with a zone of histopathologic changes that was characterized by viable cells exhibiting signs of cellular injury, the significance of which is difficult to discern from the preliminary studies. Follow-up temperature mapping studies in patients undergoing full-gland (i.e. six probes) cryo-ablations demonstrated that the effect of multiple probe placement produces a larger effective freezing zone than that predicted by simply adding single-probe freezing characteristics. The arcuate peripheral placement of cryoprobes 1.2–1.4 cm apart consistently produced temperatures lower than −100°C at points 8–10 mm medial to the probe arc. Interestingly, temperatures measured at 7–8 mm peripheral to the arc rarely were lower than the targeted threshold of −50°C, presumably because no additive effect was being produced. These preliminary data strongly indicate that for many patients, (especially those with larger glands) the originally suggested five-probe distribution may have been inadequate to reliably produce an area of coagulative necrosis that was large enough to cover all viable tissue in the prostate. Moreover, these data begin to define critical elements of probe placement for individual glands. These features may include keeping probes within 7–8 mm of the capsule, placing probes no less than 1.2–1.4 mm apart (i.e.6–7 mm radii/probe) around the gland, and using as many probes within these guidelines as the volume or shape of the prostate requires. Moreover, treatment efficiency will probably be maximized by restricting cryo-ablation to patients with gland volumes of approximately 40 cm³ or less. Whether such a treatment design will produce reliable targeted ablation in all patients will require additional study, but it is interesting that Lee has demonstrated a clear clinical improvement in results with six vs. five cryoprobes (47).

Thus although there has been significant technical variation in published reports on cryo-ablation of the prostate, the essential elements of an effective treatment are starting to emerge (Fig. 18.2). Ideally, candidate prostate glands should be between 30–40 cm³. The targeted temperatures are −40° to −50°C at the periphery of the prostate, with a minimum of six peripherally loaded cryoprobes. Urethral warming using approved devices has to be employed in order to ensure a minimized TUR slough rate. A minimum of two freezes should be used, and the entire procedure should be done under real-time temperature monitoring in order to maximize the likelihood of achieving large areas of coagulative necrosis throughout the prostate.

Cryo-ablation: clinical results

Because the first reported results with contemporary cryo-ablation of the prostate were published 1993, standard criteria for treatment efficacy, such as 10–15-year cause-specific survival data, are lacking for this procedure. However surrogate outcomes, which are increasingly being used to assess treatment efficiency, are available from many centers using this modality. The three primary surrogate outcomes in this regard are post-treatment PSA results, post-treatment biopsy results (occult local control), and post-treatment morbidities. These will be briefly summarized below.

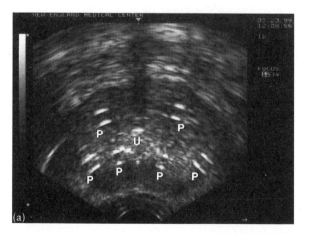
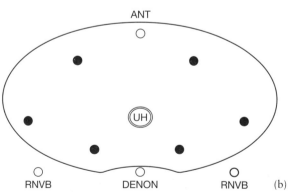

Fig. 18.2 Transverse transrectal ultrasound image depicting the six-probe cryo-ablation technique. Double echoes at each of the probe positions are characteristic of the teflon sheaths in place just prior to the actual cryoprobe placements. P denotes each of six sheaths in position. U denotes urethral warming catheter. (a) Thermocouples have not been placed yet. (b) Graphic illustration corresponding to the actual probe postitions in (a). *Filled circles* represent standard six-probe distribution; more can be added for selected glands. *Open circles* represent thermocouple positions for monitoring (ANT: anterior and just subcapsular; DENON: Denovillier's layer in the midline; R/LNVB: just extracapsular at levels of neurovascular bundles). Occasionally a fifth is placed at the apical level. UH refers to urethral heater.

PSA results

The post-cryo-ablation PSA results that have appeared in the literature have been reported variably. A number of early studies tended to document post-cryo PSA outcomes by reporting crude PSA rates at fixed post-operative time points; for example, post-cryo PSA values of < 0.5 ng/ml ranged from 41% to 74% (18, 21, 40, 48, 49). Unfortunately this early literature lacked a consensus on how best to report PSA-related outcomes post-cryo-ablation. Longer projections of PSA-based disease-free survivals from single-institution post-cryo-ablation are few; only a small number of programs have sufficient follow-up combined with an adequate number of patients treated to calculate actuarial 5-year biochemical-free survivals at any PSA threshold definition. In this regard, Long reported an overall actuarial biochemical progression-free rate at 5 years of 56% (49). Cohen recently reported 5-year biochemical-free survivals of 42% for PSA < 0.4 ng/ml and 58% for PSA < 1.0 among patients with Gleason grade 7 or higher PCA, or PSA > 10 ng/ml for pateints who undergo cryo-ablation (17, 50) Similar data from other institutions are lacking.

More recently a retrospective multi-institutional database, designed to stratify patients and outcomes in order to minimize selection bias inherent in single-institutional reporting, was constructed. One of the objectives of this study was to address the dearth of valid mid-term PSA outcomes following cryo-ablation mentioned above. Data from this analysis was instrumental in inducing the Health Care Financing Association in the US to reverse its policy and begin re-imbursing for cryo-ablation for its medicare subscribers as of July 1999. In this study, 975 patients were identified among five institutions performing cryo-ablation over the course of 5 years. For these patients the overall 5-year actuarial biochemical-free survival (BFS) post-cryo-ablation was 51% and 63% for the thresholds PSA < 0.5 ng/ml and PSA < 1.0 ng/ml, respectively (51). When patients were stratified by factors predicting higher risks of progression, the 5-year BFS rates not surprisingly declined according to increasing risk (Table 18.1). Notably, for PSA < 1.0 ng/ml, the %-year BFS rates were 76%, 67%, and 41% for patients at low, medium, and high risks for progression, respectively. A brief synopsis of contemporary radiotherapeutic techniques, including 3-dimensional conformal modifications as well as interstitial brachytherapy results, reported in the last 3 years suggest that these results are fairly comparable to what has been reported by other institutions (8–10, 52–58). For example, patients with low risk of progression undergoing these therapies have 5-year BFS rates ranging from 67% to 87%, depending on the selection criteria; those with higher risks have 5-year BFS rates ranging from 0% to 60%. The PSA results were noted to be comparable to those reported after radiotherapy, despite the fact that the data from this study are likely to reflect a 'least common denominator' effect among the institutions studied, since no attempt to segregate patients based on the actual technique used during the procedure for each patient in the database was made.

Post-cryo-ablation biopsy results

The value of post-treatment biopsy results continues to be a subject of some debate (59). What is clear is that with any type of ablative approach to the prostate

Table 18.1   Five-year actuarial biochemical success rate post-cryo stratified by risk category

	n	PSA < 0.5		PSA < 1.0	
		% rate (S.E.)	% 5-year at risk	% rate (S.E.)	% 5-year at risk
Overall	975	51.1 (2.7)	67	63 (2.7)	81.5
Low risk[†]	238	59.5 (4.7)*	26	76 (4.2)	34
Medium risk[‡]	321	61 (4.3)	23	71 (4.3)	25.5
High risk[§]	385	36 (5.0)	16.5	45 (5.2)	20.5
No AD	613	55 (2.9)	49	69 (2.7)*	61.5
AD	307	40 (5.8)	18	47 (6.0)	20

* $P < 0.05$ across groups, Logrank.
[†] PSA < 10, **and** GG < 7, **and** stage < cT2b.
[‡] Any 1:PSA > 10 **or** GG > 6 **or** stage > cT2a.
[§] Two or more: PSA > 10 **or** GG > 6 **or** stage > cT2a.

Prostate cancer

there still remains a sonographically evident residuum of tissue within which persistent or resistant foci of carcinoma have an opportunity to progress. Usually radiographic evaluations such as TRUS are not helpful in demonstrating the presence or absence of residual disease, although spectroscopically enhanced MRI may have some value (60, 61). In this context the value of random biopsies following these treatments, particularly for patients who have a rising PSA, seems obvious.

Numerous authors have reported fairly low positive biopsy rates following cryo-ablation ranging from 8% to 35%, with rates dependent on operator experience, patient selection factors, and duration of follow-up (17–21, 40, 48, 50, 62). Biopsies have been done either at predetermined time points post-treatment or in response unfavorable clinical developments such as a rising PSA, and usually 6–12 core techniques have been cited. In the retrospective multi-institutional study noted previously, the overall positive biopsy rate was only 18% (Table 18.2). Among patients at low risk for progression, the positive biopsy rate was even lower at 10%. These results are very comparable, if not superior to, positive biopsy rates following both external-beam radiotherapy or brachytherapy (8–10, 52–54). Thus, it would appear that these data suggest that, at least insofar as post-treatment biopsy sampling can indicate, cryo-ablation can produce fairly impressive degrees of local control with a very small risk of harboring occult persistent disease in the residuum.

Post-cryo morbidities

As with cancer-related outcomes, morbidities post-cryo are also variably reported. (Table 18.3). Prior radiation appears to be a significant risk factor for post-cryo-ablation related side-effects, and this will be discussed separately. The reported rates of recto-urethral fistulae have been fairly low, ranging from 0% to 3% (17–19, 21, 40–42, 48, 63, 64). Urethral drainage alone will resolve most of these fistulae, although colonic diversion and primary repair may be needed in rare instances. Reported rates of urethral sloughing in reports cited above range from 4% to 38%. As noted above, alternate urethral warming is clearly the chief risk factor among these studies for developing post-treatment sloughing. For patients with no prior therapies undergoing cryo-ablation with standard warming catheters, the slough rate can be as low as 4–8% (17, 42). Typically, sloughing is best managed with a TURP, limited only to the removal of obviously necrotic material, as extensive resections may decrease ultimate continence (19, 20). Overall the reported rates of incontinence in non-radiated patients following cryo-ablation range widely from 3% to 27% (17–19, 21, 40–42, 48, 63, 64). Again, as with urethral sloughing, factors that contribute to incontinence post-cryo include operator inexperience and inadequate urethral warming. In fact it is probably accurate to note that in the absence of tissue sloughing or prior radiation treatment, pad-dependent incontinence post-cryo occurs in < 3% of cases (17, 20, 42).

Currently, reported rates of potency following cryo-ablation are generally low, ranging from 0% to 20% (17, 18, 19, 41, 42). As with other therapies for managing PCA, it is difficult to provide objective determinations of erective function post-cryo, yet these low potency rates have been noted both in physician-based, as well as patient-based, outcomes assessment studies (42). The etiology of erectile dysfunction following cryo-ablation is poorly understood. One recent report

Table 18.2 Post-cryo positive biopsy rates (of patients biopsied)

	Post-cryo		Post-radiation				
	n	%	Ragde *et al.* (8)	Stock *et al.* (9)	Zelefsky *et al.* (10)	Laverdiere *et al.* (53)	Crook *et al.* (54)
Overall	141/779	18			43%	65%	44%
Low risk†	25/198	12*	22%	26%			
Medium risk‡	31/255	12*	22%	26%			
High risk§	82/305	27					

* $P < 0.05$ across groups, Logrank.
† PSA < 10, **and** GG < 7, **and** stage < cT2b.
‡ Any 1:PSA > 10 **or** GG > 6 **or** stage > cT2a.
§ Two or more: PSA > 10 **or** GG > 6 **or** stage > cT2a.

Table 18.3 Reported morbidity rates following cryoablation of the prostate

	Non-radiated/previously radiated, where reported									previously radiated only		
	Shinohara et al. (18)	Lee et al. (20)	Cox et al. (63)	Long et al. (17)	Wong et al. (19)	Cohen et al. (21)	Sosa et al. (64)	Coogan and McKiel (40)	Weider et al. (41)	Miller et al. (66)	Bales et al. (67)	Pisters et al. (39)
No. patients	92/10	301/46	51/12	127/18	83/7	239	1,467	95	83	33	23	150
Complications (%)												
rectourethral fistula	0/10	0.33/8.7	3.0	0/17.0	0	0.4	1.4	1	0	0	0	1.5
slough requiring TURP	23.0	NR	19.0	3.0/50.0	19	9.8	9.9/38*	10	3.8	15	52	17
bladder outlet obstruction	NR	3.2	29.0	17.2	NR	3	6.8	6	13	18	41	44
incontinence	15.0	0.3/8.7	27.0	2.0/83.0	6	4	11	3.5	2.5	10	95	73
impotence	86.0	92.0	NR	88.0	94	NR	100	47	80	NR	100	72
urethral stricture/BNC	NR	NR	3.0	3.4	11	2.2	5	1	3.8	5	14	NR
UTI/epididymitis	4.0	NR	NR	3.0/40	NR	4	9.1	4	9	NR	59	NR
perineal pain	3.0	NR	11.0	2.0/37.0	NR	0.4	9.4	1	NR	NR	37	8
sepsis	3.0	NR	3.0	1.0	NR	0.7	2.3	0	NR	0	9	NR
other (hematoma, bladder injury, ureteral obstruction, etc.	4.0	NR	13.0	5.0	1	2	NR	2	2.6	2	13	4
Total complications	NR	NR	46/82	17/89	NR	NR	NR	NR	NR	NR	NR	NR

*Approved/non-approved warmer
NR, not reported.

suggests that it is likely due to vasculogenic rather than exclusively neurogenic changes following the procedure, although this would need further study to be corroborated (65). At the moment there are few data documenting the effectiveness of different treatment strategies for post-cryo ED, although anecdotal experience suggests that intracavernous injection can be effective for most patients in this setting.

Overall the rates of developing lower urinary tract infections following cryo-ablation of the prostate range from 4% to 9% (17, 18, 21, 63). These are invariably easily managed with antibiotics. Other, more rare potential complications following this procedure that have been reported include sepsis, venous thrombosis, ureteral obstruction/hydronephrosis, and chronic penile pain. In the aggregate these more serious problems typically have occurred in < 10% of cases, and are noted to occur infrequently in institutions with large experiences performing this procedure.

Thus based on the clinical evidence available from the literature presented above, cryo-ablation seems to be a potentially effective treatment option for patients with new diagnoses of PCA. Unfortunately, the technical features that comprise a reliably effective treatment for individual patients have been evolving since its re-introduction in 1992. This lack of a genuinely validated method of applying cryo-ablation technology to adequately treat PCA has probably been the main reason hindering a broader acceptance of this procedure, as unfavorable outcomes following cryo-ablation of the prostate were noted following the initial experiences of a number of urologists with this technology (25, 63, 64). However, the currently recommended method is considerably different from that used during the initial marketing of this technique, and is based on carefully controlled clinical studies in humans. It seems reasonable to conclude that using six or more cryoprobes, standard urethral warming, multiple freeze-thaw cycles, and thermocouple monitoring will produce clinical outcomes that are comparable to those reported for other non-surgical therapies, such as external-beam radiation or brachytherapy.

Salvage cryo-ablation radiation failures

Upon its introduction in 1993 there was a fair degree of enthusiasm for cryo-ablation as a salvage option for patients who had failed radiotherapy. However, clinical outcomes from several programs examining this select patient group have been suboptimal. The rates of attaining undetectable PSA nadirs post-cryo in these patients range from 36% to 38%, but the likelihood of maintaining an undetectable PSA 12–18 months post-treatment drops to between 11% and 28% (39, 66–68). Post-cryo positive biopsy results for these patients have been a bit more encouraging, ranging between 14% and 27%, with lower rates noted in patients receiving more than one freeze-thaw cycle (39). Yet in most of these studies the biopsies were done fairly early (i.e. < 1 year) after the treatment. Longer follow-ups demonstrating the rate of maintaining a negative biopsy status in this group are lacking. Regardless of the mixed cancer-related outcomes, the primary concern with using cryo-ablation in managing these difficult patients has to do with the attendant morbidities. The side-effect profile for patients undergoing cryo-ablation after radiotherapy clearly appears to be higher than that seen in patients without prior radiation (Table 18.3). Incontinence rates range anywhere from 10% to 95% (17, 39, 64, 66–68), with all but one study noting very high rates of poor urinary control. Recto-urethral fistula rates ranged between 0% and 17%, and tissue sloughing has been noted in between 15% and 52% of cases, with somewhat lower rates for approved urethral-warmer use (68). More severe side-effects, such as chronic and unrelenting pelvic pain (17, 39, 64) and osteitis pubis (69), may be specific to previously radiated patients, as these outcomes are much less common following cryo-ablation used as primary therapy. Given these data it is not clear that with the availability of androgen deprivation (which involves a minimal effect on quality of life) the use of cryo-ablation in this patient population will provide any significant benefit to these difficult to manage patients. In fact a recent review by the Health Care Financing Agency concluded that the results available in the current medical literature, pertaining to the use of cryo-ablation as a salvage treatment option for previously radiated patients, were inadequate to justify coverage for these patients. At the moment the use of cryo-ablation for radiation therapy salvage remains experimental. The patients in this setting have to be advised that biochemical-free survivals to date have only been modest, and that the risks of post-cryoablation morbidities are higher than those who have not been previously radiated.

Conclusions

While the current results with percutaneous transrectal ultrasound-guided cryo-ablation for managing patients with localized PCA presented in this chapter are promising, they are nonetheless somewhat preliminary. It is only over the past 12–24 months that a consensus on technique has begun to be established for cryo-ablation, and whether the encouraging results seen in several institutions skilled in this procedure can be successfully transferred to other programs, will require further study. The rates of surrogate cancer-related outcomes following cryo-ablation can only be projected out to 5 years in a small number of institutional experiences, and no prospective technique-controlled data have been reported as of yet. In the absence of randomized prospective comparisons with other treatments for localized prostate carcinoma, it is particularly difficult to determine clear indications for when cryo-ablation would be preferable to more established therapies. An ongoing prospective comparison between cryo-ablation and external-beam radiotherapy for patients with localized PCA, being conducted by the Canadian National Cancer Institute, should provide very useful information in this regard over the next 5 years. Yet despite these limitations it is quite evident that there are ample data supporting the contention that using current techniques cryo-ablation of the prostate is a safe and effective treatment for localized prostate cancer, and that it will produce clinical outcomes that are comparable to established radiotherapeutic techniques. Both identifying the characteristics that constitute the ideal patient who is most likely to benefit from this procedure, as well as determining how prevalent cryo-ablation of the prostate will become as a treatment option for patients with prostate carcinoma, awaits further and ongoing investigations.

References

1. Morton RA Jr. Prostate cancer in ethnic groups. In: *Comprehensive textbook of genitourinary oncology* (ed. NJ Vogelzang. Williams and Wilkins, Baltimore, 1996, 573–8.
2. Landis SH, Murray T, Bolden S *et al*. Cancer statistics. *CA Cancer* 1998, **48**, 6–29.
3. Partin AW, Pound CR, Clemens JQ *et al*. Serum PSA after anatomic radical prostatectomy. The Johns Hopkins experience after 10 years. *Urol Clin N Am* 1993, **4**, 713–9.
4. Lerner SE, Blute ML, Bergstrahl EJ *et al*. Analysis of risk factors for progression in patients with pathologically confined prostate cancers after radical retropubic prostatectomy. *J Urol* 1996, **156**, 137–43.
5. Zelefsky MJ, Leibel SA, Wallner KE *et al*. Significance of normal serum prostate-specific antigen in the follow-up period after definitive radiation therapy for prostate cancer. *J Clin Oncol* 1995, **13**, 459–63.
6. Zietman AL, Coen JJ, Dallow KC *et al*. The treatment of prostate cancer by conventional radiation therapy: An analysis of long-term outcome. *Int J Rad Oncol Biol Phys* 1995, **32**, 287–92.
7. Mettlin C. The American Cancer Society National aprostate cancer Detection Project and national patterns of prostate cancer detection and treatment. *CA Cancer J Clin* 1997, **47**, 265–72.
8. Ragde H, Elgamal AA, Snow PB *et al*. Ten-year disease-free survival after transperineal sonography-guided inodine-125 brachytherapy with or without 45-gray external beam irradiation in the treatment of patients with clinically localized, low to high Gleason grade prostate carcinoma. *Cancer* 1998, **83** (5), 989–1001.
9. Stock G, Stone NN, Tabert A *et al*. A dose-response study for I-125 prostate implants. *Int Rad Oncol Phys* 1998, **41** (1), 101–8.
10. Zelefsky MJ, Leibel SA, Gaudin PB *et al*. Dose escalation with three-dimensional conformal radiation therapy affects the outcome in prostate cancer. *Int Rad Oncol Phys* 1998, **41** (3), 491–500.
11. Seung SK, Kroll S, Wilder RB *et al*. Candidates for prostate radioactive seed implantation treated by external-beam radiiotherapy. *Ca J Sci Am* 1998, **4** (3), 168–74.
12. Zeitlin SI, Sherman J, Raboy A *et al*. High dose combination radiotherapy for the treament of localized prostate cancer. *J Urol* 1998, **160** (1), 91–5.
13. Borghede G, Hedelin H, Holmang S *et al*. Combined treatment with temporary short-term high dose rate iridium-192 brachytherapy and external-beam radiotherpay for irradiation of localized prostatic carcinoma. *Radiotherapy & Oncology* 1997, **44** (3), 237–44.
14. Mate TP, Gottesman JE, Hatton J *et al*. High dose-rate afterloading 192 iridium prostate brachytherapy: feasibility report. *Int Rad Oncol Phys* 1998, **41** (3), 525–33.
15. Shipley WU, Verhey LJ, Munzenrider JE *et al*. Advanced prostate cancer:The results of a radomized comparative trial of high dose irradiation boosting with conformal protons compared witih conventional dose irradiation using photons alone. *Int Rad Oncol Phys* 1995, **32** (2), 3–12.
16. Gelet A, Chapelon JY, Bouvier R *et al*. Local control of prostate cancer by treansrectal high intensity focused ultasound therapy:preliminary results. *J Urol* 1998, **161** (1), 156–62.
17. Long JP, Fallick ML, LaRock DR *et al*. Preliminary outcomes following cryosurgical ablation of the prostate in patients with clinically localized prostate carcinoma. *J Urol* 1998, **159** (2),477–84.
18. Shinohara K, Connolly JA, Presti JC Jr *et al*. Cryosurgical treatment of localized prostate cancer

(stages T1 to T4): preliminary results. *J Urol* 1996, **156** (3), 115–21.

19. Wong WS, Chinn DO, Chinn M *et al.* Cryosurgery as a treament of prostate carcinoma: results and complications. *Cancer* 1997, **79** (5), 963–74.

20. Lee F, Bahin DK, McHugh TA *et al.* Cryosurgery of prostate cancer. Use of adjuvant hormonal therapy and temperature monitoring-a one year follow-up. *Anticancer Res* 1997, **17** (3A), 1511–5.

21. Cohen JK, Miller RJ, Rooker GM *et al.* Cryosurgical ablation of the prostate: two-year prostate-specific antigen and biopsy results. *Urology* 1996, **47** (3), 395–401.

22. Zietman AL, Shipley WU and Coen JJ. Radical prostatectomy and radical radiation therapy for clinical Stages T1 to 2 adenocarcinoma of the prostate: New insights into outcome from repeat biopsy and prostate specific antigen follow-up. *J Urol* 1994, 152, 1806–1812.

23. Vicini FA, Horvitz EM, Kini VR *et al.* Radiotherapy options for localized protate cancer based upon pretreatment serum prostate-specific antigen levels and biochemical control: a comprehensive review of the literature. *Int Rad Oncol Phys* 1998, **40** (5), 1101–10.

24. Cohen JK. Cryosurgical ablation of the prostate: pro (edit). *Urology* 1996, **48** (2), 178–80.

25. Cox RL, Crawford ED. Cryosurgical ablation of the prostate: con (edit). *Urology* 1996, **48** (2), 181–3.

26. Gonder MJ, Soanes WA, Shulman S. Cryosurgical treatment of the prostate. *Invest Urol* 1966, **3** (4), 372–8.

27. Soanes WA, Gonder MJ. Use of cryosurgery in prostatic cancer. *J Urol* 1968, **99**, 793–7.

28. Flocks RH, Nelson CMK and Boatman DL. Perineal cryosurgery for prostatic carcinoma. *J Urol* 1972, **108**, 933–5.

29. Bonney WW, Fallon B, Gerber WL *et al.* Cryosurgery in prostatic carcinoma:survival. *Urology* 1982, **19** (1), 37–42.

30. Bonney WW, Fallon B, Gerber WL *et al.* Cryosurgery in prostatic carcinoma:elimination of local lesion. *Urology* 1983, **22** (1), 8–15.

31. Onik G, Cobb C, Cohen JK *et al.* US characteristics of frozen prostate. *Radiology* 1988, **168**, 629–31.

32. Onik G, Porterfield B, Rubinsky B *et al.* Percutaneous transperineal prostate cryosurgeryusing transrectal ultrasound guidance:animal model. *Urology* 1991, **37** (3), 277–81.

33. Onik GM, Cohen JK, Reyes GD *et al.* Transrectal ultrasound-guided percutaneous radical cryosurgical ablation of the prostate. *Cancer* 1993, 72, 1291–9.

34. Gage AA, Baust J. Mechanisms of tissue injury in Cryosurgery. *Cryobiology* 1998, **37**, 171–86.

35. Tatsutani K, Rubinsky B, Onik G *et al.* Effect of thermal variables on frozen human primary prostatic adenocarcinoma cells. *Urology* 1996, **48** (3), 441–7.

36. Larson TR, Corica AP, Robertson DW. What cryotherapy temperture really kills tissue:*in vivo* temperture mapping correlated to pathological changes in human prostates. *J Endourol* 1998, **12** (1), 87, BS3–3A.

37. Miller GJ, Cygan JM. Morphology of prostate cancer: the effects of multifocality on histological grade, tumor volume, and capsular penetration. *J Urol* 1994, **152** (5 part. 2), 1709–13.

38. Turk TM, Ries MA, Pietrow P *et al.* Determination of optimal freezing parameters of human prostate cancer in a nude mouse model. *Prostate* 1999, **38** (2), 137–43.

39. Pisters LL, vonEschenbach AC, Scott SM *et al.* The efficacy and complications of salvage cryotherapy of the prostate. *J Urol* 1997, **157**, 921–5.

40. Coogan CL, McKiel CF. Percutaneous cryo-ablation of the prostate: Preliminary results after 95 procedures. *J Urol* 1995, **154**, 1813–7.

41. Wieder J, Schmidt JD, Casola G *et al.* Transrectal ultrasound-guided transperineal cryo-ablation in the treatment of prostate carcinoma: Preliminary results. *J Urol* 1995, **154**, 435–41.

42. Badalament RA, Bahn DK, Kim H *et al.* Patient-reported compliations after cryo-ablation therapy for prostate cancer. *Urology* 1999, **54** (2), 295–300.

43. Grampsas SA, Miller GJ, Crawford ED. Salvage radical prostatectomy after failed transperineal cryotherapy: histologic findings from prostate whole-mount specimens correlated with intraoperative transrectal ultrasound images. *Urology* 1995, **45** (6), 936–41.

44. Steed J, Saliken JC, Donnelly BJ *et al.* Correlation between thermosensor temperature and transrectal ultrasonography during prostate cryo-ablation. *Can Assoc Radiol J* 1997, **48** (3), 186–90.

45. Lee F, Bahn DK and McHugh TA. US-guided percutaneous cryo-ablation of prostate cancer. *Radiology* 1994, **192**, 770–6.

46. Chang Z, Finkelstein JJ, Ma H *et al.* Development of a high-performance multiprobe cryosurgical device. *Biomed Instr Tech* 1994, **28** (5), 383–90.

47. Lee F, Bahn DK, Badalament RA *et al.* Cryosurgery/ prostate cancer: Can more than five cryoprobes ablate the prostate gland? *Urology* 1999, **54** (1), 135–40.

48. Wake RW, Hollabaugh RS, Bond KH. Cryosurgical ablation of the prostate for localized adenocarcinoma: A preliminary experience. *J Urol* 1996, **155**, 1663.

49. Long JP. Is there a role for cryo-ablation of the prostate in the management of localiized prostate carcinoma? *Hematol/Oncol Clin N Am* 1996, **10** (3), 675–90.

50. Cohen JK, Miller RJ, Benoit RM *et al.* Cryosurgical ablation of the prostate in men with an unfavorable presentation of clinically localized prostate cancer. *J Urol* 1999, **161** (4), 1378A.

51. Long JP, Bahn DK, Lee F. Five-year retrospective, multi-institutional pooled analysis of cancer-related outcomes following cryosurgical ablation of the prostate. (Submitted for publication)

52. Scardino PT, Wheeler TM. Local control of prostate cancer with radiotherapy: Frequency and prognostic significance of positive results of postirradiation prostate biopsy. *NCI Monographs* 1988, **7**, 95.

53. Laverdiere J, Gomez JL, Cusan L *et al.* Beneficial effect of combination hormonal therapy administered prior and following external-beam radiation therapy in localized prostate cancer. *Int Rad Oncol Phys* 1997, **37** (2), 247–52.

54. Crook JM, Bahadur YA, Bociek RG *et al.* Radiotherapy for localized prostate carciinoma. The correlation of pretreatment prostate specific antigen and nadir prostate specific antigen with outcome as assessed by systematic biopsy and serum prostate specific antigen. *Cancer* 1997, **79** (2), 328–36.

55. D'Amico AV, Whittington R, Malkowicz SB *et al.* Biochemical outcome after radical prostatectomy, external-beam radiation therapy or interstitial radiation therapy for clinically localized prostate cancer. *JAMA* 1998, **280**, 969–74.

56. Beyer DC, Priestly JB Jr. Biochemical disease-free survival following I125 prostate implantation. *Int Rad Oncol Phys* 1997, **37** (3), 559–63.

57. Fukunaga-Johnson N, Sanadler HM, McLaughlin PW *et al.* Results of 3D conformal radiotherapy in the treatment of localized prostate cancer. *Int Rad Oncol Phys* 1997, **38** (2), 311–17.

58. Corn BW, Valicenti RK, Mulholland SG *et al.* Stage T3 prostate cancer: a nonrandomized comparison between definitive irradiation and induction hormonal manupulation plus prostatectomy. *Urology* 1998, **51** (5), 782–7.

59. Zietman AL, Shipley WU and Willett CG. Residual disease after radical surgery or radiation therapy for prostate cancer. *Cancer* 1993, **71** (Suppl), 959–69.

60. Parivar F, Hricak H, Shinohara K *et al.* Detection of locally recurrent prostate cancer after cryosurgery: evaluation by transrectal ultrasound, magnetic resonance imaging, and 3-dimensional proton magnetic resonance spectroscopy. *Urology* 1996, **48** (4), 594–9.

61. Salomon CG, Kalbhen CL, Dudiak CM *et al.* Prostate carcinoma:transrectal US after cryosurgical ablation. Radiology 1998, **206** (2), 533–8.

62. Cohen JK, Miller RJ, Benoit R *et al.* Five-year outcomes of PSA and biopsy following cryosurgery as primary treatment for localized prostate cancer *J Urol* 1998, **159** (5), 976A

63. Cox RL, Crawford ED. Complications of cryosurgical ablation of the prostate to treat localized adenocarcinoma of the prostate. *Urology* 1995, **45**, 932.

64. Sosa RE, Martin T, Lynn K. Cryosurgical treatment of prostate cancer: A multicenter review of complications. *J Urol* 1996, **155**, 361.

65. Aboseif S, Shinohara K, Borirakchanyavant S *et al.* The effect of cryosurgical ablation of the prostate on erectile function. *Br J Urol* 1997, **80** (6), 918–2l.

66. Miller RJ, Cohen JK, Shuman B *et al.* Percutaneous, transperineal cryosurgery of the prostate as salvage therapy for postradiation recurrence of adenocarcinoma. *Cancer* 1996, **77** (3), 1510–4.

67. Bales GT, Williams MJ, Sinnner M *et al.* Short-term outcomes after cryosurgical ablation of the prostate in men with recurrent prostate carcinoma following radiation therapy. *Urology* 1995, **46** (5), 676–80.

68. Cespedes RD, Pisters LL, von Eschenbach AC *et al.* Long-term follow-up of incontinence and obstruction after salvage cryosurgical ablation of the prostate: results in 143 patients. *J Urol* 1997, **157**, 237–40.

69. Seigne JD, Pisters LL, von Eschenbach AC. Osteitis pubis as a complication of prostate cryotherapy. *J Urol* 1996, **156** (1), 182.

19 | High-intensity focused ultrasound (HIFU) in the treatment of prostate carcinoma

Harrie P. Beerlage and Jean J. M. C. H. de la Rosette

Introduction

Prostate carcinoma has become the leading cancer site in men in the United States and the second cause of death in men (1). In the early days of PSA, the incidence in the USA rose from 113 per 100 000 in 1989 to 190 per 100 000 in the peak year 1992 (2), to fall to 144 per 100 000 in 1994. In the National Cancer Data Base Report on Prostate Carcinoma, Mettlin *et al.* compared the basic characteristics of prostate carcinoma data of 1992 and 1995 and found that the age at time of diagnosis decreased by 2 years. The proportion of patients with clinically localized disease rose from 69.3% to 76.7%. Although considerable regional variations could be observed overall more patients were treated with radical prostatectomy at the expense of radiation therapy (3). Another most interesting development, reported by Wingo *et al.*, is the fact that prostate cancer annual death rate declined with an average of 1% per year since 1990 (4). In Europe a similar trend is noted (5, 6). The expected increase in localized prostate cancer and diagnosis at younger age will lead to an increasing number of men requiring treatment.

In spite of the fact that it has not (yet) been proven that screening or case-finding for prostate carcinoma effectively reduces morbidity and mortality of prostate cancer, more men opt for a digital rectal examination (DRE) and prostate-specific antigen (PSA) measurement. Screening results in a higher incidence of prostate carcinoma (7) but also in detection at an earlier stage of the disease (8). Whereas in the past most cases were disseminated on diagnosis, nowadays in the USA up to 80% of patients are found to have a localized prostate carcinoma. The cost for diagnosis and treatment will thus increase considerably and will put high pressure on health services in the coming years (9).

The recommended treatment for patients with a T1–2 N0 M0 prostate carcinoma, who have a life-expectancy exceeding 10 years, is radical prostatectomy (10–12). Although this operation can be performed safely and a better understanding of the anatomy has improved the overall functional results, it remains a major surgical procedure associated with a considerable morbidity, erectile dysfunction and urinary incontinence being the most common complication. This is, amongst others, the reason for the development of less invasive treatment alternatives. We can define three groups of patients in whom alternative treatments for localized prostate carcinoma may at this moment already be an acceptable treatment option. The first group are patients with locally advanced disease, who have a tumor penetrating the prostatic capsule. They are generally considered not to be good candidates for radical prostatectomy, since the probability of cure by means of operation is very low (13). The second group are those patients who have a life-expectancy less than 10 years but have a significant tumor (large volume and/or high grade). The third group of patients are those who are good candidates for radical prostatectomy but who do not accept the morbidity associated with this operation and seek for an alternative treatment.

In the wave of new technologies, many different energy sources are used in the treatment of benign or malignant prostate conditions including electrosurgery, laser, microwaves, radiofrequency, cryotherapy, and brachytherapy. After initial experience in the treatment of benign prostatic hyperplasia (BPH), for which it has already been abandoned again, high-intensity focused ultrasound (HIFU) was also introduced in the treatment of prostate carcinoma. HIFU consists of focused ultrasound waves emitted from a transducer that are capable of inducing tissue damage by physical principles leading to mechanical effects, cavitation, and thermal effects (14).

In the process of evaluating and improving the treatment, however, we believe that it is crucial to obtain exact histological data on the effect of any treatment on human prostate *in vivo*. The only reliable approach is to do radical prostatectomy after the treatment. This was never performed in any of the other alternative treatments, like radiotherapy, brachytherapy, and CSAP. Many patients have been treated with the aforementioned modalities, even though their precise effects on prostatic tissue *in vivo* were not known. This has left us with a number of failures of these treatments that could possibly have been predicted had the result of the treatments been assessed accurately before embarking on them in large series.

In this chapter we will elaborate on a number of different issues concerning HIFU. First of all we will address the technical aspects of the procedure, physical as well as medical. Second, we will review the clinical and pathological outcome. Finally, we will discuss the future perspectives of this technique and the efforts to be made before widespread clinical use can be considered.

Principles of HIFU treatment

Physical principles

HIFU consists of focused ultrasound waves emitted from a transducer that are capable of inducing tissue damage by three physical principles leading to mechanical effects, cavitation, and thermal effects (14). An ultrasound field causes particle motion, which results in mechanical stress and strain. These mechanical interactions between ultrasound and tissue, which include radiation force, radiation torque, and streaming, can cause direct changes in a biological system. At high-intensity level, the biological effects are associated with the formation of cavitation bubbles. This type of interaction can cause complete destruction of the tissue located next to these bubbles. The lesion, which can be distinguished from coagulation necrosis easily, is characterized by a haemorrhagic cellular lysis with cavitation formation. In an absorbent medium the ultrasonic energy is continuously absorbed and converted into heat. The thermal effects produced by ultrasound have been utilized for many years in hyperthermia as a cancer therapy. Similar to any other type of hyperthermia treatment, its effectiveness depends on the temper-

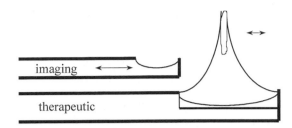

Fig. 19.1 Schematic drawing of HIFU treatment.

ature achieved and the length of the exposure. At cellular level, protein coagulation may occur resulting in irreversible cell damage.

The aim of HIFU is to heat pathological tissue to temperatures above 65°C thus destroying these tissues by means of coagulative necrosis (15). With a very sharply focused beam, the ultrasound intensity becomes high in the focal area and decreases rapidly in the sonic field lying between the focus point and the anterior face of the transducer (Fig. 19.1). So, focused ultrasound waves are capable of inducing sharp increases in temperature (70–100°C) in tissue within the focal area in a few seconds or less and consequently induce considerable tissue damage in the tissue segment. The volume of tissue destroyed by such a burst of ultrasound (shot) is termed an ultrasonically induced elementary lesion. In contrast with hyperthermia blood flow, it only minimally affects the temperature rise in such short time periods. Outside the focal region the second intensity is so low that the tissues in the intervening and immediate vicinity of the focal area remain entirely intact. To create an adequate lesion size, the elementary lesion comprising only a few millimeters is moved linearly under computer control by transducer movement.

Techniques of HIFU treatment

Standard pre-operative work-up should be performed including PSA, transrectal ultrasound, ultrasound guided prostate biopsies, and bone scan in case of PSA > 10 ng/ml. Patients receive colorectal preparation as for bowel surgery the day before HIFU treatment. The procedure is performed under general or spinal anesthesia with the patient in the lateral position. A suprapubic catheter will have to be inserted pre-operatively in all patients in order to guarantee adequate urinary drainage.

Two devices are currently available, the Ablatherm™ device (EDAP-Technomed, Lyon, France) and the Sonablate™ device (Focus Surgery USA). The

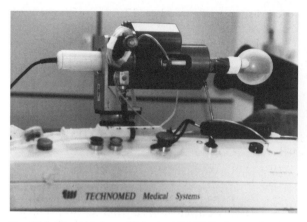

Fig. 19.2 The Ablatherm™ device (EDAP-Technomed, Lyon, France).

Ablatherm™ device is equipped with a rectangular 2.25 MHz therapy transducer and a 7.5 MHz endorectal biplane ultrasound scan probe (Kretz, Ziph, Austria) (Fig. 19.2). Focus peak is at 40 mm and lesions with a diameter of 1.6 mm and a variable length between 13 and 18 mm can be created. The Sonablate™ device has a 4 MHz therapy transducer with a focal peak at 3, 3.5, or 4 cm. With the patient in the lateral position, a treatment as well as an imaging probe are positioned rectally (Fig. 19.3). To create an adequate lesion size the elementary lesion comprising only a few millimeters is moved linearly step by step under computer control by transducer movement. One of the piezo-ceramic elements on the applicator operates as a rectum wall distance controlunit and avoids accidentally focusing on the rectum wall. A continuous flow of a fluid, with a temperature of approximately 18°C, through the balloon located around the probe should be accomplished in order to protect the rectal wall against too high temperatures. The procedure takes approximately 1 h/10 g prostate tissue treated. Patients can generally be dismissed the day after the treatment. During treatment, as well as post-operatively, generally no blood loss or other serious events occur. In most studies rectoscopy was performed post-operatively to assess possible damage to the rectal wall.

Results of HIFU treatment

Animal experiments

In several animal studies since 1956, the anti-tumor effect of HIFU alone (16, 17) or in combination with chemotherapy (18, 19) has been demonstrated. Chapelon *et al.* studied the effects of HIFU in the Dunning R3327 system on the MatLyLu and AT-2 sublines (20). Complete tumor destruction could be obtained in 61% of the MatLyLu tumors and 96% of the AT-2 tumors. These studies suggest that HIFU is capable of destroying completely certain tumors. Margonari *et al.* described a cure rate of 64% in a rat model of prostate cancer with the tumor exteriorized and treated at 80°C (21). Foster *et al.*, using the Sonablate™ (Focus Surgery USA), demonstrated the possibility of performing subtotal prostatic ablation with the present technology, destroying 90–95% of a canine (beagle) prostate (22, 23). However, even when a complete destruction could be seen in some studies, this was not obtained in all tumors treated. It may very well be that certain tumor cells are resistant to high temperatures. Another explanation may be that the tumor is not always exposed completely to the HIFU pulses or the effectiveness of each pulse may vary: the penetration of the ultrasound could be reduced by the cavitation phenomena (15).

Human studies: clinical and histopathological results

The first clinical trials using HIFU in the treatment of benign prostatic hyperplasia began in 1992 at the University of Vienna, Austria (24, 25), followed by the Indiana University in 1993 performed by Bihrle and in Paris by Vallancien. Simultaneously, the first treatments of organ-confined prostate cancer were carried out by Gelet at Edouard Herriot Hospital in Lyon.

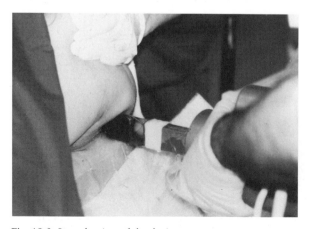

Fig. 19.3 Introduction of the device.

However, HIFU is nowadays no longer recommended for the treatment of benign prostatic hyperplasia. Although the subjective outcome was good, the objective results were moderate only and a relatively long anesthesia time is required to achieve this.

For use in prostate cancer, technical adaptations were necessary: an imaging probe with higher frequency and thus higher resolution was used and a more strongly focusing (larger) transducer. Vallancien *et al.* exposed human superficial bladder tumors to HIFU treatment with an extracorporeal firing head containing multiple piezoelectric elements focused at 320 mm (26, 27). After 6 months four patients were free of tumor and two had a partial response. There were no side-effects noted from the treatment.

Gelet *et al.* were the first to expose locally confined prostate cancers transrectally to 2.25 MHz HIFU in 14 patients with T1–2 prostate tumors (15, 28). Patients were treated in two or three sessions under general or spinal anesthesia with two different transducers (35 mm or 45 mm focus). Treatment was performed using the Ablatherm® device (Technomed Medical System). The device combines a 2.25 MHz therapy transducer with a 7.5 MHz transrectal biplane ultrasound scanning probe. Complications were seen in the first three patients treated with the 35 mm transducer, who developed a rectal burn. This complication did not occur in any of the patients treated with the 45 mm focused transducer. Three patients developed a temporary stress incontinence and one a bladder neck stenosis, managed endoscopically. Of 14 patients only four had normal sexual function before treatment, but this was lost after bilateral treatment. The patients were followed with PSA monitoring and prostate biopsies. The mean PSA level before treatment was 12 ng/ml (Hybritech) and 9 months after HIFU exposure 2.4 ng/ml. In seven of 14 patients no tumor was found at repeat biopsies. In two patients HIFU treatment was repeated after positive control biopsy.

Very important work was done by Madersbacher *et al.* who generated marker lesions in 55 human prostates with transrectal HIFU using the Sonablate® prior to surgical removal (29, 31). All specimens were analyzed by whole-mount histological sections with volumetrical analysis of the area of the necrosis. In all specimens, a HIFU-induced thermonecrosis was identified and the cross-sectional area of necrosis was directly correlated to the power input and HIFU beam focal length (29). In 10 cases, HIFU was targeted at the hypoechogenic lesion and in three of 10 cases all malignant prostate tissue was destroyed. In the remaining

seven cases a mean of 53% (37–78%) of cancer was destroyed.

To obtain a more detailed insight on the effect of HIFU-induced thermoablation on prostatic cells, the impact of heat on heat-shock protein (HSP) 27 expression of normal and malignant prostatic cells *in vitro* and *in vivo* was studied (32). This clearly demonstrated that benign and malignant human prostatic cells respond to heat by an increased expression of HSP27 *in vivo*. Beerlage *et al.* (33) reported on 14 patients treated with HIFU using the Ablatherm® device (EDAP-Technomed, France) prior to radical prostatectomy. The mean age of the patients was 62 (range 55–69) and PSA levels ranged from 3.5 to 20 ng/ml, with a mean of 10.8 ng/ml. The goal of the study was evaluation of the effect of HIFU and not complete treatment of the prostate, and therefore one (part of one) lobe was treated only. In cases of unilateral tumor on biopsies, the lobe in which the tumor was confirmed was treated. Most procedures could be performed within 3 h, depending on the volume of the prostate. After 1–2 weeks a radical retropubic prostatectomy was performed and the post-operative course was comparable to that of patients not pretreated with HIFU. In six patients biopsies of the pelvic floor were taken to assess possible damage. No intra-operative complications occurred during the HIFU treatments. Of the 14 patients treated, eight reported urgency complaints after the treatment, four of whom needed spasmolytics. In the early post-operative phase, minor anal discomfort was reported by all patients. On rectoscopy no serious side-effects could be noted and no rectal fistula was seen. Histology report revealed a pT2C in seven patients, a pT3A/B in three, and a pT4A in three patients. In one patient no tumor could be detected at all but diagnostic needle biopsy of this last patient was revised and undoubtedly showed a localization of adeno carcinoma (Gleason sum 3 + 3 = 6). In 13 out of 14 cases vital tumor was seen outside the treatment area; moreover in four of 14 cases a small focus of vital tumor was seen on the dorsal side of the lobe that was treated with HIFU. Nevertheless a problem was noted concerning the dorsal aspect of the prostate of all patients on meticulous histological analysis of the specimen. In these patients small areas of incomplete necrosis could be identified at the dorsal side of the prostate where vital glandular tissue and in fur cases even vital tumor was seen (Fig. 19.2). Extension of HIFU effect into the proximal part of the seminal vesicles was frequently seen, also indicating that treatment beyond the anatomical borders of the prostate is feasible. In nine out of 14 cases, extensive necrosis was seen in the lateral prostatic capsule and even beyond in the periprostatic tissue. In six cases biopsies of the pelvic floor were taken to establish any damage that might be inflicted on the pelvic floor. In one of these cases clear necrosis was seen, the other five showed vital muscular tissue. After the first report of the necrosis of the pelvic floor we decided to set the margin at 1 cm from the apex in order not to damage the pelvic floor. On histology, the distance between the HIFU effect and the resection margin however was 3–4 mm only, indicating that the HIFU effect is spreading beyond the target area probably due to heat conduction.

The pathological aspects of these series were extensively studied as well. The prostatectomy specimens were formalin fixed and cut in 6–10 slices of 0.4 cm. Slides of 4 μm were stained with haematoxylin and eosin (HE). The HIFU effect, which could accurately be recognized on macroscopy as a dark-red discoloration, was mainly located at the dorsal side of the treated lobe, which was the target area, and a sharp delineation could be noted between the necrotic and the adjacent vital tissue. This discoloration correlated very well with the coagulative and hemorrhagic necrosis that was seen on microscopy in the areas treated with HIFU, with desquamation of epithelium into gland-lumina. The overlap between the HIFU 'shots' was complete, since no areas of vital tissue embedded in the haemorrhagic necrosis were seen. In six prostates, glands without histologically apparent necrosis were seen within the HIFU treated area. These glands reacted with antibodies to pancytokeratin, PSA, and Ki67. However, they did not express cytokeratin 8, indicating severe cellular damage. Ultrastructural examination revealed desintegration of cellular membranes and cytoplasmatic organells. In four patients, vital appearing prostatic glands were demonstrated at the dorsal side of the prostate within the treated area, indicating incomplete tissue destruction.

Two centers have now started to offer HIFU treatment to patients with localized prostate carcinoma who are unfit for surgery. In Münich, Germany, 143 HIFU treatments have been reported on 111 patients with biopsy proven prostate carcinoma, clinical stage T1–3, Nx, M0, and a PSA < 25 ng/ml (Abott IMX) (34, 35). All patients were not fit for radical prostatectomy or were not willing to undergo the operation but had a life-expectancy exceeding 5 years. The main goal in this group of patients was to prevent local problems and to defer hormonal treatment. An informed consent was acquired in every case. The first 65 treatments in 49

patients were performed selectively, meaning that a unilateral or bilateral treatment in one or two sessions was fulfilled depending on findings on transrectal ultrasound and biopsies. After analysis of the results of the first group during the second 78 treatments, in 62 patients the whole prostate was treated (global treatment) and in 60% of cases PSA < 4 ng/ml and a negative control biopsy was achieved (Table 19.1). No serious intra-operative problems arose but 13 patients developed a complication post-operatively. Three patients acquired a recto-urethral fistula that could be solved with transurethral fibrine gluing in two cases. In another patient, a urethral stenosis occurred for which a urethral stent was inserted. Nine patients developed stress incontinence that could be managed successfully by pelvic floor exercise or with collagen injection. Most patients were over 70 years of age and had erectile dysfunction already. Only a very small minority had intact erections. Of this last group, patients who were treated unilaterally all regained their erections, whereas patients who were treated globally all lost their erectile function. Response to treatment was divided into four categories. A (complete responder): negative biopsies and a PSA < 4 ng/ml; B (partial responder): patients with PSA > 4 ng/ml and negative biopsies; C (partial responder): patients with PSA < 4 ng/ml and positive biopsies; and D (failure): patients with PSA > 4 ng/ml and positive biopsies. All patients treated have undergone at least one complete follow-up evaluation, including biopsies, digital rectal examination, transrectal ultrasound, and PSA measurement. The mean follow-up is 12 months up to now (range 6–27). The results are summarized in Table 19.1.

In areas with negative biopsies pre-HIFU, which were excluded from treatment in the beginning (selectively treated group), control biopsies showed cancer

Table 19.1 Clinical results of HIFU treatment

	Selective	Global
Biopsy negative PSA < 4 ng/ml (A)	25%	60%
Biopsy negative PSA > 4 ng/ml (B)	3%	8%
Biopsy positive PSA < 4 ng/ml (C)	37%	26%
Biopsy positive PSA > 4 ng/ml (D)	35%	6%
Local control (A + B + C)	65%	94%

spots in 58%. This was considered to be a diagnostic failure (understaging) and the patients were treated with a second HIFU session. Biopsies performed 1 and 3 month post-HIFU showed (residual) cancer spots in the selectively treated group in 72% of cases and in the completely treated group in 32%. The biopsies clearly showed that in the most dorsal, as well as in the ventral, parts of the prostate no complete necrosis could be achieved. Patients with complete treatment had significantly better results than the partially treated patients. Local control of prostate cancer, meaning complete or partial response, could be achieved in the group with complete treatment in 94%, in the partially treated patients in 65%. It is obvious that the results of the completely treated group are much better than the selectively treated group, with a PSA nadir < 0.5 ng/ml in 55% versus 19%, respectively.

Gelet *et al.* performed a total of 113 transrectal high-intensity focused ultrasound sessions in 50 patients with localized prostate cancer, who were not suitable candidates for radical prostatectomy (36). Of these patients, two underwent salvage ultrasound treatment for locally recurrent cancer following definitive radiation therapy. Median followup was 24 months (range 3–46). Control parameters were changes in PSA and random control sextant biopsies at 1–3, 3–12, 12–24, 24–36 and 36–48 months. Group 1 (complete response) included 28 patients (56%) with no residual cancer and PSA less than 4 ng/ml. (mean 0.93), group 2 (biochemical failure) included three patients (6%) with no residual cancer and PSA greater than 4 ng./ml. (mean 6.22), group 3 (biochemical control) included nine patients (18%) with residual cancer (mean positive biopsy 1.1 of 6) and PSA less than 4 ng./ml. (mean 0.90), and group 4 (failures) had 10 patients (20%) with residual cancer (mean positive biopsies 1.9 of 6) and PSA greater than 4 ng./ml. (mean 8.9). Of the 10 cases in group 4, hormone therapy was required in three and radiotherapy in five. They concluded that morbidity associated with high-intensity focused ultrasound treatment is currently minimal and local control of the localized prostate cancer was observed in groups 80% of cases.

Discussion

The question arises why we need alternative (minimally invasive) treatment options for localized prostate carcinoma when we have a very good treatment at hand,

namely radical prostatectomy. Radical prostatectomy nevertheless is a considerable surgical procedure requiring a relatively long hospital admission. In general urological practice, incontinence rate after radical prostatectomy will be 5–10%, while impotence rates will exceed 50% (37, 38). Another problem is the fact that due to difficulties in pre-operative staging, roughly 50% of patients with clinically localized prostate cancer are found to have locally advanced disease on final pathology (39). The latter group can not be considered to be operated curatively and progression will occur often in spite of the major surgery they endured. In search of alternative treatment options for localized prostate carcinoma, two critical issues concerning treatment safety are at stake. First of all the safety of the procedures in the sense of efficacy, meaning cancer control, is critical and it should at least be comparable to the results of the 'gold standard'. Second, the side-effects of the treatment will have to be considerably fewer than those caused by radical prostatectomy.

In the process of evaluating and improving the treatment, however, it is crucial to acquire exact histological data of the effect of HIFU on human prostate *in vivo*. The only reliable way to achieve this, in our view, is to do radical prostatectomy after the treatment and it is of the utmost importance to perform a meticulous analysis of the pathology specimen. In other alternative treatments, like radiotherapy, brachytherapy, and cryosurgical ablation of the prostate, this was never done. Before embarking on a new therapeutic modality, its precise effects on prostatic tissue *in vivo* should absolutely be known.

Because prostate carcinoma is a multi-focal disease by nature, the whole prostate has to be treated always, and treating the hypoechoic lesion or the peripheral zone only is insufficient by definition. Hormonal pre-treatment may be useful in larger prostates, especially since reduction of target volume may increase the efficacy of the procedure. Ideally in these alternatives one should be able to predict the lesion size and to monitor the effects during treatment. Beerlage *et al.* (33) demonstrated in their study the critical issues at stake. The histological data show that extensive and complete coagulative necrosis of prostatic tissue can be achieved in the treated area, indicating that overlap between 'shots' is sufficient. When aiming at curative treatment, however, the whole prostate has to be treated, since multi-focality is very frequently a feature. In order to achieve complete treatment of the ventral part, technical modifications of the device like increased focal length or development of a multi-focus treatment probe is required. On the other hand, down-sizing the prostate in cases of large volume gland by hormonal pretreatment may be helpful as well. A number of important problems, however, have to be solved and questions remain to be answered. The present inability of HIFU to treat the dorsal part of the prostate completely, as the histological as well as clinical data of Beerlage *et al.* (33) clearly demonstrated, is a major drawback. This is very worrying since vital prostatic tissue was seen here, which is obviously unacceptable. The explanation for this phenomena is multiple: the software was developed to deliver the energy with such a safety margin that changes of damage to the rectal wall are minimal to prevent rectal fistulas; the configuration of the focus is 'cigar like' and the energy is maximal in the center of the 'cigar' leaving small areas between the 'cigar tips' at risk for incomplete destruction; finally, the rectal wall was cooled with a fluid inside the balloon covering the treatment device. Because of the cooling effect, the conduction of heat may not be as good as in the rest of the prostate causing less 'overlap' leading to persisting vital tissue. However, adjusting the cooling temperature theoretically increases the risk for rectal injury. The distance between prostatic capsule and rectal mucosa is minimal and it may very well be that complete treatment of the dorsal part of the prostate without rectal damage is possible only when this distance is enlarged, for instance by injection of fluid or placement of a balloon to be filled with fluid, between Denonvilliers layers. It is probably the combination of the three effects that causes the incomplete tissue destruction. On the one hand, the safety of the rectum is of course very important but, on the other hand, we should be absolutely sure that no vital prostatic tissue remains after the treatment. A solution for this problem would be an overlap of the treated areas in such a way that the dorsal aspect could be treated completely without compromising the rectal wall. Further software adaptation will be necessary to achieve this. Another possibility is increasing the distance between prostate and rectal wall, as was mentioned above, allowing more complete treatment of the dorsal part of the prostate without damaging the rectal wall.

Another important problem is the fact that the ventral part of the prostate cannot be reached at this moment due to a restricted focal length. Although most tumors will be located in the dorsal part, in a considerable number of cases the ventral part is affected also and should absolutely be treated as well. The develop-

ment of a multi-focal probe will have to provide the solution for this problem.

An other major concern, finally, is the issue of targeting. In all patients, an attempt was made to destroy the lateral border of the prostate, but in only six out of nine was this completely achieved, and in three patients, with prostates larger than 40 cm³, only partly (33). This means that the effect with respect to the lateral border is in some cases smaller than was planned during treatment. On the other hand, in three patients in which they intended to treat with a margin of 10 mm from the apex on pathology, a 3-mm margin only was found in one case and a 4-mm margin in two. This means that the effect of HIFU was more profuse than planned, probably due to heat conduction. The fact that necrosis was found in pelvic floor biopsies in one of the patients points in the same direction. It is of course very important that the planned target and the HIFU effect on histopathology match exactly in order to destroy all prostatic tissue completely without unwanted damage to the neighboring structures.

Conclusions

The trend toward minimal invasive treatment that can be seen in the management of BPH, has merged in the approach of localized prostate carcinoma since early clinical stages are more frequently detected. HIFU provides a very interesting concept in the treatment of prostate carcinoma. The advantages of the technique in the treatment of prostate carcinoma are that it is relatively non-invasive, requires a short hospital stay only, can be repeated easily, and another form of therapy can be applied should this treatment fail. Preliminary results of HIFU treatments in patients unfit for surgery suggest a rather high failure rate but a larger series of patients and better patient selection is mandatory before definite conclusions can be drawn. Exact targeting is imperative in order to treat the whole prostate without damaging the rectal wall and this ultimate goal provides a truly technical challenge. At the moment improvements to HIFU are made in two ways. First, a multi-focal probe is under development, enabling treatment of the ventral part of the prostate as well. Second, injection of fluid in the layer between the rectal wall and the prostate will make adequate treatment of the dorsal border of the prostate possible without damaging the rectum.

HIFU may provide a valuable alternative in the treatment of prostate carcinoma but should for now be considered as a promising therapy that needs more evaluation. A longer follow-up is mandatory before determining its place in the treatment of localized prostate carcinoma. Until then HIFU should be considered experimental and should be performed in strictly controlled trials with accurate follow-up only.

References

1. Silverberg E, Lubera JA. Cancer statistics, 1989. *CA Cancer J Clin* 1989, **39**, 3–20.

2. Generic Ries LA, Kosary CL, Hankey BF *et al. Anonymous SEER cancer statistics review, 1973–1994.* National Cancer Institute 1997 NIH Pub No 97-2789.Anonymous.

3. Mettlin CJ, Murphy GP, Rosenthal DS *et al.* The National Cancer Data Base report on prostate carcinoma after the peak in incidence rates in the U.S. The American College of Surgeons Commission on Cancer and the American Cancer Society. *Cancer* 1998, **83**, 1679–84.

4. Wingo PA, Ries LA, Rosenberg HM *et al.* Cancer incidence and mortality, 1973–1995: a report card for the US. *Cancer* 1998, **82**, 1197–207.

5. Giard RW, Coebergh JW, Casparie-van VI. [A marked increase in the rate of diagnosed prostate cancer in the Netherlands during 1990–1996]. Sterke stijging van de detectiefrequentie van prostaatkanker in Nederland gedurende de periode 1990–1996. *Ned Tijdschr Geneeskd* 1998, **142**, 1958–62.

6. Menegoz F, Black RJ, Arveux P *et al.* Cancer incidence and mortality in France in 1975–95. *Eur J Cancer Prev* 1997, **6**, 442–66.

7. Meikle AW, Smith JA J. Epidemiology of prostate cancer. *Urol Clin North Am* 1990, **17**, 709–18.

8. Adolfsson J, Steineck G, Whitmore WF J. Recent results of management of palpable clinically localized prostate cancer. *Cancer* 1993, **72**, 310–22.

9. Optenberg SA, Thompson IM. Economics of screening for carcinoma of the prostate. *Urol Clin North Am* 1990, **17**, 719–37.

10. Catalona WJ, Bigg SW. Nerve-sparing radical prostatectomy: evaluation of results after 250 patients. *J Urol* 1990, **143**, 538–43.

11. Frohmuller H, Theiss M, Wirth MP. Radical prostatectomy for carcinoma of the prostate: long-term follow-up of 115 patients. *Eur Urol* 1991, **19**, 279–83.

12. Walsh PC. Radical prostatectomy, preservation of sexual function, cancer control. The controversy. *Urol Clin North Am* 1987, **14**, 663–73.

13. Paulson DF. Radiotherapy versus surgery for localized prostatic cancer. *Urol Clin North Am* 1987, **14**, 675–84.

14. Hill CR, ter Haar GR. Review article: high intensity focused ultrasound–potential for cancer treatment. *Br J Radiol* 1995, **68**, 1296–303.

15. Gelet A, Chapelon JY, Margonari J *et al.* Prostatic tissue destruction by high-intensity focused ultrasound: experimentation on canine prostate. *J Endourol* 1993, **7**, 249–53.

16. Fry FJ, Johnson LK. Tumor irradiation with intense ultrasound. *Ultrasound Med Biol* 1978, **4**, 337–41.

17. Moore WE, Lopez RM, Matthews DE *et al.* Evaluation of high-intensity therapeutic ultrasound irradiation in the treatment of experimental hepatoma. *J Pediatr Surg* 1989, **24**, 30–3.

18. Yang R, Reilly CR, Rescorla FJ *et al.* High-intensity focused ultrasound in the treatment of experimental liver cancer. *Arch Surg* 1991, **126**, 1002–9.

19. Loverock P, ter Haar G, Ormerod MG *et al.* The effect of ultrasound on the cytotoxicity of adriamycin. *Br J Radiol* 1990, **63**, 542–6.

20. Chapelon JY, Margonari J, Vernier F *et al. In vivo* effects of high-intensity ultrasound on prostatic adeno-carcinoma Dunning R3327. *Cancer Res* 1992, **52**, 6353–7.

21. Margonari J, Gorry F, Blanc E *et al.* Effects of high intensity focused ultrasound on healthy and tumoral tissues. *Int Soc Urol* 1994, **46** (Abstract), 86–6.

22. Foster RS, Bihrle R, Sanghvi N *et al.* Production of prostatic lesions in canines using transrectally administered high-intensity focused ultrasound. *Eur Urol* 1993, **23**, 330–6.

23. Kincaide LF, Sanghvi NT, Cummings O *et al.* Noninvasive ultrasonic subtotal ablation of the prostate in dogs. *Am J Vet Res* 1996, **57**, 1225–7.

24. Madersbacher S, Kratzik C, Szabo N *et al.* Tissue ablation in benign prostatic hyperplasia with high-intensity focused ultrasound. *Eur Urol* 1993, **23** (Suppl 1) 251.

25. Ebert T, Graefen M, Miller S *et al.* High-intensity focused ultrasound (HIFU) in the treatment of benign prostatic hyperplasia (BPH). *Keio J Med* 1995, **44**, 146–9.

26. Vallancien G, Chartier KE, Chopin D *et al.* Focussed extracorporeal pyrotherapy: experimental results. *Eur Urol* 1991, **20**, 211–9.

27. Vallancien G, Chartier KE, Harouni M *et al.* Focused extracorporeal pyrotherapy: experimental study and feasibility in man. *Semin Urol* 1993, **11**, 7–9.

28. Gelet A, Chapelon JY, Bouvier R *et al.* Treatment of prostate cancer with transrectal focused ultrasound: early clinical experience. *Eur Urol* 1996, **29**, 174–83.

29. Madersbacher S, Pedevilla M, Vingers L *et al.* Effect of high-intensity focused ultrasound on human prostate cancer *in vivo. Cancer Res* 1995, **55**, 3346–51.

30. Susani M, Madersbacher S, Kratzik C *et al.* Morphology of tissue destruction induced by focused ultrasound. *Eur Urol* 1993, **23** (Suppl 1), 34–38.

31. Madersbacher S, Kratzik C, Susani M *et al.* Tissue ablation in benign prostatic hyperplasia with high intensity focused ultrasound. *J Urol* 1994, **152**, 1956–60.

32. Madersbacher S, Grobl M, Kramer G *et al.* Regulation of heat shock protein 27 expression of prostatic cells in response to heat treatment. *Prostate* 1998, **37**, 174–81.

33. Beerlage HP, van Leenders G, Oosterhof GO *et al.* High-intensity focused ultrasound (HIFU) followed after one to two weeks by radical retropubic prostatectomy: results of a prospective study. *Prostate* 1999, **39**, 41–6.

34. Thüroff S, Chaussy C, Zimmermann R. Global versus selective treatment of localized prostate cancer gy high intensive focused ultrasound (HIFU). *J Endourol* 1998, **12** (Suppl 1), 141.

35. Chaussy C, Thüroff S, Zimmermann R. Transrectal high intensive focused ultrasound (HIFU) a new therapy option for localized prostate cancer. *J Endourol* 1998, **12** (Suppl 1), 140.

36. Gelet A, Chapelon JY, Bouvier R *et al.* Local control of prostate cancer by transrectal high intensity focused ultrasound therapy: preliminary results. *J Urol* 1999, **161**, 156–62.

37. Fowler-FJ J, Barry MJ, Lu YG *et al.* Patient-reported complications and follow-up treatment after radical prostatectomy. The National Medicare Experience: 1988–1990 (updated June 1993). *Urology* 1993, **42**, 622–9.

38. Murphy GP, Mettlin C, Menck H *et al.* National patterns of prostate cancer treatment by radical prostatectomy: results of a survey by the American College of Surgeons Commission on Cancer. *J Urol* 1994, **152**, 1817–9.

39. Jager GJ, Ruijter ET, Oosterhof GO *et al.* Dynamic TurboFLASH subtraction technique for contrast-enhanced MR imaging of the prostate: correlation with histopathologic results. *Radiology* 1997, **203**, 645–52.

20 | *Neoadjuvant hormonal therapy prior to radical prostatectomy: promises and pitfalls*

Martin E. Gleave and S. Larry Goldenberg

Introduction

The goal of radical prostatectomy is complete removal of all cancer cells. Unfortunately, even in carefully selected patients, up to two-thirds of clinically-confined tumors are understaged, and positive margin rates of 30–60% are reported following radical prostatectomy (1–3). Although higher tumor stage, grade, and preoperative serum PSA levels correlate with higher pathologic stage and risk of disease recurrence, prognostic variables are limited in their ability to independently and individually predict pathologic stage and risk of recurrence (4–6). In order to optimize outcomes from radical prostatectomy, only men with low-risk tumors (T1 or T2a, Gleason score < 6, serum PSA < 10 μg/l) were traditionally considered ideal for cure by surgical intervention. Thus, ideal candidates for radical prostatectomy are men with the highest probability of being cured by the operation. Indeed, cure rates following radical prostatectomy alone exceed 80% in men with low-risk tumors (7, 8). However, radical therapy may represent overtreatment in some of these men because of the indolent natural history of low risk disease (9). In contrast, most men with high-risk localized tumors (> T2b, Gleason score > 7, PSA > 10 μg/l) and life expectancies > 10 years will die of their disease if they are not treated with curative intent (9). High-risk tumors exhibit a more aggressive natural history and have higher positive margin and recurrence rates after radical prostatectomy or radiotherapy alone, where unimodality therapy likely represents undertreatment (4–9). Paradoxically, the therapeutic ratio (patients who actually realize a survival benefit from a therapeutic intervention) may therefore be greater in high-risk disease if its natural history can be altered by multimodality therapy. It is important, therefore, to investigate therapies that optimize complete extirpation of all cancer cells and reduce the incidence of positive surgical margins and disease recurrence.

The term adjuvant therapy refers to the use of systemic therapy after management of localized disease when risk for recurrence is known to be high. Chemotherapy regimens can cure some patients when used in the adjuvant setting, even though the same regimen fails to alter the natural history of established metastatic disease. Experimental animal model and early clinical trial data suggest that administration of systemic therapy is more likely to affect cure when tumor burden is low (10). Neoadjuvant therapy extends this logic further by applying systemic therapy earlier in the course of the disease prior to definitive locoregional therapy. The aim of neoadjuvant hormonal therapy (NHT) prior to radical prostatectomy is reduction of positive margins rates and ultimately decreased disease recurrence. The role of NHT prior to radical prostatectomy is controversial, as some clinicians argue that down-sizing occurs without downstaging and any apparent downstaging results from difficulty in pathologic evaluation of the neoadjuvantly-treated prostatectomy specimen (11, 12). Others further argue that short-term follow-up from randomized studies comparing 3 months of neoadjuvant therapy to surgery alone show no difference in biochemical recurrence rates (13). However, NHT has many attractive theoretical features and research in this area is justified and important. The purpose of this chapter is to review the rationale behind NHT, critique the randomized studies of 3 months of therapy, and examine the optimal duration of therapy.

Rationale behind neoadjuvant therapy prior to radical prostatectomy

High positive margin rates following radical prostatectomy.

Although higher tumor stage, grade and pre-operative serum PSA levels correlate with higher pathologic stage, no prognostic variable exists that can be applied independently and individually to predict pathologic stage (4). Up to two-thirds of clinically-confined tumors are understaged, and positive margin rates of 30–60% are reported following radical prostatectomy (1–3). Incomplete excision places the patient at higher risk of disease recurrence (5–8). Selection of patients who are most likely to benefit from NHT remains critical; NHT is less likely to alter outcome in most low-risk tumors (PSA < 10 μg/l, Gleason score < 6, stage T1C), since most of these patients do well with surgery alone. In contrast, men with high-risk localized tumors (PSA > 10 μg/l, Gleason grade > 7) are at significant risk for positive margins and PSA recurrence. Patients with positive margins are often offered post-operative radiation therapy to consolidate local therapy, which is associated with increased risk of urinary incontinence, impotence, and anastomotic strictures. It is therefore important to investigate combinations of therapies that optimize complete extirpation of all cancer cells and reduce the incidence of positive surgical margins.

Reversible androgen-suppression therapy

The development of potent, well-tolerated, and reversible agents for androgen-ablation therapy provides a safe method for inducing prostate cancer cell death and tumor regression prior to radical prostatectomy. Several classes of drugs induce castrate levels of testosterone through suppression of LH release from the pituitary gland. Diethylstilbestrol (DES) suppresses hypothalamic release of LHRH, and also increases testosterone binding globulin (TeBG), which decreases free serum testosterone. DES is the least expensive of the synthetic estrogens and castrate testosterone levels are achieved at doses of 1 mg daily (14). Its main advantage is its low cost, but this must be weighed against increased risk of thromboembolic and cardiovascular complications. Luteinizing-hormone-releasing hormone (LHRH) agonists include goserelin and leuprolide (available as 1 or 3 months depot injec-

tions), and buserelin (2 months depot formulation). Pulsatile release of LHRH from the hypothalamus normally stimulates LH release from the pituitary but when this periodicity is effaced by continuous administration of LHRH-agonists, the pituitary becomes refractory to hypothalamic regulation. LHRH-agonists produce a biphasic response with an initial rise in LH and testosterone, termed the 'flare phenomenon', followed in 2 weeks by a fall in LH and testosterone. Although LHRH-agonists appear equivalent to DES and orchiectomy, the presence of the flare compromises the efficacy of LHRH-agonist monotherapy (15, 16). The flare reaction is prevented by cyproterone acetate or DES one week prior to the LHRH-analogue, or blocked by non-steroidal anti-androgens like flutamide or bicalutamide.

Prostate tumor cell death, not just tumor shrinkage, occurs following medical castration. Apoptosis, or programmed cell death, occurs in normal, benign hyperplastic, and malignant prostatic epithelial cells by any procedure that results in castrate levels of testosterone (17–19). Apoptotic cell death appears to be a 'genetic suicide' process that requires activation of a series of genes and is characterized morphologically by shrunken cells with condensed and fragmented nuclei (apoptotic bodies). Initiation of apoptosis may, in part, be cell-cycle specific or regulated by epigenetic factors and may therefore begin at different times in different populations of cells. Maximal apoptotic regression of ventral rat prostate glands and Shionogi tumors is complete within 1–2 weeks following castration (19); however, timing of apoptosis has not been well characterized in benign or malignant human prostate tissue and likely takes place over a longer period of time.

Sensitivity of soft tissue disease to androgen withdrawal

Clinical observations suggest that soft-tissue metastases respond more favorably to androgen ablation with more frequent and durable complete responses than do osseous metastases (20–22). Patients with stage D2 lymph node-only disease have a median survival more than twice that of patients with D2 osseous disease (21). Adjuvant androgen-ablation therapy following radical prostatectomy in patients with regional lymph node metastases results in long-term (15 year) survival in 30%, which suggests that a significant proportion of patients with low-volume soft-tissue metastases may be cured with surgery and immediate androgen ablation

(22). One would anticipate that a similar proportion of patients with pathologically localized tumors and unrecognized subclinical metastases, which would ultimately recur after radical prostatectomy alone, may also be cured by NHT as long as the course of therapy is long enough.

Availability of PSA as a marker of tumor regression

PSA gene expression is androgen-regulated and serum PSA levels are dependent on both androgen levels and tumor volume (23, 24). After institution of androgen-ablation therapy, serum PSA levels decrease rapidly and dramatically due to cessation of androgen-regulated PSA gene expression and apoptosis. Although significant down-sizing occurs after 3 months of therapy, serum PSA does not reach undetectable levels after 3 months in most patients, which suggests that optimal duration of NHT may be longer than 3 months. Maximal tumor regression is likely signaled by PSA when it reaches its nadir level. Changes in serum PSA following NHT provide objective biochemical information that reflects tumor response and may identify patients not responding favorably.

Animal-model studies

Androgen withdrawal in the Shionogi tumor model precipitates apoptosis and tumor regression in a highly reproducible manner with up to a 2-log cell kill, but despite undergoing complete regression, androgen-independent tumors recur after 1 month (22). Conceptually, the ideal time to implement curative therapy is after maximal castration-induced tumor involution but before outgrowth of androgen-resistant clones. Experiments were designed to determine whether local recurrence rates after tumor excision were reduced by neoadjuvant compared to adjuvant androgen ablation (25). Group 1 underwent tumor excision with wide margins and castration upon tumor recurrence, while Group 2 were treated with neoadjuvant castration for 10 days followed by wide excision of the regressed tumor. Tumor-free survival was significantly greater in Group 2 (56% vs. 20%, $P < 0.05$; Fig. 20.1). These animal studies demonstrate that neoadjuvant therapy reduces local recurrence and positive margin rates by 50%. Although this model cannot address the issue of affect of NHT on subclinical metastases, extrapolation of these results to the clinical

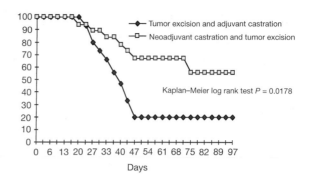

Fig. 20.1 Neoadjuvant castration reduces local recurrence rates in the Shionogi tumor model. Tumors were allowed to grow to 1–2 g before mice were randomized to either tumor excision with wide margins and castration upon tumor recurrence (Group 1), or neoadjuvant castration for 10 days followed by wide excision of the regressed tumor (Group 2). The study endpoint was androgen-independent tumor recurrence, which occurred in 80% of Group 1 after a median of 36 days and 44% of mice in Group 2 after a median of 42 days.

disease suggests that NHT may help to reduce not only the positive margin rates but also the subsequent risk of local recurrence following radical prostatectomy.

Clinical studies with short-term neoadjuvant therapy

Most studies have chosen, somewhat empirically, 3 months of NHT. Useful surrogate endpoints to assess the efficacy of NHT prior to radical prostatectomy include serum PSA nadir levels prior to surgery, pathologic stage and positive margin rates, and most importantly, serum PSA recurrence rates following surgery.

Non-randomized clinical studies

Most non-randomized studies report decreases in serum PSA, prostatic volume, and positive margin rates following 3 months of NHT (Table 20.1). These studies do not report on time to PSA nadir or absolute PSA nadir levels. Soloman *et al.* (26) reported on the largest phase II series of 156 patients with T2/T3 tumors treated with between 3 and 6 months of an LHRH agonist plus flutamide. Positive margin rates were 11.5%, compared to 35% in historical controls, but no post-operative follow-up data has been reported. Investigators at Memorial Sloan Kettering Cancer Center have conducted a series of studies begin-

Table 20.1   Nor-randomized studies of short-term neoadjuvant hormone therapy

Investigator (Ref)	Sample size	Clinical stage	Serum PSA*	Duration of NHT (months)	Positive margin rate	Follow-up
Soloman et al. 1993 (26)	156	T2/T3	NA	3–6	11.5%	NA
Aprikian et al. 1994 (27)	55	T3/T2b	20.4 (median)	3 (median)	33%	62%/26 months
Häggman et al. 1993 (32)	40	T2/T3	NA	3	31%	15%/3 months
Schulman 1993 (31)	40	T2/T3	NA	3 (mean)	32%	NA
Fair et al. 1993, 1997 (28, 29)	74	T2	8.7 (median)	3	10%	18%/48 months
Soloway 1993 (34)	37	T3/T2b	NA	3 (median)	40%	26%/33 months
McFarlane 1993 (11)	22	T3/T2b	14.8	3	32%	NA
Oesterling 1993 (12)	22	T3/T2b	30	1.5	68%	NA

* Pretreatment serum PSA (μg/l).

ning with a report by Aprikian et al. (27), which suggested that most patients with locally advanced cT3 tumors did not benefit from between 2 and 8 months of neoadjuvant DES. A subsequent phase II study of 141 patients with cT1 or cT2 tumors reported significant decreases in serum PSA (> 98%) and a 38% decrease in prostatic volume after 3 months of LHRH agonist with flutamide (28). Pathologic staging revealed increased organ-confined rates (74% vs. 49%) and decreased positive margin rates (10% vs. 33%) when compared to a group of 72 concurrent controls who did not receive NHT. However at 48 months follow-up, no differences in PSA recurrence rates were apparent (29). Several smaller non-randomized studies by Sassine and Schulman (30, 31) and by Häggman et al. (32) also reported 40–50% decreases in positive margin rates when groups of patients pretreated with 3 months of NHT were compared to historical controls. In contrast, reports on small cohorts of patients with cT2 or cT3 tumors by McFarlane et al. (12) and

Oesterling et al. (13) suggested no improvement in pathologic outcome following short-term NHT. It is apparent from these non-randomized studies (reviewed in Table 20.1) that outcome (pathologic stage, positive margin rates, and risk of PSA recurrence) is dependent on many factors including proportion of T3 tumors and other high-risk features, length of post-operative follow-up, and time-period during which the study accrued (stage migration towards earlier diagnosis began in early 1990s). Conclusions from such studies must be drawn with caution, but taken together, the results suggest that 3 months on NHT results in encouraging pathologic effects and led to initiation of phase III randomized studies.

Randomized clinical studies

To date, seven phase III randomized studies comparing 0 vs. 3 months of NHT have been published (Table 20.2) (33–39). The primary endpoint in all these

Table 20.2   Randomized studies of short-term neoadjuvant hormone therapy

Investigator	Sample size	Clinical Stage	Type of NHT	Change in serum PSA	Change in TRUS volume	Positive margin rate
Labrie et al. 1995 (33)	161*	T2/T3	3 month L + F	NA	NA	8% vs. 34%†
Soloway et al. 1995 (34)	303	T2b	3 month L + F	14.3 to < .5 in 70%	44 to 35 cm³	18% vs. 48%†
Van Poppel et al. 1995 (35)	130	T2b/T3	6 week E.P.	14 to 1.0 μg/l	43 to 29 cm³	20% vs. 46%‡
Goldenberg et al. 1996 (36)	213	T1/T2	3 month CPA	13 to 1.1 μg/l	43 to 33 cm³	28% vs. 65%†
Fair and Kara et al. 1997 (37)	148	T1/T2	3 month G + F	8.9 to	NA	18% vs. 37%†
Witjes et al. 1997 (38)	354	T2/T3	3 month G + F	20 to 0.8 μg/l	38 to 27 cm³	27% vs. 46%†
Hugosson et al. 1996 (39)	111	T1–T3a	3 month T + C	NA	NA	23% vs. 41%†

* 30 patients refused randomization and were included in the NHT arm.
† Statistically significant difference in primary endpoint.
‡ Statistically significant difference only in T2 patients.
L + F = leuprolide acetate plus flutamide; G + F = goserelin plus flutamide; CPA = 300 mg cyproterone acetate daily;
E.P. = estramustine phosphate; T = triptorelin plus cyproterone acetate 50 mg bid.

trials was incidence of positive margin disease. All seven of these studies demonstrate significant decreases in positive surgical margins after 3 months of NHT, reporting decreases ranging from 34–65% to 8–28%. These studies do not report on time to PSA nadir or absolute PSA nadir levels. Soloway *et al.* (34) published the results of a multicenter randomized study comparing 0 vs. 3 months of leuprolide and flutamide prior to radical prostatectomy. Positive margin rates decreased from 42% in the control group, to 17% in the NHT group. Organ-confined disease (pT2) was reported twice as frequently in the NHT group (53%), compared to the surgery alone group (22%). Similarly, a randomized multicenter trial by the Canadian Uro-Oncology Group (CUOG) using 3 months of cyproterone acetate, also reported a 50% reduction in positive margin rates (65% vs. 28%) and doubling of the organ-confined rate (20% vs. 42%) (36). Fair and Kava (37) reported results of a recent randomized trial comparing 0 vs. 3 months of neoadjuvant therapy (LHRH plus flutamide) in 148 patients with clinically confined prostate cancer. Overall, the incidence of positive margins decreased from 37% to 18% (*P* < 0.05). The decrease in positive margins was even greater in high-risk patients with pretreatment PSA levels > 10 μg/l (63% vs. 18%), suggesting that these men may be the most likely to benefit from noeadjuvant therapy. In the Belgian study, no difference in positive margin rates was observed using only 6 weeks of estramustine phosphate when all patients were considered (40.5% vs. 46.5%); however, when only T2 patients were considered, there was a statistically significant decrease in positive margin disease (35).

Consistent observations from these randomized studies using 3 months of NHT include > 90% decrease in serum PSA levels, 30% decrease in prostatic volume, 50% decrease in positive margin rates in cT1 or cT2 (but not cT3) disease, higher organ-confined rates, and no difference in incidence of seminal vesicle involvement or positive lymph nodes.

Caution is required, however, when interpreting studies using pathologic stage as an endpoint despite apparent encouraging results reviewed above. The ability of NHT to reduce biochemical and local recurrence is the ultimate goal and this has not yet been determined because of lack of long-term follow-up of the randomized studies. Soloway *et al.* (40) recently reported 24-month follow-up data on 256 evaluable patients in the US Intergroup Study and found that 21% of the NHT group compared to 21.6% of the surgery alone group had PSA levels > 0.4 μg/l (*P* = 0.473). Similarly, the CUOG study has not demonstrated any difference in PSA recurrence rates at 24 months follow-up, with recurrence rates of 22% and 25% in the control and NHT arms, respectively (41). There are several possible reasons for lack of apparent difference in PSA recurrence rates despite favorable changes in positive margin rates. First, and most important, the sample size of these studies was based on detecting differences in positive margin rates (where the number of *events* in the control arm is > 40%), and therefore the studies are not large enough to have the statistical power necessary to detect significant differences in biochemical recurrence rates (where the number of *events* in the control arm is < 25%). Second, follow-up is short and any benefit from NHT may only become apparent after longer follow-up. Patterns of failure following radical prostatectomy suggest that early failures (i.e. < 2 years) are more often distant, while most local failures (i.e. those most likely to be affected by NHT), do not become manifest until 3 or more years after surgery. Third, approximately half the patients in these studies had low-risk tumors (Gleason < 6, PSA < 10 μg/l) with a very low risk of PSA recurrence after radical prostatectomy (10–20%), which could dilute any potential benefit from NHT. Finally, there may be a true lack of benefit from 3 months of NHT, either because of an error in application (i.e. the duration of NHT was too short), or concept (i.e. no matter how NHT is applied, it will not alter recurrence rates).

Clinical studies with long-term neoadjuvant therapy

Serum PSA levels decrease rapidly and dramatically after institution of androgen withdrawal therapy due to cessation of androgen-regulated PSA gene expression and apoptosis (23, 24). Although the molecular events regulating apoptosis are becoming better understood, the timing (in terms of initiation at the molecular/cellular level and completion at the tumor population level) of castration-induced apoptosis of prostate carcinoma cells remains poorly defined, but is likely to be an asynchronous event initiated at variable times in a heterogeneous tumor population. Timing of apoptosis is difficult to characterize in human prostatic tumors because of the absence of appropriate animal-model systems, and because serial or comparative immunostaining of biopsies for apoptotic bodies inconsistently detects uncommon events that exist for relatively short periods of time. Although down-sizing occurs after 3

months of NHT, serum PSA has not reached undetectable levels in most patients after this period of time.
Ongoing decreases in serum PSA after the second
month of therapy are not due to further decreases in
PSA gene expression and synthesis because changes in
gene expression occur rapidly and reach basal levels
shortly after testosterone reaches castrate levels (42).
Therefore, decreases in serum PSA after the second
month are likely to reflect an ongoing imbalance
between apoptotic prostate epithelial-cell death and
decreased tumor-cell proliferation, which leads to
further reduction in tumor volume. These observations
suggest that optimal duration of NHT may be longer
than 3 months.

To study the optimal duration of NHT, a prospective, phase II trial was initiated to determine the duration of NHT required for PSA to reach its nadir, and to
characterize the pathologic effects of 8 months of
androgen-withdrawal therapy (43). To date, 150
patients with clinically localized prostate cancer have
been treated, and the results of the first 100 patients
have been previously reported (44). Surrogate endpoints used to assess the effects of longer duration
NHT include changes in serum PSA levels, effects on
pathologic stage, positive margin rates, and proliferation marker immunostaining, and most importantly,
serum PSA recurrence rates following surgery.

Changes in serum PSA

Different rates of PSA decline after institution of
therapy produces two distinct slopes: a precipitous
drop during the first month and a more gradual subsequent decrease, which continued into the eighth month
of therapy (Fig. 20.1). Serum PSA decreases an average
of 80–90% during the first month of therapy and a
further 50% between the third and eighth months of
NHT. The initial rapid decrease in PSA results from
cessation of androgen-regulated PSA synthesis and
apoptosis, while the ongoing slower decline likely
reflects decreasing tumor volume. When the data are
plotted on a log-scale, decreases in PSA follow first-
order kinetics with exponential decline to nadir levels
(Fig. 20.2(a)). Serum PSA decreases to undetectable
levels or reaches nadir levels in 34% of patients after 3
months, 60% after 5 months, and 84% after 8 months.
Using an ultrasensitive assay (Abbott IMX) that detects
PSA levels as low as 0.07 μg/l, time to PSA nadir was
delayed even further with only 22% of patients reaching their PSA nadir at 3 months, 42% at 5 months, and
84% after 8 months of therapy (Fig. 20.2(b)). After 8
months of neoadjuvant therapy, serum PSA levels were
> 0.5 μg/l in 18% of patients, < 0.4 μg/l in 82% of
patients, < 0.3 μg/l in 76% of patients, and < 0.2 μg/l
in 66%.

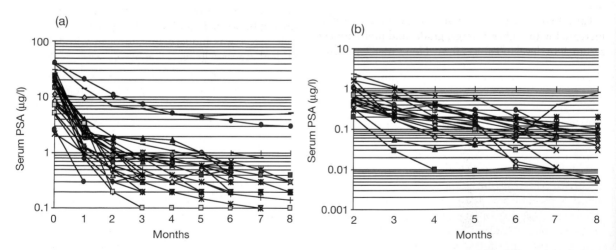

Fig. 20.2 (a) After initiation of androgen-withdrawal therapy, serum PSA levels decrease exponentially, falling 80% after the
first month of therapy and a more gradual 50% between the third and eighth months of neoadjuvant therapy. Mean time to
PSA nadir was 5.4 months. (b) Ongoing exponential decreases in serum PSA were observed after the third month of therapy,
with serum PSA continuing to fall into the undetectable range < 0.1 μg/l in many patients.

Table 20.3 Pathologic stage vs. pretreatment PSA and grade after 8 months of NHT

Pathologic	Overall		Serum PSA (μg/l) (%)*			Gleason grade (%)*		
stage	n (%)	< 4	4–9.9	10–20	> 20	<4	5, 6	> 7
P–0	17 (11)	3 (18)	10 (12)	3 (9)	1 (5)	7 (15)	9 (13)	1 (3)
P2a	53 (35)	7 (44)	30 (37)	11 (34)	5 (24)	19 (41)	20 (29)	14 (41)
P2b	49 (33)	6 (38)	26 (33)	10 (28)	7 (33)	14 (30)	26 (37)	9 (26)
P3 M–	20 (13)	0	13 (16)	3 (11)	4 (20)	5 (11)	11 (16)	4 (12)
P3 M+	8 (5)	0	0	5 (16)	3 (14)	1 (2)	3 (4)	4 (12)
PxN+	3 (2)	0	1 (1)	1 (3)	1 (5)	0	1 (1)	2 (6)

* Pretreatment.

Changes in pathology

After 8 months of NHT, most patients in this study had organ-confined, stage pT2 tumors (79%), and one-half of these had micro-foci or small-volume tumors occupying less than 5% of the prostate (Table 20.3). Microscopic extension through prostatic capsule with negative margins (pT3M-) was reported in 13% of the patients. The positive margin rate was 5%, lower than that reported after 3 months of NHT in similar cohorts of patients (34, 36, 37) (Fig. 20.3). Although patients with organ-confined tumors tended to have lower mean PSA nadir levels, the nadir PSA value was not predictive of pathologic stage in individual patients; however, patients whose PSA nadir was > 0.3 μg/l were more likely to have extracapsular disease, with 50% having pT3 tumors. Patients with serum PSA nadir levels < 0.1 μg/l were less likely to have extracapsular extension or positive margins (4%) compared to those with nadir levels > 0.1 μg/l (27%).

Pathologic stage and risk of positive margins increased with higher T-stage, grade, and pretreatment serum PSA levels (Table 20.3). None of 62 patients with T1c or T2a tumors had positive margins compared to 6% of 78 with T2b and 30% of 10 patients with T3a disease. Positive margins were identified in 2% of patients with Gleason scores < 4, 5% with scores of 5 or 6, and 16% with Gleason scores of > 7. None of 96 patients with PSA levels < 10 μg/l had positive margins, compared to 18% of 54 with PSA levels > 10 μg/l.

Because of possible risk for progression and outgrowth of androgen-independent clones during prolonged NHT, immunostaining with proliferation markers (PCNA and Ki-67) and the oncoprotein Bcl-2 was performed (43, 45). Neither proliferation marker showed increased staining in radical prostatectomy specimens post-NHT compared to pretreatment biopsy specimens. In particular, Ki-67 staining remained suppressed in patients who completed 8 months of NHT (43). Other investigators also reported that immunostaining for the cyclin-dependent kinase inhibitor, p27, increased in prostate cancer specimens after NHT ranging between 3 and 8 months (45), suggesting cell-cycle arrest was induced by androgen withdrawal in residual cancer cells surviving NHT. Levels of the anti-apoptotic oncoprotein, Bcl-2, increase beginning during the first 3 months of NHT (46), and remain elevated after 8 months of therapy (45), consistent with its role in prevention of castration-induced apoptosis (47). Taken together, ongoing decreases in serum PSA, the high percentage of organ-confined and small-volume tumors, and the absence of increased PCNA and Ki-67, immunostaining suggests that progression from outgrowth of androgen-independent clones during prolonged NHT is unlikely.

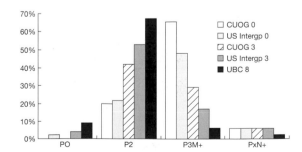

Fig. 20.3 Pathologic stage in patients treated with no NHT or 3 months of NHT in the US Intergroup (34) and CUOG (36) studies, compared to patients treated with 8 months of NHT in the Vancouver (43) study.

Post-operative PSA recurrence rate

After a mean 28 months post-operative followup (range: 3–79 months) and 36 months from time of ini-

Prostate cancer

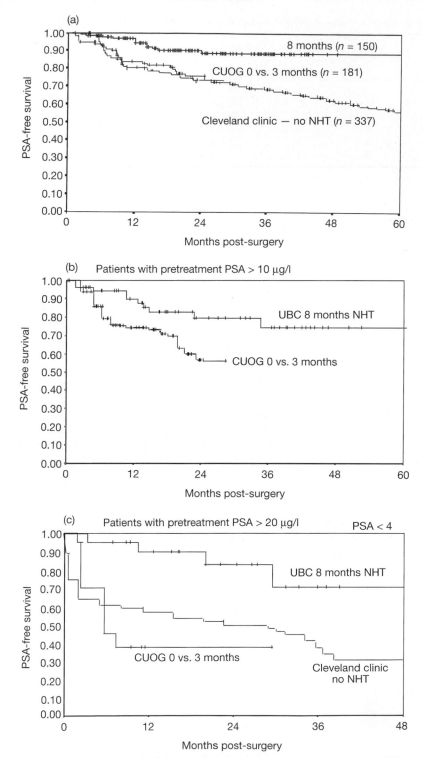

Fig. 20.4 Kaplan–Meier survival curves for 150 patients treated with 8 months of NHT and radical prostatectomy, with mean follow-up post-surgery of 28 months. (a) Overall, compared to CUOG 0 vs. 3-month NHT study (36) and Cleveland Clinic series (7). (b) Stratified by pretreatment serum PSA levels > 10 μg/l and compared to CUOG 0 vs. 3-month NHT study (36) and Cleveland Clinic series (7). (c) Stratified by pretreatment serum PSA levels > 20 μg/l and compared to CUOG 0 vs. 3-month NHT study (36) and Cleveland Clinic series (7). *continued*

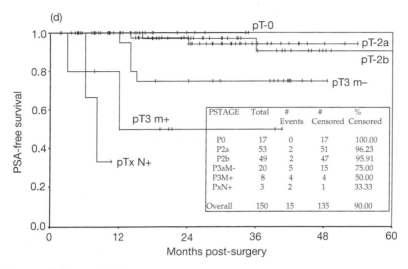

Fig. 20.4 *continued* (d) Stratified by pathologic stage.

tiation of NHT, biochemical recurrences occurred in 15 patients (10%), most within the first 2 years of surgery (Fig. 20.4(a)). Risk of biochemical recurrence after 8 months of NHT remains proportional to known risk factors for recurrence, including pretreatment serum PSA and Gleason score, and pathologic stage (Table 20.4). The low PSA recurrence rate in this phase II study using 8 months of NHT compares favorably against recurrence rates reported by the US Intergroup (40), the Canadian Uro-Oncology Group (41), the Cleveland Clinic (7), and Baylor University (8) (Table 20.4). Differences in PSA recurrence rates are most pronounced when only patients with high-risk features are considered (Figs 20.4(b) and 20.4(c), Table 20.4). For example, 2-year PSA recurrence rates in patients

with pretreatment serum PSA > 10 μg/l were 20% in the 8-month NHT study compared to 40% in the CUOG study and Baylor series, and 20% in patients with PSA levels > 20 μg/l, compared to 48% in the Cleveland Clinic series, 56% in the Baylor series, and 60% in the CUOG study. Apparent improvement in recurrence rates between uncontrolled studies from different centers must, however, be interpreted with caution. The potential benefit of longer term NHT can only be evaluated by phase III studies, one of which has been recently initiated by the Canadian Uro-Oncology Group. CUOG-P95A was initiated in 1995 and will randomize 540 men with clinically confined prostate cancer to either 3 or 8 months of leuprolide acetate and flutamide prior to radical prostatectomy. Accrual will

Table 20.4 Biochemical-free survival after radical prostatectomy in contempory series

	Baylor (8)	Cleveland Clinic (7)	CUOG (36, 41) 0 vs 3 NHT	Vancouver (43, 44) 8 months NHT
Overall	79%	74%	78 vs 75%	90%
Mean follow-up	38 months	36 months	24 months	28 months
Biopsy Gleason				
2–4	92%	92%	100 vs. 100%	96%
5,6	84%	77%	83 vs. 81%	91%
7–10	46%	48%	64 vs. 53%	83%
Pretreatment PSA				
<4	93%	93%	92 vs. 100%	100%
4–10	76%	78%	93 vs. 85%	94%
10.1–20	69%	65%	73 vs. 67%	83%
> 20.1	44%	30%	29 vs. 62%	82%

be complete early in 1998 and the study will have adequate power to detect a 30% reduction in PSA recurrence rates (assuming a 30% recurrence rate in the 3 month arm).

Potential pitfalls of neoadjuvant therapy

Does NHT result in artifactual pathological understaging?

Following NHT, residual foci of atrophic glands can be difficult to identify with H&E staining, raising the possibility that pT-0 staging or low positive margin rates may be an artifact resulting from pathological understaging. Some authors argue that down-sizing occurs without downstaging and any apparent downstaging results from difficulty in pathologic evaluation of the NHT-treated prostatectomy specimen (11–13). Evidence thus far, however overwhelming, suggests that the NHT-induced decrease in positive margin rates is a real, rather than an artifactual, phenomenon. First, all randomized studies using a single central and experienced pathologist report similar (50%) decreases in positive margin rates (34, 36, 37). Second, re-evaluation of prostatectomy specimens using prostatic acid phosphatase (PAP) and cytokeratin immunostaining to help identify foci of cancer difficult to see with H&E prepared sections, did not significantly increase positive margin rates (40, 41). Although PAP and cytokeratin staining helps identify residual carcinoma cells inside and outside of the prostate, and may upstage occasional pT0 specimens, positive margin rates remain unchanged (41). Third, animal-model studies using androgen-dependent Shionogi tumors demonstrate that NHT reduces local recurrence and positive margin rates by 50% (25). Finally, pathologic stage remains proportional to pretreatment risk factors (serum PSA, T-stage, and Gleason grade), and an important prognostic predictor for biochemical relapse (36, 37, 42). Taken together, these observations suggest that the favorable pathologic features induced by NHT are real and not artifactual.

Is surgery more difficult following neoadjuvant therapy?

Concerns have been raised by some urologists that NHT makes surgery more difficult by increasing peri-prostatic adhesions. However, this does not appear to be the case. Randomized series that have documented surgical difficulty, blood loss, length of procedure, and post-operative complications, found no significant difference in these parameters between neoadjuvantly-treated and untreated groups (23, 24). Apoptosis initiated by androgen withdrawal (or other stimuli elsewhere throughout the organism) is a controlled cellular event that is not associated with acute inflammation or scarring. However, one technical factor after 8 months of NHT is that the prostate can decrease to a small, fusiform swelling of the urethra, which can make it more difficult to palpate the prostatic apex and decide where to take the dorsal bundle.

Does tumor progression occur during prolonged NHT?

This concern has been expressed by some investigators who argue against the use of NHT. However, 8 months is a relatively short time-period in the natural history of a clinically-confined prostate cancer, where local or distant progression is not apparent for often longer than 5 years or 10 years (9). Furthermore, as outlined above, the ongoing decreases in serum PSA, the high percentage of organ-confined and small-volume tumors, and the absence of increased proliferation marker immunostaining suggests that progression from outgrowth of androgen-independent clones during prolonged NHT is unlikely.

Will recurrence rates be altered by neoadjuvant therapy?

With the exception of testis, low ano-rectal, and Wilm's tumors, most data do not support use of neoadjuvant therapies for most solid tumors when survival outcomes are compared to local therapy alone or followed by adjuvant therapy. Indeed, it remains possible that delay in definitive local therapy by neoadjuvant treatments may be detrimental. Lack of benefit of neoadjuvant chemotherapy in other solid tumors such as cervix (48), small cell lung (49), and bladder (50), illustrates that use of therapies capable of inducing complete responses may not have positive effects on survival when used in a neoadjuvant setting. Whether NHT reduces recurrences after radical prostatectomy will have to await maturation of the recently completed phase III studies (33–39) (Table 20.2). However, it is critical to realize that the sample size of these studies was based on detecting differences in positive margin rates, and therefore they have insufficient statistical power to detect significant differences in biochemical recurrence rates. The question of optimal duration of NHT is being evaluated by phase-III studies recently initiated by the CUOG and SWOG. Until recurrence rates have been demonstrated to decrease in randomized studies, NHT should be considered investigational and studied in the context of controlled clinical studies.

References

1. Rosen MA, Goldstone L, Lapin S *et al.* Frequency and location of extracapsular extension and positive surgical margins in radical prostatectomy specimens. *J Urol* 1992, **148**, 331–7.
2. Jones EC. Resection margin status in radical prostatectomy specimens: relationship to type of operation, tumor size, tumor grade and local tumor extension. *J Urol* 1990, **144**, 89–93.
3. Trapasso JG, deKernion JB, Smith RB *et al.* The incidence and significance of detectable levels of serum PSA after radical prostatectomy. *J Urol* 1994, **152**, 1821–5.
4. Partin AW, Yoo J, Carter HB *et al.* The use of prostate specific antigen, clinical stage, and Gleason score to predict pathologic stage in men with localized prostate cancer. *J Urol* 1993, **150**, 110–4.
5. Lange PH, Ercole CJ, Vessella RL. Serum prostatic specific antigen in the management of patients after radical prostatectomy. *J Urol* 1988, **139**, 607–10.
6. Frazier HA, Robertson JE, Humphrey PA *et al.* Is PSA of clinical significance in evaluating outcome after radical prostatectomy. *J Urol* 1993, **149**, 516–8.
7. Kupelian P, Katcher J, Levin H *et al.* Correlation of clinical and pathologic factors with rising prostate-specific antigen profiles after radical prostatectomy alone for clinically localized prostate cancer. *Urology* 1996, **48**, (2), 249–60.
8. Dillioglugil O, Leiban BD, Kattan MW *et al.* Hazard rates for progression after radical prostatectomy for clinically localized prostate cancer. *Urology* 1997, **50**, 93–9.
9. Chodak GW, Thisted RA, Gerber GS *et al.* Results of conservative management of clinically localized prostate cancer. *New Engl J Med* 1994, **330**, 242–8.
10. Skipper HE, Schabel FM Jr, Wilcox WS. Experimental evaluation of potential anticancer agents. XII: On the criteria and kinetics associated with 'curability' of experimental leukemia. *Cancer Chemother Rep* 1964, **35**, 1–111.
11. Macfarlane MT, Abi-aad A, Stein A *et al.* Neoadjuvant hormonal deprivation in patients with locally advanced prostate cancer. *J Urol* 1993, **150**, 132–4.
12. Oesterling JE, Andrews PE, Suman VJ *et al.* Pre-operative androgen deprivation therapy: Artificial lowering of serum prostate specific antigen without downstaging the tumor. *J Urol* 1993, **149**, 779–82.
13. Paulson DF. Neoadjuvant androgen deprivation therapy prior to radical prostatectomy: Con. *Urology* 1996, **48**, 539–40.
14. Cox RL, Crawford ED. Estrogens in the treatment of prostate cancer. *J Urol* 1995, **154**, 1991–8.
15. The Leuprolide Study Group. Leuprolide versus diethylstilbesterol for metastatic prostate cancer. *N Engl J Med* 1984, **311**, 1281–6.
16. Mahler C. Is disease flare a problem? *Cancer* 1993, **72**, 3799–802.
17. Bruchovsky N. The metabolism of testosterone and dihydrotestosterone in an androgen-dependent tumor. A possible correlation between dihydrotestosterone and tumor growth in vivo. *Biochem J* 1972, **127**, 561–75.
18. Tenniswood M. Apoptosis, tumour invasion and prostate cancer. *Br J Urol* 1997, **79**, 27–34.
19. Bruchovsky N, Rennie PS, Coldman AJ *et al.* Effects of androgen withdrawl on the stem cell population of the Shionogi carcinoma. *Cancer Res* 1990, **50**, 2275–82.
20. Goldenberg SL, Bruchovsky N, Gleave ME *et al.* Intermittent androgen suppression in the treatment of prostatic carcinoma: a preliminary report. *Urology* 1995, **45**, 839–45.
21. Sayer J, Ramirez EI, von Eschenbach AC. Retrospective review of prostate cancer patients with lymph node metastases. *J Urol* 1992, **147**, 52A.
22. Cheng CWS, Bergstralh EJ, Zincke H. Stage D1 prostate cancer. A non-randomized comparison of conservative treatment options versus radical prostatectomy. *Cancer* 1993, **71**, 996–1004.
23. Gleave ME, Hsieh JT, Wu HC *et al.* Serum PSA levels in mice bearing human prostate LNCaP tumors are determined by tumor volume and endocrine and growth factors. *Canc Res* 1992, **52**, 1598–605.
24. Stamey TA, Kabalin JN, Ferrari M *et al.* Prostate specific antigen in the diagnosis and treatment of adenocarcinoma of the prostate. IV. Anti-androgen treated patients. *J Urol* 1989, **141**, 1088–90.
25. Gleave ME, Sato N, Bowden M *et al.* Neoadjuvant androgen ablation reduces local recurrence rates after tumour excision in the Shionogi tumour model. *J Urol* 1997, **157**, 1727–30.
26. Soloman MH, McHugh TA, Dorr RP *et al.* Hormone ablation treatmetns as neoadjuvant therapy prior to radical prostatectomy. *Clin Invest Med* 1993, **16**, 532–8.
27. Aprikian AG, Fair WR, Reuter VE *et al.* Experinece with neoadjuvant diethylstibesterol and radical prostatectomy in patients with localy advanced prostate cancer. *Br J Urol* 1994, **74**, 630–6.
28. Fair WR, Aprikian A, Sogani P *et al.* The role of neoadjuvant hormonal manipulation in localized prostate cancer. *Cancer* 1993, **71**, 1031–8.
29. Kava BR, Vlamis V, Rabbani F *et al.* Interim follow-up of patients receiving neoadjuvant hormonal therapy prior to radical prostatectomy at Memorial Sloan-Kettering Cancer Center: Tumor designation as organ-confined and specimen-confined does not appear to result from pathologic understaging. *Mol Urol* 1997, **1**, 141–8.

30. Sassine AM, Sculman CC. Neoadjuvant hormonal deprivation before radical prostatectomy. *Eur Urol* 1993, **24**, 46–50.

31. Schulman CC. Neoadjuvant androgen blockade prior to prostatectomy: a retrospective study and critical review. *Prostate* 1994, **5**, 9–14.

32. Häggman M, Hellstrom M, Aus G *et al.* Neoadjuvant GnRH agonist treatment and total prostatectomy. *Eur Urol* 1993, **24**, 456–60.

33. Labrie F, Cusan L, Gomez JL *et al.* Downstaging of early stage prostate cancer: the first randomized trial of neoadjuvant combination therapy with flutamide and a luteinizing hormone-releasing hormone agonist. *Urology* 1995, **44**, 29.

34. Soloway MS, Sharifi R, Wajsman Z *et al.* Randomized prospective study compring radical prostatectomy alone versus radical prostatectomy preceded by androgen blockade in clinical stage B2 (T2bNxM0) prostate cancer. *J Urol* 1995, **154**, 424–8.

35. Van Poppel H, De Ridder D, Elgamal A *et al.* Neoadjuvant hormonal therapy before radical prostatectomy decreases the number of positive surgical margins in stage T2 prostate cancer: Interim results of a prospective randomized trial. *J Urol* 1995, **154**, 429–34.

36. Goldenberg SL, Klotz LH, Jewitt MAS and the Canadian Urologic Oncology Group. Randomized controlled study of neoadjuvant reversible androgen withdrawal therapy with cyproterone acetate in the surgical management of localized prostate cancer. *J Urol* 1996, **156**, 873–7.

37. Fair WR, Kava B. Neoadjuvant Hormonal Therapy: Update on Memorial Sloan-Kettering Cancer Center Trials. Molecular *Urology* 1997, **1**, 135–40.

38. Witjes W, Schulman CC, Debruyne MJ and the European Study Group on Neoadjuvant Treatment for Prostate Cancer. Preliminary results of a prospective randomized study copartin radical prostatectomy versus radical prostatectomy associated with neoadjuvant hormonal combination therapy in T2–3N0M0 prostatic carcinoma. *Urology* 1997, **49**, 65–9.

39. Hugosson J, Abrahamsson PA, Ahlgren G *et al.* The risk of malignancy in the surgical margin at radical prostatectomy reduced almost 3-fold in patients given neo-adjuvant hormone treatment. *Eur Urol* 1996, **29**, 413–9.

40. Bazinet M, Zheng W, Begin LR *et al.* Morphologic changes induced by neoadjuvant androgen ablation may result in underdetection of positive surgical margins and capsular involvement by prostatic adenocarcinoma. *Urology* 1997, **49**, 721–5.

40. Soloway MS, Sharifie R, Wajsman Z *et al.* and the Lupron Depot Neoadjuvant Study Group. Radical prostatectomy alone vs. radical prostatectomy preceeded by androgen blockade in cT2b prostate cancer: 24 month results. *J Urol* 1997, **157**, 160A.

41. Klotz L, Goldenberg SL, Bullock MJ *et al.* and the Canadian Urologic Oncology Group. Neoadjuvant cyproterone acetate therapy prior to radical prostatectomy reduces tumour burden and margin positivity without altering 6 and 12 month post-treatment PSA: results of a randomized trial. *J Urol* 1996, **155**, 399A.

42. Sato N, Gleave ME, Bruchovsky N *et al.* Intermittent androgen suppression delays time to non-androgen regulated prostate specific antigen gene expression in the human prostate LNCaP tumour model. *J Steroid Biochem Mol Biol* 1996, **58**, 139–46.

43. Gleave ME, Goldenberg SL, Jones EC *et al.* Biochemical and pathological effects of eight months of androgen withdrawal therapy prior to radical prostatectomy in clinically confined prostate cancer. *J Urol* 1996, **155**, 213–9.

44. Gleave ME, Goldenberg SL, Jones E *et al.* Longer duration of neoadjuvant androgen withdrawal therapy prior to radical prostatectomy in clinically localized prostate cancer: Biochemical and pathological effects. *Mol Urol* 1997, **1**, 199–204.

45. Zubovitis JT, Paterson RF, Gleave ME *et al.* The effect of neoadjuvant hormone therapy on prostatic adenocarcinoma in radical prostatectomy specimens: an analysis of tumor cell proliferation. *Am J Pathology* 1998, **157**, 290 (Abstract).

46. McDonnell TJ, Navone NM, Troncoso P *et al.* Expression of bcl-2 oncoprotein and p53 protein accumulation in bone marrow metastases of androgen independent prostate cancer. *J Urol* 1997, **157**, 569–74.

47. Reed JC. Bcl-2 and the regulation of programmed cell death. *J Cell Biol* 1994, **124**, 1–6.

48. Souhami L, Gil RA, Allan SE *et al.* A randomized trial of chemotherapy followed by pelvic radiation therapy in stage IIIB carcinoma of the cervix. *J Clin Oncol* 1991, **9**, 970–7.

49. Murray N, Coy P, Pater J *et al.* Importance of timing for thoracic irradiation in the combined modality treatment of limited stage small cell lung cancer. *J Clin Oncol* 1993, **11**, 336–44.

50. Hall RR for the MRC Study Group. Neoadjuvant CMV chemotherapy and cystectomy or radiotherapy in muscle-invasive bladder cancer. First analysis of MRC/EORTC Intercontinental trial. *Proc Am Soc Clin Oncol* 1996, **15**, 244A.

21 | *Therapeutic decision-making in localized prostate cancer*

Louis J. Denis

Introduction

The incidence of prostate cancer had a steady increase worldwide for some time but dramatic increases have been recorded in the US up till 1992, when a remarkable downward swing led to a revision in incidence and mortality expectations in 1997 (1). Multiple causes may explain this rise and fall of which increased life expectancy of males is the most pleasant and the introduction of prostate-specific antigen (PSA) the most important. The parallel decline in mortality has been rather small but follows a constant decline in annual prostate death rate of 1% per year (2). It is tempting to attribute this decline to increased PSA testing. However the historical nature of the event and a number of uncontrolled variables make it impossible to prove any particular theory of causation and further research is needed to quantify the association between early detection, treatment, and declining mortality (3).

The fact remains that there is a clear decrease in incidence of advanced-stage disease at initial diagnosis. Comparable data from 1992 and 1995 in the US National Cancer Data Base (NCDB) show that the average age at diagnosis declined by 2 years, that the proportion of patients with localized disease increased from 69.3% to 76.7%, and that the treatment patterns showed an increase in radical prostatectomy procedures (34.1%) at the expense of external-beam radiation treatment (26.3%) in the 1995 figures. Brachytherapy increased from 1.4% to 2.2%, while endocrine (11.7%), other treatment (4.1%), and no treatment (21.6%) remained essentially unchanged (4). The full impact of the shift in treatment is emphasized when the treatment percentages are compared to the 1974 figures. Then radical prostatectomy was performed on 9.2% and external-beam treatment on 5.5% of all prostate cancer patients (5). While these changes clearly herald the era of increasing cure rates for prostate cancer, caution is indicated since these data are derived from hospital-based information and wide variations are registered in regional comparisons of treatment. Extra caution in final interpretation is the balance between over-treatment following overdiagnosis (10–20%) and insufficient treatment (20–35%) if the cancers are too advanced to be cured (6).

Still, more than half of the screen-detected cancers can be cured—a concept that was enthusiastically accepted by the medical community and endorsed by the general public. This optimistic mood led to a rush to early detection studies in prostate cancer, with the realization that primary prevention is in the research stage and that cure of metastatic prostate cancer looks distant at the moment. This rush created the controversy about screening for prostate cancer, where experts state that half of the screening detected and histologically confirmed cases are false-positives (7) and overenthusiastic organizers claim that screening and early treatment permits a 69% decrease in deaths from prostatic cancer (8).

Is there a 'best' treatment?

Radical surgery and radiation treatment both practiced in the beginning of this century for treatment of local prostate cancer remained the only choice of active treatment for more than 80 years. Both treatments have been refined in the last decades and innovative research is performed in both fields.

The complete list of options for the patient with localized prostate cancer is presented in Table 21.1. Explaining the procedures and their outcome results takes time, not all technology is available, all procedures can be combined with neoadjuvant or adjuvant endocrine treatment, and last but not least conservative treatment, which in general stands for delayed

Table 21.1   List of available treatment options with the intention to cure. HIFU and RITA are in investigational stage

Curative treatment options for localized prostate cancer	
Surgery:	Retropubic
	Perineal
	Laparoscopic
Radiation:	External beam
	Conformal
	Brachytherapy (I 125-Pd 103)
	Protons Neutrons
Cryosurgery:	High-intensive focused ultrasound (HIFU)
	Transperineal radiofrequency ablation (RITA)

endocrine treatment, should be considered as a viable option.

The counseling of the patient is subject to bias from the provider of the services. A number of years ago a questionnaire was published on the preferred personal treatment from urologists and radiation oncologists, if they happened to have localized prostate cancer. The answers were revealing: 80% of the urologists preferred surgery, while 92% of the radiation oncologists preferred radiotherapy (9). The choice in a structured debate between surgery and radiation at the 1999 annual EAU meeting in Stockholm was simple. More than 80% of the urologists prefer surgery as first-choice treatment. Facing the lack of appropriately analyzed randomized trials, the American Urological Association convened the Prostate Cancer Clinical Guidelines Panel (10) to analyze the literature regarding available methods to treat locally confined cancer and make practice policy recommendations.

A number of interesting observations came out of a Medline search from all publications in English between 1966 and 1993. The panel reviewed 12 501 articles. On the basis of this review, 1453 were retrieved. After detailed review, 396 were found relevant of which 231 articles were rejected because of incomplete data, leaving 166 papers with outcome data for analysis. More sobering was the conclusion that the outcome data were inadequate for valid comparisons of treatment. Differences in age, tumor grade and stage were too great, and treatments were presented as options identifying advantages and disadvantages recommending that the patient should be informed of all commonly available options. Selected data are presented in Tables 21.2 and 21.3 from this important paper, knowing that small numbers of patients were analyzed for brachytherapy and conservative treatment. The conclusions from this review point to the importance of the prognostic factors that determine the outcome of the treatment. This leads us to prognostic factors.

Prognostic factors

The untreated natural history of prostate cancer takes from 15 to 20 years to develop into a clinical cancer with a limited window of opportunity to search for the clinical relevant cancers that are locally confined. Moving upfront with invasive treatment results in over-treatment, which may occur in a number of patients depending on the definition of a relevant clinical cancer. Most urologists will agree that a well-differentiated cancer involves more than one core of

Table 21.2   Range of survival/no evident disease (NED) after 5 and 10 years of radical prostatectomy vs. external-beam treatment

Survival/NED after treatment PCA*				
Radical prostatectomy			Radiation	
	Min%	Max%	Min%	Max%
5 years				
Alive	68.9	95.0	51.4	93.0
NED	81.9	92.0	32.0	93.0
10 years				
Alive	44.4	88.0	41.4	70.0
NED	82.0	82.0†	40.0	64.0

* Adapted from table 2, ref. 10.
† Only one publication available.

Table 21.3   Range of survival/no evidence of disease (NED) after 5 and 10 years of brachytherapy vs. conservative treatment

Survival/NED after treatment PCA*	Brachytherapy		Conservative treatment	
	Min%	Max%	Min%	Max%
5 years				
Alive	75.0	93.0	67.0	920
NED	38.0	90.0	68.0	68.0
10 years				
Alive	—	—†	34.0	70.7
NED	50.0	90.0	53.0	53.0†

* Adapted from table 2, ref. 10.
† No or only one publication available.

the six-core biopsy and includes a simple focus measuring more than 3 mm (11). The other side of the coin includes the understaged cancers that show locally advanced disease, where stage, size, and poorly differentiated disease present with a poor prognosis.

Histological differentiation for similar stages and volume provide the most important prognostic factor in the routine clinic. This is clearly demonstrated in Table 21.4 where 10-year survival after treatment for

Table 21.4   RP (radical prostatectomy), RT (radiation treatment) and CT (conservative treatment) % survival after 10 years according to histological grade. Note decrease in RP and greater decrease in RT and CT

Ten-year survival in localized PCA (%)			
	RP	RT	CT
G1	94	90	93
G2	87	76	77
G3	67	53	45

Adapted from table 3, ref. 12.

localized disease is presented by grade (12). Histological grade is now frequently expressed in the Gleason score (13) and once again the differences in outcome are striking. In a selected series of 652 patients treated for localized disease by radical prostatectomy, extra-prostatic extension was present in 30.6%, 56.9%, and a whopping 90.8%, respectively, with Gleason score 6, 7, and 8 or more. This resulted in NED survival of 91.2%, 75.0%, and 34.5% of the same patients (14). Clinical stage, tumor volume, PSA levels, and of course grade contribute to the prognostic index that can be used for survival estimate, therapy selection, evaluation of response, and data comparison between different populations. Clinical decisions are taken on biopsy grading, which leave a margin of error. Serious consideration should be given to all relevant prognostic factors as presented in Table 21.5. Further research in this area is badly needed and artificial neural network analysis (ANNA) could provide a more reliable prognosis (15). Do we have updated information on treatment choice?

Table 21.5   Prognostic factors in advanced prostate cancer

Summary table advanced prostate cancer			
Prognostic factors	Tumor	Host	Environment
Essential	T4,N,M stage	Age	Socio-economic
	Grade	Co-morbidity	
	PSA	Performance status	
	Pain		
Additional	No bone mets	Hemoglobin	Access
	Alk. Phosphatase	Creatinine	Expertise
	Endocrine response		
Promising	Artificial neural networks		
	PSMA		
	Epidermal growth factors		
	Androgen receptors		

Treatment innovation and choice

Conservative treatment

One of the therapeutic dilemmas, especially in males over 70 or males with serious co-morbidity, is the question to defer treatment. From a number of terms, including watchful waiting, intentional neglect, or deferred treatment, we prefer conservative treatment.

This term implies that treatment is considered with active in follow-up methodology, usually a digital rectal (DRE) and PSA test at regular intervals. We like to note that in some cases with high co-morbidity, in the absence of any prostate cancer-related symptoms, the wise approach will be to avoid diagnostic tests leading to documentation of prostate cancer. Considerations of age are in consensus related to 10-year lifetime expectancy as a base to decide on active treatment. Pursuing the diagnosis including prostate biopsy is justified since low grade and low volume allow conservative treatment to be included in the patient's options.

A few relevant studies on conservative treatment show it as a reasonable option. These observations point to grade of differentiation as the most important factor in predicting survival. Well-differentiated cancers have a low cumulative mortality of less than 10%, similar to the average population in a 10–15 year follow-up. These low-grade cancers constitute about 10% of all the prostate cancers detected. In contrast, patients with moderately differentiated cancer and poorly differentiated cancers showed cancer-specific mortality from one-quarter to a half of the patients (16, 17). The clinical decision for conservative treatment should in any case focus on complete evaluation including staging. The biopsy pathology is not always representative of the specimen pathology after surgery and 30% of cancer on biopsy tissue has an unfavorable prognosis (18). There should be no confusion in the deferred treatment assigned to patients with locally advanced or metastatic but asymptomatic cancer. This clinical question relates to the impact and drawback of endocrine treatment. No surprise of course, that only low-grade tumors seem to be the best choice for deferred treatment (19).

The decision to chose conservative treatment is more complex than choosing invasive treatment and frequently a burden to the patient and physician alike. The most frequent hurdles to consider are the calendar and biological age of the patient. Are the biopsies representative of the tumor in the specimen? Is the lack of immediate treatment complications not balanced by the late complications of tumor progression beyond the hope of cure? And last but not least, how much quality of life is lost independent of the choice? The bottom line is that physicians make errors by omission and commission, confounded many times by the perception of the patient based on medical and extramedical information. Unfortunately, most available information based on study designs, biases, outcome variables, and statistical techniques to guide prostate cancer management, suffer from selection biases that confuse the issues. Examples in the literature abound and 10–15 years cancer-specific survival in cohorts of patients treated by radical surgery, external-beam radiation, and conservative treatment relate the efficacy of the procedure to the over-riding nature of the histology in well and moderately well-differentiated localized prostate cancers (20, 21, 22). Other more practical biases include the availability of the treatment, the skill of the surgeon, the expertise and quality control of the radiation department, the diagnostic technique and biopsy interpretation, comparisons to historical cohorts (mainly the pre-PSA era), outcome metrics on survival and disease-specific survival, statistical techniques, health-related quality of life, and the economic condition of the patient. The International Consultation on Urological Diseases (ICUD) tries to overcome these problems by organizing regular consultation/consensus meetings with the support of the major urological organizations, the World Health Organization (WHO), and the International Union against Cancer (UICC), where multi-professional collaboration is the credo to the recommendations. We hope by improved data reporting, based on evidence, to assemble a database that could provide more accurate risk assessment by the ANN analysis (15).

One of the many examples for improving data reporting would be a pathology review to assign Gleason scores not only of 2–4 (well-differentiated) and 8–10 (poorly differentiated) to a division of moderately well-differentiated, counting 5 and 6, and reserve Gleason score 7 to a separate category (14, 22, 23).

Radical prostatectomy

The better term for radical prostatectomy should be a total, anatomical prostatectomy. The surgery is conceived not only as a chance for cure but due to the life-long dedication of Walsh towards perfecting the surgery by the reducing of blood loss, saving continence, and preserving potency if feasible, to maintain quality of life (24). Control of dorsal vein complex preservation of the neurovascular bundles and access to the pelvic nodes in the same setting increased the popularity of the classic radical retropubic prostatectomy. There are no prospective studies available but the general feeling is that surgeons experienced, in the perineal-exposure approach, equivalent results in terms of cancer control and complication rates (25). The latest technical innovation is the laparoscopic radical prostatectomy. When an experienced team is available, the surgery is feasible with low morbidity. It is too soon to report on cancer control but the preliminary reports of 87.7% of negative margins and 85.7% of undetectable PSA require confirmation after the learning curve (26).

The large well-documented series of radical surgery from a number of centers, especially in the US and more recently in Europe, have contributed enormously to our insight into the natural history of prostate cancer and have provided procedures in diagnosis, prognosis, and staging of the scientific databases to evaluate risk for diagnosis, prognosis, and staging, which are vital for correct recommendations (27, 28). One of the pivotal questions remains the complication rates of the surgery. Just as for cancer control, the reported outcomes are difficult to compare with other treatment modalities, and even between surgical series. It is fair to believe that the complication rates should oscillate between the results reported for population-based data and the results of one surgeon in a specialized referral center. A study of 101 604 radical prostatectomies, of which 93 986 (92.8%) via the retropubic approach, was performed by urologists in community hospitals recorded for Medicare in the period 1991–94. Complications were common and affected 25% of the patients. The 30-day mortality rate approached 1% in males aged 75–79 (29). Late complications, such as incontinence and impotence, reduce the loss of quality of life. The reported prevalence of urinary incontinence after surgery varied between 5% and 50%, but was related to a number of factors such as the age of the patient, the definition of incontinence, the surgical techniques, and the absence of complications. Persistent and continuous incontinence could be expected in 1–6% of the radical prostatectomies even in experienced centers (30).

In contrast, a report from 1870 patients, operated for radical retropubic prostatectomy by the same urologist between 1983 and 1997 and followed for a minimum of 18 months, shows a different picture. Post-operative complications still occurred in 10% of

patients overall and were associated with age but declined significantly with surgical experience. There was no post-operative mortality. Anatomic structures of the bladder neck, thrombo-embolic events, inguinal hernia, and infection constitute the bulk of complications. Recovery of urinary continence occurred in 92% of the patients and recovery of erections in 858 potent patients before surgery occurred in 71–48% patients < 70 years and 48–40% patients over 70, depending on a bilateral or unilateral nerve-sparing surgery (31). Comparing reported rates of permanent incontinence of 23% and a post-operative potency rate of 11% without reporting of the nerve-sparing technique, contrasts the expectations of the patients between specialized centers and community hospitals (32).

Unfortunately no valid randomized prospective studies are available to compare the outcome results of conservative treatment to the two most prevalent treatments of surgery or radiotherapy. A few trials are in progress but the randomization will be a major problem in the statistical analysis. Our bias is that age, co-morbidity, the perception of the patient, and the histological grade of the tumor, guides the decision to conservative treatment resulting in deferred endocrine treatment after 5–10 years. However the majority of the prostate cancers are moderately well-differentiated and an active treatment decision could be based on short- and long-term complications. Our second bias is that Gleason score 7 and certainly poorly differentiated tumors Gleason score 8–10 deserve aggressive treatment. Fortunately the latter grade category usually covers a maximum 5% of all detected cancers, since these tumors are usually outside the prostate at the time of diagnosis. The indication for surgery in clinical practice is usually based on younger age, absence of co-morbidity, and the combination of clinical stage, PSA serum values, and Gleason score, to anticipate the prediction of organ-conferred disease (33). The ideal candidates for surgery are patients with T1b, T1c, and T2 disease, according to the TNM classification (34). Surgery in patients with poorly differentiated tumors that started with a PSA < 10 and finished with negative margin status showed a disease-free survival of 56.2% for PSA < 10 and 55.0% for specimen-confined disease with a median follow-up of 36.2 months with surgery as monotherapy (14). Still the disease-free survival for non-specimen-confined tumors was 26.6% over the same period. This has introduced a trend among surgeons having operated on a great number of patients with T3 (extracapsular) disease to establish this procedure as a clinical indication with acceptable disease-free status for a number of years (35).

A small, randomized prospective trial involving T2b (cancer in both lobes of the prostate) and T3 compared radical prostatectomy versus external-beam radiotherapy, preceded and concomitant with endocrine therapy. With a median follow-up of 58.5 months, progression-free survival and disease-specific survival was 90.5% and 96.6% in the surgery group and 81.2% and 84.6% in the radiated group (36). Adding endocrine therapy to surgery reduces the positive margins but so far in follow-up studies shows equal biochemical recurrence and no proof or trends to extended survival (37, 38).

External-beam radiation

The use of neoadjuvant and adjuvant endocrine treatment on the contrary has become a norm in the radiation therapy even since the EORTC 22.863 trial on increased survival and local control in patients with locally advanced cancer as presented in Ttable 21.6 (39). A number of innovations to the external-beam treatment have been introduced since its application to prostate cancer in the 1960s. One of the most important was the introduction of the linear accelerator, producing high-energy X-rays for treating deep tumors. Radiation can also be given directly into the prostatic tissue, a technique used since the beginning of this century, by the implantation of radioisotopes, a procedure referred to as brachytherapy.

Radiation techniques over the last 3 decades have improved the cure rates with changing the field size and treatment planning. Quality control and simulated images are now routine to include the entire prostatic volume and respecting the critical surrounding tissues including bladder and rectum. The introduction of the three dimensional conformal radiation therapy (3DCRT) resulted in excellent treatment results for clinically localized prostate cancer (T1 and T2) with durable disease free survival (DFS) including biochemical remission with no evidence of disease (b NED) at 5 years and a reduction of radiation morbidity in patients

treated with dose escalations (40, 41, 42, 43). Improved local control by increasing the dose by delivering photon irradiation for early stage cancer or treating with neutron irradiation is in progress (44).

Comparing radiation to surgery proved to be impossible to match in terms of patient populations and prognostic indicators while outcome results are presented in clinically staged radiated patients and pathology staged surgical patients. It is evident from the surgical series that a great number of T2 tumors are in reality T3 tumors. The 1988 National Cancer Institute Consensus Conference concluded that the long-term results of radiation therapy for early stage cancer were comparable to surgery (45). Rather than hoping to live through an appropriate randomized prospective trial including some 1200 patients one should insist on reporting the prognostic factors relevant to outcome results. Next to the stage and grade it is evident that PSA, despite its shortcomings in many aspects, can serve as a prognostic surrogate marker for local recurrence or any other relapse of tumor growth in clinical practice.

Correcting mistakes in comparing outcome results of treatment can follow a few simple rules. The subdivision of T2 tumors into T2a, T2b, and T2c, coupling palpation, and biopsy information relates to the predicted outcome and should be routinely used in clinical practice (46). It is evident that the PSA declines with a half-life of 3 days after successful surgery cannot be reproduced by radiation, since it does not eliminate the prostate and PSA slowly declines with the irradiation of the tumor. The kinetics are not precisely known but in general PSA nadir values of < 1 after 3 years predict the most favorable outcome (47). The correlation of pretreatment PSA to outcome is evident in this paper as presented in Table 21.7. External-beam therapy with minimal volume cancer (T1b and T2a) has a favorable long-term outcome as monotherapy, while higher stages should be staged by a pelvic lymphadenectomy for proper selection assignment (48). This observation

Table 21.6 Results of 401 patients with adjunctive endocrine treatment for 3 years with median follow-up of 45 months in locally advanced prostate cancer (ref. 39)

EORTC 22.836: RxT vs. RxT and LHRHA		
	Survival	Disease-free survival
RxT mono	62% (CI 52–72)	48% (CI 38–58)
RxT LHRHA	79% (CI 72–86)	85% (CI 78–92)

Table 21.7 Adaptation from ref. 47 to link pretreatment PSA and disease free survival

Pretreatment PSA and disease-free survival	
Pre-treatment PSA/ng/ml	Five-year disease-free survival
< 4.0	90%
4.0–20	60%
> 20	45%

is definitely confirmed by the analysis of four prospective phase-III randomized trials conducted by the Radiation Therapy Oncology group between 1975 and 1992 with a long-term follow-up. Of the T1–T2 tumors, 36% had positive lymph nodes while the bulk of 1557 patients were staged as T3. The 10-year disease-specific survival for patients with a Gleason score of 2–5, 6–7, and 8–10 was, respectively, 87%, 75%, and 44% (49).

These studies suggest, but do not prove, that monotherapy of external-beam radiation is better than conservative treatment, which explains the popularity of the combined use of radiation and androgen ablation. The endocrine treatment decreases the local tumor and we know that larger tumors are more radio-resistant and control tumor sites elsewhere. This also allows cessation of pelvic lymph node irradiation, which was never proven to have a survival advantage in a randomized trial. Despite the lack of increased survival in other combination randomized trials, the impact on other factors such as clinical control of local tumor, metastases, disease-free survival, and biochemical remission brings it into clinical practice as neoadjuvant or adjuvant treatment of androgen ablation to radiotherapy (50). The optimal timing, duration, and dose of the endocrine treatment are under clinical investigation in these patients.

Further research can help to distinguish patients with localized prostate cancer who will respond to radiotherapy. Positive BCL2 and P53 expressions are independent prognostic variables for treatment failure (51). More research should be given to quality of life outcome, which may influence the understanding and choice of the patient for a certain treatment. A comparison between a surgical and a radiated group has revealed more urinary and sexual complaints after prostatectomy, while more bowel dysfunction was noted after radiation (52). Both treatments achieve respectable care rates in localized disease and can achieve cure in locally advanced disease with good prognostic factors. However, cancer occurrence forms a definite part of the clinical picture and certainly in the patients under conservative treatment who are prone to cancer progression. Salvage prostatectomy is the exception, while salvage radiotherapy remains an option after PSA recurrence following surgery. Patients with high Gleason grades, seminal vesicle or lymph node invasion, and immediate PSA recurrence after surgery rarely benefit from salvage radiation, while PSA late recurrence has a 44% chance to respond to radiotherapy (53).

Brachytherapy

From the external-beam experience it looks desirable to deliver more radiation to the prostate and less to the surrounding tissues. Brachytherapy is the answer to this hope by the implantation of radioactive sources. Modern brachytherapy for prostate cancer was popularized by Whitmore in 1972 (54). The initial reports of local control and survival were favorable but were followed by a high number of late local failures. Holm provided a second chance to prostate implantation by the development of needle placement under visual transrectal ultrasound control (55). This procedure is now standard in brachytherapy for prostate cancer utilizing primarily I125 for well-differentiated cancers up to Gleason score 6, while Pd103 is used in patients with Gleason 7 or greater. Experience with external-beam treatment led to a number of strategies that adapt the total treatment to the prognostic factors leading to a choice of implant alone, implant with neoadjuvant endocrine treatment, and finally for the high-risk cases adding a boost of peripheral external-beam irradiation (56).

The new technique is developed in the PSA era and executed by physicians with extensive experience in ultrasound evaluation. The resulting patient selection, expertise of the procedure, minimal invasive treatment, few complications, and excellent efficacy results attract the attention of the medical community and a number of positive reports have been published. The most complete report with a long term (10-year) follow-up on 152 patients presented results with low complication rates that are comparable in β Ned to most surgical or radiation series (57). Overall survival was 65% and 64% had clinical and biochemical NED with an average PSA of 0.18 ng/ml without resorting to endocrine treatment. Higher risk patients received an extra dose of 45 Gy to the pelvis. The early quality of life-assessment in patients treated by brachytherapy showed a decrease in the first 3 months after treatment but restored to baseline levels after that period (58). The results are less spectacular for salvage brachytherapy after external-beam radiation, failure being determined as two successive rising PSA values, where about half achieved a post-treatment nadir of < 0.5 ng/ml and 6% of complete urinary incontinence (59).

Cryosurgical ablation of the prostate (CSAP)

Looking for a better risk–benefit equation for treatment of localized disease, cryosurgical ablation of the prostate (CSAP) has been renovated to control local-ized cancer by a minimal invasive treatment with few complications. The technology is new, regularly inno-vated, the application carries a learning curve, and long-term outcome results are not available.

A series of 176 patients who underwent 207 cryosur-gical procedures for localized disease with neoadjuvant endocrine treatment in 101 patients were followed for 3 years. Nadir PSA was undetectable or < 0.5 ng/ml in 70% of the patients and follow-up biopsy was positive in 38% of patients. Most of the patients had T3 tumors (60). Patient satisfaction, despite an impotency rate of 85%, rested on 4.3% incontinence and a subse-quent resection of necrotic tissue in 10% of cases (61). Salvage cryotherapy after radiotherapy failure fared no better than salvage prostatectomy (62). The role of CSAP is still being defined. The hope is that it will be able to deal with high-grade, high-stage (T2b or higher) localized disease or as a salvage procedure after unsuc-cessful radiotherapy. A report on 475 men with unfa-vorable diagnosis reports low serum PSA of 0.4 ng/ml in 42,3% after 5 years. The learning curve and techni-cal innovations are a point of caution (63).

High-intensity focused ultrasound (HIFU) and transperineal radiofrequency ablation (RITA) are under clinical investigation but exact targeting is needed for further development of these techniques.

Conclusions

The role of active treatment in early prostate cancer is dependent on the prognostic factors that define outcome more than the treatment itself. These factors relate to the patient in age, co-morbidity, and percep-tion, and to the tumor in grade and stage, tumor mass, as well as a pre-operative value of PSA. Cure or control are obtained in the great majority of patients with a Gleason score of > 6, a PSA lower than 10 ng/ml, and a stage up to T2a or b.

Clinical choice depends on the perception of the patient and for surgery a 10-year life-expectancy on what is considered quality of life loss over continence and sex. For the high-risk tumors, surgery seems a logical choice if one deals with localized disease, while extra-prostatic disease calls for a multi-modality treat-ment of some type of radiation and endocrine treat-ment where brachytherapy can play a role in the future.

There are still a number of open questions, especially on the treatment of locally advanced disease. It is our

bias that in the absence of randomized trials all patients can benefit from proper data recording to establish possible guidelines on how to treat localized prostate cancer (64).

References

1. Stanford JL, Damber JE, Fair WR *et al.* Epidemiology in prostate cancer. In: *Second international consultation on prostate cancer* (ed. GP Murphy, P Eckman, Y Homma *et al.*) (In pess)
2. Landis SH, Murray T, Bolden S *et al.* Cancer Statistics 1998. *Cancer J Clin* 1998, **48**, 6–29.
3. Smart CR. The results of prostate carcinoma screening in the US is reflected in the Surveillance, Epidemiology and End Results program. *Cancer* 1997, **80**, 1835–44.
4. Mettlin C, Murphy GP, Rosenthal DS *et al.* The National Cancer Data Base Report on Prostate Carcinoma after the Peak in Incidence Rates in the US. *Cancer* 1998, **83**, 1679–84.
5. Mettlin C, Murphy GP, Menck HR. Changes in Patterns of Prostate Cancer Care in the United States: results of American College of Surgeons Commission on Cancer Studies, 1974–1993. *J Urol* 1996, **156**, 1084–91.
6. Rietbergen JBW, Hoedemaeker RF, Boeken Kruger AE *et al.* The changing pattern of prostate cancer at the time of diagnosis: characteristics of prostate cancers detected in a population-based screening study (ERSPC Data, Rotterdam Region). *J Urol* 1999 (In press).
7. Weyler J. Prostate Cancer: screening or watchful waiting? *Annals of Oncology* 1998, **9**, 9–11.
8. Labrie F, Candas B, Dupont A *et al.* Screening decreases prostate cancer death: first analysis of the 1988 Quebec prospective randomized controlled trial. *Prostate* 1999, **38**, 83–91.
9. Moore MJ, O'Sullivan B, Tannock IF. How expert physicians would wish to be treated if they had geni-tourinary cancer. *J Clin Oncol* 1988, **11**, 1736–45.
10. Middleton RG, Thompson IM, Austenfeld MS *et al.* Prostate Cancer Clinical Guidelines Panel Summary Report on the Management of Clinically Localized Prostate Cancer. *J Urol* 1995, **154**, 2144–48.
11. Bassler TJ Jr, Orozco R, Bassler IC *et al.*, UroCor Inc, Edmond, OK, USA. Most prostate cancers missed by raising the upper limit of normal prostate-specific antigen for men in their sixties are clinically significant. *Urology* 1998, **52**, 1064–9.
12. Lu-Yao GL, Long-Yao S. Population-based study of long: term survival in patients with clinically localized prostate cancer. *The Lancet* 1997, **349**, 906–10.
13. Gleason DF, Mellinger GT. The Veterans Administration Cooperative Urological Research Group: prediction of prognosis for prostatic carcinoma by combined histological grading and clinical staging. *J Urol* 1974, **111**, 58–64.
14. Tefilli MV, Gheiler EL, Tiguert R *et al.* Should Gleason score 7 prostate cancer be considered a unique grade category? *Urology* 1999, **53**, 372–77.

15. Snow P, Altinein J, Andersson L *et al.* Use of artificial neural networks for diagnosis, staging and prognosis prediction for prostate cancer. In: *Second international consultation on prostate cancer* (ed. GP Murphy, P Eckman, Y Homma *et al.*) (In pess)

16. Chodak GW, Thisted RA, Gerber GS *et al.* Results of conservative management of clinically localized prostate cancer. *New Engl J Med* 1994, **330**, 242–8.

17. Albertsen PC, Hanley JA, Gleason DF *et al.* Competing risk analysis of men aged 55 to 74 years at diagnosis managed conservatively for clinically localized prostate cancer. *JAMA* 1998, **280**, 975–80.

18. Ravery V, Schmid HP, Toublanc M *et al.* Is the percentage of cancer in biopsy cores predictive or extracapsular disease in T–T2 prostate cancer? *Cancer* 1996, **78**, 1079–84.

19. Adolfsson J, Steineck G, Hedlund PO. Deferred treatment of locally advanced nonmetastatic prostate cancer: a long-term follow-up. *J Urol* 1999, **161**, 505–8.

20. Gerber GS, Thisted RA, Scardino PT *et al.* Results of radical prostatectomy in men with clinically localized prostate cancer. *JAMA* 1996, **276**, 615.

21. Bagshaw MA, Cox RS, Hancock SL. Control of prostate cancer with radiotherapy: long-term results. *J Urol* 1994, **152**, 1781.

22. Albertsen PC, Hanley JA, Murphy-Setzko M. Statistical considerations when assessing outcomes following treatment for prostate cancer. *J Urol* 1999, **162**, 439–44.

23. Partin AW, Pound CR, Clemens J *et al.* Serum PSA after anatomic radical prostatectomy. The Johns Hopkins Experience after 10 years. *Urologic Clinics of North America* 1993, **20**, 713–25.

24. Radical retropubic prostatectomy. In: *Campbells urology* (3rd edn) (ed. PC Walsh, AB Retik, TA Stamey *et al.*). WB Saunders, Philadelphia, 1992, 2865–86.

25. Gibbons RP. Radical perineal prostatectomy: definitive treatment for patients with localized prostate cancer. *AUA update series* 1994, **XIII**, 34–43.

26. Guillonneau B, Vallancien G. Laparoscopic radical prostatectomy: initial experience and preliminary assessment after 65 operations. *Prostate* 1999, **39**, 71–5.

27. Partin AW, Pound CR, Eisenberger MA *et al.* Prostate-specific antigen doubling time (PSADT), Gleason score and the time to PSA recurrence following radical prostatectomy predicts time to distant progression. *AUA Annual Meeting*, 1999 (Abstract) (In press).

28. Horninger W, Rogatsch H, Reissigl A *et al.* Correlation between preoperative predictors and pathologic features in radical prostatectomy specimens in PSA-based screening. *Prostate* 1999, **40**, 56–61.

29. Lu-Yao GL, Albertsen P, Warren J *et al.* Effect of age and surgical approach on complications and short-term mortality after radical prostatectomy – a population-based study. *Urology* 1999, **54**, 301–7.

30. Feneley MR, Walsh PC. Incontinence after radical prostatectomy. *The Lancet* 1999, **353**, 2091.

31. Catalona WJ, Carvalhal GF, Mager DE *et al.* Potency, continence and complication rates in 1,870 consecutive radical retropubic prostatectomies. *J Urol* 1999, **162**, 433–8.

32. Fowler JE Jr, Barry MJ, Lu-Yoa G *et al.* Patient reported complications and follow-up treatment after radical prostatectomy. the national Medicare experience: 1988–1990 (updated June 1993). *Urology* 1993, **42**, 622–8.

33. Partin AW, Yoo JK, Carter HB *et al.* The use of prostate-specific antigen, clinical stage and Gleason score to predict pathological stage in men with localized prostate cancer. *J Urol* 1993, **150**, 110.

34. Sobin LH, Wittekind C. *TNM classification of malignant tumours* (5th edn). Wiley Liss Inc, New York, 1997.

35. Van den Ouden D *et al.* Radical prostatectomy as a monotherapy for locally advanced (stage T3) prostate cancer. *J Urol* 1994, **151**, 646–51.

36. Akakura K, Isaka S, Akimoto S *et al.* Long-term results of a randomized trial for the treatment of stages B2 and C prostate cancer: radical prostatectomy versus external beam radiation therapy with a common endocrine therapy in both modalities. *Urology* 1999, **54**, 313–8.

37. Bonney WW, Schned AR, Timberlake DS. Neo-adjuvant androgen ablation for localized prostatic cancer: pathology methods, surgical end points and meta-analysis of randomized trials. *J Urol* 1999, **160**, 1754–60.

38. Witjes WPJ, Schulman CC, Debruyne FMJ and the European Study Group on Neo-adjuvant Treatment of Prostate Cancer. Results of a European randomized study comparing radical prostatectomy and radical prostatectomy plus neo-adjuvant hormonal combination therapy in stage T2–3 N0M0 prostatic carcinoma. *Molecular Urology* 1998, **2**, 181–7.

39. Bolla M, Gonzales D, Warde PG *et al.* Improved survival in patients with locally advanced prostate cancer treated with radiotherapy and Goserelin. *N Engl J Med* 1997, **337**, 295–300.

40. Horwitz EM, Hanlon AL, Hanks GE, Fox Chase Cancer Cent Philadelphia, PA, USA. Update on the treatment of prostate cancer with external beam irradiation. *Prostate* 1998, **37**, 195–206.

41. Hubert J, Rossi D, Beckendorf V. Radiothérapie conformationnelle. *Progrès en Urologie* 1999, **9**, 544–51.

42. Dearnaley DP, Khoo VS, Norman AR *et al.* Comparison of radiation side-effects of conformal and conventional radiotherapy in prostate cancer: a randomized trial. *The Lancet* 1999, **353**, 267–72.

43. Zelefsky MJ, Cowen D, Fuks Z *et al.* Long term tolerance of high dose three-dimensional conformal radiotherapy in patients with localized prostate carcinoma. *Cancer* 1999, **85** (11), 2460–68.

44. Hodgson D, Warde P, Gospodarowicz M. The management of locally advanced prostate cancer. *Urologic Oncology* 1998, **4**, 3–12.

45. The Management of Clinically Localized Prostate Cancer: National Institute of Health Consensus Development Conference. *J Urol* 1989, **13**, 1369–373.

46. Iyer RV, Hanlon AL, Pinover WH *et al.* Outcome evaluation of the 1997 American Joint Committee on Cancer Staging System for Prostate Carcinoma Treated by Radiation Therapy? *Cancer* 1999, **85**, 1816–20.

47. Zagars GK, Pollack A, Karadi VS *et al.* Prostate specific antigen and RT for clinically localized prostate cancer. *Int J Radiat Oncol Biol Physics* 1995, **32**, 293–306.

48. Akakura K, Furuya Y, Suzuki H *et al.* External Beam Radiation Monotherapy for prostate cancer. *International Journal of Urology* 1999, **6**, 408–13.

49. Roach M III, Lu J, Pilepich MV *et al.* Long-term survival after radiotherapy alone: radiation therapy oncology group prostate cancer trials. *J Urol* 1999, **161**, 864–8.

50. Pilepich MV, Caplan R, Byhardt RW *et al.* Phase III trial of androgen suppression using goserelin in unfavorable-prognosis carcinoma of the prostate treated with definitive radiotherapy. Report of the Radiation Therapy Oncology Group Protocol 85–31. *J Clin Onc* 1997, **15**, 1013–21.

51. Scherr DS, Vaughan ED Jr, Wei J *et al.* BCL2 and P53 expression in clinically localized prostate cancer predicts response to external beam radiotherapy. *J Urol* 1999, **162**, 12–7.

52. Shrader-Bogen CL, Kjellberg JL, McPherson CP *et al.* Quality of life and treatment outcomes. *Cancer* 1997, **79** (10), 1977–86.

53. Cadeddu JA, Partin AW, deWeese TL *et al.* Long-term results of radiation therapy for prostate cancer recurrence following radical prostatectomy. *J Urol* 1998, **159**, 173–8.

54. Whitmore WF Jr, Hilans B, Grabstald H. Retropubic implantation of I125 in the treatment of carcinoma of the prostate. *J Urol* 1972, **108**, 1918–20.

55. Holm JJ, Juul N, Pederen JF. TP I125 seed implantation in prostate cancer guided by transrectal sound. *J Urol* 1983, **130**, 283–6.

56. Stone NN, Stock RG. Prostate brachytherapy: treatment strategies. *J Urol* 1999, **162**, 421–6.

57. Ragde H, Elgamal A-AA, Snow PB *et al.* Ten-year disease free survival after transperineal sonography-guided Iodine-125 brachytherapy with or without 45-Gray external beam irradiation in the treatment of patients with clinically localized, low to high Gleason grade prostate carcinoma. *Cancer* 1998, **83**, 989–1001.

58. Lee WR, McQuellon RP, Case LD *et al.* Early quality of life assessment in men treated with permanent source interstitial brachytherapy for clinically localized prostate cancer. *J Urol* 1999, **162**, 403–6.

59. Grado GL, Collins JN, Kriegshauser JS *et al.* Salvage brachytherapy for localized prostate cancer after radiotherapy failure. *Urology* 1999, **53**, 2–10.

60. Koppie TM, Shinohara K, Grossfeld GD *et al.* The efficacy of cryosurgical ablation of prostate cancer: the University of California, San Francisco experience. *J Urol* 1999, **162**, 427–32.

61. Badalament RA, Bahn DK, Kim H *et al.* Patient-reported complications after cryoablation therapy for prostate cancer. *Urology* 1999, **54**, 295–300.

62. Perrotte P, Litwin MS, McGuire EJ *et al.* Quality of life after salvage cryotherapy: the impact of treatment parameters. *J Urol* 1999, **162**, 398–402.

63. Cohen JK, Miller RJ Jr, Benoit RM *et al.* Cryosurgical ablation of the prostate in men with an unfavorable presentation of clinically localized prostate cancer. *J Urol* 1999, **161** (356) (Abstract), 1378.

64. Van Erps P, Van Den Weyngaert D, Denis L. Surgery or radiation: is there really a choice for early prostate cancer. *Oncology/Hematology* 1998, **27**, 11–27.

Section V

22 | Hormonal therapy in the management of prostate cancer

Fernand Labrie

Introduction

Prostate cancer is the most frequently diagnosed cancer and is the second cause of cancer death in men in North America and Europe (1). One in eight men will be diagnosed with prostate cancer during his lifetime. At the present rate of the living male population in the United States, prostate cancer will kill more than 3 000 000 men. Prostate cancer is thus a major medico-social problem comparable to that of breast cancer in women. In fact, it is predicted that 37 800 men will die from prostate cancer in the United States in 1999 while 43 700 or only 15.6% more deaths are estimated from breast cancer during the same time period (1). Prostate cancer is thus a major challenge in urgent need of significant improvement in diagnosis and treatment.

Without male hormones or androgens, there is no prostate and no prostate cancer. The most important factor that permits the development, growth, and function of the prostate is thus the androgens. In fact, the male hormones are absolutely required for the growth and normal functioning of the prostate. When a normal prostatic cell becomes cancerous, this newly developed cancer cell, as well as its daughter cells, retain this fundamental property of depending upon androgens for their growth. If these cancer cells, alike the normal prostatic cells, are deprived of androgens, the cells become smaller and smaller and eventually die by a process called apoptosis.

Knowing this essential property of the prostatic cells, which completely depend upon male hormones for their growth, the logical treatment for prostate cancer is to starve the cancer cells of male hormones. It is also reasonable to suggest that the removal or blockade of androgens should be as complete as possible. It is now recognized that male hormones acting in the human prostate are from two sources, namely, the testicles and the adrenals. These two sources of male hormones must be blocked simultaneously at the start of treatment in order to achieve the best result. In fact, the more complete the blockade of androgens is achieved, and the earlier this blockade is performed in the evolution of the disease, the more successful the treatment will be and cure thus becomes a clear possibility when the treatment is started before the cancer spreads to the bones.

The role of testicular antrogens

The first observation of the role of male hormones in prostate cancer was made by Huggins and his colleagues in 1941 (2, 3). They then observed some dramatic responses in metastatic prostate cancer patients treated by castration or estrogens. During the next 50 years that followed the introduction of the concept of androgen dependency of prostate cancer by Huggins, orchiectomy (surgical castration) and high doses of estrogens have remained the gold standard for the treatment of advanced prostate cancer (Fig. 22.1).

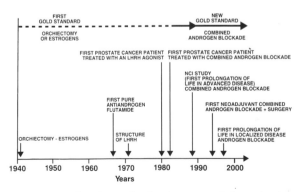

Fig. 22.1 Landmarks in the development of the endocrine therapy of prostate cancer.

Professor Charles Huggins received the Nobel Prize in Medicine for this important discovery in 1966.

Although this treatment or monotherapy discovered by Huggins is limited to blockade of the androgens of testicular origin, reports from many groups have shown that such treatment achieves a positive response in as many as in 60–70% of patients, although for a limited period of time (4–8). As indicated by such a high proportion of positive responses observed after only partial blockade of androgens, prostate cancer is highly sensitive to endocrine therapy. In fact, prostate cancer is the most sensitive of all hormone-sensitive cancers to endocrine therapy.

The serious and frequently lethal cardiovascular and cerebrovascular complications of estrogens (5, 9, 10) on one hand, and the psychological (11, 12) as well as physical limitations of surgical castration on the other hand, have generally delayed endocrine treatment until late stages of the disease when pain and debility had developed. Typically, at such a late stage, the large and disseminated tumors show poor and short-lived responses, thus limiting the success of endocrine therapy. In fact, in analogy with all other types of cancers, androgen blockade looses its effectiveness with increasing size of the tumors (13).

The discovery that LHRH agonists could achieve medical castration, or completely block the activity of the testicles, was a completely unexpected scientific finding. In fact, treatment of adult male animals for a few days with LHRH agonists led to variable degrees of inhibition of serum testosterone levels accompanied by a relatively smaller but usually significant inhibition of ventral prostate, seminal vesicle, and testis weight (14–19). This unexpected finding did not fit the well-established dogma in whole medicine, where the synthesis of an analog more potent than the natural hormone is always found to induce a higher greater biological response. The studies that followed demonstrated that man is the most sensitive of all species to the castration effect of LHRH agonists, thus facilitating the development of this uniquely efficient and well-tolerated method of castration, which is now widely used worldwide. Thus, prostate cancer patients treated with an LHRH agonist (Buserelin), the 500 μg dose of the LHRH agonist administered intranasally, caused 70% and 85% inhibitions of the serum levels of testosterone and dihydrotestosterone (DHT), respectively, as early as 2 weeks after the start of therapy (Fig. 22.2) (20). This marked inhibition of the serum concentration of both testosterone and DHT followed an initial period of stimulation that lasted approximately 1 week. It was

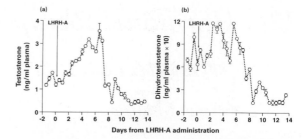

Fig. 22.2 Effect of twice daily intranasal administration of the LHRH agonist Burerelin on the serum levels of (a) testosterone and (b) DHT in the first prostate cancer patient treated with an LHRH agonist (20).

concluded that medical castration with LHRH agonists, easily achieved in men (20–23), has eliminated all the limitations described above, including the serious and even life-threatening side-effects of previous therapies, especially estrogens (5, 9, 10).

The availability of a safe and highly efficient method of medical castration with LHRH agonists free of the side-effects of estrogens and surgical castration has generated renewed interest in the treatment of prostate cancer and has stimulated an unprecedented number of clinical studies, which rapidly led to the worldwide commercialization of a series of LHRH agonists having equivalent characteristics, mechanisms of action, and efficacy.

The role of the androgens of adrenal origin

Following the discovery of the castration effect of LHRH agonists summarized above, the next most important advance made in our understanding of the biology and endocrinology of prostate cancer and its impact on cancer treatment is probably the observation that humans and some other primates are unique among animal species in having adrenals that secrete large amounts of the inactive precursor steroids dehydroepiandrosterone (DHEA), its sulfate DHEA-S, and some androstenedione, which are converted into potent androgens in a large series of peripheral tissues, including the prostate (Fig. 22.3). In fact, the plasma concentration of DHEA-S secreted by the adrenals in adult men is 100–500 times higher than that of testosterone (24), the main secretory product of the testicles. Such high circulating levels of DHEA-S (and also DHEA) provide high amounts of the prehormones or

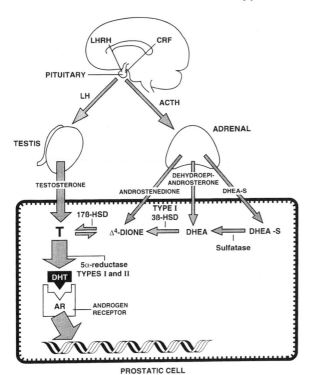

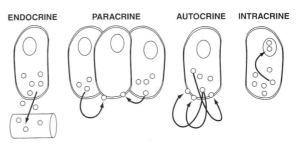

Fig. 22.4 Schematic representation of endocrine, paracrine, autocrine, and intracrine secretion. Classically, endocrine activity refers to the hormones secreted in specialized glands (endocrine glands) for release into the general circulation and transport to the distant target cells. In addition, hormones released from one cell can influence neighboring cells (paracrine activity) or can exert a positive or negative action on the same cell (autocrine activity). Intracrine activity describes the formation of active hormones from inactive precursors in the same cells where these exert their action without significant release into the extracellular compartment and the general circulation.

Fig. 22.3 Intracrine activity of the human prostate or biosynthetic steps involved in the formation of the active androgen dihydrotestosterone (DHT) from testicular testosterone as well as from the inactive adrenal precursors dehydroepiandrosterone (DHEA), DHEA-sulfate (DHEA-S), and androstenedione in human prostatic tissue. 17β-HSD = 17β-hydroxysteroid dehydrogenase; 3β-HSD = 3β-hydroxysteroid dehydrogenase/Δ^5 Δ^4-isomerase. The widths of the arrows indicate the relative importance of the sources of DHT in the human prostate: 60% originating from the testes and 40% from the adrenals in a 65-year-old men. The testis secretes testosterone (T), which is transformed into the more potent androgen DHT by 5α-reductase in the prostate. Instead of secreting T or DHT directly, the adrenal secretes very large amounts of DHEA and DHEA-S, which are transported in the blood to the prostate and other peripheral tissues. These inactive precursors are then transformed locally into the active androgens T and DHT. The enzymatic complexes DHEA sulfatase, 3β-HSD, 17β-HSD, and 5α-reductase are all present in the prostatic cells, thus providing 40% of total DHT in this tissue.

precursors required for conversion into active androgens in the prostate, as well as in other peripheral intracrine tissues.

Intracrinology

The local synthesis of active steroids in peripheral target tissues has been called intracrinology (25, 26)

(Fig. 22.4). The active androgens made locally in the prostate exert their action by interacting with the androgen receptor in the same cells, where their synthesis takes place without being released in the extracellular environment. Contrary to the previous belief that the testes are responsible for 95% of total androgen production in men (as suggested by simple measurement of circulating serum testosterone), it is now well demonstrated that the prostatic tissue efficiently transforms the inactive steroid precursors DHEA-S and DHEA, into the active androgens testosterone and DHT. In fact, the prostate synthesizes its own androgens to a level comparable to the androgens of testicular origin (24, 27–29).

Combined androgen blockade

A series of prospective, randomized, and controlled clinical trials have demonstrated that life could be prolonged in prostate cancer, with combined androgen blockade. Although the clinical data are not yet available for bicalutamide, the two anti-androgens flutamide and nilutamide have been shown, in prospective and randomized studies, to prolong life, to increase the number of complete and partial responses, to delay progression, and to provide better pain control (thus improving quality of life) in metastatic prostate cancer when added to surgical or medical castration compared to castration alone (30–36). In the first large-scale randomized study, patients who were treated with flutamide and lupron lived, on average, 7.3 months longer than those who received lupron plus placebo (30). Analysis of all the studies performed with flutamide and nilutamide associated with medical or surgical castration, compared to castration plus placebo, shows that overall survival is increased by an average of 3–6 months (30–38). Since about 50% of patients at that age die from causes other than prostate cancer, this difference in overall survival translates into an average of 6–12 months of life gained for cancer-specific survival, which are obtained by adding flutamide or nilutamide to castration. These data demonstrate the particularly high level of sensitivity of prostate cancer to androgen deprivation, even at the very advanced stage of metastatic disease.

Using the trials where sufficient information published in scientific journals was available to permit rigorous statistical analysis of the data, Caubet *et al.* (34) have shown a relative risk of approximately 0.8 in favor of combination therapy for both time to progression and survival. In other words, the addition of a pure anti-androgen to castration decreases by approximately 20% the risk of progression of disease and overall death compared to castration alone in advanced metastatic prostate cancer. In a meta-analysis, which included all published as well as unpublished trials of variable size and quality in addition to a short median follow-up of only 40 months, the difference in survival in favor of combination therapy did not quite reach the level of statistical significance in a two-sided test, the *P* value being 0.09 for flutamide (37–40). The conclusion, however, was misleading and almost suggested the absence of effect while, in fact, the difference was almost statistically significant. Another problem with the meta-analysis is the absence of recognition that the steroidal anti-androgen, cyproterone acetate, is different from the pure anti-androgens which, in turn, are all different from each other. An analysis (38) of the same but more mature data, with the addition of some new data, performed 2 years later, showed a statistically significant benefit on overall survival by adding a pure anti-androgen, especially Flutamide, to castration compared to castration alone.

Bennett *et al.* (36) have performed a meta-analysis of all peer-reviewed published randomized controlled trials comparing treatment with flutamide in association with medical (LHRH agonist) or surgical castration with castration alone in advanced prostate cancer. Nine studies with 4128 patients were included in the analysis, which demonstrated a statistically significant

10% improvement in overall survival with the combination therapy using flutamide compared to castration alone (Figs 22.5 and 22.6) (Table 22.1). As mentioned above and predicted (40), the difference has also become statistically significant in the most recent PCTCG analysis (41, 42).

With the clinical data summarized above, the controversy concerning combined androgen blockade should be part of history and the addition of a pure anti-androgen should be recognized by all, as providing an advantage of 3–6 months of life in metastatic disease. When considering cancer-specific survival, life is prolonged by 6–12 months when flutamide is added. Comparable

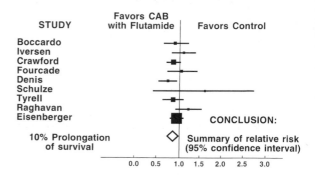

Fig. 22.5 Relative risk for Flutamide plus medical or surgical castration vs. medical or surgical castration alone from nine individual phase III randomized trials. Bennet *et al. Prostate Cancer and Prostatic Disease* 1999, **2**, 4–8.

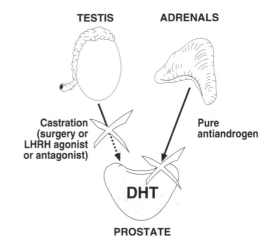

Fig. 22.6 Combined androgen blockade or the blockade of androgens of both testicular and adrenal origins should be achieved at start of treatment.

Table 22.1 Hazard ratios and 95% of confidence intervals using alternative methods for estimating hazard ratios for survival data (this study) and comparison with results from the 1995 and 1999 PCTCG analyzes

Year of analysis	Method meta-analysis	RR	95%	Number of studies
(36)	Literature-based	0.90	0.79	9
PCTCG (1995)	Patient-level	0.91	0.84	10
PCTCG (1999)	Patient-level	0.92	0.89	12

In favor of Flutamide + castration versus castration alone

benefits are obtained with nilutamide (Anandron) (33). Combined androgen blockade is thus the only opportunity to prolong life for men with advanced prostate cancer. This is the only means of gaining months of life of good quality. Moreover, combined androgen blockade leads to a greater proportion of positive and more complete responses, causes a more rapid and more complete decrease of pain and it delays the progression of the disease. Finally, recent data clearly suggest that combined androgen blockade might well be the best treatment for localized prostate cancer (as already recognized for advanced disease). With long-term treatment of localized prostate cancer, the evidence obtained even suggests cure of the disease for a large proportion of patients (43).

Early diagnosis and treatment

As part of the prospective, randomized, and controlled Laval University Prostate Cancer Detection Program (LUPCDP), men aged 45–80 years were randomly selected for screening tests from the electoral rolls of Quebec City and its vicinity. Men in the control group not invited for screening and treatment were followed according to current medical practice for diagnosis of prostate cancer and were identified during follow-up in the Quebec Cancer Death Registry, while the men selected for screening were invited to participate by letter and were followed by annual visits at the prostate cancer clinic. To minimize bias, no public announcement was made through the media. From November 1988 to December 1994, a total of 7195 men (> 99% Caucasians) in the invited group of the electoral rolls were examined at first visit; and 30 891 follow-up visits were performed. The number of men selected in each age group was proportional to that in the general male population. Other men (4616), not invited for screening as part of the LUPC Detection Program, received the same screening tests at first visit, while 15 860 follow-up visits were performed in this group of not-invited men.

Since the population of invited men is exclusively composed of previously unscreened men, we have the opportunity to obtain information specific for each visit, and thus compare the findings at first visit with those obtained at annual follow-up visits. Since no difference was found between the men invited for screening and those who come to our clinic for screening on their own, the data were pooled. It can be seen that 16.6% of 11 811 men at first visit had abnormal PAS, while at 46 751 follow-up visits PSA was abnormal in 15.6% of cases (Fig. 22.7). The distribution of serum PSA at all first and follow-up visits can be more easily visualized on the same Figure, which shows that at first (11 811) and follow-up (46 751) examinations, 83.4% and 84.4% of men have serum PSA within normal limits or below 3.0 ng/ml. It can also be seen on this Figure that serum PSA was at or below 2.0 ng/ml in 72.5% of men at first visits and 73.6% of them at follow-up visits (Fig. 22.8). Because the goal of detection of prostate cancer is to find cancer at a curable stage, it is of major interest that of the 206 cancers found among invited men where clinical staging could be performed at first visit, 151 (73.3%) were at stage A/B, 42 (20.4%) were at stage C, and 13 (6.3%) were at stage D. At follow-up visits, of the 124 evaluable cancers, 110 (88.7%) were at stage B, 13 (10.5%) were at stage C, and only one (0.8%) was at stage D. Similar values were observed in invited and not-invited men. Figure 22.9 shows the results obtained when all data are pooled for a total of 337 cancers at first visit and 215 cancers at follow-up visits. As it has been demonstrated, the diagnosis of metastatic prostate cancer can practically be eliminated by screening (44 and the present data), thus offering a unique opportunity to use curative therapies and decrease death from prostate cancer. If every man simply follows the recommendations of the American Cancer Society (45) and of the American Urological Association (46), namely annual screening starting at the age of 50 years in the general population and at 40 years for men at high

DISTRIBUTION OF SERUM PSA IN 45-80 YEAR-OLD MEN

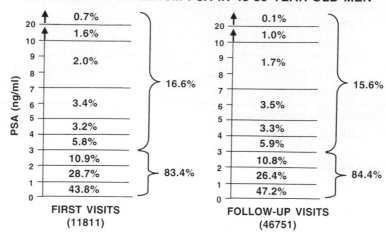

Fig. 22.7 Distribution of serum PSA at first and follow-up visits in 45–80-year-old men.

Prevalence (first visits) and incidence (follow-up visits) in men invited (□) or not invited (▨) for screening

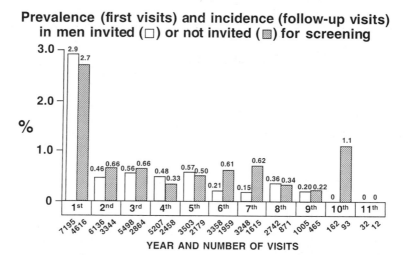

Fig. 22.8 Prevalence (first visits) and incidence (follow-up visits) of prostate cancer in men invited or not invited for screening.

risk, the proportion of localized or potentially curable prostate cancer can be increased from approximately 40% in the absence of screening (47–50) to close to 100% (44 and present data).

Early hormonal treatment

The major source of controversy concerning early diagnosis and early treatment of prostate cancer is that, until recently, no prospective and randomized trial had shown statistically significant benefits of treatment of localized prostate cancer on survival (51,

52). Such an absence of studies and consequently such as absence of results have been erroneously interpreted as being equivalent to the availability of negative data, despite the fact that negative data have never been obtained.

Two prospective randomized trials have recently demonstrated for the first time that not only quality of life but, most importantly, prolongation of life was observed in localized prostate cancer patients treated with androgen blockade. In the EORTC (European Organization for Research and Treatment of Cancer) trial performed in stage T_3-patients, overall survival at 5 years was increased from 62% in the group of

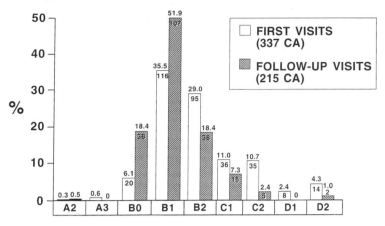

Stage distribution at first and follow-up visits

Fig. 22.9 Distribution of clinical stages of 337 and 215 (327 and 206 staged) prostate cancers diagnosed at first and follow-up screening visits, respectively. Data are expressed as percentage of total number of staged cancers in each group to facilitate comparison.

patients who received radiation therapy alone to 79% (45% difference) in the group of patients who received androgen blockade using an LHRH agonist for 3 years and an anti-androgen for 1 month in association with radiotherapy (51). Death from prostate cancer at 5 years was decreased by 77% by androgen blockade. A 20% improvement in overall survival at 5 years has also been found in RTOG trial 08351 in the subgroup

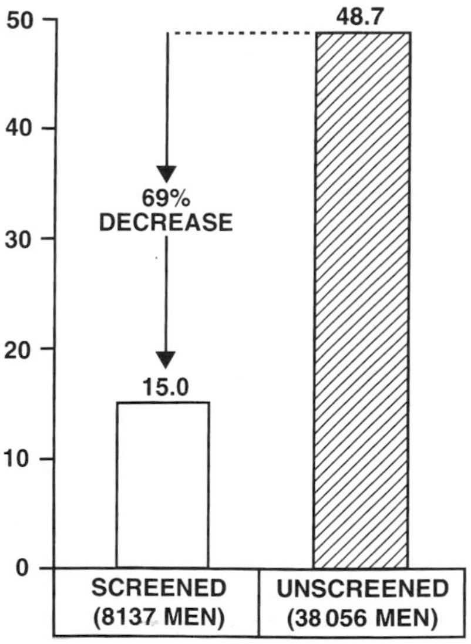

of high Gleason score patients who received androgen blockade (LHRH agonist) indefinitely or until progression (53).

Following a long controversy, a large prospective and randomized clinical trial performed by the Medical Research Council Prostate Cancer Working Party Investigators Group (54) has shown the benefits of early androgen blockade in a study of 938 patients with locally advanced or asymptomatic metastatic disease. The patients were randomized to immediate androgen blockade (orchiectomy or LHRH agonist) versus treatment deferred until symptoms developed. Marked benefits of early treatment were observed on time to progression and development of pain. Complications from metastatic disease were twice as frequent in the deferred group and, most importantly, a 21% decrease in cancer-specific death was observed in patients who had early androgen blockade. It can be added that the 69% decrease in the incidence of death from prostate cancer observed during the first 8 years of our randomized and prospective study on prostate cancer screening can only be due to the treatments used (Fig. 22.10).

Watchful waiting

While deferred treatment or watchful waiting can sometimes be an approach that can be considered in men having a short life-expectancy and diagnosed with low-grade localized disease, the data summarized above clearly limit the indication of this approach to a

Fig. 22.10 Effect of screening on the incidence of death from prostate cancer. Screening permits a 69% decrease in prostate cancer death compared to the group of men followed by standard medical practice.

small proportion of patients who should, in any case, be well informed about the recently available data and the risks involved in deferring treatment. In fact, the controversy over screening largely results from the publication of a few but much publicized reports on the potential value of deferred treatment for localized prostate cancer in selected men older than 70 years. The questionable conclusions derived from case reports have been erroneously extended to prostate cancer in general. In fact, all these reports are from uncontrolled studies, which simply describe data obtained from small series of highly selected patients. These patients were selected for deferred treatment because of a more favorable prognosis. Moreover, almost all such patients were treated at first sign of progression (55–63).

Long-term combined androgen blockade for localized prostate cancer

Prostate cancer growing in the prostate or in the tissue surrounding the prostate is very different from cancer growing in the bones. Localized prostate cancer is exquisitely sensitive to combined androgen blockade and can apparently be cured by long-term treatment. On the other hand, when prostate cancer has reached the bones, life can only be prolonged but cure is rare and can, at best, be expected in only 10–20% of patients.

Prostate cancer does spread selectively from the prostatic area to the cancellous bones of the axial skeleton where it produces osteoblastic lesions (64). The fact that prostate cancer grows preferentially in the bones could be related to the paracrine secretion by bone cells of growth factors, which stimulate prostate cancer thus facilitating the proliferation of prostatic cancer cells in this tissue (65, 66). In fact, bone fibroblasts were the most potent stimulators of human prostate cancer LNCaP cell growth. This may well explain why prostate cancer growing in the bones progressively becomes independent from androgens.

The fact that localized prostate cancer responds much better than bone metastases to androgen blockade is a well-known fact recognized by all urologists and physicians treating prostate cancer. Typically, when a patient suffering from metastatic prostate cancer receives combined androgen blockade, there is a

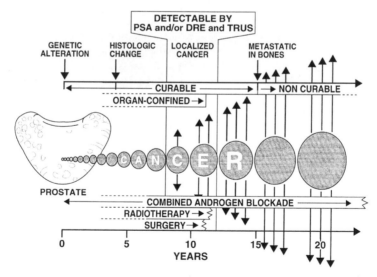

Fig. 22.11 Schematic representation of the evolution of prostate cancer from appearance of the first genetic change which following other mutations, will lead to a cancer cell. For years, the cancer cells can be seen by histology or gene markers but it is only when the tumor reaches a relatively large volume (0.3 cm) that diagnosis can be made by screening using PSA, digital rectal examination, and transrectal echography of the prostate. At that stage of possible diagnosis by screening, approximately 50% of the cancers have already migrated outside the prostate and are not organ-confined. Radical prostatectomy can cure the disease when the cancer is organ-confined. Radiotherapy and brachytherapy (seed implants) are believed to have about equal efficacy. Combined androgen blockade can also cure the disease if treatment is started before the cancer migrates to the bones. At the advanced stage of bone metastasis, only combined androgen blockade is active against the disease and can prolong life compared to monotherapy although the possibility of a cure is minimal. Much remains to be understood about the treatment of localized disease but this diagram is drawn according to the best knowledge available today.

much more rapid regression of the cancer at the prostatic compared to the metastatic level. Most importantly, when the cancer progresses again, after a period of remission, the site of cancer progression is almost always in the bones and rarely at the prostatic level. Thus, the degree of androgen-dependency of prostate cancer growing in the prostatic area is much higher than the cancer growing in the bones. All available means should thus be taken to prevent prostate cancer from migrating to the bones where treatment becomes extremely difficult and cure, or even long-term control of the disease, is an exception. The only way to prevent prostate cancer from migrating to the bones and becoming incurable is treatment of localized disease. It is also clear from the data summarized below that combined androgen blockade could well be the most efficient treatment of localized disease, thus adding to the recognition dating back for almost 60 years, that androgen blockade was already recognized as the best therapy for metastatic disease (Fig. 22.11).

In 26 patients diagnosed with clinically localized prostate cancer who received Flutamide and an LHRH agonist as only treatment for up to 12 years (median = 7.1 years), the first and still only rise of PSA when patients were under combined androgen blockade treatment occurred in one patient after 7 years and 4 months of treatment (Fig. 22.12). At 7.3 years of com-

bined androgen blockade (n = 10), the estimated response rate is thus 90% with a 95% confidence interval of 74–100%.

The side-effects of combined androgen blockade are well tolerated, namely hot flushes usually lasting for a few months at start of therapy, impotence, and loss of libido (24, 30, 32). It can be mentioned that the combination of Flutamide and an LHRH agonist leads to an improved lipid profile compared to orchiectomy (67).

The role of surgery and radiotherapy

Although the number of patients is limited, the present data clearly indicate that combined androgen blockade alone is very efficient for the treatment of clinically localized prostate cancer, its ability to control the disease being apparently superior to that of radical prostatectomy and radiation therapy alone (Fig. 22.13). In fact, although a 15-year follow-up is required to assess the long-term effect of treatment of localized prostate cancer, it is recognized that local recurrence and especially serum PSA can be used as a surrogate parameter to evaluate efficacy (68, 69). Without a randomized study, however, it is not possible to strictly compare one clinical series with another. Despite these limitations, it is of interest to see in Fig. 22.13 that the 5-year actuarial rate of recurrence in a similar category of patients who had radical prostatectomy was 24% at the Johns Hopkins Hospital (70), while it was 57% at the Boston University Medical Center (71), and 31% in a comparable series at the UCLA Medical Center (72). In a series of stage T1–2

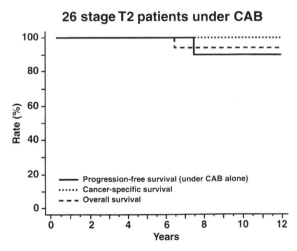

Fig. 22.12 Progression-free survival, cancer-specific survival, and overall survival in 26 previously untreated patients diagnosed with clinical localized prostate cancer who received as single treatment the anti-androgen flutamide and the LHRH agonist [d-trp6], des-gly-nh210] LHRH ethylamide (tryptal) for the indicated time intervals (median = 7.1 years, from 2.8 to 11.7 years). These data are those obtained when patients were under continuous CAB.

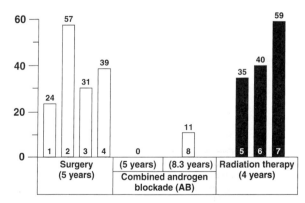

Fig. 22.13 Comparison of the failure rate after combined androgen blockade (first failure at 7.3 years in this study) versus the failure rates of 24%, 57%, 31%, and 39% at 5 years after radical prostatectomy and 35%, 40%, and 59%, 4 years after the start of radiation therapy.

prostate cancers at the Cleveland Clinic Foundation, the 5-year recurrence rate was calculated at 39% (73). Similarly, PSA failure after radiation therapy has identified a high level of cancer recurrence. Thus, following radical irradiation for T1 and T2 disease, the 4-year % actuarial rate of recurrence has been reported at 35% for the Boston University Hospital (68) and 59% for Baylor University (74). A 5-year recurrence rate of disease-free survival has been calculated at 40% at the M. D. Anderson Hospital (75). The only patient who died from prostate cancer showed biochemical progression (PSA elevation) of his cancer 9 months after arrest of combined androgen blockade. Prior to cessation of combined androgen blockade, this patient had received combined androgen blockade for 5.0 years. Since serum PSA had remained undetectable during continuous treatment with combined androgen blockade alone for as long as 11.7 years (median: 7.2 years) in 25 of the 26 patients (96%), treatment has been stopped in 20 patients of this group. Of the group of 20 patients who stopped combined androgen blockade after a median duration of 7.2 years (from 2.8 to 11.7 years), and who have been followed for a median duration of 3.9 years (from 0.0 to 5.9 years), progression has occurred in only two patients (Fig. 22.14). In both cases, progression occurred within 1 year after cessation of combined androgen blockade. In one patient, no treatment

was given because of poor general health, while the second patient died from prostate cancer nearly 4 years after stopping combined androgen blockade received continuously for 5 years. This patient was first treated with Lupron alone when PSA reached 1.7 ng/ml with no significant PSA response. Anandron was then added to Lupron approximately 1 year later when PSA had reached 6.6 ng/ml. Serum PSA continued to increase and the patient died from prostate cancer 2 years later. Two patients died from lung cancer, while two died from a cardiac infarct.

Very different results are seen when combined androgen blockade is administered for only 1 year in a similar group of patients (Fig. 22.15). Of the 11 clinical stage B2/T2 patients who stopped combined androgen blockade after only 1 year of treatment, PSA increased within 1 year in all of them except one patient who died early from cardiac failure. Serum PSA rapidly returned to undetectable levels in the six patients when combined androgen blockade was restarted.

As summarized in Fig. 22.16, the present data show a dramatic effect of duration of treatment with combined androgen blockade on the PSA failure rate after cessation of endocrine therapy. In fact, while serum PSA did not remain undetectable for 1 year after cessation of combined androgen blockade in any of the 11 patients who had received combined androgen

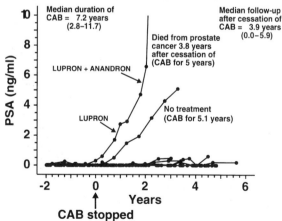

Fig. 22.14 Illustration of the duration of treatment with continuous CAB in the 26 stage T3 patients who stopped CAB after a median duration of 9.9 years of treatment and follow-up after cessation of CAB in these patients.

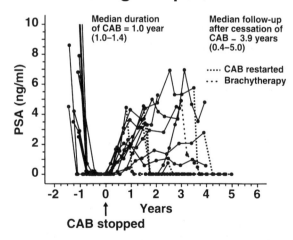

Fig. 22.15 Changes in serum PSA after cessation of CAB (LHRH agonist + Flutamide) in 20 patients with stage T2 disease, who had received CAB alone, continuously for a median of 7.2 years. Serum PSA increased in only two patients during a median follow-up of 3.9 years.

Undetectable PSA after cessation of continuous combined androgen blockade: stages T2-T3 (0.0–7.0 years of follow-up)

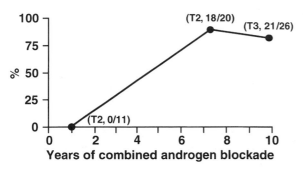

Fig. 22.16 Percentage of patients where serum PSA remained undetectable following cessation of CAB in 57 stage T2 or T3 prostate cancer patients who received combined androgen blockade for median duration of 1 year (0%: 0/11 stage T2 patients), 7.2 years (90%: 18/20 stage T2 patients), or 9.9 years (81%: 21/26 stage T3 patients).

blockade for only 1 year (Fig. 22.15), 90% of the same category of patients (stage T2) who had received combined androgen blockade for a median duration of 7.2 years remained with undetectable PSA for a median follow-up of 3.9 years (Fig. 22.14). Moreover, 81% of stage T3 patients treated for a median duration of 9.9 years with continuous combined androgen blockade had undetectable PSA during a median 4.4-year follow-up period following cessation of combined androgen blockade (Fig. 22.16). Although the maintenance of serum PSA at undetectable levels after cessation of combined androgen blockade cannot be considered equivalent to cure or complete apoptosis of the tumors, it certainly indicates that chronic treatment with continuous combined androgen blockade has a major impact on the viability of the cancer.

Intermittent hormonal therapy

Intermittent androgen blockade has become widely used recently by urologists without any valid support from randomized clinical trials. The main argument for intermittent therapy is the possibility of regaining libido and sexual potency between the periods of treatment. The return of libido and sexual potency takes months after the arrest of androgen blockade, thus seriously limiting the value of this argument. Indeed, after a single administration of a 3-month depot

formulation of an LHRH agonist, the median duration of castrated levels of testosterone in 13 patients was 6 months and the median duration of hypogonadal symptoms was 13.6 months, in parallel with the return of serum testosterone towards baseline levels (76). In fact, at 6 months, castrated levels of testosterone were maintained in 10 (77%) of 13 patients. In patients who had received an LHRH agonist for a mean of 38.6 months (range 25–82 months) before discontinuation of treatment (77), no significant increase in serum testosterone or LH occurred up to 6 months. Four of the 14 patients continued to have suppression of testosterone at 12 months. Similarly, a few reports have described the prolonged inhibition or the persistent loss of recovery of testosterone after long-term estrogen administration (9, 78). It is clear from the above-summarized data that one of the arguments for intermittent therapy, namely a return of libido and sexual potency during the intermittent period of no treatment, does not occur in many, and probably in the majority of patients. In fact, in most men, libido and sexual potency are unlikely to return before PSA rises again and treatment must be started.

References

1. Landis SH, Murray T, Bolden S *et al.* Cancer Statistics, 1999. *CA Cancer J Clin* 1999, **49**, 8–31.
2. Huggins C, Hodges CV. Studies of prostatic cancer. I. Effect of castration, estrogen and androgen injections on serum phosphatases in metastatic carcinoma of the prostate. *Cancer Res* 1941, **1**, 293–307.
3. Huggins C, Stevens RE, Hodges CV. Studies on prostatic cancer. II. The effects of castration on advanced carcinoma of the prostate gland. *Arch Surg* 1941, **43**, 209–23.
4. Nesbit RM, Baum WC. Endocrine control of prostatic carcinoma: clinical and statistical survey of 1818 cases. *JAMA* 1950, **143**, 1317–20.
5. VACURG. Treatment and survival of patients with cancer of the prostate. *Surg Gynecol Obstet* 1967, **124**, 1011–7.
6. Staubitz WJ, Oberkircher OJ, Lent MH. Clinical results of the treatment of prostatic carcinoma over a ten-year period. *J Urol* 1954, **72**, 939–45.
7. Mettlin C, Natarajan N, Murphy GP. Recent patterns of care of prostatic cancer patients in the United States: results from the surveys of the American College of Surgeons Commission on Cancer. *Int Adv Surg Oncol* 1982, **5**, 277–321.
8. Murphy GP, Beckley S, Brady MF *et al.* Treatment of newly diagnosed metastatic prostate cancer patients with chemotherapy agents in combination with hormones versus hormones alone. *Cancer* 1983, **51**, 1264–72.

9. Robinson MR, Thomas BS. Effect of hormone therapy on plasma testosterone levels in prostatic cancer. *Br Med J* 1971, **4**, 391–4.

10. Peeling WB. Phase III studies to compare goserelin (Zoladex) with orchiectomy and with diethylstilbestrol in treatment of prostatic carcinoma. *Urology* 1989, **33**, 45–52.

11. Lunglmayr G, Girsch E, Meixner EM *et al.* Effects of long-term GnRH analogue treatment on hormone levels and spermatogenesis in patients with carcinoma of the prostate. *Urol Res* 1988, **16**, 315–9.

12. Cassileth BR, Soloway MS, Vogelzang NJ *et al.* Patient's choice of treatment in stage D prostate cancer. *Urology* 1989, **33**, 57–62.

13. Chen C, Poulin R, Labrie F. Large Shionogi tumors lose their responsiveness to Flutamide treatment. *J Steroid Biochem Mol Biol* 1996, **48**, 489–94.

14. Auclair C, Kelly PA, Labrie F *et al.* Inhibition of testicular luteinizing receptor level by treatment with a potent luteinizing hormone-releasing hormone agonist of human chorionic gonadotropin. *Biochem Biophys Res Commun* 1977, **76**, 855–62.

15. Auclair C, Kelly PA, Coy DH *et al.* Potent inhibitory activity of [D-Leu^6, des-Gly -NH$_2$^{10}] ethylamide on LH/hCG and PRL testicular receptor levels in the rat. *Endocrinology* 1977, **101**, 1890–3.

16. Labrie F, Auclair C, Cusan L *et al.* Inhibitory effects of LHRH and its agonists on testicular gonadotropin receptors and spermatogenesis in the rat. *Int J Androl* 1978, **112**, 303–18.

17. Rivier C, Rivier J, Vale W. Chronic effects of [D-Trp6-Pro9-NEt]luteinizing hormone-releasing factor on reproductive processes in the female rat. *Endocrinology* 1978, **103**, 2299–305.

18. Rivier C, Rivier J, Vale W. Chronic effects of [D-Trp6,Pro9-NEt]luteinizing hormone-releasing factor on reproductive processes in the male rat. *Endocrinology* 1979, **105**, 1191–201.

19. Rivier C, Vale WW. Hormonal secretion in male rats chronically treated with [D-Trp6,Pro9-NEt]-LRF. *Life Sci* 1979, **25**, 1065–74.

20. Labrie F, Bélanger A, Cusan L *et al.* Antifertility effects of LHRH agonists in the male. *J Androl* 1980, **1**, 209–28.

21. Faure N, Labrie F, Lemay A *et al.* Inhibition of serum androgen levels by chronic intranasal and subcutaneous administration of a potent luteinizing hormone-releasing hormone (GNRH) agonist in adult men. *Fertil Steril* 1982, **37**, 416–24.

22. Labrie F, Dupont A, Bélanger A *et al.* New hormonal therapy in prostatic carcinoma: combined treatment with an LHRH agonist and an antiandrogen. *Clin Invest Med* 1982, **5**, 267–75.

23. Tolis G, Ackman D, Stellos A *et al.* Tumor growth inhibition in patients with prostatic carcinoma treated with LHRH agonists. *Proc Natl Acad Sci* 1982, **79**, 1658–62.

24. Labrie F, Dupont A, Bélanger A. Complete androgen blockade for the treatment of prostate cancer. In: *Important advances in oncology* (ed. VT de Vita, S Hellman, SA Rosenberg). JB Lippincott, Philadelphia, 1985, 193–217.

25. Labrie C, Bélanger A, Labrie F. Androgenic activity of dehydroepiandrosterone and androstenedione in the rat ventral prostate. *Endocrinology* 1988, **123**, 1412–7.

26. Labrie F. Intracrinology. *Mol Cell Endocrinol* 1991, **78**, C113–C118.

27. Labrie F, Dupont A, Simard J *et al.* Intracrinology: the basis for the rational design of endocrine therapy at all stages of prostate cancer. *Eur Urol* 1993, **24** (Suppl 2), 94–105.

28. Labrie F, Simard J, Luu-The V *et al.* Structure, function and tissue-specific gene expression of 3b-hydroxysteroid dehydrogenase/5-ene-4-ene isomerase enzymes in classical and peripheral intracrine steroidogenic tissues. *J Steroid Biochem Mol Biol* 1992, **43**, 805–26.

29. Labrie F, Simard J, Luu-The V *et al.* The 3b-hydroxysteroid dehydrogenase/isomerase gene family: lessons from type II 3b-HSD congenital deficiency. In: *Signal transduction in testicular cells Ernst Schering Research Foundation Workshop* (ed. V. Hansson, F.O. Levy, K. Taskén). Springer-Verlag, Berlin, Heidelberg, New York, 1996, 185–218.

30. Crawford ED, Eisenberger MA, McLeod DG *et al.* A controlled trial of leuprolide with and without flutamide in prostatic carcinoma. *N Engl J Med* 1989, **321**, 419–24.

31. Janknegt RA, Abbou CC, Bartoletti R *et al.* Orchiectomy and Nilutamide or placebo as treatment of metastatic prostatic cancer in a multinational double-blind randomized trial. *J Urol* 1993, **149**, 77–83.

32. Denis L, Carnelro de Moura JL, Bono A *et al.* Goserelin acetate and flutamide vs bilateral orchiectomy: a phase III EORTC trial (30853). EORTC GU Group and EORTC Data Center. *Urology* 1993, **42**, 119–29.

33. Dijkman GA, Janknegt RA, Dereijke TM *et al.* Long-term efficacy and safety of nilutamide plus castration in advanced prostate-cancer, and the significance of early prostate specific antigen normalization. *J Urol* 1997, **158**, 160–3.

34. Caubet JF, Tosteson TD, Dong EW *et al.* Maximum androgen blockade in advanced prostate cancer: a meta-analysis of published randomized controlled trials using nonsteroidal antiandrogens. *Urology* 1997, **49**, 71–8.

35. Denis LJ, Keuppens F, Smith PH *et al.* Maximal androgen blockade: final analysis of EORTC Phase III trial 30853. *Eur Urol* 1998, **33**, 144–51.

36. Bennett CL, Tosteson TD, Schmitt B *et al.* Maximum androgen-blockade with medical or surgical castration in advanced prostate cancer: a meta-analysis of nine published randomized controlled trials and 4128 patients using flutamide. *Prostate Cancer and Prostatic Diseases* 1999, **2**, 4–8.

37. Prostate Cancer Triallists' Collaborative Group. Maximum androgen blockade in advanced prostate cancer: an overview of 22 randomized trials with 3283 deaths in 5710 patients. *Lancet* 1995, **346**, 265–9.

38. Prostate Cancer Triallists' Collaborative Group. Update of data 1997.

39. Taubes G. Epidemiology faces its limits. *Science* 1995, **269**, 164–9.

40. Labrie F, Crawford D. Anti-androgens in treatment of prostate cancer. *Lancet* 1995, **346**, 1030–1.

41. Prostate Cancer Triallists' Collaborative Group. Update of data 1999.

42. Raghavan D. Systemic therapy for advanced prostate cancer. *J Clin Oncol* 1999, **17**, 494–501.

43. Labrie F, Cusan L, Gomez JL *et al*. Long-term combined androgen blockade alone for localized prostate cancer. *Mol Urol* 1999, **3**, 217–25.

44. Labrie F, Candas B, Cusan L *et al*. Diagnosis of advanced or noncurable prostate cancer can be practically eliminated by prostate-specific antigen. *Urology* 1996, **47**, 212–7.

45. American Cancer Society. *Guidelines for the cancer-related checkup: an update*. Atlanta (GA). American Cancer Society 1993.

46. American Urological Association. *Executive Committee Report*. Baltimore (MD). American Urological Association 1992, January.

47. Murphy GP, Natarajan N, Pontes JE *et al*. The national survey of prostate cancer in the United States by the American College of Surgeons. *J Urol* 1982, **127**, 928–34.

48. Schmidt JD, Mettlin CJ, Natarajan N *et al*. Trends in patterns of care for prostatic cancer, 1974–1983: results of surveys by the American College of Surgeons. *J Urol* 1986, **136**, 416–21.

49. Mettlin C, Murphy GP, Lee F *et al*. Characteristics of prostate cancers deteted in a multimodality early detection program. The Investigators of the American Cancer Society National Prostate Cancer Detection Project. *Cancer* 1993, **72**, 1701–8.

50. Labrie F, Dupont A, Suburu R *et al*. Serum prostatic specific antigen (PSA) as prescreening test for prostate cancer. *J Urol* 1992, **147**, 846–51.

51. Bolla M, Gonzalez D, Warde P *et al*. Improved survival in patients with locally advanced prostate cancer treated with radiotherapy and goserelin. *N Engl J Med* 1997, **337**, 295–300.

52. Kolata G. Prostate cancer consensus hampered by lack of data. *Science* 1987, **236**, 1626–7.

53. Pilepich MV, Caplan R, Byhardt RW *et al*. Phase III trial of androgen suppression using Goserelin in unfavorable prognosis carcinoma of the prostate treated with definitive radiotherapy: report of radiation therapy oncology group protocol 85–31. *J Clin Oncol* 1997, **15**, 1013–21.

54. The Medical Research Council Prostate Cancer Working Party Investigators Group. Immediate versus deferred treatment for advanced prostatic cancer: initial results of the Medical Research Council trial. *Br J Urol* 1997, **79**, 235–46.

55. Johansson JE, Adami HO, Andersson SO *et al*. High 10-year survival rate in patients with early, untreated prostatic cancer. *JAMA* 1992, **267**, 2191–6.

56. Whitmore Jr WF, Warner JA, Thompson IM. Expectant management of localized prostatic cancer. *Cancer* 1991, **67**, 1091–6.

57. Goodman CM, Busuttil A, Chisholm GD. Age, and size and grade of tumour predict prognosis in incidentally diagnosed carcinoma of the prostate. *Br J Urol* 1988, **62**, 576–80.

58. Adolfsson J, Carstensen J, Lowhagen T. Deferred treatment in clinically localized prostatic carcinoma. *Br J Urol* 1992, **69**, 183–7.

59. Jones GW. Prospective, conservative management of localized prostate cancer. *Cancer* 1992, **70**, 307–10.

60. Orestano F. Problems of wait-and-see policy in incidental carcinoma of the prostate. In: *Incidental carcinoma of the prostate* (ed. F Altwein, W Schneider). Springer Verlag, Berlin-Heidelberg, 1991, 162–6.

61. Moskovitz B, Nitecki S, Richter-Levin D. Cancer of the prostate: is there a need for aggressive treatment? *Urol Int* 1987, **42**, 49–52.

62. Larsson A, Norlen BJ. Five-year follow-up of patients with localized prostatic carcinoma initially referred for expectant treatment. *Scand J Urol Nephrol* 1985, **19**, 30.

63. Chodak GW, Thisted RA, Gerber GS *et al*. Results of conservative management of clinically localized prostate cancer. *New Engl J Med* 1994, **330**, 242–8.

64. Jacobs SC. Spread of prostatic cancer to bone. *Urology* 1983, **21**, 337–44.

65. Gleave ME, Hsieh JT, von Eschenbach AC *et al*. Prostate and bone fibroblasts induce human prostate cancer growth *in vivo*: implications for bidirectional tumor-stromal cell interaction in prostate carcinoma growth and metastasis. *J Urol* 1992, **147**, 1151–9.

66. Chackal-Roy M, Niemeyer C, Moore M *et al*. Stimulation of human prostatic carcinoma cell growth by factors present in human bone marrow. *J Clin Invest* 1989, **84**, 43–50.

67. Moorjani S, Dupont A, Labrie F *et al*. Changes in plasma lipoproteins during various androgen suppression therapies in men with prostatic carcinoma: effects of orchiectomy, estrogen, and combination treatment with LHRH agonist and Flutamide. *J Clin Endocrinol Metab* 1988, **66**, 314–22.

68. Zietman AL, Shipley WU, Coen JJ. Radical prostatectomy and radical radiation therapy for clinical stages T1 to 2 adenocarcinoma of the prostate. New insights into outcome from repeat biopsy and prostate specific antigen follow-up. *J Urol* 1994, **152**, 1806–12.

69. Zagars GK, von Eschenbach AC. Prostate-specific antigen. An important marker for prostate cancer treated by external beam radiotherapy. *Cancer* 1993, **72**, 538–48.

70. Morton RA, Steiner MS, Walsh PC. Cancer control following anatomical radical prostatectomy: an interim report. *J Urol* 1991, **145**, 1197–200.

71. Zietman AL, Edelstein RA, Coen JJ *et al*. Radical prostatectomy for adenocarcinoma of the prostate: the influence of preoperative and pathologic findings on biochemical disease-free outcome. *Urology* 1994, **43**, 828–33.

72. Trapasso JG, deKernion JB, Smith RB *et al*. The incidence and significance of detectable levels of serum prostate specific antigen after radical prostatectomy. *J Urol* 1994, **152**, 1821–5.

73. Kupelian P, Katcher J, Levin H *et al*. Correlation of clinical and pathological factors with rising prostate-specific antigen profiles after radical prostatectomy alone for clinically localized prostate cancer. *Urology* 1996, **48**, 249–60.

74. Goad JR, Chang SJ, Ohori M *et al*. PSA after definitive radiotherapy for clinically localized prostate cancer. *Urol Clin North Am* 1993, **20**, 727–36.

75. Kaplan ID, Cox RS, Bagshaw MA. Prostate specific antigen after external beam radiotherapy for prostatic cancer: followup. *J Urol* 1993, **149**, 519–22.

76. Oefelein MG. Time to normalization of serum testosterone after 3-month luteinizing hormone-releasing hormone agonist administered in the neoadjuvant setting: implications for dosing schedule and neoadjuvant study consideration. *J Urol* 1998, **160**, 1685–8.

77. Hall M, Fritzsch S, Sagalowsky AI *et al*. Prospective determination of the hormonal response after cessation of luteinizing hormone-releasing hormone agonist treatment in patients with prostate cancer. *Urology* 1999, **53**, 898–903.

78. Tomic R, Bergman B. Hormonal effects of cessation of estrogen treatment for prostatic carcinoma. *J Urol* 1987, **138**, 801–5.

23 | Management of hormone-resistant prostate cancer

Cora N. Sternberg and Fabio Calabrè

Introduction

The incidence of prostate cancer has increased dramatically over the past few years due to heightened public awareness, screening programs, more widespread use of prostatic-specific antigen (PSA), and advanced imaging techniques. Prostate cancer is the most common cancer (excluding skin cancer) in American men, and the second leading cause of death from cancer in men, exceeded only by lung cancer. The American Cancer Society estimates that there will be about 179 300 new cases of prostate cancer in the United States this year, and about 37 000 men will die of this disease (1). Although men of any age can get prostate cancer, it is found most often in men over 50. Eight of ten of the men with prostate cancer are over the age of 65. Prostate cancer is about twice as common among African-American men as it is among white American men. It is also most common in North America and northwestern Europe. It is less common in Asia, Africa, Central America, and South America.

Of men with prostate cancer, 89% live at least 5 years, and 63% survive at least 10 years. Once cancer has spread, 5-year survival is around 31% (2). Discovery of the HPC1 gene has yielded information about inherited risk of prostate cancer (3, 4). Controversy surrounds the advisability and effectiveness of screening, the most appropriate staging evaluations, and the optimal management of patients with all stages of prostate cancer. For metastatic disease, hormonal therapy is clearly indicated. Uncertainty exists about the optimal therapy and timing. For the patients who have become refractory to hormonal therapy, new therapeutic strategies are needed.

Advanced disease

Approximately 30–35% of patients with prostate cancer will present with regional or metastatic tumors, while an additional 25% will develop metastases in the course of the disease. Metastases are commonly to bone, where the lesions can be seen on X-ray as osteosclerotic lesions or on a bone scan as areas of increased activity 'hot spots'. In patients presenting with metastatic disease and receiving androgen ablation, median survival is 2.5 years (5).

Hormone-naive disease

The mainstay of therapy is androgen ablation, which is palliative rather than curative. Hormonal therapy can produce objective tumor regression in soft-tissue sites in upwards of 80% of cases, normalization of an abnormal PSA in 70%, and an improvement in the bone scan in 30–50% of cases (6). With monotherapy such as orchiectomy, estrogens, or luteinizing hormone-releasing agonists, 50% will live less than 2 years, and 90% will die within 3 years (5). Orchiectomy has been the gold standard endocrine therapy for many years. However, in most parts of Europe and the world, medical therapy is more acceptable to patients than surgical castration, both for psychological and cultural reasons. Non-steroidal anti-androgens such as, flutamide, bicalutamide, and nilutamide act directly on prostatic cells and avoid loss of sexual potency. Bicalutamide, another non-steroidal anti-androgen, has a longer half-life, making once a day administration suitable. There may be fewer side-effects than with flutamide (7). Three-monthly depots have become available, which require less frequent administration (8).

Combined androgen blockade (CAB) was conceived as a means of blocking the adrenal androgens. The main advantages to the combination of a LHRH analog and an anti-androgen is blockade of the LHRH agonist flare. Many investigators with contradictory results have evaluated CAB compared to androgen suppression (AS) alone.

In the NCI Intergroup trial, androgen blockade with leuprolide and flutamide resulted in a longer progression-free survival and over-all survival than with leuprolide alone in patients with minimal disease and good performance status (9). In the EORTC study, treatment with goserelin and flutamide was associated with a longer time to objective progression and longer survival than orchiectomy alone (10). Nilutamide plus orchiectomy proved to be more effective than orchiectomy alone for metastatic prostate cancer (11).

A meta-analysis of 22 trials with 5425 patients, 2720 treated with CAB and 2705 with monotherapies, revealed 5-year survival of 20% with CAB and 17% with monotherapy. Although the risk of death was reduced by 7%, the standard deviation for this observation was 4%, which was not statistically significant (12)

This collaborative meta-analysis was recently updated to include 8275 men; 98% of men being randomized between CAB and AS alone. Five-year survival was 25.4% with CAB versus 23.6% with AS alone, a non-significant gain of 1.8% (13). The results of cyproterone acetate (CPA) seemed slightly unfavorable; 27.6% CAB versus 24.7% AS alone, a difference of 2.9%. Addition of AS appeared to improve 5-year survival by about 2–3%.

For patients with widespread bone or soft-tissue metastases and a poor performance status, responses are characteristically short, and CAB appears not to provide a significant advantage over LHRH agonists or orchiectomy alone. The major disadvantage of CAB is that available LHRH analogs and pure anti-androgens are expensive. Nonetheless, CAB has been widely accepted as standard first-line therapy in many countries, particularly in younger patients (14).

Hormone refractory prostate cancer

Hormone-refractory prostate cancer is defined as progressive disease despite castration serum levels of testosterone. The development of hormonal resistance predictably occurs after androgen deprivation. The median time to progression is 18 months, with median survival of approximately 6 months (15). Following disease progression, some remaining androgen-sensitive cells may respond to second-line hormonal therapy.

Bone is the primary and only site of metastases in 65% of patients who present with metastatic prostatic cancer. For this reason, objectively measurable criteria

for response evaluation are often lacking. In many patients, bone pain and decreased performance status are predominant, and relief of these symptoms may be as important as prolongation of survival. Contemporary trials seem to suggest that prostate cancers are not as resistant to therapy as previously believed. This is due in part to the change in reporting of results in prostate cancer. Many older trials did not use PSA and included patients with stable disease as responders.

Use of surrogate endpoints, such as reduction in PSA or improvement in pain, has been useful in the evaluation of new agents. An evaluation of quality of life has become a fundamental part of many prostate cancer studies. Although the value of PSA decline as a measure of therapeutic benefit has not been definitively established, studies have shown that a > 50% to > 80% decrease in PSA may be associated with prolonged survival (16).

There are problems in the interpretation of post-therapy PSA. PSA expression is modulated by a number of agents, including androgens, retinoids, and vitamin D, as well as growth factors. A drug may decrease PSA release without killing cells. This can be accounted for in the clinic by requiring a given degree of decline be documented more than once, and be maintained for a defined period of time before classifying a patient as having a 'benefit'. For instance, after cis-retinoic acid or other differentiating agents, an increase in PSA may proceed a decline.

Second-line hormonal therapy

Second-line hormonal treatment works by diminishing circulating adrenal androgens, which may cause tumor regression by suppressing any remaining hormone dependent prostatic cancer cells. Symptom relief often occurs rapidly, suggesting a mechanism other than adrenal suppression. A variety of hormonal therapies, such as flutamide, have been used as second-line therapy with modest results that have been well-documented (5). It appears that there is a modulation of the testosterone receptor that may be clinically useful after patients no longer seem to respond to hormonal therapy.

One of the most interesting observations has been called the 'flutamide withdrawal syndrome'. This was first described at Memorial Hospital in New York by Scher et al. (17). Up to 40% of patients failing CAB may respond when the anti-androgen is discontinued.

This seemingly paradoxical response was first documented with flutamide withdrawal, but was subsequently shown to occur with two other non-steroidal anti-androgens, bicalutamide and nilutamide (17).

Addition of a higher dose of bicalutamide, 150 mg daily, has also shown to be efficacious as second-line therapy in this setting (18). Megace and dexamethasone are less expensive secondary hormonal therapies. Steroids, in particular, may produce symptomatic improvement and disease regression. There are undoubtedly objective responses in 10–30% of patients (5, 19).

Other hormonal therapies

Ketoconazole

Ketoconazole is an oral imidazole derivative with anti-fungal properties that works through a hormonal-adrenal mechanism and by inhibiting the cytochrome P450 enzyme system. It totally blocks all steroid production, including that of the adrenal glands, making endogenous steroid replacement a necessity for patients in treatment with ketoconazole. In one study, ketoconazole in combination with hydrocortisone, produced a > 50% decline in PSA in 30 of 48 (63%) patients treated with the combination of ketoconazole and hydrocortisone, for a median of 3.5 months. In addition, 48% had > 80% decline in PSA, with 23/48 having responses ranging from 3.25 to 12.75+ months (20).

In combination with adriamycin > 50% decrease in PSA was seen in 57% of patients. Cardiac and important mucocutaneous toxicity was seen (21). It is unknown whether or not ketoconazole may act by modulation of retinoic acid breakdown. It has also been postulated that ketoconazole functions as a hormonal agent, which serves to enhance intracellular adriamycin exposure through an effect on multidrug resistance gene product.

Estramustine

Estramustine (estracyt), the combination of nornitrogen mustard and estradiol inhibits microtubules by a different mechanism of action than the vinca alkaloids. Overall response rates in the United States have been low, 0–4%, while in Europe response rates have been 30–50% (22). Advantages include oral administration and lack of myelosuppression. It possesses no overlap-

ping toxicities with other cytotoxic agents, as its primary toxicity is gastro-intestinal.

There is evidence of synergism with of estracyt with vinca alkaloids, epidophyllotoxins, and taxanes in experimental models. It is not cross-resistant with these agents, and bypasses the multi-drug-resistance (*p*-glyco-protein) phenotype. Its toxicity is primarily gastro-intestinal, than myelosuppressive.

Estracyt was combined with vinblastine in three separate trials illustrated in Table 23.1. Cumulative data revealed a > 50% decrease in PSA in 46–61% of patients, with measurable disease regression in 24% (23–25). Two comparative randomized studies of the combination were published (Table 23.2).

An American study revealed a benefit in terms of progression free-survival, although not in overall survival ($P = 0.08$) with the combination as compared to vinblastine alone (26). Overall median survival was 11.9 months for the combination versus 9.2 months for vinblastine alone. The combination was superior to single agent vinblastine for secondary endpoints of time to progression ($P < 0.001$) median 3.7 vs. 2.2 months, respectively, and for the proportion of patients with > 50% (PSA) decline sustained for at least 3-monthly measurements (25.2% vs. 3.2%, respectively; $P < 0.0001$). Granulocytopenia was less for the combination compared to vinblastine alone. However, grade > 2 nausea

Table 23.1 Phase II Trials of Estracyt plus Vinblastine in HRPC

Institution	Year	Ref No	>50% ↓PSA	Measurable Disease (CR+PR)
MDAH	1991	28	13/28 (46%)	3/13 (23%)
MSKCC	1992	25	13/24 (54%)	2/5 (40%)
Fox Chase	1992	36	22/6 (61%)	1/7 (14%)
Total		89	48/88 (55%)	6/25 (24%)

Table 23.2 Phase III Trials of Estracyt plus Vinblastine in HRPC

	Fox Chase Hudes 1999 (26)		EORTC Albrecht 1999 (28)	
Treatment	E+V	V	E+V	E
N	95	98	35	36
>50% ↓PSA	25.2%	3.2%	34%	22%
PFS/TTP	3.7 mos	2.2 mos	7.2 mos	8.1 mos
OS/MDS	11.9 mos	9.2 mos	10.2 mos	10.9 mos

(26% vs. 7%) and extremity edema (22% vs. 8%) were more frequent for combination therapy.

An EORTC study attempted to compare the combination to estracyt alone. This study was stopped due to toxicity and found no overall difference in time to progression or overall survival (27, 28).

Chemotherapy

Despite the wide disparity in reports suggesting efficacy of 40–80%, hormone-refractory prostate cancer is resistant to most chemotherapy. Objective tumor regression occurs in less than 10–20% (29), and no standard chemotherapy regimen has been defined. Median survival from study to study is similar, 30–40 weeks. No agent or regimen has shown a consistent impact on survival.

Low-dose weekly adriamycin 20 mg/m^2 was considered by many oncologists in the United States as first-line therapy in hormone refractory prostate cancer. In Europe, an adriamycin analog, epirubicin, was often used. Response rates for adriamycin have ranged from 0 to more than 50%, depending upon the response criteria utilized (30, 31). Mitoxantrone, another anthracycline, has modest activity as a single agent. Two randomized trials with mitoxantrone plus prednisone have been reported (32, 33). Both trials employed crossover designs, which may explain why palliation was observed with no survival benefit. The primary endpoint was a palliative response described as a decrease in analgesic use. The combination was approved by the FDA for the palliation of pain, and some consider this regimen as the new standard against which other approaches should be compared.

Etoposide (Vp-16), a podophyllotoxin derivative, is known to inhibit topoisomerase II at the nuclear matrix level. Although not active as a single agent, the combination with estracyt has shown a synergistic effect (34–37). The combination of estracyt and etoposide was first introduced in 1994, with updated results reported in 1997 (35). Although estracyt is best known as an antimicrotubule agent, it appears to act synergistically with etoposide. The mechanism of action may be different from that in combination with vinblastine. Of 95 patients, the first 52 were treated with a dose of 15 mg/kg/day estracyt and oral etoposide 50 mg/m^2/day (1 capsule bd in most) for 21 days every 28 days. The remaining 43 patients were treated with a reduced dose of estracyt 10 mg/kg/day and allowed prior chemotherapy. Fifty of 95 (53%) had a > 50%

decline in PSA, with no difference in the two groups in response or median survival. The authors concluded that the 10 mg/kg/day dose was equally effective and, of importance, was associated with less nausea. These results are of interest in view of the limited activity of etoposide as a single agent.

The taxoids are a new class of anti-neoplastic drugs. Paclitaxel (taxol) and Docetaxel (taxotere) share a similar mechanism of action: the promotion of microtubule assembly and inhibition of microtubule disassembly. Taxol is the active ingredient of the bark. Taxotere was prepared from the needles of *Taxus baccata*. Single-agent taxol has not shown to be very effective in HRPC. A phase II trial of the Eastern Cooperative Oncology Group evaluated 24-h taxol 135–170 mg/m^2, given as a continuous infusion, every 21 days. Of 23 measurable patients, PR was achieved in only 1 (14.3%) patients for 9 months 41. However, in combination with estracyt taxol and taxotere have shown activity in phase-II trials (34–39).

The combination of estracyt and taxol, as a 96-h infusion showed responses in over 50% of cases (34). Estracyt 280 mg PO tid plus taxotere was administered at escalated doses from 40 to 80 mg/m^2 on day 2 (39). Dose-limiting myelosuppression was reached at 80 mg/m^2. Twenty of 33 patients (61%) had a > 50% reduction in PSA. Of 18 patients with bidimensionally measurable disease, five (28%) achieved a partial response. At the time of entry onto the study, 15 patients required narcotic analgesics for bone pain; after treatment, eight (53%) discontinued their pain medications.

In a similar study, estracyt 14 mg/kg was given concurrent taxotere every 21 days with dexamethasone 8 mg and then orally bd for 5 days (38). The taxotere dose was escalated from 40–80 mg/m^2. PSA decreases greater than 50% from baseline were seen in 14/17 (82%), and one patient had a partial response in lung and liver lesions. These combinations clearly show some activity in men with androgen-independent prostate cancer. Future trials will explore different schedules of administration (Table 23.3).

Palliation of pain with decline in PSA has been shown with the growth factor inhibitor suramin in combination with hydrocortisone. In published studies, approximately 40–70% of patients have a > 50% decrease in PSA, and a 20–40% objective response rate. There is a wide variability in schedules, conflicting response rates, and a high rate of neurotoxicity. Trials were difficult to interpret due to the concomitant use of corticosteroids, and failure to recognize regression due

Table 23.3   Estracyt Combination Therapies in HRPC

Author	Year	Ref No	Chemotherapy	>50% ↓PSA	OR
Hudes (34)	1997	34	R+T	17/32 (53%)	4/9 (44%)
Pienta (35)	1997	62	E+Vp16	24/62 (39%)	8/15 (53%)
Smith (36)	1999	40	E+T+Vp16	24/38 (63%)	10/16 (63%)
Dimopolous (37)	1997	56	E+T+Vp16	30/52 (58%)	15/33 (45%)
Kreis (38)	1999	17	E+Taxotere	14/17 (82%)	1PR
Petrylak (39)	1999	33	E+Taxotere	20/33 (61%)	5/18 (28%)

E = Estracyt, T = Taxol, Vp16 = Etoposide

to flutamide withdrawal. A large co-operative group trial of suramin plus hydrocortisone versus hydrocortisone and placebo was undertaken (40–42). The mechanisms of suramin-mediated anti-tumor activity still need to be clarified. Suramin, unlike mitoxantrone, did not receive FDA approval, although it also showed an effect on palliative endpoints.

Radiation therapy

Bone pain is often a debilitating component of metastatic prostate cancer and should be approached systematically. Focal irradiation to palliate bone pain for solitary painful bone metastases may be supplemented by hemibody irradiation for the palliation of widespread metastases. After allowing for adequate recovery, the alternate half-body can be irradiated. Side-effects include nausea, vomiting, diarrhea, hematologic abnormalities, and pneumonitis. In one study, 82% receiving upper hemibody and 67% receiving lower half-body irradiation remained pain-free until death (43). Strontium-89 has been found to be effective in palliating bone pain, with subjective response in more than 75–80% of patients. This bone-seeking radionuclide, has high uptake in osteoblastic metastases, and remains in the tumor sites up to 100 days, decaying by beta-particle emission (44). It may be most useful in combination with RT in delaying development of new lesions (6, 44). Other radionuclides such as Rhenium-186 and Samarium-153 conjugated to ligands with affinity to bone emit both gamma energies that provide images and beta energies that are therapeutic (6). CYT-356, conjugated with Yttrium-90, a beta-emitter has been increasingly used in the US for diagnosis of occult metastatic disease (45).

Small-cell carcinoma of the prostate

An advance has been the recognition of a neuroendocrine component of cells in the prostate. Cells with neuroendocrine features may produce a variety of neuropeptides such as serotonin, bombesin, and others, which regulate tumor growth and metastatic potential. Small-cell carcinoma of the prostate is a subtype of prostate cancer that often presents with advanced disease and does not respond to hormones. It is also the most frequently acquired phenomenon in patients who initially present with adenocarcinoma of the prostate. This entity should be considered in patients who have rapidly progressing disease, visceral metastases and a disproportionately low PSA. Patients should be treated with chemotherapy, using regimens for small cell carcinoma of other sites, such as etoposide and cisplatin (46).

Dietary fat and vitamins

An expanding body of evidence has implicated particular nutrients in carcinogenesis and cancer progression. Prostate cancer has been associated with dietary factors, including fat. The incidence of prostate cancer is much lower in Japan than in the United States. Animals with prostate cancer that are fed a high-fat diet have a higher growth rate of their tumors. Research in the United States is focusing upon modifying fat intake in individuals with prostate cancer (47, 48). Vitamin and mineral supplement use has also been associated with reduced risk of prostate cancer(49). Further study is needed to investigate the direct role of these dietary supplements, as well as the role of lifestyle variables associated with supplement use, on prostate cancer risk.

Gene therapy and vaccine therapy

There is a surge of interest in gene therapy with vaccines in the treatment for prostate cancer and other tumors. Gene therapy usually involves the transfer of genetic probes. There are many different approaches to gene therapy. Genetic immunization (polynucleotide vaccination, DNA vaccines) is a process whereby gene therapy methods are used to create vaccines and immunotherapies. The hypothesis is that genomic alteration causes the malignant phenotype, and that tumorogenesis is a multi-step pathway. A number of different gene therapy strategies are currently being evaluated.

The *ex vivo* and many of the *in vivo* therapies involve stimulating a specific anti-tumor immune response. Autologous vaccines involving interleukin-2 (IL-2)- or granulocyte-macrophage colony-stimulating factor (GM-CSF)-transduced whole tumor cells have shown promise in animal models. Clinical trials of these and other vaccine strategies are underway. *In vivo* gene therapies involving the replacement of mutant tumor-suppressor genes, antisense strategies, and the insertion of suicide genes are also being evaluated in prostate cancer (50).

Another novel strategy is through suicide gene approaches in which a medication is given that is not toxic too the patient and cells. For example, at Baylor University, a replication-deficient adenovirus (ADV) containing the herpes simplex virus thymidine kinase gene (HSV-tk) was injected directly into the prostate, and followed by intravenous administration of the prodrug ganciclovir (GCV) (51).

Growth factors are responsible for inducing tumor growth. To produce a tumor cell vaccine, one may remove the primary tumor and make a suspension that is kept in culture and transfected with various cytokine genes (such as GM-CSF) and then irradiated and proliferated and re-injected into the host. A wide spectrum of possibilities is available. Potential vehicles for gene therapy are:

- plasmid DNA vectors
- viral vectors (of which there are 2 types).

With plasmid vectors, a piece of DNA is extracted to a plasmid. It is taken out of the cell and used for target DNA. The problem with plasmid DNA vectors is that they are rapidly degraded. There is virtually no time to reach the tumor cells. They have very low efficacy therefore, DNA coating with lipids may be used to enhance their potential.

Viral vectors may be more effective. However there are safety issues to be considered, and it is not known whether or not they can generate tumors themselves. Retroviral vectors: require diving cells, 8 Kb is the maximum sized gene that can be inserted. There is genomic integration (random), and therefore, they have the potential to become oncogenes, and are stable for long periods of time. Adenoviral vectors: do not require diving cells, 8 Kb is the maximum sized gene insert, genomic integration is not required. The potential for oncogesis exists, and the length of time is transient.

At Johns Hopkins University, vaccination with irradiated GM-CSF-secreting gene-transduced cancer vaccines induced tumoricidal immune responses in a phase I human gene therapy trial in eight patients. GM-CSF-secreting, irradiated tumor vaccines were prepared from *ex vivo* retroviral transduction of surgically harvested cells. Expansion of primary cultures of autologous vaccine cells was successful in 8 of 11 patients. The yield of the primary culture cell limited the number of courses of vaccination. These data showed that both T-cell and B-cell immune responses to human prostate cancer could be generated by treatment with irradiated, GM-CSF gene-transduced PCA vaccines (52).

Genetic immunization may works indirectly via a bone marrow derived cell, probably a type of dendritic antigen presenting cell (APC). Direct targeting of genetic vaccines to these cells may provide an efficient method for stimulating cellular and humoral immune responses to infectious agents and tumor antigens. Initial studies have provided monocytic-derived dendritic cell (DC) isolation and culture techniques, simple methods for delivering genes into these cells, and have also uncovered potential obstacles to effective cancer immunotherapy which may restrict the utility of this paradigm to a subset of patients (53).

Administration of dendritic cells pulsed with prostate-specific membrane antigen (PSMA) induces cellular immune responses against tumor. In Seattle, a phase-II trial involving infusions of autologous dendritic cells (DC) and two human histocompatibility antigen (HLA-A2)-specific prostate-specific membrane antigen (PSMA) peptides, was completed. Some 30% of the patients, including those with hormone-refractory disease and patients with local recurrences, had partial responses according to NPCP criteria, alkaline phosphatase, prostate markers, physical examination, performance status, bone scan, ProstaScint scan, as well as other assays to monitor cellular and humoral immune responses (54–56).

At Memorial Hospital, peptide and carbohydrate vaccines have been evaluated in relapsed prostate cancer (57). Monovalent carbohydrates and glycoprotein-conjugated vaccines were studied, using the patients' immune system to generate an anti-tumor response. These synthetic vaccines were conjugated to keyhole limpet hemocyanin (KLH) and given with the immunologic adjuvant QS21. All patients generated specific high-titer immunoglobulin M (IgM) and/or IgG antibodies, some of which were able to mediate complement lysis.

In Philadelphia, investigators have tried to induce anti-tumor immunity by enriching the cytokine environment within the tumor by intra-prostatic injection of leukocyte interleukin, a mixture of natural cytokines that includes interleukin-1β (IL-1β), IL-2, granulocyte-macrophage colony-stimulating factor (GM-CSF), interferon γ (IFN-γ), and tumor necrosis factor α (TNF-α) (58). The same investigators have also used OncoVax-P, a vaccine consisting of liposome-encapsulated recombinant PSA and lipid A, given as an emulsion or with BCG/cyclophosphamide or GM-CSF with or without IL-2/ cyclophosphamide. Humoral and cellular immunity was enhanced (58).

At the University of Michigan, a clinical study was undertaken to evaluate the safety and biologic effects of vaccinia-PSA (PROSTVAC) given to patients with recurrent prostate cancer, to assess the feasibility of interrupted androgen-deprivation in modulating expression of the vaccine target antigen, as well as detecting vaccine bioactivity *in vivo*. These authors reported that immune responses against PSA may be present among some patients with prostate cancer at baseline and may be induced in others through vaccinia-PSA immunization (59).

No gene-therapy vector or method of administration is ideal. There are many strategies and new technologies under research. Which is the best method? It is not known whether adeno or retroviral vectors or liposomes, systemic, IA, topical, or intratumoral techniques are best. The long-term side-effects, for example of retroviral vectors, which require incorporation into the host genome for therapeutic effect, are unknown.

Unfortunately there is no known gene product that is uniformly associated with the occurrence of the malignancy. There is no ideal gene sequence that can be used

to treat all urologic tumors. There is no tumor-specific gene promoter sequence that limits the effects to the cancer cells targeted. Several gene-therapy trials are ongoing. Most trials are still in the initial phase of research. This approach is highly interesting, and must be pursued. It will ultimately provide us with some important answers. However, some time is needed.

Conclusions

After failure of initial hormonal therapy, various treatment options are available that provide objective remissions and palliation of symptoms. Hormone refractory prostate cancer remains a challenge, but may not be as resistant as previously believed. A trial of anti-androgen withdrawal should be offered to patients progressing on CAB. An increased understanding of the biology of the disease will undoubtedly direct future therapeutic strategies.

References

1. American Cancer Society. *Prostate cancer.* 1999. (GENERIC) Ref Type: Internet Communication.
2. Santi DV, McHenry CS, Summer H. Mechanisms of interaction of thymidylate synthetase with 5-fluorodeoxyuridylate. *Biochemistry* 1974, **13**, 471–81.
3. Smith JR, Freije D, Carpten JD *et al.* Major susceptibility locus for prostate cancer on chromosome I suggested by a genome-wide search. *Science* 1996, **274**, 1371–4.
4. Walsh PC. Early stage at diagnosis in families providing evidence of linkage to the hereditary prostate cancer locus (HPC) on chromosome 1. *Urology* 1998, **265**, 266
5. Sternberg C. Hormone refractory metastatic prostate cancer. *Ann.Oncol* 1992, **3** (5), 331–5.
6. Scher HI, Chung LWK. Bone metastases: improving the therapeutic index. *Sem Oncol* 1994, **21** (5), 630–56.
7. Schellhammer PF, Sharifi R, Block NL *et al.* Clinical benefits of bicalutamide compared with flutamide in combined androgen blockade for patients with advanced prostatic carcinoma: a final report of a double-blind, randomized, multicenter trial. Casodex Combination Study Group. *Urology* 1997, **50** (3), 330–6.
8. Dijkman GA, Fernandez del Moral P, Plasman JWHME. A new extra long acting depot preparations of the LHRH analog Zoladex. First endocrinological and pharmacokinetic data in patients with advanced prostate cancer. *J Steroid Biochem.Mol.Biol* 1990, **37**, 933–6.
9. Crawford ED. Combined androgen blockade. *Eur Urol* 1996, **29**(2), 54–61.
10. Denis LJ, Carneiro de Moura JL, Bono A *et al.* Goserelin acetate and flutamide versus bilateral orchiec-

tomy: a phase III EORTC trial (30853). *Urology* 1993, **42**, 119–30.

11. Dijkman GA, Fernandez del Moral P, Debruyne FMJ, Janknegt RA, on behalf of the International Anandron Study Group. Improved subjective response to orchiectomy plus nilutamide (anandron) in comparison to orchiectomy plus placebo in metastatic prostate cancer. *Eur Urol* 1995, **27**, 196–201.

12. Denis L. Role of maximal androgen blockade in advanced prostate cancer. *Prostate* 1994, 5, 17–22.

13. Dalesio O. On behalf of the Prostate Cancer Trialist's Group. Meta analysis on the randomized trials in prostate cancer. *Eur J Cancer* 1999, **35** (4), 1566A.

14. Eisenberger MA, Blumenstein BA, Crawford ED *et al.* Bilateral orchiectomy with or without flutamide for metastatic prostate cancer. *N Engl J Med* 1998, **339**, 1036–42.

15. Scher HI, Sternberg CN. Chemotherapy of urologic malignancies. *Semin.Urol* 1985, **3**, 239–80.

16. Kelly WK, Scher HI, Mazumdar M, Vlamis V, Schwartz M, Fossa SD. Prostate specific antigen as a measure of disease outcome in hormone-refractory prostatic cancer. *J Clin.Oncol* 1993, **11**, 607–15.

17. Scher HI, Kelly WK. The flutamide withdrawal syndrome: its impact on clinical trials in hormone-refractory prostatic cancer. *J Clin.Oncol* 1993, **11**, 1566–72.

18. Blackledge GR. High-dose bicalutamide monotherapy for the treatment of prostate cancer. *Urology* 1996, **47**, 44–7.

19. Tannock I, Gospodarowicz M, Meakin W *et al.* Treatment of metastatic prostatic cancer with low-dose prednisone: evaluation of pain and quality of life as pragmatic indices of response. *J Clin.Oncol* 1989, 7, 590–7.

20. Small EJ, Baron AD, Fippin L, Apodaca D. Ketoconazole retains activity in advanced prostate cancer patients with progression despite flutamide withdrawal. *J Urol* 1997, **157**, 1204–7.

21. Sella A, Kilbourn R, Amato R *et al.* Phase II study of ketaconazole combined with weekly doxorubicin in patients with androgen-indipendent prostate cancer. *J Clin Oncol* 1994, **12**, 683–8.

22. Konyves I, Muntzing J. Ten year experience with estramustine phosphate in the treatment of prostatic carcinoma. In: AnonymousNew trends in diagnosis and treatment of prostatic cancer. *Rome: Acta Medica S.p.A* 1987, 210–8.

23. Hudes G. Estramustine based chemotherapy. *Sem Urol Oncol* 1997, **15**, 13–9.

24. Hudes GR, Greenberg R, Krigel RL *et al.* Phase II study of estramustine and vinblastine, two microtubule inhibitors, in hormone-refractory prostate cancer. *J Clin Oncol* 1992, **10**, 1754–61.

25. Seidman AD, Scher HI, Petrylak D *et al.* Estramustine and vinblastine: use of prostate specific antigen as a clinical trial endpoint in hormone-refractory prostatic cancer. *J Urol* 1992, **147**, 931–4.

26. Hudes G, Einhorn L, Ross E *et al.* Vinblastine versus vinblastine plus oral estramustine phosphate for patients with hormone-refractory prostate cancer: a Hoosier Oncology Group and Fox Chase Network Phase III Trial. *J Clin Oncol* 1999, **17**(10), 3160–6.

27. Albrecht W, Horenblas S, Marechal JM *et al.* A randomized phase II trial assessing estramustine and vinblastine combination chemotherapy vs. estramustine alone in patients with hormone escaped progressive metastatic prostate cancer. *Eur Urol* 1998, **33** (S1) (Abstract 187), 47.

28. Albrecht W, Horenblas S, Marechal J *et al.* Randomized phase II trial assessing estramustine and vinblastine combination chemotherapy vs. estramustine alone in patients with hormone escaped prostate cancer. ECCO 10. *Eur J Cancer* 1999, **35**, 1379A.

29. Eisenberger MA, Simon R, O'Dwyer PJ *et al.* A reevaluation of nonhormonal cytotoxic chemotherapy in the treatment of prostatic carcinoma. *J Clin.Oncol* 1985, **3**, 827–41.

30. Scher H, Yagoda A, Watson RC *et al.* Phase II trial of doxorubicin in bidimensionally measurable prostatic adenocarcinoma. *J Urol* 1984, **131**, 1099–102.

31. Torti FM, Aston D, Lum B, *et al.* Weekly doxorubicin in endocrine-refractory carcinoma of the prostate. *J Clin.Oncol* 1983, **1**, 477–82.

32. Tannock IF, Osoba D, Stochler MR *et al.* Chemotherapy with mitoxantrone plus prednisone or prednisone alone for symptomatic hormone resistant prostate cancer: a Canadian randomized trial with palliative end-points. *J Clin Oncol* 1996, **14**, 1756–64.

33. Kantoff PW, Conaway M, Winer E *et al.* Hydrocortisone (HC) with or without mitoxantrone (M) in patients (pts) with hormone refractory prostate cancer (HRPC): preliminary results from a prospective randomized Cancer and Leukemia Group B Study (9182) comparing chemotherapy to best supportive care. *Proc Amer Soc Clin Onc* 1998, **14** (Abstract 2013), 1748.

34. Hudes GR, Nathan F, Khater C *et al.* Phase II trial of 96 hour paclitaxel plus oral estramustine phosphate in metastatic hormone refractory. *J Clin Oncol* 1997, **15**, 3156–63.

35. Pienta KJ, Redman BG, Bandekar R *et al.* A phase II trial of oral estramustine and oral etoposide in hormone refractory prostate cancer. *Urology* 1997, **50**, 401–6.

36. Smith DC, Pienta KJ. Paclitaxel in the treatment of hormone-refractory prostate cancer. *Sem Oncol* 1999, **26**, 109–11.

37. Dimopoulos MA, Panopoulos C, Barnia C *et al.* Oral estramustine and oral etoposide for hormone refractory prostate cancer. *Urology* 1997, **50**, 754–8.

38. Kreis W, Budman DR, Fetten J *et al.* Phase I trial of the combination of daily estramustine phosphate and intermittent docetaxel in patients with metastatic hormone refractory prostate carcinoma. *Ann Oncol* 1999, **10**, 33–8.

39. Petrylak DP, MacArthur RB, O'Connor J *et al.* Phase I trial of docetaxel with estramustine in androgen-independent prostate cancer. *J Clin Oncol* 1999, **17**, 958–67.

40. Scher HI, Sternberg C, Heston WD *et al.* Etoposide in prostatic cancer: experimental studies and phase II trial in patients with bidimensionally measurable disease. *Cancer Chemother Pharmacol* 1986, **18**, 24–6.

41. Roth B, Yeap B, Wilding G *et al.* Taxol in advanced, hormone-refractory carcinoma of the prostate. A phase

II trial of the Eastern Cooperative Oncology Group. *Cancer* 1993, **15** (72), 2457–60.

42. Small EJ, Marshall ME, Reyno L *et al.* Superiority of suramin + hydrocortisone (S+H) over placebo + hydrocortisone (P+H): results of a multi-center double-blind phase III study in patients with hormone refractory prostate cancer (HRPC). *Proc Amer Soc Clin Onc* 1998, **17**, 308.

43. Kuban DA, Delbridge T, El-Mahdi AM, Schellhammer PF. Halfbody irradiation for treatment of widely metastatic carcinoma of the prostate. *J Urol* 1989, **141**, 572–4.

44. Porter AT, McEwan AJB, Powe JE *et al.* Results of a randomized phase III trial to evaluate the efficacy of strontium-89 adjuvant to local field external beam irradiation in the management of endocrine resistant metastatic prostate cancer. *Int J Radiation Oncology Biol Phys* 1993, **25**, 805–13.

45. Babaian RJ, Sayer J, Podoloff DA *et al.* Radioimmunoscintigraphy of pelvic lymph nodes with 111-indium labeld monoclonal antibody CYT-356. *J Urol* 1994, **152**, 1952–5.

46. Logothetis CJ, Hoosein NM, Hsieh JT *et al.* The clinical and biological study of androgen indipendent prostate cancer (AIPCa). *Semin Oncol* 1994, **21**, 620–9.

47. Wang Y, Corr JG, Thaler HT *et al.* Decreased growth of established human prostate LNCaP tumors in nude mice fed a low-fat diet. *J Natl Cancer Inst* 1995, **4**, 87, 1456–62.

48. Lee CT, Fair WR. The role of dietary manipulation in biochemical recurrence of prostate cancer after radical prostatectomy. *Semin Urol Oncol* 1999, **17**, 154–63.

49. Kristal AR, Stanford JL, Cohen JH *et al.* Vitamin and mineral supplement use is associated with reduced risk of prostate cancer. *Cancer Epidemiol Biomarkers Prev* 1999, **8**, 887–92.

50. Hrouda D, Perry M, Dalgleish AG. Gene therapy for prostate cancer. *Semin Oncol* 1999, **26**(4), 455–71.

51. Herman JR, Adler HL, Aguilar-Cordova E *et al. In situ* gene therapy for adenocarcinoma of the prostate: a phase I clinical trial. *Hum Gene Ther* 1999, **10**, 1239–49.

52. Simons JW, Mikhak B, Chang JF *et al.* Induction of immunity to prostate cancer antigens: results of a clinical trial of vaccination with irradiated autologous prostate tumor cells engineered to secrete granulocyte-macrophage colony-stimulating factor using *ex vivo* gene transfer. *Cancer Res* 1999, **59**, 5160–8.

53. Berlyn KA, Ponniah S, Stass SA *et al.* Developing dendritic cell polynucleotide vaccination for prostate cancer immunotherapy. *J Biotechnol* 1999, **73**, 155–79.

54. Tjoa BA, Simmons SJ, Elgamal A *et al.* Follow-up evaluation of a phase II prostate cancer vaccine trial. *Prostate* 1999, **40**, 125–9.

55. Tjoa BA, Elgamal AA, Murphy GP. Vaccine therapy for prostate cancer. *Urol Clin.North Am* 1999, **26**, 365–74.

56. Murphy GP, Tjoa BA, Simmons SJ *et al.* Phase II prostate cancer vaccine trial: report of a study involving 37 patients with disease recurrence following primary treatment. *Prostate* 1999, **39**, 54–9.

57. Slovin SF, Scher HI. Peptide and carbohydrate vaccines in relapsed prostate cancer: immunogenicity of synthetic vaccines in man-clinical trials at Memorial Sloan-Kettering Cancer Center. *Semin Oncol* 1999, **26**, 448–54.

58. Harris DT, Matyas GR, Gomella LG *et al.* Immunologic approaches to the treatment of prostate cancer. *Semin Oncol* 1999, **26**, 439–47.

59. Sanda MG, Smith DC, Charles LG *et al.* Recombinant vaccinia-PSA (PROSTVAC) can induce a prostate-specific immune response in androgen-modulated human prostate cancer. *Urology* 1999, **53**, 260–6.

24 | Gene therapy for prostate cancer

Kevin J. Harrington and Richard G. Vile

Introduction

Gene therapy for cancer can be defined as the transfer to, and expression of, genetic material in malignant human cells for a therapeutic purpose (1). However, this narrow definition can be enlarged to encompass gene delivery to normal immune cells for the purpose of immunomodulatory gene therapy. In the last decade, which has seen rapid progress in our understanding of the molecular basis of cancer, this treatment approach has moved from the status of theoretical possibility to the reality of preliminary phase I/II clinical trials, albeit with little evidence, as yet, of therapeutic effect. A large number of trials are currently in progress or planned and the next decade will probably bring considerable clarification of the potential value of gene therapy in the treatment of cancer.

Prostate cancer represents an attractive target for gene therapy since there are limited treatment options available to the clinician. For localized prostate cancer, radical surgery or radiotherapy (with or without the use of neoadjuvant androgen deprivation) represent the only effective curative therapies. However, a significant number of patients treated for apparently localized disease will later present with disseminated metastatic disease. Adjuvant therapy with cytotoxic chemotherapy has not been shown to reduce the frequency of this event. For those patients who present with metastatic disease, the prognosis is bleak despite initial responses to hormonal manipulation in the form of androgen deprivation. Disseminated prostate cancer is essentially resistant to systemic cytotoxic chemotherapy. Radiotherapy (external beam and radioisotopic) can achieve nothing more than palliation. Therefore, if a significant impact is to be made on the outcome of prostate cancer, novel therapies are required to act in the adjuvant setting and to effect responses in patients with metastatic disease.

The term gene therapy encompasses a broad range of therapeutic approaches and can usefully be subdivided into the following categories:

(1) corrective gene therapy in which the aim is to restore to normal the function of a deleted or mutated gene (usually a tumor-suppressor gene);

(2) cytoreductive gene therapy in which delivery of an exogenous gene results in cell death either through metabolism of a prodrug to a cytotoxic agent (suicide), or by means of an alternative cytotoxic mechanism;

(3) ablative gene therapy in which the aim is to negate the effect of a tumor-promoting gene (oncogene);

(4) immunomodulatory gene therapy in which induction of gene expression in a targeted tissue renders it susceptible to clearance by the immune system.

Each of these different approaches may have relevance to the treatment of prostate cancer and will be reviewed in detail below.

Vectors for gene therapy

The identification and elaboration of sophisticated selective gene-therapy systems will amount to nothing unless genes can be delivered to tumors in sufficient quantities to target a significant fraction of the clonogenic cells. It is in this arena that the success or failure of gene therapy will be decided and, for this reason, the development of vectors for the delivery of therapeutic genes represents an extremely active field of investigation (2, 3). Thus far, most work has focused on locoregional gene delivery by means of direct injection or infusion. Whilst this technique is useful for the assessment of candidate therapeutic systems, it has limited relevance to clinical situations, such as disseminated metastatic disease, in which a systemic delivery system will be required. Immunomodulatory gene therapy is an exception to this rule in that the purpose of treatment is to use loco-regional gene delivery to prime a systemic immune response, which will be capable of dealing with both local and distant metastatic cancer (4). Vectors for gene therapy can be considered under the broad headings of non-viral and viral systems.

Non-viral vectors

Naked DNA

Physical injection of DNA, in the form of an expression plasmid, into the target-cell population represents the simplest and most direct form of gene-delivery system. In this situation, the therapeutic gene is delivered as part of a circular piece of DNA (plasmid or naked DNA), which also contains promoter/enhancer elements to drive transcription (Fig. 24.1). These promoters can be selected to be permanently (constitutively) active (e.g. cytomegalovirus immediate/early CMV I/E or Rous sarcoma virus RSV promoters) or can come under the control of tissue-specific promoters (e.g. prostate-specific antigen or probasin promoter in the case of prostate cancer), which may add a level of selectivity to gene expression. This approach relies on plasmid DNA uptake into the cell by undefined mechanisms. This process can be enhanced *in vivo* by permeabilization of the target-cell membrane by exposing it to an electric field (electroporation) (5). Once plasmid DNA has been taken into a cell, it must be translocated to the nucleus before the genes it encodes can be expressed, either transiently from an extra-chromosomal episomal location or in a sustained fashion if integration into the host genome occurs. This process of gene transfer into cells is known as transfection or transduction.

There have been no published studies to date of direct intraprostatic injection of naked DNA, although it has been shown to be feasible in other tumor types (6). Intratumoral naked DNA delivery has been shown to result in rapid clearance from the tumor (7). This process can be delayed by encapsulating the DNA in liposomes (see below) but these complexes do not diffuse far from the injection site and are unlikely to transduce a significant number of cells. At present, for reasons which remain obscure, skeletal muscle is the tissue most efficiently transduced by injection of naked DNA. Therefore, for the foreseeable future, this approach is likely to be of use only in situations in which synthesis and release of a protein into the circulation will be of therapeutic benefit (e.g. hemophilia) (8). Another potential use of this technique might be as a means of delivering (prostate)-specific antigens as part of vaccination strategies (see below).

DNA-coated gold particles

The efficiency of transduction of tumor cells *in vivo* can be increased by administering the DNA in a form in which it is adsorbed onto gold particles and injected using a 'gene gun' (9). The precise mechanism by which this procedure improves DNA delivery to cells is unknown. Responses have been seen in animal tumor models following intratumoral gene-gun delivery of therapeutic cytokine genes (10). There have been no reports of gene-gun delivery of therapeutic genes to the prostate, either in animal models or in patients. The ease of access of this organ to direct injection and the wealth of clinical experience with intraprostatic delivery of brachytherapy implants (11) suggests that this route may be worthy of exploration in the future.

Cationic liposomes

Liposomes are vesicles composed of phospholipid bilayer membranes (12), which are capable of enclosing a wide range of substances including DNA. Preparations of lipids and DNA are capable of forming complexes

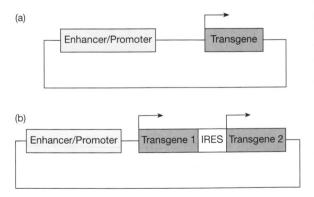

Fig. 24.1 Diagrammatic representation of expression of therapeutic transgenes from plasmids. (a) an enhancer/promoter element drives expression of a single transgene. The promoter can be a non-specific viral promoter (RSV or CMV promoter) or can be a tissue specific promoter (PSA or probasin promoter); (b) a single promoter drives expression of two separate genes which are linked by an IRES internal ribosome entry site) sequence in a so-called bi-cistronic vector.

(lipoplexes) (13), which can deliver DNA in to cells and lead to gene expression both *in vitro* and *in vivo* (14–16). Lipid-mediated gene delivery has the following potential advantages over viral systems (see below):

(1) the ability to transfect a variety of different cells without the need for interaction with specific receptors;

(2) minimal immunogenicity of the lipid components, which facilitates multiple administrations;

(3) high-capacity vectors with the ability to deliver large DNA sequences;

(4) ease of production.

However, they are not without their potential drawbacks, which can be considered to be as follows:

(1) relatively low efficiency of transfection;

(2) they mediate only transient expression of DNA;

(3) release of plasmid DNA from the lipoplex can mediate inflammatory and/or immune reactions;

(4) the lipid components used to complex the DNA may have distinct toxicity profiles against normal tissues (17).

A wide variety of lipid formulations have been described, with varying abilities to deliver DNA to cells. Although these agents are effective *in vitro* in a number of cell lines, including prostate cancer (18), major problems have been encountered when they are administered *in vivo*. Standard liposomal preparations suffer from the fact that they are cleared from the circulation very rapidly after intravenous injection, mainly by the lungs, reticuloendothelial system (liver and spleen), and the heart. As a result, their use has been largely restricted to intralesional injection. The insertion of polyethylene glycol (PEG) derivatives in to the lipid membrane (pegylation) has been shown to increase the circulation half-life of liposomes after intravenous administration and, hence, their ability to localize to tumors (19, 20). Unfortunately, pegylated liposomes are poorly fusogenic by virtue of their coating of PEG, which significantly reduces their ability to deliver DNA (21). The pharmacokinetics, biodistribution, and fusogenicity of liposomes can be varied by altering the composition of the lipid membrane. In particular, incorporation of certain cationic lipids (e.g. DMRIE, DOSPA, and DOTAP), along with neutral or helper co-lipids (choles-

terol or DOPE) in liposomes has been shown to increase markedly their ability to fuse with cell membranes and deliver their contents in to cells. Phase I/II trials have confirmed the ability of these agents to transfect human tumors *in vivo* (22, 23). Further development of both conventional and pegylated liposomes is likely to yield improved therapeutic vectors in the future.

Polymer–DNA complexes

A number of non-lipid polymers have the ability to form complexes with DNA (polyplexes). These polyplexes have also been shown to deliver DNA in to cells. Examples include polycationic compounds such as poly-L-lysine, polyethylenimine, polyglucosamines, and peptoids (24–27). Goldman *et al.* (1997) (26) have shown that polyglucosamine polymer-based delivery of genes into intracranial tumors can yield levels of gene expression comparable with viral systems. This arena of vector development is a rapidly expanding field of study and in the next few years may yield a number of new products with attractive pharmacokinetics and biodistribution profiles.

Viral vectors

Viruses are an extremely attractive vehicle for the delivery of therapeutic genes, since they have evolved specific and efficient means of gaining entry to human cells and securing expression of their genes. The challenge in the field of viral vector development lies in harnessing the efficiency of viruses while, at the same time, abrogating their ability to cause infection and disease in the patient. In addition, the activities of the immune system of the host lead to generation of specific immune response (cell-mediated and humoral) against viral vectors, which preclude repeated dosing with the same vector. The most commonly used means of achieving these objectives has been by modification of the viral genome to remove sequences required for viral replication and pathogenicity. This leaves space in the viral genome, which may be replaced with exogenous therapeutic genes. Such genetically engineered viral vectors will theoretically retain the wild-type viral cellular tropism and ensure expression of the transgene in the desired population of cells without being propagated as an ongoing infection. In an attempt to improve on the natural tropisms of viruses, studies are under way to manipulate the viral components that mediate cell-binding and internalization as a means of directing viruses specifically to chosen target cells (28, 29).

Thus far, the development of viral vectors has focused on the use of three classes of viruses: retroviruses (RV), adenoviruses (AV), and adeno-associated viruses (AAV). Other viruses are also being investigated, including vaccinia (30), reovirus (31), herpes virus (32, 33), canarypox (ALVAC) virus (34), and Newcastle disease virus (35, 36). However, a detailed discussion of all of the viruses that are currently under active development is beyond the scope of this review, which will be restricted to RV, AV, and AAV.

Retroviral vectors

RV are single-stranded diploid RNA viruses the basic structure of which is illustrated in Fig. 24.2. The group of viruses that has been most intensely investigated is the C-type RV, based on the Moloney murine leukemia

virus (MoMLV). They gain entry to certain cells through binding of surface envelope proteins (encoded by the *env* genes) to specific cellular receptors. Upon entry to the cell, the viral enzyme reverse transcriptase (encoded by the *pol* gene) transcribes the viral genome into a double-stranded DNA copy. This DNA sequence can enter the nucleus of dividing cells (because the nuclear membrane has broken down) and can be randomly integrated into the genome of the host by the viral integrase enzyme. It is this step that accounts for a significant advantage of RV vectors, namely that of stable integration and expression of genes carried in the viral particle. In the case of wild-type RV, gene expression results in viral replication, assembly, and packaging with subsequent propagation of the viral infection. Clearly, if RV-targeted gene therapy were associated with an ongoing RV infection, this would have serious

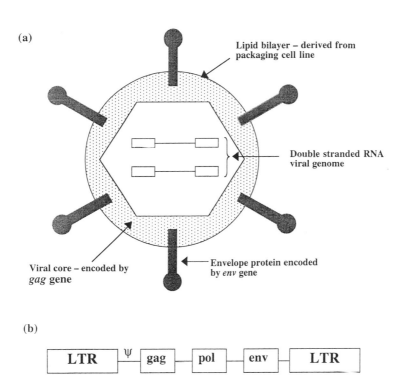

Key
LTR – long terminal repeat, important in replication and transcriptional control
Ψ – packaging signal
gag – encodes the viral core proteins
pol – encodes the reverse transcriptase enzyme
env – encodes the viral envelope protein

Fig. 24.2 Structure of a typical retrovirus (RV). (a) viral morphology: RV are double-stranded RNA viruses that have a lipid bilayer membrane surrounding the viral core. (b) Viral genome: the viral genome consists of a packaging sequence (*Y*) and three genes (gag, pol, and env).

consequences for the safety of this approach. Therefore, the RV used for gene therapy protocols have been manipulated to render them replication deficient. This is achieved by producing RV from so-called packaging cell lines, which have been engineered stably to express the RV *gag*, *pol*, and *env* genes from plasmids lacking the packaging sequence (*v*). Delivery of the therapeutic gene in a construct containing the RV long terminal repeats (LTR) and *v* into such a packaging cell line, permits assembly, packaging, and release of infectious but non-replicative RV, which can be harvested from the supernatant. In recent years it has been appreciated that RV have a number of potential disadvantages compared with their rivals. Their production from RV packaging cell-lines yields relatively low titres (10^7 infectious units/ml), which may seriously restrict the ability to scale-up production for clinical trials. The RV genome is relatively small, which places constraints on the size of the genetic construct that they can effectively carry. Since the process of integration into the host genome is random, it has the ability to disrupt the function of cellular genes (insertional mutagenesis). In addition, their life-cycle requires entry of the viral genome into the nucleus of the host cell, which can only occur in actively dividing cells because RV core particles lack a nuclear localization signal (NLS).

These perceived problems with the use of C-type RV vectors have resulted in a significant shift towards the development of AV and AAV vectors (see below). However, the lentiviruses (a subtype of RV) may represent a potentially valuable alternative. Lentiviruses, such as human, simian, and feline immunodeficiency viruses (HIV, SIV, and FIV, respectively), have the ability to infect non-dividing cells (37) and integrate in the same way as other RV. Clearly, the development of lentiviral vectors will need special emphasis on the safety aspects of the viral constructs, in view of the serious nature of the clinical syndromes caused by these agents. However, irrespective of these considerations, further development of these agents could prove to be useful.

Adenoviral vectors

AV are double-stranded DNA viruses composed of non-enveloped icosahedral proteins capsids enclosing an inner core made up of DNA and protein cores (38) (Fig. 24.3). The outer viral capsid is formed by a mosaic of 240 hexones and 12 pentone bases at the vertices of the icosahedron. Antenna-like fibers, which terminate in a knob protein, protrude from each

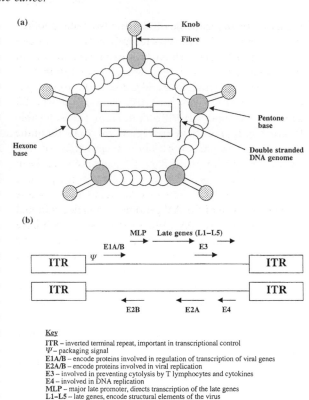

Fig. 24.3 Structure of a typical adenovirus (AV). (a) Viral morphology: AV are double-stranded DNA viruses composed of non-enveloped icosahedral proteins capsids (hexones and pentones), which bind to the CAR receptor through the knob domain of the fiber. (b) Viral genome: the AV genes are divided into early (E) and late (L) genes.

pentone base. These knob proteins are responsible for the binding of the virus to its receptor. Most adenoviruses bind to the coxsackie and adenovirus receptor (CAR), a cellular membrane protein with no presently known function. Binding of the virus to the CAR receptor facilitates interaction of viral arginine-glycine-aspartate (RGD) sequences with cellular integrins of the $\alpha_v\beta_3$ and $\alpha_v\beta_5$ type and subsequent internalization within clathrin-coated pits. The virus evades degradation within cellular endosomes and, once in the cytoplasm, it disassembles and is translocated to the nucleus under the influence of NLS within the capsid proteins. Upon entry to the nucleus, expression of the viral genes can begin. Clearly, the administration of replicating adenoviruses to patients with malignant disease, and its associated immune suppression, raises a number of important safety concerns. For this reason, strenuous efforts have been made to render AV safe by rendering them incapable of division (so-called replication-defective AV). This was initially achieved by deletion of the E1 gene, which has an important role in regulating the transcription of the viral genome. A further level of control was added by generating replication-defective AV with selective deletion of the E3 gene, which, amongst other functions, is responsible for the ability of virally infected cells to evade immune destruction. In addition, later generations of AV vectors, in which the E2 and E4 genes have been disrupted, have been described. More recently, these processes have been extended to remove the whole coding sequence of the AV genome – so-called minimal sequence or 'gutless' AV (39). Such viruses, which have residual ITR sequence and the packaging signal, have enormous potential to package therapeutic genes but need to be grown in producer cell-lines in the presence of helper viruses, which are unable to package themselves but which can supply all the necessary viral gene functions to facilitate packaging of infectious, replication-incompetent AV containing the therapeutic transgene.

In excess of 40 adenoviral serotypes have been identified and these have been subdivided into six groups (Groups A to F). Viruses from Group C (serotypes 2 and 5, Ad2, and Ad5) have been most extensively evaluated as candidates for gene delivery (38). However, since adenoviral infections are extremely common in the general population, as many as 70% of the population will have circulating neutralizing antibodies to Ad2 and Ad5. Such pre-existing antibodies are likely to accelerate clearance of these viruses at the time of first administration and the immunogenicity of these serotypes will tend to preclude repeated dosing, even in patients who have previously not been exposed. In the context of prostate cancer, Lu *et al.* (1999) (40) reported the effect of route of administration of an adenovirus expressing the *Escherischia coli* lacZ (β-galactosidase) gene on the site and extent of gene expression. This gene acts as a so-called reporter gene in that, in areas where it is expressed, addition of a specific substrate yields a blue colour. Not surprisingly, higher levels of expression were seen after intraprostatic rather than intravenous or intra-arterial injection.

Replication-defective AV have a number of potential advantages as vectors for targeted gene delivery. In contrast to RV, AV are capable of infecting non-dividing cells since their DNA is able to cross the intact nuclear membrane under the direction of viral NLS. They can be produced in high titers (10^{10}–10^{11} infectious units/ml) from available producer cell-lines. Their life-cycle does not require integration of their DNA into the host genome, which circumvents the risk of insertional mutagenesis. In addition, the recent development of gutless AV has opened the door to the development of vectors with vastly expanded capacity for therapeutic transgenes.

In recent years, there has been a move towards the investigation of replication-competent AV (RCAV) for gene therapy of cancer. In view of the obvious concerns about the safety of RCAV, these agents have been engineered to have additional levels of control to reduce the potential risk associated with their use in patients. The best known example of a RCAV is the E1B-deleted ONYX-015 (dl1520) virus (41). Since the viral E1B gene product is responsible for binding and inactivating cellular p53, E1B-deleted viruses are unable to replicate in normal p53 wild-type cells. In contrast, the virus replicates very effectively in p53-deficient cells (such as tumor cells). This agent has entered phase I/II studies in head and neck, colorectal, pancreatic, and ovarian cancers (42) but has not yet been used in prostate cancer. In addition, two so-called 'prostate-specific' RCAV have been developed (43–45). Rodriguez *et al.* (1997) (43) have developed an attenuated virus (CN706) in which the expression of the E1A gene is under tight transcriptional control by the prostate-specific antigen (PSA) promoter (see below). As a consequence, E1A is expressed in PSA-positive cell lines at significantly higher levels than in PSA-negative prostate and non-prostate cell-lines, permitting efficient viral replication and cytotoxicity only in PSA-expressing cells. Tumor responses were seen after *in vivo* intratumoral administration of this agent in a prostate cancer cell line. In a similar approach, Yu *et al.* (1999) (44) have constructed a RCAV in which the E1A and E1B genes are under the transcriptional control of two separate prostate tissue specific promoters. Further studies have shown that by adding the E3 region of Ad5, the resulting virus (CV787) replicates 100 000 times more effectively in PSA-positive as compared with PSA-negative cells. Significantly, single intravenous injections of CV787 were capable of eradicating subcutaneous deposits of LNCaP tumors in nude mice (45).

Adeno-associated viral vectors

AAV are single-stranded DNA viruses composed of non-enveloped icosahedral proteins capsids. They belong to the parvovirus group and are native human viruses, which are not known to cause any disease (46). They may, in fact, suppress the development of tumors induced by other viruses (47). They require co-infection with another virus (a so-called 'helper virus') in order to replicate. The helper virus can be an AV or a herpes virus. In the absence of a helper virus, AAV infection of a cell leads to latency in which the viral genome persists either in an integrated from (see below) or as episomal DNA. Subsequent infection of the cell with a virus capable of providing the necessary helper functions allows replication to proceed.

AAV vectors have a number of potential advantages over RV and AV vectors. They are capable of infecting non-dividing cells and are stably integrated/maintained in the host genome, although this issue is of lesser importance in cancer gene therapy where transient expression of cytotoxic genes will be adequate. An additional benefit is that, in contrast to RV, the process of integration occurs preferentially at a site-dependent locus in chromosome 19. This characteristic of AAV reduces the risk of insertional mutagenesis. However, in AAV vectors this characteristic integration is largely lost due to deletion of rep proteins (in an attempt to reduce the risk of the emergence of replication competent AAV). AAV have a number of potential drawbacks as vectors for gene therapy. They have limited packaging capacity (approximately 5 kbp) and gene expression may be slow to reach its peak. Production requires the use of helper viruses, which means that preparations for pre-clinical and clinical use may be contaminated with these entities.

Strategies for gene therapy of prostate cancer

The pathogenesis of prostate cancer is a multi-step process involving the sequential accumulation of a number of genetic defects. A diagrammatic (and by no means comprehensive) representation of this process is shown in Fig. 24.4. It is likely that further study will elucidate other genes involved in the development and progression of prostate cancer. Each of these abnormalities (both loss- and gain-of-function mutations) may be seen as potential targets for gene therapy approaches (48).

In addition to this panoply of possible targets, the fact that a number of genes are expressed in prostatic tissue in a tissue-specific fashion means that prostatic cancer may be very useful model system for the

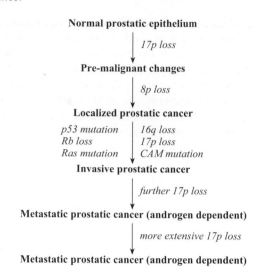

Fig. 24.4 Representation of the possible sequence of genetic changes involved in the pathogenesis of prostate cancer (adapted from Hrouda and Dalgleish 1999).

development of gene-therapy approaches (49–53). Genes such as PSA, probasin, and relaxin H2 are expressed almost exclusively in prostatic tissue and each of these genes is under tight control by a tissue-specific promoter (TSP). Therefore, the expression of therapeutic genes under the control of prostate TSP offers the prospect of selectively increasing anti-tumor efficacy and reducing normal tissue toxicity. Steiner *et al.* (1999) (54) have demonstrated the potential of TSP-driven gene therapy in a canine model. Dogs received intraprostatic injections of adenoviral vectors expressing the lacZ reporter gene under the control of one of three TSP (PSA, probasin, or murine mammary tumor virus promoters) or the non-specific RSV promoter. The highest levels of expression were seen with the RSV promoter but all three TSP directed prostate-specific expression of lacZ, despite the fact that the viral genome was detected in other tissues.

Corrective gene therapy

A number of tumor-suppressor genes (TSG) have been implicated in the etiology and pathogenesis of prostatic cancer (Fig. 24.4). Therefore, restitution of normal TSG function has been seen as a legitimate target for *in vivo* corrective gene therapy aimed at a variety of different molecular targets, including p53, Rb, cell-cycle control genes (p16 and p21), and certain cell-adhesion molecules (CAM). Although preliminary studies have confirmed that delivery of TSG can have an impact on the malignant phenotype, both *in vitro* and *in vivo*, the central weakness in this strategy lies in the fact that TSG-directed gene therapy must be delivered to every cell in order for it to eradicate a tumor. However, it is much more feasible to imagine strategies in which TSG will be given as part of a multi-modality approach, for instance in combination with cytotoxic chemotherapy or radiotherapy.

p53

p53 contributes to a bewildering array of control processes within human cells, the central theme of which is to protect the integrity of the genome against genotoxic stress (55). This function has earned p53 the title of 'guardian of the genome' (56). Normal wild-type p53 protein is largely responsible for the G1/S cell-cycle arrest that is observed in response to DNA damage. This delay allows time for the cell to attempt to repair the DNA before entry to the DNA synthetic S phase of the cell-cycle or, if the damage exceeds the repair capacity of the cell, p53 acts to push the cell in to the apoptotic pathway (57). Mutations of the p53 gene can lead to expression of a non-functioning protein incapable of triggering these processes. Consequently, the cell can proceed through the cell-cycle in the presence of unrepaired DNA damage, which, if the abnormality is not lethal, will be passed on to the progeny of cell division. There have been reports that p53 mutations in prostate cancers are relatively uncommon at a frequency of only 3% of primary tumors (58), although they are seen with greatly increased frequency in prostate cancer cell lines *in vitro* (59) and in patients with metastatic disease (60, 61). More recently, however, conflicting data have demonstrated p53 mutations in 79% of cases (62).

A number of studies have been performed in an attempt to rectify aberrant p53 expression *in vitro* and *in vivo*. The vast majority of these studies have focused on the use of adenoviral vectors to deliver a wild-type p53 transgene (Ad-p53). *In vitro* suppression of growth and induction of apoptosis in both androgen-dependent and independent prostate cancer cell lines (Tsu-pr1, C4-2, DU145, and PC-3) has been reported following delivery of Ad-p53 (63–65). Such cell lines have also been shown to be less tumorigenic *in vivo*. These observations have also been extended to primary cultures of radical prostatectomy samples with evidence of significant efficacy of Ad-p53 in comparison to control virus (66). Inhibition of the growth of subcu-

taneous xenograft and syngeneic tumors in nude and immunocompetent mice has also been demonstrated after intratumor injection of Ad-p53 (63, 65, 66). In addition to the above studies, adenovirus-mediated restitution of wild-type p53 function has been shown to sensitise prostate cancer cell lines to the effects of genotoxic chemotherapy (paclitaxel, cisplatin, doxorubicin, 5-fluorouracil, methotrexate, and etoposide) both *in vitro* and *in vivo* (67, 68).

Rb

The retinoblastoma (Rb) gene product acts to regulate transition of cells across the G1/S boundary of the cell-cycle. Loss of normal Rb function removes this cell-cycle checkpoint and serves to confer on cells a growth advantage. Rb mutations are relatively common in primary and metastatic prostate cancers (69, 70). As yet, there have been no published reports of the use of Rb gene therapy in prostate cancer cells lines either *in vitro* or *in vivo*. However, there have been a number of reports that delivery of wild-type Rb to lung, bladder, pituitary, and neuroendocrine tumors yields tumor responses in animal models (71–73).

p21

p21 (waf1/cip1) protein is a cyclin-dependent kinase inhibitor able to arrest the cell cycle at the G1 phase by inhibiting DNA replication. Its abnormal expression in prostate cancer has been shown to be associated with poor prognosis (74). Eastham *et al.* (1995) (63) have reported the effect of transducing prostate cancer cells with adenoviral vectors carrying a p21 transgene both *in vitro* and *in vivo*. Treatment with Ad-p21 was associated with significant growth delay *in vitro* and *in vivo*. In fact, in these studies the activity of Ad-p21 exceeded that of Ad-p53.

CAM

Restoration of normal CAM expression represents a potentially valuable target for gene therapy of prostate cancer. These molecules act as more than simple anchors to hold cells steady in their environment but, rather, are capable of mediating cell–matrix and cell–cell signaling (75). CAM are frequently mutated in prostate cancers and such abnormalities are associated with disease progression (75, 76). Reduced cell–matrix adhesion allows neoplastic cells to ignore the signals from the normal extracellular environment, which promote differentiation, while loss of normal cell–cell adhesion allows malignant cells to escape from their site of origin, degrade the extracellular matrix, acquire a more motile and invasive phenotype, and, finally, to invade and metastasise. The androgen-regulated cell adhesion molecule (C-CAM1), a member of the immunoglobulin superfamily, has been shown to function as a tumor suppressor in prostate cancer (77). It has been reported that adenoviral vectors encoding C-CAM1 were able to reduce tumor growth *in vivo*. In further studies, Lin *et al.* (1999) (78) demonstrated that this effect was significantly increased by the use of multiple injections in PC-3 tumors and that most tumors underwent complete regression. The same group has reported that the human homolog of C-CAM1 (CD66a) is able to reduce the tumorigenicity of the human cell-line DU145. Furthermore, intratumoral injection of CD66a into established DU145 tumors significantly retarded their growth (79). Other studies have shown that transduction of prostate cancer cells with wild-type E-cadherin (an important CAM) reduces their invasive potential and decreases their expression of matrix metalloproteinase 2, an important marker associated with invasive and metastatic potential (80).

Other TSG

The promyelocytic leukaemia gene (PML) is another putative TSG for prostate cancer (81). PML appears to exert its growth suppressing effects by modulating several key cell-cycle regulatory proteins, including p53, p21, cyclins, and cyclin-dependent kinases (82). These authors have reported that adenoviral-mediated delivery of PML (Ad-PML) reduced *in vitro* growth and *in vivo* tumorigenicity of prostate cancer cell-lines. Furthermore, direct intratumoral injection of Ad-PML significantly slowed the growth of established DU145 tumors in mice. Matsubara *et al.* (1998) (83) have reported that transient transfection of malignant prostate cell-lines with the wild-type fibroblast growth factor (FGF) receptor 2IIIb gene restores their response to FGF-7 and reduces their tumorigenicity.

Cytoreductive gene therapy

A number of strategies fall under this umbrella term, including gene-directed enzyme prodrug therapy (GDEPT), which is otherwise known as 'suicide' gene therapy. In the case of such systems, the aim is to avoid the systemic toxicity and lack of tumor specificity of existing cytotoxic agents by ensuring that they are

formed in high concentrations only at the tumor site. Essentially, the ideal elements of a GDEPT system are as follows:

(1) a gene that is not expressed in human cells and encodes an active enzyme that catalyses the conversion of a prodrug to an active cytotoxic agent;

(2) a means of restricting the expression of the gene to tumor tissue;

(3) an enzyme that elicits a minimal host immune-response (although in the context of immunomodulatory gene therapy an immune response might be beneficial);

(4) a prodrug with little or no inherent cytotoxicity and well-established pharmacokinetics;

(5) an active drug that kills cycling and non-cycling cells;

(6) an active agent that is capable of diffusing to adjacent tumor cells to mediate a bystander effect (Fig. 24.5).

A number of candidate suicide genes have been proposed and are in various stages of pre-clinical and clinical development (see Table 24.1) (84, 85).

The two most widely studied examples of GDEPT are:

(1) the herpes simplex virus thymidine kinase (HSVtk) and ganciclovir (GCV) system in which the viral enzyme thymidine kinase directs the conversion of the nucleoside analog prodrug GCV into its toxic phosphorylated metabolite; and

(2) the *Escherischia coli* bacterial cytosine deaminase (CD) and 5-fluorocytosine (5-FC) system in which the antifungal agent 5-FC is converted to the pyrimidine analog 5-fluorouracil.

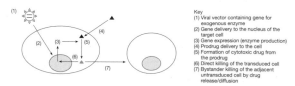

Fig. 24.5 Components of a typical GDEPT system. Delivery of a vector containing a transgene for an exogenous enzyme followed by delivery of an innocuous prodrug results in local generation of a toxic agent, which is capable of killing both the cell in which it was formed and adjacent bystander cells.

Table 24.1 Examples of GDEPT systems that are currently the subject of pre-clinical and clinical investigation (modified from Connors 1995)

Enzyme	Prodrug	Active drug
HSVtk	Ganciclovir	Ganciclovir triphosphate
Cytosine deaminase	5-Fluorocytosine	5-Fluorouracil
DT diaphorase	CB 1954	5-(Aziridin-1-yl)-4-hydroxylamino-2-nitrobenzamide
Nitroreductase	CB 1954	5-(Aziridin-1-yl)-4-hydroxylamino-2-nitrobenzamide
Azoreductase	Azobenzene mustards	Phenylenediamine-mustards
Glucose oxidase	Glucose	Hydrogen peroxide
Xanthine oxidase	Hypoxanthine	Superoxide, hydrogen peroxide
Plasmin	Peptidyl-p-phenylenediamine-mustard	Phenylenediamine-mustard
α-Galactosidase	N-[4-(α-D-galactopyranosyl)benzyloxycarbonyl]-daunorubicin	Daunorubicin
β-Glucosidase	Amygdalin	Cyanide
β-Lactamase	Vinca-cephalosporin	4-Desacetylvinblastine-3-carboxyhydrazide
	Phenylenediamine mustard-cephalosporin	Phenylenediamine-mustard
	Nitrogen mustard-cephalosporin	Nitrogen mustard
Carboxypeptidase Al	Methotrexate-α-peptides	Methotrexate
Carboxypeptidase G2	Benzoic acid mustard glutamates	Benzoic acid mustards
Alkaline phosphatase	Doxorubicin phosphate	Doxorubicin
	Mitomycin phosphate	Mitomycin
	Etoposide phosphate	Etoposide
Cytochrome P-450 (CYP2B6)	Cyclophosphamide, Ifosfamide	Phosphoramide mustard

In the context of prosate cancer, the HSVtk/GCV system has been most extensively evaluated. The activity of adenoviral vectors delivering HSVtk (Ad-HSVtk) followed by GCV treatment has been confirmed *in vitro* (52, 86) and *in vivo* in murine models of subcutaneous xenograft (52, 86, 87) and orthotopic (88) tumors. Another potential advantage of the HSV/tk is that it has the potential to sensitize cells incorporating phosphorylated GCV derivatives to the effects of ionizing radiation (89–91). Atkinson and Hall (1999) (89) have reported *in vitro* evidence that Ad-HSVtk and GCV can enhance the effect of single-fraction doses of radiotherapy in what might be either an additive or synergistic fashion. Similarly, Ad-HSVtk has been shown to co-operate with castration-induced androgen withdrawal in mouse models of subcutaneous and orthotopic prostate cancer (92). In contrast, there have been few studies evaluating the effects of the CD/5FC system in prostate cancer, perhaps due to the knowledge that conventional cytotoxic agents have little activity against this tumor. Blackburn *et al.* (1999) (90) have recently reported that adenoviral delivery of a fusion gene encoding CD and HSVtk significantly increased the killing of PC-3 cells *in vitro* on exposure to the respective prodrugs. In addition, as discussed

above, this system was also shown to yield an increased response to ionizing radiation.

HSVtk is generally considered to be the gold-standard against which other GDEPT systems are compared. Lockett *et al.* (1997) (93) have described a system based on the purine nucleoside phosphorylase (PNP) and 9-(β-M-2-deoxyerythropento-furanosyl) 6-methylpurine (6MPDR) prodrug. HSVtk/GCV and PNP/6MPDR were compared directly in prostate cancer cell lines *in vitro* using identical adenoviral vectors. *In vitro*, the PNP/6MPDR system demonstrated a clear 5–10-fold greater activity but this difference was not apparent in subsequent *in vivo* studies in mice bearing PC-3 xenograft tumors (87).

There has been one report of a clinical study using GDEPT in patients with prostate cancer (94). They conducted a phase-I evaluation, in which 18 patients with locally recurrent prostate cancer received intraprostatic injections of Ad-HSVtk at doses between 10^8 and 10^{10} infectious units followed by systemic GCV. There was minimal (grade 1–2) toxicity in four patients but one patient, at the highest dose level, developed self-limiting grade 3 hepatotoxicity and grade 4 thrombocytopenia. Interestingly, there were three objective responses, as determined by a 50% reduction in the serum PSA level.

Other gene-delivery approaches can be considered under the definition of cytoreductive gene therapy. Spitzweg *et al.* (1999) (53) have reported a novel strategy based on the successful treatment of thyroid cancer with radioactive ^{131}I. The basis of this therapy is that benign and malignant thyroid cells express very high levels of the sodium iodide symporter (NIS) in a tissue-specific fashion. This accounts for their prodigious ability to concentrate iodine, which acts as a cytotoxic agent when it is administered as a β-particle emitting radioisotope (^{131}I). Therefore, transduction of prostate cancer cells with the NIS gene, under the control of the PSA promoter, has been shown specifically to confer on them the ability to concentrate ^{131}I. As yet, no data have been presented dealing with the feasibility of this approach *in vivo*. Marcelli *et al.* (1999) (95) have targeted the apoptotic machinery of the cell directly by delivering an adenoviral vector encoding the caspase 7 gene. Caspase 7 is a key control element in directing cells towards apoptosis. These authors demonstrated that expression of caspase 7 in parental LNCaP cells, and in the same cell line engineered to over-express the anti-apoptotic gene bcl-2, resulted in an increase in apoptosis.

Ablative gene therapy

In contrast to the TSG, a number of mutations may lead to direct activation of oncogenes, which confer upon the tumor a growth advantage or the ability to avoid normal apoptotic pathways. Examples of such oncogenes, which are frequently mutated in cancers, including prostate cancers, are the ras, myc, erbB2, and bcl-2 oncogenes (96–99). In such situations, gene therapy faces the challenge of negating the activating function of these mutated genes. Again, the potential limitation of such an approach is that it must target every cell in a tumor in order to eradicate the disease. This consideration has led a number of investigators to examine the effect of ablative gene therapy in combination with other conventional cytotoxic agents. Two main strategies for ablative gene therapy have been described:

(1) anti-sense oligonucleotides; and

(2) catalytic ribozymes.

Anti-sense oligonucleotides (AO) are nucleic acid sequences, which are complementary to the sequences of the genes whose functions are to be negated. They are able specifically to inhibit the activities of oncogenes either by binding to the DNA sequence and preventing transcription or by binding to the messenger RNA (mRNA) transcripts and preventing them from being translated. As yet, the precise mechanisms by which AO act have not been defined clearly. Balaji *et al.* (1997) (100) reported that delivery of an AO against the c-myc oncogene was able to reduce the growth of prostate cancer cells *in vitro*. These results have been confirmed using RV-mediated delivery of anti-c-myc AO, which was able to reduce the growth of xenograft tumors in nude mice, although it did not affect the growth of tumor cells *in vitro* (101). Over-expression of the bcl-2 oncogene, which protects cells against being directed into apoptotic pathways, has been observed in prostate cancer cells after androgen withdrawal and has been associated with the development of androgen independence and chemoresistance. Treatment with AO against bcl-2 has been shown to delay the progression of prostate cancer to an androgen-independent state and to increase its sensitivity to cytotoxic chemotherapy (102, 103). The ras family of oncogenes (Ha-ras, Ki-ras, and N-ras, and their downstream signalling component raf) has also been assessed as a potential target for AO therapy. The ability to reverse the malignant phenotype by delivery of a dominant negative ras gene has been reported and has given impetus to this approach (104). Geiger *et al.* (1997) (105) reported that direct administration of AO against raf significantly increased the effect of cytotoxic chemotherapy agents against subcutaneous prostate xenograft tumors in nude mice. As yet, there have been no reports of gene-directed delivery of anti-ras AO, although from the above data it would appear to be an appropriate target. Lee *et al.* (1996) (106) have demonstrated *in vitro* activity of an AO under the control of the PSA promoter against DNA polymerase-α and topoisomerase-IIα in prostate cancer cell-lines. Significantly, this activity was restricted to prostate cancer cell-lines by virtue of the relatively tight transcriptional control of the PSA promoter.

Ribozymes are RNA molecules with specific catalytic activities, which confer on them the ability to degrade certain mRNA molecules. The most clearly defined molecules in this class are the hammerhead ribozymes (HR) (so-called because of their molecular shape). Dorai *et al.* (1997) (107) have reported the ability of a specific HR to degrade bcl-2 mRNA both in LNCaP *in vitro* and *in vivo*. In addition, expression of this ribozyme was able to induce apoptosis of prostate cancer cells with low levels of bcl-2 expression.

Another cell line with high level bcl-2 expression was rendered susceptible to the effects of an apoptosis inducing agent. In a further study, the same group reported that adenoviral delivery of this HR construct was effective in bcl-2 over-expressing cell lines (108). The activity of HR in non-prostate cancer cell lines with ras mutations has also been reported (109, 110). There have been no reports of ribozyme activity against the myc or c-erbB2 oncogenes.

A variation on the theme of using AO or HR to inactivate mRNA has been proposed by Kim *et al.* (1997) (111). In this situation, delivery of an adenovirus expressing an intracellular single-chain antibody against c-erbB2 was shown to reduce significantly the growth of c-erbB2 positive, but not negative, cell lines.

Immunomodulatory gene therapy

The development of cancer in the context of an apparently immune-competent patient can be seen as a paradox. While many tumors express so-called tumor-associated antigens (TAA), which can be recognized by both the humoral and cellular arms of the immune system, verifiable clinically relevant anti-tumor immune responses are exceedingly rare. This observation has resulted in the notion that the tumor is capable of evading the immune system, both by reducing its own immunogenicity and by blunting the effectiveness of any immune response that is activated against it (112). A number of mechanisms, which play a part in the ability of tumors to evade immune recognition, have been identified. Total or partial loss of expression of the major histocompatibility complex (MHC) Class I (113) and co-stimulatory B7.1/B7.2 (114) molecules have been documented in many cancer types, including prostate cancer, and serves to reduce the efficiency of presentation of TAA to cytotoxic T lymphocytes (CTL). Mutations in the pathways controlling the transport and presentation of peptides at the surface of tumor cells may also mask them from detection by CTL (115). CTL, which infiltrate prostate cancers, may be killed by means of release of soluble Fas ligand (FasL) from the tumor cells (116), while the malignant cells appear to be relatively resistant to this important pathway of cell killing (117).

The presence of these documented immune defects has fuelled interest in approaches aimed at delivering genes that enhance the immunogenicity of tumors and the ability of the immune system to mount an effective response (4, 118, 119). Attempts to mobilize the immune system against cancer have a number of theoretical advantages:

(1) the specificity of recognition inherent in immune reactions should limit the occurrence of normal tissue toxicity;

(2) the generation of an immune response at one site should prime the immune system against other distant deposits of disease;

(3) the nature of the immune system involves significant signal amplification, such that a small stimulus can lead to a much larger response;

(4) once established, anti-tumor immunity should be permanent and protect against disease recurrence.

The organization of the immune system is extremely complex and a detailed analysis of the cellular and humoral components involved in generation of an effective immune response against cancer is beyond the scope of this review. The contribution of the cellular arm of the immune system has been most actively studied and certainly appears to be the most fruitful avenue for further development of immunomodulatory gene therapy. The role of humoral immunity in the form of production of specific anti-tumor antibodies is less clear and will not be considered further. Figure 24.6 represents a simplified version of the key players involved in generating an immune response against a tumor. The central theme is one of activating specific CD8+ CTL capable of recognizing TAA and endowing them with the power to kill those cells. A number of steps in this process are deranged in the tumor milieu and are, therefore, targets for immunomodulatory gene therapy. Figure 24.7 illustrates some of the means by which delivery of a therapeutic gene could be used to generate or enhance the immune response against tumors. These approaches can be divided as follows:

(1) delivery of cytokine genes with the aim of increasing localization and immunoreactivity of antigen-presenting cells (APC), most notably dendritic cells (DC) and macrophages, and T cells (120);

(2) delivery of genes encoding co-stimulatory molecules with the intention of improving the ability of CTL to recognize, engage, and destroy tumor cells (121);

(3) expression of exogenous foreign immunogens (e.g. allogeneic tumor cells or MHC molecules), which will generate a potent local immune and inflammatory reaction and generate an environment conductive to APC acquiring TAA (so-called cross-priming of an immune response) (119, 122);

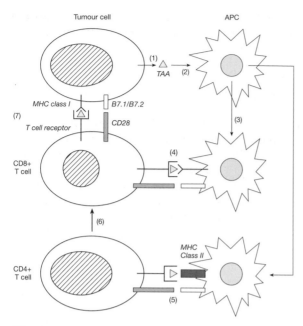

Key
(1) Release of tumor-associated antigen (TAA) from tumor cell (physiological or induced by cytocine therapy)
(2) Phagocytosis of TAA by immature antigen-presenting cell (APC)
(3) Processing and presentation of TAA by APC to CD⁺+ T cell in the context of MHC Clas: B7.1/B7.2 co stimulatory molecules. This interaction serves to activate the CD8+ cytot((CTL)
(5) Presentation of TAA by APC to CD4+ T cell in the context of MHC Class II and B7.1/B7 stimulatory molecules. this interaction serves to activate CD4+ cellsto help the CD8+ c becoming a CTL
(6) Secretion of cytokines from CD4+ T cell (T helper cell) to stimulate CD8+ T cell
(7) recognition of TAA presented in context of MHC Class I molecule with appropriate co-stimulatory molecules (B7.1/B7.2) by CTL. Tumors frequently have down-regulated expression of MHC Class I and/or co-stimulatory molecules, which result in poor T cell response

Fig. 24.6 Simplified representation of the steps involved in generating an effective immune response to a tumor cell. A number of these processes are targets for immunomodulatory gene therapy (see text for details).

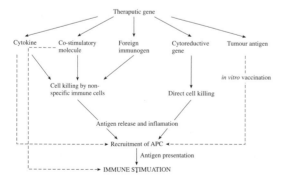

Fig. 24.7 Strategies for immunomodulatory gene therapy of cancer: delivery of a number of therapeutic genes has the potential to prime an immune response against cancer (modified from Melcher *et al.* 1999).

(4) delivery of a cytoreductive gene therapy (e.g. HSV-tk/GCV) with release of TAA which is phagocytosed by APC and presented to immune effector cells (123, 124);

(5) delivery of cloned TAA as intramuscular injections of naked DNA with the generation of an immune response by means of mechanisms which are, as yet, unclear but which probably involve local uptake and expression by APC (125, 126).

Most studies of immunomodulatory gene therapy have been conducted in tumor types other than prostate cancer, although the lessons learned from these studies may be applicable to a broad range of malignancies. A great deal of work has been conducted in animal models using transfer of cytokine genes in an attempt to stimulate APC, CD4+, and CD8+ immune effector cells to localize to tumors and kill tumor cells. Particular attention has focused on the use of granulocyte-macrophage colony stimulating factor (GM-CSF) and interleukin-2 (IL-2), although work has also been conducted using IL-4, IL-6, IL-7, IL-12, interferons beta (IFN-β) and gamma (IFN-γ) and tumor necrosis factor alpha (TNF-α) (120). In the context of prostate cancer, it has been shown that rats bearing hormone refractory prostate cancers (Dunning rat model) vaccinated with irradiated, non-viable prostate cancer cells engineered to express and secrete GM-CSF, had prolonged survival when compared to animals vaccinated with irradiated cells alone or with the same cells mixed with soluble GM-CSF (127). The same authors went on to show that it was possible to engineer fresh cultures of human prostate cancer cells taken from radical prostatectomy samples to express GM-CSF. Following on from this, a phase I trial was conducted in which eight immunocompetent patients with prostate cancer received autologous, GM-CSF-secreting, irradiated tumor vaccines prepared from *ex vivo* RV transduction of surgically harvested cells with GM-CSF. The side-effects of the treatment were local and limited to pruritis, erythema, and swelling at the vaccination sites, biopsy of which revealed infiltrates of DC and macrophages among prostate tumor vaccine cells. New T-cell and B-cell immune responses against prostate cancer TAA were documented. Further studies of this approach are in progress (128). The results of a phase II clinical trial have suggested that local secretion of GM-CSF from the vaccine cells is important, since systemic adjuvant administration of GM-CSF during a DC-based vaccination study appeared not to alter the generation of immune responses or clinical outcomes (129). The effect of IL-2, GM-CSF, and IFN-γ secreting irradiated tumor-cell vaccines has been compared in the Dunning rat model (130). The IL-2 vaccine was capable of curing animals with established subcutaneous tumors and protected them from subsequent tumor challenge. The GM-CSF vaccine was less effective and the IFN-γ vaccine had only a minimal effect. Other cytokine-based gene therapy approaches that have been reported in prostate cancer models *in vitro* and *in vivo* include adenoviral delivery of IL-12, which enhanced both natural killer (NK) and T-cell activity against orthotopic prostate tumors (131), enhancement of the effect of radiotherapy by expression of TNF-α in prostate tumor xenografts (132), expression of IFN-β as a means of reducing tumorigenicity, metastatic potential and tumor-induced angiogenesis (133), and adenoviral delivery of Fas ligand, which resulted in increased apoptosis *in vitro* and growth retardation *in vivo* (134).

Although not directly involving gene transfer, vaccination strategies using APC that have been exposed to TAA *in vitro* (*ex vivo*) is generally considered as a form of gene therapy. This technique has enormous potential and is currently the subject of intense research activity. As can be seen from Fig. 24.6, such approaches represent a means of improving the ability of APC to present TAA to T cells and prime an immune response. The prospect of using DC isolated from patients to present prostate cancer TAA was initially reported by Tjoa *et al.* (1995) (135). Subsequently, this group has reported a number of phase I/II clinical studies of the administration of autologous DC exposed to prostate-derived peptides (prostate-specific membrane antigen, PSMA) in patients with prostate cancer (129, 136–138). Response rates in the order of 30% have been reported in these studies, which have included patients with locally recurrent and metastatic prostate cancer.

Summary

As can be seen from this brief review of gene therapy for prostate cancer, work is proceeding actively on a number of fronts. In fact, such is the range of potential therapeutic interventions that there is a very real danger that the effort to produce effective clinical strategies will be diluted. Clearly, the first major challenge to be addressed is the question of efficient gene delivery by optimized, systemically administered vectors. If this step can be achieved, the next decision will be the selection of the most appropriate target of therapy. In this regard, it is likely that cytoreductive therapies will be most advantageous since, in the setting of cancer, transient-gene expression may be sufficient to achieve cell kill. In addition, immunomodulatory gene therapy represents an extremely attractive therapeutic target in that local administration of potent genes may be sufficient to recruit and mobilize the immune system to reject disseminated disease. In contrast, the elegant approaches aimed at correcting aberrant expression of TSP or tumor oncogenes may be less well-suited to cancer gene therapy. Such approaches would either need to achieve prolonged (permanent) gene expression or would have to be given in combination with standard anti-cancer treatment modalities, which have already been shown to have limited efficacy against prostate cancer. As is apparent from the large number of studies that have been published within the last 2–3 years, the pace of research into gene therapy for prostate cancer is likely to accelerate in the coming years. Hopefully, this work will define a number of novel therapeutic modalities which will have a significant impact on the outcome of this disease.

References

1. Sikora K, Pandha H. Gene therapy for prostate cancer. *British Journal of Urology* 1997, **79**, 64–8.
2. Verma IM, Somia N. Gene therapy – promises, problems and prospects. *Nature* 1997, **389**, 239–42.
3. Peng KW, Vile RG. Vector devlopment for cancer gene therapy. *Tumor Targeting* 1999, **4**, 3–11.
4. Melcher A, Gough M, Todryk S, Vile R. Apoptosis or necrosis for tumor immunotherapy: what's in a name? *Journal of Molecular Medicine* 1999, **77**, 824–33.
5. Goto T, Nishi T, Tamura T *et al.* Highly efficient electro-gene therapy of solid tumor by using an expression plasmid for the herpes simplex virus thymidine kinase gene. *Proceedings of the National Academy of Science of the USA* 2000, **97**, 354–9.
6. Yang JP, Huang L. Direct gene transfer to mouse melanoma by intratumor injection of free DNA. *Gene Therapy* 1996, **3**, 542–8.
7. Nomura T, Nakajima S, Kawabata K *et al.* Intratumoral pharmacokinetics and *in vivo* gene expression of naked plasmid DNA and its cationic liposome complexes after direct gene transfer. *Cancer Research* 1997, **57**, 2681–6.
8. Herzog RW, Yang EY, Couto LB *et al.* Long-term correction of canine hemophilia B by gene transfer of blood coagulation factor IX mediated by adeno-associated viral vector. *Nature Medicine* 1999, **5**, 56–63.
9. Fynan EF, Webster RG, Fuller DH *et al.* DNA vaccines: protective immunizations by parenteral, mucosal, and gene-gun inoculations. *Proceedings of the National Academy of Science of the USA* 1993, **90**, 11478–82.

10. Sun WH, Burkholder JK, Sun J *et al*. *In vivo* cytokine gene transfer by gene gun reduces tumor growth in mice. *Proceedings of the National Academy of Science of the USA* 1995, **92**, 2889–93.

11. Charyulu K, Block N, Sudarsanam A. Preoperative extended field radiation with I-125 seed implant in prostatic cancer: a preliminary report of a randomized study. *International Journal of Radiation Oncology Biology Physics* 1979, **5**, 1957–61.

12. Bangham AD, Standish HM, Watkins JC. Diffusion of univalent ions across the lamellae of swollen phospholipids. *Journal of Molecular Biology* 1965, **13**, 238–52.

13. Felgner PL, Gadek TR, Holm M *et al*. Lipofection: a highly efficient, lipid-mediated DNA-transfection procedure. *Proceedings of the National Academy of Science of the USA* 1987, **84**, 7413–17.

14. Hug P, Sleight RG. Liposomes for the transformation of eukaryotic cells. *Biochimica Biophysica Acta* 1991, **1097**, 1–17.

15. Zhu N, Liggitt D, Liu Y *et al*. Systemic gene expression after intravenous DNA delivery into adult mice. *Science* 1993, **261**, 209–11.

16. Li S, Huang L. *In vivo* gene transfer via intravenous administration of cationic lipid-protamine-DNA (LPD) complexes. *Gene Therapy* 1997, **4**, 891–900.

17. Clark PR, Hersh EM. Cationic lipid-mediated gene transfer: current concepts. *Current Opinion in Molecular Therapeutics* 1999, **1**, 158–76.

18. Vieweg J, Boczkowski D, Roberson KM *et al*. Efficient gene transfer with adeno-associated virus-based plasmids complexed to cationic liposomes for gene therapy of human prostate cancer. *Cancer Research* 1995, **55**, 2366–72.

19. Klibanov AL, Maruyama K, Torchilin VP *et al*. Amphipathic polyethyleneglycols effectively prolong the circulation times of liposomes. *FEBS Letters* 1990, **268**, 235–37.

20. Papahadjopoulos D, Allen TM, Gabizon A *et al*. Sterically stabilised liposomes: improvements in pharmacokinetics and anti-tumour therapeutic efficacy. *Proceedings of the National Academy of Science of the USA* 1991, **88**, 11460–4.

21. Lasic DD, Vallner JJ, Working PK. Sterically stabilised liposomes in cancer therapy and gene delivery. *Current Opinion in Molecular Therapeutics* 1999, **1**, 177–85.

22. Rini BI, Selk LM, Vogelzang NJ. Phase I study of direct intralesional gene transfer of HLA-B7 into metastatic renal carcinoma lesions. *Clinical Cancer Research* 1999, **5**, 2766–72.

23. Galanis E, Hersh EM, Stopeck AT *et al*. Immunotherapy of advanced malignancy by direct gene transfer of an interleukin-2 DNA/DMRIE/DOPE lipid complex: phase I/II experience. *Journal of Clinical Oncology* 1999, **17**, 3313–23.

24. Boussif O, Lezoualch F, Zanta MA *et al*. A versatile vector for gene and oligonucleotide transfer into cells in culture and *in vivo*: polyethylenimine. *Proceedings of the National Academy of Science of the USA* 1995, **92**, 7297–301.

25. Godbey WT, Wu KK, Mikos AG. Poly(ethylenimine) and its role in gene delivery. *Journal of Controlled Release* 1999, **60**, 149–60.

26. Goldman CK, Soroceanu L, Smith N *et al*. *In vitro* and *in vivo* gene delivery mediated by a synthetic polycationic amino polymer. *Nature Biotechnology* 1997, **15**, 462–6.

27. Murphy JE, Uno T, Hamer JD *et al*. A combinatorial approach to the discovery of efficient cationic peptoid reagents for gene delivery. *Proceedings of the National Academy of Science of the USA* 1998, **95**, 1517–22.

28. Krasnykh VN, Mikheeva GV, Douglas JT *et al*. Generation of recombinant adenovirus vectors with modified fibers for altering viral tropism. *Journal of Virology* 1996, **70**, 6839–46.

29. Kasono K, Blackwell JL, Douglas JT *et al*. Selective gene delivery to head and neck cancer cells via an integrin targeted adenoviral vector. *Clinical Cancer Research* 1999, **5**, 2571–9.

30. Gnant MF, Puhlmann M, Alexander HR Jr *et al*. Systemic administration of a recombinant vaccinia virus expressing the cytosine deaminase gene and subsequent treatment with 5-fluorocytosine leads to tumor-specific gene expression and prolongation of survival in mice. *Cancer Research* 1999, **59**, 3396–403.

31. Coffey MC, Strong JE, Forsyth PA *et al*. Reovirus therapy of tumors with activated Ras pathway. *Science* 1998, **282**, 1332–4.

32. Krisky DM, Marconi PC, Oligino TJ *et al*. Development of herpes simplex virus replication-defective multigene vectors for combination gene therapy applications. *Gene Therapy* 1998, **5**, 1517–30.

33. Walker JR, McGeagh KG, Sundaresan P *et al*. Local and systemic therapy of human prostate adenocarcinoma with the conditionally replicating herpes simplex virus vector G207. *Human Gene Therapy* 1999, **10**, 2237–43.

34. Kawakita M, Rao GS, Ritchey JK *et al*. Effect of canarypox virus (ALVAC)-mediated cytokine expression on murine prostate tumor growth. *Journal of the National Cancer Institute* 1997, **89**, 428–36.

35. Plaksin D, Porgador A, Vadai E *et al*. Effective antimetastatic melanoma vaccination with tumor cells transfected with MHC genes and/or infected with Newcastle disease virus (NDV). *International Journal of Cancer* 1994, **59**, 796–801.

36. Schirrmacher V, Haas C, Bonifer R *et al*. Human tumor cell modification by virus infection: an efficient and safe way to produce cancer vaccine with pleiotropic immune stimulatory properties when using Newcastle disease virus. *Gene Therapy* 1999, **6**, 63–73.

37. Naldini L, Blomer U, Gallay P *et al*. *In vivo* gene delivery and stable transduction of nondividing cells by a lentiviral vector. *Science* 1996, **272**, 263–7.

38. Zhang WW. Development and application of adenoviral vectors for gene therapy of cancer. *Cancer Gene Therapy* 1999, **6**, 113–38.

39. Hay RT. The origin of adenovirus DNA replication: minimal DNA sequence requirement *in vivo*. *European Molecular Biology Organisation Journal* 1985, **4**, 421–6.

40. Lu Y, Carraher J, Zhang Y *et al*. Delivery of adenoviral vectors to the prostate for gene therapy. *Cancer Gene Therapy* 1999, **6**, 64–72.

41. Heise C, Sampson-Johannes A, Williams A *et al.* ONYX-015, an E1B gene-attenuated adenovirus, causes tumor-specific cytolysis and antitumoral efficacy that can be augmented by standard chemotherapeutic agents. *Nature Medicine* 1997, **3**, 639–45.

42. Kirn D, Hermiston T, McCormick F. ONYX-015: clinical data are encouraging. *Nature Medicine* 1998, **4**, 1341–2.

43. Rodriguez R, Schuur ER, Lim HY *et al.* Prostate attenuated replication competent adenovirus (ARCA) CN706: a selective cytotoxic for prostate-specific antigen-positive prostate cancer cells. *Cancer Research* 1997, **57**, 2559–63.

44. Yu DC, Sakamoto GT, Henderson DR. Identification of the transcriptional regulatory sequences of human kallikrein 2 and their use in the construction of calydon virus 764, an attenuated replication competent adenovirus for prostate cancer therapy. *Cancer Research* 1999, **59**, 1498–504.

45. Yu DC, Chen Y, Seng M *et al.* The addition of adenovirus type 5 region E3 enables calydon virus 787 to eliminate distant prostate tumor xenografts. *Cancer Research* 1999, **59**, 4200–3.

46. Flotte TR, Carter BJ. Adeno-associated viral vectors. In: *Gene therapy technologies, applications and regulations*, (ed. A Meagen). John Wiley & Sons Ltd, Chichester, UK, 1999.

47. Cukor G, Blacklow NR, Kibrick S, Swan IC. Effect of adeno-associated virus on cancer expression by herpesvirus-transformed hamster cells. *Journal of the National Cancer Institute* 1975, **55**, 957–9.

48. Hrouda D, Perry M, Dalgleish AG. Gene therapy for prostate cancer. *Seminars in Oncology* 1999, **26**, 455–71.

49. Israeli RS, Grob M, Fair WR. Prostate-specific membrane antigen and other prostatic tumor markers on the horizon. *Urologic Clinics of North America* 1997, **24**, 439–50.

50. Pang S, Dannull J, Kaboo R *et al.* Identification of a positive regulatory element responsible for tissue-specific expression of prostate-specific antigen. *Cancer Research* 1997, **57**, 495–9.

51. Brookes DE, Zandvliet D, Watt F *et al.* Relative activity and specificity of promoters from prostate-expressed genes. *Prostate* 1998, **35**, 18–26.

52. Gotoh A, Ko SC, Shirakawa T *et al.* Development of prostate-specific antigen promoter-based gene therapy for androgen-independent human prostate cancer. *Journal of Urology* 1998, **160**, 220–9.

53. Spitzweg C, Zhang S, Bergert ER *et al.* Prostate-specific antigen (PSA) promoter-driven and rogen-inducible expression of sodium iodide symporter in prostate cancer cell lines. *Cancer Research* 1999, **59**, 2136–41.

54. Steiner MS, Zhang Y, Carraher J *et al. In vivo* expression of prostate-specific adenoviral vectors in a canine model. *Cancer Gene Therapy* 1999, **6**, 456–64.

55. Agarwal ML, Taylor WR, Chernov MV *et al.* The p53 network. *Journal of Biological Chemistry* 1998, **273**, 1–4.

56. Lane DP. Cancer. p53, guardian of the genome. *Nature* 1992, **358**, 15–6.

57. Schwartz D, Rotter V. p53-dependent cell cycle control: response to genotoxic stress. *Seminars in Cancer Biology* 1998, **8**, 325–36.

58. Voeller HJ, Sugars LY, Pretlow T *et al.* p53 oncogene mutations in human prostate cancer specimens. *Journal of Urology* 1994, **151**, 492–5.

59. Carroll AG, Voeller HJ, Sugars L *et al.* p53 oncogene mutations in three human prostate cancer cell lines. *Prostate* 1993, **23**, 123–34.

60. Chi SG, deVere White RW, Meyers FJ *et al.* p53 in prostate cancer: frequent expressed transition mutations. *Journal of the National Cancer Institute* 1994, **86**, 926–33.

61. Dinjens WN, van der Weiden MM, Schroeder FH *et al.* Frequency and characterization of p53 mutations in primary and metastatic human prostate cancer. *International Journal of Cancer* 1994, **56**, 630–3.

62. Gumerlock PH, Chi SG, Shi XB *et al.* p53 abnormalities in primary prostate cancer: single-strand conformation polymorphism analysis of complementary DNA in comparison with genomic DNA. The Cooperative Prostate Network. *Journal of the National Cancer Institute* 1997, **89**, 66–71.

63. Eastham JA, Hall SJ, Sehgal I *et al. In vivo* gene therapy with p53 or p21 adenovirus for prostate cancer. *Cancer Research* 1995, **55**, 5151–5.

64. Yang C, Cirielli C, Capogrossi MC *et al.* Adenovirus-mediated wild-type p53 expression induces apoptosis and suppresses tumorigenesis of prostatic tumor cells. *Cancer Research* 1995, **55**, 4210–3.

65. Ko SC, Gotoh A, Thalmann GN *et al.* Molecular therapy with recombinant p53 adenovirus in an androgen-independent, metastatic human prostate cancer model. *Human Gene Therapy* 1996, **7**, 1683–91.

66. Asgari K, Sesterhenn IA, McLeod DG *et al.* Inhibition of the growth of pre-established subcutaneous tumor nodules of human prostate cancer cells by single injection of the recombinant adenovirus p53 expression vector. *International Journal of Cancer* 1997, **71**, 377–82.

67. Nielsen LL, Lipari P, Dell J *et al.* Adenovirus-mediated p53 gene therapy and paclitaxel have synergistic efficacy in models of human head and neck, ovarian, prostate, and breast cancer. *Clinical Cancer Research* 1998, **4**, 835–46.

68. Gurnani M, Lipari P, Dell J *et al.* Adenovirus-mediated p53 gene therapy has greater efficacy when combined with chemotherapy against human head and neck, ovarian, prostate, and breast cancer. *Cancer Chemotherapy Pharmacology* 1999, **44**, 143–51.

69. Kubota Y, Fujinami K, Uemura H *et al.* Retinoblastoma gene mutations in primary human prostate cancer. *Prostate* 1995, **27**, 314–20.

70. Ittmann MM, Wieczorek R. Alterations of the retinoblastoma gene in clinically localized, stage B prostate adenocarcinomas. *Human Pathology* 1996, **27**, 28–34.

71. Xu HJ, Zhou Y, Scigne J *et al.* Enhanced tumor suppressor gene therapy via replication-deficient adenovirus vectors expressing an N-terminal truncated retinoblastoma protein. *Cancer Research* 1996, **56**, 2245–9.

72. Riley DJ, Nikitin AY, Lee WH. Adenovirus-mediated retinoblastoma gene therapy suppresses spontaneous pituitary melanotroph tumors in Rb+/− mice. *Nature Medicine* 1996, **2**, 1316–21.

73. Nikitin AY, Juarez-Perez, MI Li S *et al*. RB-mediated suppression of spontaneous multiple neuroendocrine neoplasia and lung metastases in Rb+/− mice. *Proceedings of the National Academy of Science of the USA* 1999, **96**, 3916–21.

74. Aaltomaa S, Lipponen P, Eskelinen M *et al*. Prognostic value and expression of p21 (waf1/cip1) protein in prostate cancer. *Prostate* 1999, **39**, 8–15.

75. Syrigos KN, Harrington KJ, Pignatelli M. Role of adhesion molecules in bladder cancer: an important part of the jigsaw. *Urology* 1999, **53**, 428–34.

76. Umbas R, Isaacs WB, Bringuier PP *et al*. Decreased E-cadherin expression is associated with poor prognosis in patients with prostate cancer. *Cancer Research* 1994, **54**, 3929–33.

77. Kleinerman DI, Zhang WW, Lin SH *et al*. Application of a tumor suppressor (C-CAM1)-expressing recombinant adenovirus in androgen-independent human prostate cancer therapy: a preclinical study. *Cancer Research* 1995, **55**, 2831–6.

78. Lin SH, Pu YS, Luo W *et al*. Schedule-dependence of C-CAM1 adenovirus gene therapy in a prostate cancer model. *Anticancer Research* 1999, **19**, 337–40.

79. Luo W, Tapolsky M, Earley K *et al*. Tumor-suppressive activity of CD66a in prostate cancer. *Cancer Gene Therapy* 1999, **6**, 313–21.

80. Luo J, Lubaroff DM, Hendrix MJ. Suppression of prostate cancer invasive potential and matrix metalloproteinase activity by E-cadherin transfection. *Cancer Research* 1999, **59**, 3552–6.

81. He D, Mu ZM, Le X *et al*. Adenovirus-mediated expression of PML suppresses growth and tumorigenicity of prostate cancer cells. *Cancer Research* 1997, **57**, 1868–72.

82. Le XF, Vallian S, Mu ZM *et al*. Recombinant PML adenovirus suppresses growth and tumorigenicity of human breast cancer cells by inducing G1 cell cycle arrest and apoptosis. *Oncogene* 1998, **16**, 1839–49.

83. Matsubara A, Kan M, Feng S *et al*. Inhibition of growth of malignant rat prostate tumor cells by restoration of fibroblast growth factor receptor 2. *Cancer Research* 1998, **58**, 1509–14.

84. Moolten FL. Drug sensitivity ('suicide') genes for selective cancer chemotherapy. *Cancer Gene Therapy* 1994, **1**, 279–87.

85. Connors TA. The choice of prodrugs for gene directed enzyme prodrug therapy of cancer. *Gene Therapy* 1995, **2**, 702–9.

86. Eastham JA, Chen SH, Sehgal I *et al*. Prostate cancer gene therapy: herpes simplex virus thymidine kinase gene transduction followed by ganciclovir in mouse and human prostate cancer models. *Human Gene Therapy* 1996, **7**, 515–23.

87. Martiniello-Wilks R, Garcia-Aragon J, Daja MM *et al*. *In vivo* gene therapy for prostate cancer: preclinical evaluation of two different enzyme-directed prodrug therapy systems delivered by identical adenovirus vectors. *Human Gene Therapy* 1998, **9**, 1617–26.

88. Hall SJ, Mutchnik SE, Chen SH *et al*. Adenovirus-mediated herpes simplex virus thymidine kinase gene and ganciclovir therapy leads to systemic activity against spontaneous and induced metastasis in an orthotopic mouse model of prostate cancer. *International Journal of Cancer* 1997, **70**, 183–7.

89. Atkinson G, Hall SJ. Prodrug activation gene therapy and external beam irradiation in the treatment of prostate cancer. *Urology* 1999, **54**, 1098–104.

90. Blackburn RV, Galoforo SS, Corry PM *et al*. Adenoviral transduction of a cytosine deaminase/thymidine kinase fusion gene into prostate carcinoma cells enhances prodrug and radiation sensitivity. *International Journal of Cancer* 1999, **82**, 293–7.

91. Rogulski KR, Zhang K, Kolozsvary A *et al*. Pronounced antitumor effects and tumor radiosensitization of double suicide gene therapy. *Clinical Cancer Research* 1997, **3**, 2081–8.

92. Hall SJ, Mutchnik SE, Yang G *et al*. Cooperative therapeutic effects of androgen ablation and adenovirus-mediated herpes simplex virus thymidine kinase gene and ganciclovir therapy in experimental prostate cancer. *Cancer Gene Therapy* 1999, **6**, 54–63.

93. Lockett LJ, Molloy PL, Russell PJ *et al*. Relative efficiency of tumor cell killing *in vitro* by two enzyme-prodrug systems delivered by identical adenovirus vectors. *Clinical Cancer Research* 1997, **3**, 2075–80.

94. Herman JR, Adler HL, Aguilar-Cordova E *et al*. In situ gene therapy for adenocarcinoma of the prostate: a phase I clinical trial. *Human Gene Therapy* 1999, **10**, 1239–49.

95. Marcelli M, Cunningham GR Walkup M *et al*. Signaling pathway activated during apoptosis of the prostate cancer cell line LNCaP: overexpression of caspase-7 as a new gene therapy strategy for prostate cancer. *Cancer Research* 1999, **59**, 382–90.

96. Konishi N, Hiasa Y, Tsuzuki T *et al*. Comparison of ras activation in prostate carcinoma in Japanese and American men. *Prostate* 1997, **30**, 53–7.

97. Jenkins RB, Qian J, Lieber MM *et al*. Detection of c-myc oncogene amplification and chromosomal anomalies in metastatic prostatic carcinoma by fluorescence in situ hybridization. *Cancer Research* 1997, **57**, 524–31.

98. Gu K, Mes-Masson AM, Gauthier J *et al*. Overexpression of Her-2/neu in human prostate cancer and benign hyperplasia. *Cancer Letters* 1996, **99**, 185–9.

99. McDonnell TJ, Troncoso P, Brisbay SM *et al*. Expression of the protooncogene bcl-2 in the prostate and its association with emergence of androgen-independent prostate cancer. *Cancer Research* 1992, **52**, 6940–4.

100. Balaji KC, Koul H, Mitra S *et al*. Antiproliferative effects of c-myc antisense oligonucleotide in prostate cancer cells: a novel therapy to prostate cancer. *Urology* 1997, **50**, 1007–15.

101. Steiner MS, Anthony CT, Lu Y *et al*. Antisense c-myc retroviral vector suppresses established human prostate cancer. *Human Gene Therapy* 1998, **9**, 747–55.

102. Gleave M, Tolcher A, Miyake H *et al*. Progression to androgen independence is delayed by adjuvant treatment with antisense Bcl-2 oligodeoxynucleotides after castration in the LNCaP prostate tumor model. *Clinical Cancer Research* 1999, **5**, 2891–8.

103. Miyake H, Tolcher A, Gleave ME. Chemosensitization and delayed androgen-independent recurrence of prostate cancer with the use of antisense Bcl-2 oligodeoxynucleotides. *Journal of the National Cancer Institute* 2000, **92**, 34–41.

104. Ogiso Y, Sakai N, Watari H *et al.* Suppression of various human tumor cell lines by a dominant negative H-ras mutant. *Gene Therapy* 1994, **1**, 403–7.

105. Geiger T, Muller M, Monia BP *et al.* Antitumor activity of a C-raf antisense oligonucleotide in combination with standard chemotherapeutic agents against various human tumors transplanted subcutaneously into nude mice. *Clinical Cancer Research* 1997, **3**, 1179–85.

106. Lee CH, Liu M, Sie KL *et al.* Prostate-specific antigen promoter driven gene therapy targeting DNA polymerase-alpha and topoisomerase II alpha in prostate cancer. *Anticancer Research* 1996, **16**, 1805–11.

107. Dorai T, Olsson CA, Katz AE *et al.* Development of a hammerhead ribozyme against bcl-2. I. Preliminary evaluation of a potential gene therapeutic agent for hormone-refractory human prostate cancer. *Prostate* 1997, **32**, 246–58.

108. Dorai T, Perlman H, Walsh K *et al.* A recombinant defective adenoviral agent expressing anti-bcl-2 ribozyme promotes apoptosis of bcl-2-expressing human prostate cancer cells. *International Journal of Cancer* 1999, **82**, 846–52.

109. Kashani-Sabet M, Funato T, Florenes VA *et al.* Suppression of the neoplastic phenotype *in vivo* by an anti-ras ribozyme. *Cancer Research* 1994, **54**, 900–2.

110. Scherr M, Maurer AB, Klein S *et al.* Effective reversal of a transformed phenotype by retrovirus-mediated transfer of a ribozyme directed against mutant N-ras. *Gene Therapy* 1998, **5**, 227–34.

111. Kim M, Wright M, Deshane J *et al.* A novel gene therapy strategy for elimination of prostate carcinoma cells from human bone marrow. *Human Gene Therapy* 1997, **8**, 157–70.

112. Diaz RM, Vile RG. Molecular immunotherapy by gene transfer. In: *Blood cell biochemistry. Vol. 8: Hematopoiesis and gene therapy* (ed. LG Fairbairn, NG Testa. Kluwer Academic/Plenum Publishers, New York, USA, 1999.

113. Bander NH, Yao D, Liu H *et al.* MHC class I and II expression in prostate carcinoma and modulation by interferon-alpha and -gamma. *Prostate* 1997, **33**, 233–9.

114. Kwon ED, Hurwitz AA, Foster BA *et al.* Manipulation of T cell costimulatory and inhibitory signals for immunotherapy of prostate cancer. *Proceedings of the National Academy of Science of the USA* 1997, **94**, 8099–103.

115. Sanda MG, Restifo NP, Walsh JC *et al.* Molecular characterization of defective antigen processing in human prostate cancer. *Journal of the National Cancer Institute* 1995, **87**, 280–5.

116. Liu QY, Rubin MA, Omene C *et al.* Fas ligand is constitutively secreted by prostate cancer cells *in vitro*. *Clinical Cancer Research* 1998, **4**, 1803–11.

117. Rokhlin OW, Bishop GA, Hostager BS *et al.* Fas-mediated apoptosis in human prostatic carcinoma cell lines. *Cancer Research* 1997, **57**, 1758–68.

118. Nabel GJ, Chang AE, Nabel EG *et al.* Immunotherapy for cancer by direct gene transfer into tumors. *Human Gene Therapy* 1994, **5**, 57–77.

119. Nabel GJ, Chang AE, Nabel EG *et al.* Clinical protocol: immunotherapy of malignancy by *in vivo* gene transfer into tumors. *Human Gene Therapy* 1992, **3**, 399–410.

120. Tepper RI, Mule JJ. Experimental and clinical studies of cytokine gene-modified tumor cells. *Human Gene Therapy* 1994, **5**, 153–64.

121. Dohring C, Angman L, Spagnoli G, Lanzavecchia A. T-helper-and accessory-cell-independent cytotoxic responses to human tumor cells transfected with a B7 retroviral vector. *International Journal of Cancer* 1994, **57**, 754–9.

122. Dalgleish A. The case for therapeutic vaccines. *Melanoma Research* 1996, **6**, 5–10.

123. Vile RG, Nelson JA, Castleden S *et al.* Systemic gene therapy of murine melanoma using tissue specific expression of the HSVtk gene involves an immune component. *Cancer Research* 1994, **54**, 6228–34.

124. Hall SJ, Sanford MA, Atkinson G *et al.* Induction of potent antitumor natural killer cell activity by herpes simplex virus-thymidine kinase and ganciclovir therapy in an orthotopic mouse model of prostate cancer. *Cancer Research* 1998, **58**, 3221–5.

125. Pardoll DM, Beckerleg AM. Exposing the immunology of naked DNA vaccines. *Immunity* 1995, **3**, 165–9.

126. Wei C, Willis RA, Tilton BR *et al.* Tissue-specific expression of the human prostate-specific antigen gene in transgenic mice: implications for tolerance and immunotherapy. *Proceedings of the National Academy of Science of the USA* 1997, **94**, 6369–74.

127. Sanda MG, Ayyagari SR, Jaffee EM *et al.* Demonstration of a rational strategy for human prostate cancer gene therapy. *Journal of Urology* 1994, **151**, 622–8.

128. Simons JW, Mikhak B, Chang JF *et al.* Induction of immunity to prostate cancer antigens: results of a clinical trial of vaccination with irradiated autologous prostate tumor cells engineered to secrete granulocyte-macrophage colony-stimulating factor using *ex vivo* gene transfer. *Cancer Research* 1999, **59**, 5160–8.

129. Simmons SJ, Tjoa BA, Rogers M *et al.* GM-CSF as a systemic adjuvant in a phase II prostate cancer vaccine trial. *Prostate* 1999, **39**, 291–7.

130. Vieweg J, Rosenthal FM, Bannerji R *et al.* Immunotherapy of prostate cancer in the Dunning rat model: use of cytokine gene modified tumor vaccines. *Cancer Research* 1994, **54**, 1760–5.

131. Nasu Y, Bangma CH, Hull GW *et al.* Adenovirus-mediated interleukin-12 gene therapy for prostate cancer: suppression of orthotopic tumor growth and pre-established lung metastases in an orthotopic model. *Gene Therapy* 1999, **6**, 338–49.

132. Chung TD, Mauceri HJ, Hallahan DE *et al.* Tumor necrosis factor-alpha-based gene therapy enhances radiation cytotoxicity in human prostate cancer. *Cancer Gene Therapy* 1998, **5**, 344–9.

133. Dong Z, Greene G, Pettaway C *et al.* Suppression of angiogenesis, tumorigenicity, and metastasis by human prostate cancer cells engineered to produce interferon-beta. *Cancer Research* 1999, **59**, 872–9.

134. Hedlund TE, Meech SJ, Srikanth S *et al.* Adenovirus-mediated expression of Fas ligand induces apoptosis of

human prostate cancer cells. *Cell Death and Differentiation* 1999, **6**, 175–82.

135. Tjoa B, Erickson S, Barren R 3rd *et al. In vitro* propagated dendritic cells from prostate cancer patients as a component of prostate cancer immunotherapy. *Prostate* 1995, **27**, 63–9.

136. Tjoa B, Boynton A, Kenny G *et al.* Presentation of prostate tumor antigens by dendritic cells stimulates T-cell proliferation and cytotoxicity. *Prostate* 1996, **28**, 65–9.

137. Tjoa BA, Simmons SJ, Bowes VA *et al.* Evaluation of phase I/II clinical trials in prostate cancer with dendritic cells and PSMA peptides. *Prostate* 1998, **36**, 39–44.

138. Tjoa BA, Simmons SJ, Elgamal A *et al.* Follow-up evaluation of a phase II prostate cancer vaccine trial. *Prostate* 1999, **40**, 125–9.

25 | Prostate cancer in the elderly

Vicki Michalaki, Kevin J. Harrington, and Konstantinos N. Syrigos

Introduction

Due to the well-recognized changes in population in the last half-century, there has been an increase in the numbers of elderly people as a proportion of the total population. The number of people over 80 years of age is projected to increase by 135% by the year 2020. It is also important to consider that these older individuals can anticipate further years of life-expectancy, with the concomitant risk of cancer increasing (1, 2). Those who survive to 70–75 years of age can be expected to live for a further 14 years, those who survive to 80–85 years can expect 8 more years of life and those alive at 85 can expect for another 6 years (3). The risk of developing cancer increases with advancing age usually up until the age of 80–85 years and then declines. It has been estimated that in the new millennium, 70% of cancers will arise in the over 65 years age group (4, 5).

Age is the greatest risk factor for prostate cancer. In autopsy studies, the prevalence of the disease is about 30% of men over 50. The incidence increases with age and foci of adenocarcinoma occur in virtually all men over 90. As a result of improvements in life-expectancy, there are now more elderly men with prostate cancer (6, 7). Recent attention has been focused on management of prostate cancer in the elderly and in view of the increasing incidence of this disease, there is the dilemma if their management should differ from that of the younger patients.

Elderly patients and co-existing diseases

Aging is a complex biological process therefore, not only does the incidence of malignant disease increase, but also a variety of non-malignant diseases follows a similar pattern. The commonest co-existing diseases in patients with cancer are arthritis, hypertension, diseases of the digestive tract, cardiac, and respiratory disorders (8). The number of co-existing conditions is variable with many patients having a number of underlying disturbances of tissue and organ function.

Of vital importance is the patient's underlying mental state. Disturbance of mental function and depressive disorders often complicate the care of elderly patients, impairing their ability to fully understand their disease and its management, and restricting the delivery of optimal therapy. Also patients with severe co-existing disease may receive less complete diagnostic or therapeutic interventions because of their inability to tolerate these procedures.

In circumstances where treatment options are not limited by the presence of severe co-existing diseases, elderly patients should not be excluded from similar management strategies used for younger patients (9, 10, 11). Although an age of 70 is frequently a cut-off point between different management strategies, a life-expectation of 10 years is usually considered more important than a chronological age.

Diagnosis and screening of prostate cancer in the elderly

With the development of prostate-specific antigen (PSA), transrectal ultrasound (TRUS), and TRUS-guided biopsy, screening for prostate cancer is now a possibility (12, 13). Routine PSA screening for prostate cancer is highly controversial. The American Cancer Society and the American Urological Association favor screening, whereas the US Preventive Services Task Force on the Periodic Health Examination, and the Canadian Urologic Association recommend against it. While the use of PSA to diagnose subclinical prostatic carcinoma is controversial in the younger man, it is easier to be categorical in the older man (14, 15). Most authorities agree that there is no reason to routinely screen men age 75 and olde,r or other men unlikely to live long enough for prostate cancer to become symptomatic. There is a consensus that PSA should only be measured in the elderly if there is clinical evidence for prostate cancer (16, 17). Most urinary symptoms in the elderly are not due to cancer, and too often the raised PSA causes confusion. The mean size of the prostate increases with age due to development of benign prostate hyperplasia. The concept of age-related PSA is useful. Age-specific reference ranges have been proposed, since PSA values and prostatic volume normally increase with age (Table 25.1). Essentially, these propose that the level of PSA above which investigation is appropriate increases with age. The age-related range is helpful; a man 80 years old can be reassured that for him a PSA of 6.0 is normal (18). Use of such ranges would increase the test's sensitivity in younger men and its specificity in older men; it would reduce the number of biopsies performed but would also result in large numbers of organ-confined tumors being missed in older patients.

PSA has proved most helpful in the elderly men with symptoms of possible prostate cancer, notably back or other bone pain, because serum PSA is a good marker of tumor volume: the higher the level, the greater the likelihood of extra-prostatic disease. A PSA of less than 10 ng/ml rules out advanced prostate cancer and the patient could have localized early disease, which is likely to have slow progression and be of little threat. If PSA is over 100 it is diagnostic of prostate cancer and usually is associated with metastatic disease (19). PSA tests merely identify those for whom a biopsy should be considered.

Transrectal ultrasound may demonstrate lesions in the prostate not palpable on rectal examination. However its main use is in guiding a biopsy needle. Besides being an undignified and uncomfortable procedure, the contribution of TRUS-guided biopsy for the diagnosis of prostate cancer in older men is limited. The false-negative rate is about one-quarter of men with cancer and repeat biopsy is recommended for the patients for whom the initial biopsy is negative and there is strong indication of having the disease (20). Considering both the risk (significant morbidity) and discomfort of biopsy, histological confirmation is a little academic, as a negative biopsy does not in any case rule out cancer; otherwise rushing into a biopsy, with its attendant risks, is certainly not appropriate for an old man (21, 22, 23, 24). It is suggested that, if the older patient has obstructive symptoms, a transurethral resection of the prostate (TURP) is an appropriate way to deal with these and also to confirm the diagnosis, especially if the PSA is above 20 ng/ml and carcinoma is likely. In men with a PSA at this level and without symptoms, the decision is more difficult. If we could exclude the metastatic disease in such men, surveillance would be appropriate whether or not a pathologist has confirmed the diagnosis.

Staging of prostate cancer in the elderly

Staging of prostate cancer used to include in the past a bone scan, CT-scans, and an acid phosphatase measurement. With the increasing use of PSA measurement, most urologists are dropping these tests, since results are rarely positive, when PSA levels are less than 20 ng/ml. For patients with values higher than 20 ng/ml, imaging studies may be used (25, 26). PSA is a good marker for tumor volume and an important predictor of survival. Men older than 60 years with cancers smaller than 0.5 ml in volume are unlikely to live long enough for the cancer to grow large enough to metastasize (27). However volume is difficult to estimate accurately before surgery. It has been suggested that a core length of 3 mm or more on one of six cores on biopsy indicates a tumor volume of more than 0.5 ml.

A number of other molecular staging strategies are currently being tested. The reverse transcriptase-polymerase chain reaction (RT-PCR) assay, targeted against PSA or prostatic-specific membrane antigen (PSMA), can detect occult prostate cancer cells at sites far from the primary tumor. Other assays under investigation include the measurement of telomerase activity, high levels of which are frequent in men with poorly differentiated tumors. Whether this assay can differentiate between aggressive and more indolent forms of prostate cancer requires further investigation.

Table 25.1   Age-related PSA range

Age range	Reference range (ng/ml)
40–49	0–2.5
50–59	0–3.5
60–69	0–4.5
70–79	0–6.5

A chart review study was done in 242 cancer patients to determine whether the age of patients with prostate cancer influenced their physicians' staging strategies. Their model indicated that men received less intensive diagnostic evaluations as a function of age, even when symptoms, comorbidities, and hospital were controlled, so they suggested that older patients with prostate cancer appear to be less likely to receive intensive clinical staging and therapies (28).

Age and histologic grade in prostate cancer

The relationship of age to histologic grade of malignancy has received little attention in the medical literature. Studying the relationship of age to survival in 597 prostate carcinoma patients in England, Smedley *et al.* demonstrated that neither grading based on a modification of Gleason's score nor survival are related to age at diagnosis (29). The same relationship was studied in 44 300 cases in Sweden: survival was decreased by about 10% in men younger than 45 and older than 75, when compared to those aged between 46 and 74 years at diagnosis, but the effect of histologic grade on survival was not examined (30).

Borec *et al.* studied 4968 cases of prostatic carcinoma, which were stratified into age groups and classified as either well-differentiated (Grades I and II) or poorly differentiated (Grades III and IV). The 4596 graded cases were distributed by stage as follows: local 3451 (75%), regional 509 (11%), and distant 636 (14%). The findings indicated that when all stages of prostatic carcinoma are considered together, there is a direct relationship between tumor grade and patient age. In fact, it was suggested that in older men, clinically apparent prostatic carcinoma is of advanced grade. It seems that in the elderly, there are two types of prostatic cancer, which differ in their biological behavior. The well-differentiated variety may have no ability to spread beyond the prostate, while the undifferentiated type is more aggressive (31).

An alternative interpretation by the Stanford University group related differentiation directly to tumor volume and evidence of spread beyond the prostate (32). In the older patients increasing tumor volume was accompanied by an increase in the number of poorly differentiated tumors (33).

The trend toward increased grade with increased age becomes clear when all stages of disease are considered together. However, this trend is mainly seen in-patients with localized disease and not observed in-patients with distant metastases. This apparent discrepancy between patients with localized disease and patients with regional or distant spread may be due to the biological behavior of prostatic carcinoma.

Management of localized disease in the elderly

Many aspects of the management of prostate cancer are controversial. Curative treatment is only considered possible if the tumor is confined to the prostate without invasion of the capsule. Options for the management of cancer confined to the prostate include watchful observation, radical prostatectomy, and external-beam radiotherapy (34, 35). Hormone therapy is usually reserved for men whose tumor has failed primary treatment or who have evidence of metastatic disease (36).

Elderly patients are often excluded from participating in clinical trials on the basis of their age alone. However more recent studies have suggested that older patients frequently wish to be involved in the decision-making process and the treatments they chose are comparable with those chosen by younger patients (37).

Confined cancer in this age group is usually managed expectantly. Observation is the preferred approach outside the United States and is fairly common even within the US for stage A (nonpalpable) cancers. In the alternative term watchful waiting, it is the watching that is vital. The patient is being observed to ensure that an indication for treatment does not arise and, when it does, that it is treated promptly. The reason for surveillance is that the majority of cancers will not progress so rapidly as to endanger the life of the patient. With the possible exception of poorly differentiated tumors, confined disease is only considered a threat to those with a life-expectancy of more than 10 years (38). One recent study in Sweden found that survival in patients with localized disease that deferred treatment, was similar to those patients who received early treatment (39). Another study reported that men age 65–75 years with low-grade localized prostate cancer (Gleason score 2–4), who were untreated or received only hormone therapy, had the same survival as men the same age in the general population; that is, they had about a 13% risk of dying within 10 years. However the risk of dying within 10 years was 24% for men with moderate grade disease (Gleason score 5–7) and 46% for men with high-grade disease (Gleason score 8–10) (40).

Men in their mid-70s or older who have low- to moderate-grade localized prostate cancer are good candidates for observation management. The same implies for men aged 65 or over who have low-grade disease or minimal tumor volume. Men with greater risk of progression may also consider this approach since currently available treatments have not been shown to control poorly differentiated disease. Treatment outcomes for localized disease with surgery or radiation therapy are equally effective in-patients with a life-expectancy of less than 10 years. The benefit of observation is avoidance of the complications that can occur following aggressive treatment. As men live longer, their expectations change. Sexual activity remains important for many elderly men. It is important to discuss with the patient the possible options, that withholding potentially curative treatment carries the risk of tumor progression and metastasis.

Radical retropubic prostatectomy in the elderly

Elderly patients with surgically resectable prostate cancer require different considerations unique to their age group when surgery is considered for this disease. Elderly patients, even those without significant medical problems, may have a prolonged recovery period and may be at increased risk for complications from surgery; these complications must be balanced against the probability of non-cancer-related morbidity and mortality (41).

Surgical resection is considered by many surgeons to be the treatment for healthy men with prostate cancer and a life-expectancy of more than 10 years, and several studies suggested that radical therapy should be withheld from patients with life-expectancy less than 10 years. The appropriate candidates for surgery are men in reasonably good health that are about 73 or younger, with tumor confined in the prostate. Several studies have examined the morbidity and mortality of pelvic surgery in elderly patients and found that in well-selected patients, the surgical outcome is positive. In a study at the Mayo Clinic 1966–88, 191 patients who were < 55 years old and 51 elderly

patients who were > 75 years old underwent radical retropubic prostatectomy. Compared with younger patients, elderly patients had a higher stage and two-thirds of them did not have peri-operative complications. No elderly patients died within 5 years after operation. The incidence of respiratory distress and significant urinary incontinence was greater, however, in the elderly patients and only the elderly experienced delirium or confusion. The major criticism about these studies is that the older patients were well-selected, healthy older men.

Unfortunately in many patients radical surgery does not appear to improve survival. Lu-Yao and associates found that 24% of men with organ-confined disease at the time of surgery, required additional treatment within 5 years of undergoing radical prostatectomy (42). Even when the disease is confined to the prostate, radical surgery may be inappropriate for very old patients. All major pelvic surgery is associated with a high risk of deep venous thrombosis and pulmonary embolism, as well as cardiovascular and infective complications; elderly patients are more susceptible to such complications. They also benefit less from nerve-sparing techniques; 80% of patients over 70 years are impotent after radical prostatectomy (43). A chart review study was done of 216 patients with prostate cancer who had non-metastatic disease, in the registries of ten Southern California hospitals during the years 1980–82. There were significant variations in the intensity of treatment as a function of patient age. Table 25.2 shows a strong relationship between increasing age and less frequent use of treatment with surgery or radiation therapy. These data indicated that physicians and patients considered the likelihood of tolerating therapy when deciding on the therapy. The American College of Physicians has concluded that radical prostatectomy potentially adds 3 years of life for men in their 50s, 1.5 years for men in their 60s, and 0.4 years for men in their 70s.

Table 25.2   Treatment for localized prostate cancer and age

	Age (yr)		
	50–64 (n = 60)	65–74 (n = 74)	> 75 (n = 82)
Treatment			
Local therapy only	66.7	47.3	9.8
Hormonal therapy	11.7	12.2	45.1
Hormonal and local	3.3	4.0	0.0
Observation only	18.3	36.5	45.1

Radiation treatment of elderly patients with prostate cancer

One of the options of treatment presented to patients with localized prostate cancer is radiation therapy. A major concern has been the suggestion that elderly patients are unable to tolerate the conventional radiotherapy dosage treatment schedules. However, this is not necessarily the case and many elderly patients can tolerate radiotherapy treatment just as well as younger patients (44, 45).

The US national surveys in prostate cancer conducted by the Patterns of Care Study in radiation oncology and the prostate cancer database from the Department of Radiation Oncology of the Fox Chase Cancer Center (Philadelphia, PA) have been used to compare processes and outcomes of conventional radiation treatment with conformal 3-dimensional (3D) radiation treatment in elderly patients compared with younger patients (46). Their data are the result of four national surveys conducted to evaluate patients treated for prostate cancer in 1973, 1978, 1983, and 1989. There were a total of 2210 patients. The results demonstrated the dramatic shift in the median age of patients treated with radiation therapy in the United States from 65 years in 1973 to 72 years in 1979. From 1973 to 1989, the 70-years or older group increased from 28% to 63% of the population, the 75-years or older group increased from 10% to 35%, and patients older than 80 years increased from 3% to 9%. The data suggested no significant late complications of treatment between the two age groups of patients (< 70years, > 70years). There was a significant decrease of 117 cGy in dose for older patients but this not thought to be biologically significant. Conventional technique was associated with an increase in acute (during treatment) symptoms for patients older than 65. With the new 3D conformal therapy, which uses computer modeling to reconstruct the tumor and shielding to protect surrounding normal tissues, high doses can be delivered to the prostate from outside the body without causing an extensive amount of injury to skin and adjacent tissues, such as the small bowel, posterior wall of the rectum, anal canal, and urethra. When the conformal technique was used, rate of acute symptoms decreased by half, and older patients experienced the same rate of acute symptoms as younger patients (47, 48).

Cohort studies of patients with clinically localized prostate cancer treated with radiation therapy found that overall survival at 10 years was not different from that for age-matched controls. It has been shown that long-term clinical control is confirmed by a normal prostate-specific antigen in 88% of 10-year survivors of prostate cancer (49, 50, 51). Radiation therapy of localized carcinoma of the prostate it is as effective as surgery, whilst for locally advanced disease radiotherapy is preferred to surgery, because it is associated with fewer complications. As for interstitial brachytherapy, there are not studies to suggest that in the elderly.

Although some biological and molecular data indicate a rise in radiation sensitivity with growing age, appropriately selected elderly patients can realize the benefits of radiation treatments of their prostate cancers as younger patients.

Management of extra-prostatic disease in the elderly

Prostate cancer metastatic disease is treated with hormone therapy aiming to remove the sources of androgen or testosterone in the body. This can be accomplished through bilateral orchiectomy or medical castration. Diethylstilbestrol has also been used, but this non-steroidal estrogen has a higher rate of cardiovascular complications than do other approaches (52). Therapy with a luteinizing hormone-releasing analogs (e.g. leuprolide) is now favored by most clinicians. These agents greatly diminish pituitary secretion of luteinizing hormone and testicular production of testosterone; currently they are available in a suspension that needs to be injected only once every 3 months (53). Hormone treatment may be more readily accepted in the elderly. Where prostate cancer is causing troublesome bladder outflow obstruction, hormone treatment is a reasonable alternative to TURP, especially in a man unfit for surgery. Men with prostate cancer presenting with retention of urine will often be able to void urine spontaneously after a few weeks of hormone treatment (54, 55). Some clinicians favor total androgen ablation. This is achieved by therapy with anti-androgens (e.g. flutamide) whose action is to compete with circulating testosterone for androgen receptors. Adverse effects of hormone therapy include loss of libido and impotence, hot flushes, and a small weight gain. Since the introduction of LHRH analogs, the number of elderly men undergoing orchiectomy has decreased. However orchiectomy has some advantages, such as simplicity, which is very important for an old immobile man with multiple diseases who may be on a large number of drugs.

Unfortunately, androgen-deprivation therapy is not curative. After a period of time androgen-resistant cells break through and spread, eventually causing death. Recent studies indicate that a patient whose cancer has become refractory to total androgen ablation may have a temporary remission of disease if anti-androgen therapy is withdrawn, but such response is usually short-lived. The general consensus is that the majority of patients probably do not benefit from combined androgen ablation. If it has a role, it probably is in the younger patient with low-volume disease and is not an issue for a man over 75.

Because hormone therapy primarily relieves the symptoms of metastatic disease, some clinicians believe that it should be held in reserve until symptoms develop; others favor initiating treatment as soon as metastatic disease is identified. However, early hormone therapy appears to offer no survival advantage over delayed hormone therapy (56). Advanced prostate cancer is incurable, however the intervention of another disease may lead to the elderly man dying before this happens. The right decision in this case is to concentrate on prompt effective symptom palliation (57).

Analgesia and radiotherapy can usually control bone pain. In some men palliative treatment with the strontium-89 helps control pain from metastases to bone. The clinician must be alert to complications, notably spinal cord compression that can often be prevented if radiotherapy starts at the first indication. Many men suffer from local progression and urinary symptoms or hematuria can often be palliated by a low dose of radiotherapy. Ureteric obstruction in hormone refractory disease should be considered terminal event (58). While a remission with nephrostomy drainage or stents might be useful for the younger man, the imposition of these is rarely justified in the elderly.

Conclusions and recommendations

Elderly patients with prostate cancer should be carefully evaluated. The choice of therapy for localized prostate cancer is often guided by concern for patient tolerance and longevity. Patients should be informed that treatment does not guarantee that the cancer will not metastasize, and the amount by which treatment reduces the risk of metastasis is uncertain. Elderly men are more likely to be followed without additional therapy, because the potential benefits of therapy are small enough that watchful waiting is a reasonable alternative.

Older men must consider the likelihood that maybe they will die from some other cause before their cancer generates significant problems. Previous studies have not indicated clearly that older men have significant shortening of expected survival if they are just followed clinically. Future studies that retrospectively investigate the importance of patient preferences, quality of life, and survival are needed to understand the age-related variations in care for men with cancer of the prostate.

Physicians need to consider life-expectancy and the quality of life in making treatment decisions. Decisions based on age alone are likely to result in reduced potential for cure or quality in elderly men. They should always remember that they are treating not prostate cancer, but a man who has the disease and for whom no rigid formula can provide the correct solution.

References

1. Coeburg JWW. Significant trends in cancer in the elderly. *Eur J Cancer* 1996, **32A**, 569–71.
2. Golini A, Lori A. Aging of the population, demographic and social changes. *Aging* 1990, **2**, 319–36.
3. McKenna RJ. Clinical aspects of cancer in the elderly. *Cancer* 1994, **74**, 2107–17.
4. Ashkanani F, Heys SD, Eremin O. The management of cancer in the elderly. *J Roy Coll Surg Edinb* 1999, **44**, 2–10.
5. Joint NCI-EORTC consensus meeting on neoplasia in the elderly. *Eur J Cancer* 1991, **27**, 653–4.
6. Franks LM. Latent carcinoma of the prostate. *J Path Bacteriol* 1954, **68**, 603–16.
7. McNeal JE. Origin and development of carcinoma of the prostate. *Cancer* 1969, **23**, 24–34.
8. Repetto L, Granetto C, Venturino A. Comorbidity and cancer in the aged: the oncologists point of view. *Rays* 1997, **22** (Suppl 1), 17–9.
9. Mor V, Masterson-Allen S, Goldberg RJ *et al.* Relationship between age and diagnosis and treatments received by cancer patients. *J Am Geriatr Soc* 1985, **33**, 585–9.
10. Wettle VT. Age as a risk factor for inadequate treatment (editorial). *JAMA* 1987, **258**, 516.
11. Kennedy BJ. Aging and cancer. *J Clin Oncol* 1988, **6**, 1903–11.
12. Kirby RS, Kirby MG, Feneley MR *et al.* Screening for prostate cancer: a GP based study. *Br J Urol* 1994, **74**, 64–71.
13. Oesterling JE. Prostatic tumour markers: preface. *Urol Clin N Am* 1993, **20**, xv–xvi.
14. Albertsen PC. Screening for prostate cancer is neither appropriate nor cost-effective. *Urol Clin N Am* 1996, **23**, 521–30.
15. American College of Physicians. Screening for prostate cancer. *Ann Inter Med* 1997, **126**, 480.

16. Barry MJ *et al*. Should Medicare provide reimbursement for prostate-specific antigen testing for early detection of prostate cancer? Part III: Management strategies and outcomes. *Urology* 1995, **46**, 277–89.

17. Coley CM *et al*. Early detection of prostate cancer. Part I: Prior probability and effectiveness of tests. *Ann Inter Med* 1997, **126**, 394–406.

18. Oesterling JE, Cooner WH, Jacobson SJ *et al*. Influence of patient age on the serum PSA concentration. An important clinical observation. *Urol Clin N Am* 1993, **20**, 671–80.

19. Kirk D. Prostate cancer in the elderly. *Eur J Surg Oncol* 1998, **24**, 379–83.

20. Flemming C, Wasson JH, Albertsen PC *et al*. A decision analysis of alternative treatment strategies for clinically localized prostate cancer. *JAMA* 1993, **269**, 2650–8.

21. Reissigl A *et al*. Frequency and clinical significance of transition zone cancer in prostate cancer screening. Prostate 1997, 30, 130–5.

22. Brewster SF, Rooney N, Kabala J *et al*. Fatal anaerobic infection following transrectal biopsy of a rare prostatic tumour. *Br J Urol* 1993, **72**, 977–8.

23. Rabrani F, Stroumbakis N, Kaya BR *et al*. Incidence and clinical significance of false-negative sextant prostatic biopsies. *J Urol* 1998, **159**, 1247–50.

24. Kanamaru H, Arai Y, Moroi S *et al*. Long-term results of definitive treatment in elderly patients with localized prostate cancer. *Int J Urol* 1998, **5**, 546–9.

25. Albertsen P. Prostate disease in older men: 2. *Cancer. Hosp Pract* 1997, **15**, 159–76

26. Murphy GP, Natarajan N, Pontes JE. The national survey of prostate cancer in the United States by the American College of Surgeons. *J Urol* 1982, **127**, 928–34.

27. Mettlin C, Littrup P, Kane RA. Relative sensitivity and specificity of serum prostate specific antigen (PSA) level compared with age reference PSA, PSA density and PSA change. *Cancer* 1994, **74**, 1615–20.

28. Bennett CL, Greenfield S, Aronow H *et al*. Patterns of care related to age of men with prostate cancer. *Cancer* 1991, **67**, 2633–41.

29. Smedley HM, Sinnott M, Freedman LS *et al*. Age and survival in prostate carcinoma. *Br J Urol* 1983, **55**, 529–33.

30. Adami HO, Norlen BJ, Malker B *et al*. Long term survival in prostate carcinoma, with special reference to age as a prognostic factor. A nation-wide study. *Scad J Urol Nephrol* 1986, **20**, 107–12.

31. Borec D, Butcher D, Hassanein K *et al*. Relationship of age to hostologic grade in prostate cancer. *Prostate* 1990, **16**, 305–11.

32. Stamey TA, McNeal JE, Freiha FS *et al*. Morphometric and clinical studies on 68 consecutive radical prostatectomies. *J Urol* 1988, **139**, 1235–41.

33. McNeal JE, Bostwick DE, Kindrachuk RA *et al*. Patterns of progression in prostate cancer. *Lancet* 1986, I, 60–3

34. Walsh PC, Lepor HL. The role of radical prostatectomy in the management of prostate cancer. *Cancer* 1987, **60**, 526–37.

35. Dearnaley D. The way ahead for radiotherapy in prostate cancer. In: *New perspectives in prostate cancer* (ed. A Beldegrun, RS Kirby, RTD Oliver). Isis Medical, Oxford, 1998, 215–26.

36. Jacobi GH. Hormonal treatment of metastatic carcinoma of the prostate. In: *The prostate* (ed. JM Fitzpatrick, RJ Krane). Churchill Livingstone, Edinburgh, 1989, 389–99.

37. Samet J, Hunt WC, Key C *et al*. Choise of cancer therapy varies with patient age. *JAMA* 1986, **255**, 3385–90.

38. Chodac GW, Thisted RA, Gerber GS *et al*. Results of conservative management of clinically localized prostate cancer. *N Engl J Med* 1994, **330**, 242–8.

39. Johansson JE *et al*. Fifteen-year survival in prostate cancer: a prospective population-based study in Sweden. *JAMA* 1996, **277**, 467–71.

40. Albertsen PC *et al*. Long-term survival among men with conservatively treated localised prostate cancer. *JAMA* 1995, **274**, 626–31.

41. Kerr L, Zincke H. Radical retropubic prostatectomy for prostate cancer in the elderly and the young: complications and prognosis. *Eur Urol* 1994, **25**, 305–12.

42. Lu-Yao GL *et al*. Follow-up prostate cancer treatments after radical prostatectomy: a population based study. *J Natl Cancer Inst* 1996, **88**, 166–73.

43. Christopher K, Payne, Joseph W *et al*. Genitourinary problems in the eldely. *Surg Clin N Am* 1994, **74**, 401–29.

44. Huguenin PU, Bitterli M, Lutolf UM *et al*. Localised prostate cancer in elderly patients. Outcome after radiation therapy compared to matched younger patients. *Strahlenther Onkol* 1999, **175**, 554–8.

45. Olmi P, Ausili-Cefaro G. Radiotherapy in the elderly: a multicentric prospective study on 2060 patients referred to 37 Italian therapy centers. *Rays* 1997, **22** (Suppl), 53–6.

46. Hanks GE, Hanlon A, Owen JB *et al*. Patterns of radiation treatment of elderly patients with prostate cancer. *Cancer* 1994, **74** (Suppl), 2174–7.

47. Soffen EM, Hanks GE, Hunt M *et al*. Conformal static field radiation therapy treatment of early prostate cancer versus non-conformal techniques: a reduction in acute morbidity. *Int J Radiat Oncol Biol Phys* 1992, **24**, 485–8.

48. Epstein B, Peter R, Martin E *et al*. Low comlication rate with conformal radiotherapy for cancer of the prostate. *Radiother Oncol* 1992, **24** (Abstact), 394.

49. Hanks GE, Perez CA, Kozar M *et al*. PSA confirmation of cure aye 10 years of the TAB, T2, N0, M0 prostate cancer patients treated in TOG protocol 7706 with external beam irradiation. *Nit J Radiate Once Boil Phys* 1994, **30**, 289–92.

50. Hanks GE, Hanlon A, Schultheiss TE *et al*. Early prostate cancer: the national results of radiation treatment from the Patterns of Care and RTOG studies with prospects of improvement with conformal radiation and adjuvant androgen deprivation. *J Urol* 1994, **152**, 1775–80.

51. Geinitz H, Zimmermann FB and Molls M. Radiotherapy of the elderly patient. Radiotherapy tolerance and results in older patients. *Strahlenther Onkol* 1999, **175**, 119–27.

52. Prostate Cancer Trialists Collaborative Group. Maximum androgen blockade in advanced prostate cancer: an overview of 22 randomized trials with 3283 deaths in 5710 patients. *Lancet* 1995, **346**, 265–9.

53. Huggins C, Hodges CV. Studies in prostate cancer. 1. The effect of castration of oestrogen and of androgen injection on serum phosphatases in metastatic carcinoma of the prostate. *Cancer Res* 1941, **1**, 293–7.

54. Crawford ED, Eisenberger MA, McLeod DG *et al.* A controlled trial of leuprolide with and without flutamide in prostatic carcinoma. *New Engl J Med* 1989, **321**, 419–24.

55. Nesbit RM, Baum WC. Endocrine control of prostate cancer. Clinical survey of 1818 cases. *JAMA* 1950, **143**, 1317–20.

56. Beynon LL, Chisholm GD. The stable state is not an objective response in hormone-escaped prostate carcinoma of the prostate. *Br J Urol* 1984, **56**, 733–6.

57. Cherny NI, Foley KM. Management of pain associated with prostate cancer. In: *Principles and practice of genitourinary oncology* (ed. D Raghaven, HI Scher, SA Leibel *et al.*). Lippincott-Raven, Philadelphia, 1997, 613–27.

58. Paul AB, Love C, Chisholm GD. The management of bilateral ureteric obstruction and renal failure in advanced prostate cancer. *Br J Urol* 1994, **74**, 642–5.

Section VI

26 | Quality of life of prostate cancer patients

Fernando Calais da Silva

Introduction

In the past 10 years, the world has seen a rapid expansion of interest in health-related quality of life among patients with adenocarcinoma of the prostate. Driven by patients, clinicians, and researchers, this interest has led to increase of both the public awareness and the research funding. As medical science has advanced in prostate cancer, diagnosis is made earlier in the course of disease. Treatments have been improved, refined, and innovated; however, prostate cancer-related mortality remains high in the Western world. Controversy continues to surround all of the fundamental clinical questions in prostate cancer, including whether to screen the general population, whether and how to treat patients with early stage tumors, and how to manage those with advanced disease. Traditionally, the primary endpoints in most treatment evaluations have been cure and survival, but the use of 'medical' outcomes and the worldwide effort to contain the rising costs of care have underscored the importance of patient-centered outcomes, such as quality of life in prostate cancer. Health-related quality of life can even be a robust predictor of mortality in patients with prostate cancer. Contemporary interpretations of health-related quality of life (HRQOL) are based on the World Health Organization's definition of health as not merely the absence of disease, but a state of physical, emotional, and social well-being (1). HRQOL encompasses a wide range of human experience, including the daily necessities of life, such as food and shelter, personal and interpersonal responses to illness, and activities associated with professional fulfillment and personal happiness (2). HRQOL also encompasses the overall sense of satisfaction that an individual experiences in life (3). Most importantly, HRQOL involves patients' own perceptions of their health and ability to function in life. HRQOL is often confused with physi-

cal functional status (4). While physical function represents an important component of disease and treatment-related side-effects, equally important dimensions of HRQOL also include role function, vitality, mental health, and social interactions. Morbidity applies to specific complications, but HRQOL opens a wider umbrella to include the bother associated with particular dysfunctions, any impact on normal functions or social roles, and a composite of other psychosocial domains. The impact of HRQOL on therapeutic decision-making is now considered so important that some investigators consider a clinical cancer trial to be incomplete in the absence of HRQOL assessment (5, 6). HRQOL can even be a robust predictor of mortality in patients with prostate cancer (7). In broad terms, HRQOL may be conceived as the quotient of an individual's actual status over his or her expected status. For example, to the degree that a prostate cancer patient's impotence is expected, not bothersome, and not intrusive into his life or self-image, it does not impact his HRQOL. Conversely, a patient who is highly focused on his expectations of good erectile function after therapy may perceive even the slightest decrement as having a powerful effect on his quality of life (8). It is axiomatic that HRQOL applies to a patient's own self-perception, regardless of how he may be assessed by his family, friends, or physicians.

HRQOL instruments

HRQOL instruments must have the fundamental properties of reliability, validity, and responsiveness (9). Reliability refers to how reproducible the scale is. Test–retest reliability is a measure of response stability over time. It is assessed by administering scales to subjects, at two time points, typically 1 month apart. Correlation coefficients between the two scores reflect the stability of responses. Internal consistency reliability measure the similarity of an individual's responses across several items, indicating the homogeneity of a scale. The statistic used to quantify the internal consistency, or unidimensionality, of a scale is called Cronbach's coefficient alpha (10). Generally, accepted standards dictate that reliability statistics measured by these two methods should exceed 0.70 (11).

Validity refers to how well the scale or instrument measures the attribute it is intended to measure. Content validity, sometimes referred to as face validity, involves qualitative assessment of the scope, completeness, and relevance of a proposed scale (12). Criterion validity is a more quantitative approach to assessing the performance of scales and instruments. It requires the correlation of scales scores with other measurable health outcomes (predictive validity) and with results from established 'gold-standard' tests. (concurrent validity). Generally accepted standards also dictate that validity statistics should exceed 0.70 (13). Construct validity, perhaps the most valuable assessment of a survey instrument, is a measure of how meaningful the scale or survey instrument performs in a multitude of settings and populations over a number of years. Construct validity comprises two other forms of validity: convergent and divergent. Convergent validity implies that several different methods for obtaining the same information about a given trait or concept produce similar results. Divergent validity means that the scale does not correlate too closely with similar but distinct concepts or traits.

Responsiveness of a HRQOL instrument refers to how sensitive the scales are to change over time. That is, a survey may be reliable and valid, but it must also be able to detect meaningful improvements or decrements in quality of life during longitudinal studies. The instrument 'reacts' in a time frame that is relevant for patients over time.

HRQOL instruments may be general or disease-specific. General HRQOL domains address the components of overall well-being, while disease-specific domains focus on the impact of particular organic dysfunctions that affect HRQOL(14).

When studying quality of life for clinical or research purposes, it is preferable to use published instruments that have been previously validated in the relevant population. In general, one should avoid extracting single items or scales from different instruments to construct a new one unless they have been independently psychometrically validated. The development and validation of a new HRQOL instrument is an arduous task.

Hence, investigators should first examine existing instruments to determine if they adequately capture the domains of interest before developing a new instrument. Because of the well-documented impact of malignancies and their treatment on HRQOL, cancer-specific quality of life also has been investigated extensively. Numerous instruments have been developed and tested that measure the special impact of cancer on patients' routine activities. Examples include the Cancer Evaluation Rehabilitation System Short Form (CARES-SF) (15, 16), the Functional Assessment of Cancer Therapy (FACT) (17), and the European Organization for the Research and Treatment of Cancer Quality of Life Questionnaire (EORTC QLQ-C30) (18). Each has been validated and tested in patients with various types of cancer.

The EORTC QLQ-C30 was designed to measure cancer-specific HRQOL in patients with a variety of malignancies. Its 30 items address domains that are common to all cancer patients. The questionnaire includes five general scales (physical, role, emotional, cognitive, and social functioning) a global health scale, three symptom scales (fatigue, nausea/vomiting, and pain), and six single items concerning dyspnea, insomnia, appetite loss, constipation, diarrhea, and financial difficulties due to the disease. The EORTC QLQ-C30 does not include domains specific to prostate cancer, but it has performed well in this population (19). Disease-specific modules for cancers of the breast, and head and neck (20, 21), have been developed according to methodologically rigorous techniques.

Another HRQOL disease-specific instrument, presently under investigation, is the prostate cancer module of the EORTC QLQ-C30. Researchers developed this module to be used in conjunction with the EORTC QLQ-C-30 as a measure of disease-specific HRQOL in prostate cancer. Its 20 items include bowel, urinary, and sexuality symptom scales and are reliable and valid in men with localized (22, 23) or metastatic (24) prostate cancer. Its transformed scales are scored from 0 to 100 with higher scores representing worse outcomes in functional status domains.

For the localized, theoretically curable stages of prostatic cancer most literature has dealt with treatment-induced toxicity. Radical prostatectomy has historically led to sexual impotence in nearly all patients and to urinary incontinence in 30% (25). New operative techniques have decreased these percentages considerably (26), making radical prostatectomy a more acceptable treatment option. The principle side-effects following irradiation of the prostate are frequency, dysuria, diarrhea, and abdominal pain, seen in 10–30% of patients (27–29). Much of this toxicity can be avoided by the use of computed tomography-based radiation planning, optimal shielding techniques, and proper selection of the target dose. Definitive radiation treatment may also lead to decreased sexual function in 20–30% of patients (30).

The EORTC Genitourinary Tract Cancer Co-operative Group, in co-operation with the EORTC Study Group on quality of life, designed a study to evaluate the quality of life in patients with metastatic prostatic carcinoma (31). This is a randomized phase-III study comparing the therapeutic effect of orchiectomy vs. a luteinizing hormone-releasing hormone (LHRH) analog depot preparation and flutamide. The primary endpoints of the trial are the incidence and duration of response, time to progression, and overall survival. In an optional study in the overall analysis, which is reported here, a 30-item questionnaire was developed to assess the relative impact of these two therapies on the daily lives of the patients.

A total of 22 institutions entered 327 patients into the study (EORTC protocol 30853), all of whom had metastatic prostatic cancer and had not received prior treatment. Patients were randomized to receive either orchiectomy or an LHRH analog depot preparation (goserelin acetate, 3.6 mg s.c. every 4 weeks) and flutamide (250 mg t.i.d.).

The patients were asked during pretreatment and at each follow-up visit to fill in a 30-item quality-of-life questionnaire. Parameters evaluated included personal functioning (A self-report scale of physician-rated performance status), social role functioning, physical symptoms of prostate cancer (dysuria, frequency, hematuria, and metastatic pain), fatigue and malaise, sleep-disturbance psychological distress, sexual dysfunction, and disruption of social life. Most of the items and scales composing the questionnaire have been used in previous EORTC trials and have established levels of validity and reliability (32).

The doctors completed EORTC clinical forms, including clinical findings and biochemical and radiological results, before treatment and then every 3 months. The doctors' evaluation of the patients' performance status was according to the WHO guidelines, as either no impairment, slight impairment but ambulatory, less than 50% confined to a bed or a chair, more than 50% confined to a bed or a chair, or completely confined to a bed or a chair and help required for basic daily functions. Pain level was scored as either no analgesics, non-narcotic analgesics used irregularly, non-narcotic analgesics used regularly, narcotic analgesics used irregularly, or narcotic analgesics used regularly.

Only 23% of the 327 patients underwent the pretreatment quality-of-life assessment. With this limited sample size, we could only tentatively draw conclusions about the key questions highlighted by the analysis of these questionnaires. There was considerable non-compliance in completion of the questionnaires. Completion, however, was optional and represented the EORTC Genitourinary Group's first attempt to assess quality of life in patients with prostate cancer. At the start of the trial, most of the urologists were unfamiliar with systematic assessment of patient quality of life. Consequently, few clinicians were willing to regularly make the effort needed; they probably did not feel confident that this type of assessment would provide any valuable information to add to that obtained from the clinical, biochemical, and radiological evaluations. The limited number of patients makes it difficult to analyze psychological aspects. The questionnaires had no personal questions about quality of life (such as 'How would you rate your overall quality of life?'), but did include four questions about psychological well-being. The questions were 'Did you feel tense?'; 'Did you feel irritable?'; 'Did you worry?'; and 'Did you feel depressed?'. The score derived from the answers to these four questions was used to evaluate the overall quality of life.

A simple correlation analysis (Pearson's correlation coefficient) revealed that some domains were particularly well-correlated with quality of life in patients with prostate carcinoma (Table 26.1). Fatigue and reduced social and sexual life all played important roles in the overall psychological well-being of these (previously untreated) patients with prostate cancer, confirming that the patient's assessment was a better monitor of quality of life. No significant correlations were found between psychological well-being and the physician's assessment of performance status and pain.

Our reluctance to use self-administered questionnaires to assess subjective morbidity was related to the lack of validity and reliability of previously used tools. However, clinicians, psychologists and sociologists have developed questionnaires that, although still not completely satisfactory, can assess subjective morbidity and quality of life from the patient's point of view in a valid manner. It has been shown that clinically worthwhile and valid information can be obtained from patient questionnaires during the treatment of hormone-resistant prostatic carcinoma (33).

Table 26.1 Correlation coefficients (*r*) between overall psychological well-being and other domains of quality of life in prostate cancer

	Doctor assessment		Patient assessment	
	r	P	r	P
Performance status (WHO)	0.113	0.360	ND	ND
Pain	0.024	0.844	0.190	0.124
Fatigue	ND	ND	0.406	< 0.001
Reduced social life	ND	ND	0.430	< 0.001
Reduced sexual life	ND	ND	0.362	0.003
Urological problems	ND	ND	0.280	0.021
Reduced professional life	ND	ND	0.285	0.023

ND: not determined; WHO: World Health Organization.

Our results were consistent with those from another EORTC study (protocol 30865) (34) showing large variations between the patients' and the physicians' evaluations of performance status and sexual status (potency). Our data on performance status and potency support the view that these parameters should be evaluated by the patients, and that the information relevant to quality of life is insufficient when obtained directly in the clinic by the physician. This observation may have significant therapeutic consequences. If the patients' complaints are not adequately recognized, they may not be treated appropriately. Furthermore, underestimation of patient symptoms by the doctor may cause patient dissatisfaction with the health service. Finally, we recommend the development of a better scoring system for the physician's evaluation of pain. Simply recording the use of analgesics, their type and their doses, is not sufficient, since it does not indicate whether or not the treatment achieved satisfactory pain relief. Furthermore, self-administered questionnaires for this type of patients should be simple and short, but nevertheless contain significant and relevant questions to enable assessment of subjective morbidity.

Conclusions

Quality-of-life assessment obtained by self-administered questionnaires, represents a feasible approach, also providing a mean of evaluating the benefits of treatment in prostate cancer. However, an important condition for the successful application of quality-of-life assessment in clinical trials of prostatic carcinoma is the clinician's interest in quality-of-life research. We believe that quality-of-life assessment should become a mandatory part of clinical trials in prostate cancer.

Furthermore, data collection must be achieved using valid and reliable methods, which allow interstudy comparisons. When designing the questionnaire, aspects of feasibility must be considered, especially for multicenter studies. The EORTC approach, using a general quality-of-life questionnaire supplemented by disease-specific and treatment-specific questions, seems to represent a reasonable way of performing quality-of-life research in multicenter trials. This strategy, plus the questionnaires currently used, are still under investigation and must be re-evaluated regularly.

References

1. WHO. *Constitution of the World Health Organization, basic documents.* Geneva WHO, 1948.
2. Patrick DL, Erickson P. *Assessing health-related quality of life for clinical decision-making.* Kluwer Academic Publishers, Dordrecht, 1993.
3. Osoba D. *Measuring the effect of cancer on quality of life.* CRC Press, Boca Raton, 1991.
4. Gill TM, Feinstein AR. A critical appraisal of the quality of life measurements. *JAMA* 1994, **272**, 619–26.
5. Altwein J, Ekman P, Barry M *et al.* How is quality of life in prostate cancer patients influenced by modern treatment? The Wallenberg Symposium. *Urology* 1997, **49** (Suppl 4A), 66–76.
6. Fayers PM, Jones DR. Measuring and analysing quality of life in cancer clinical trials: a review. *Stat Med* 1983, **2**, 429–46.
7. Albertsen PC, Aaronson NK, Muller MJ *et al.* Health-related quality of life among patients with metastatic prostate cancer. *Urology* 1977, **49**, 207–16.
8. Fitzpatrick JM, Kirby RS, Krane RJ *et al.* Sexual dysfunction associated with the management of prostate cancer. *Eur Urol* 1998, **33**, 513–22.
9. Litwin MS. *How to measure survey reliability and validity.* Sage Publications, Thousand Oaks, CA, 1995.
10. Cronbach LJ. Coefficient alpha and the internal structure of tests. *Psychometrika* 1951, **16**, 297–334.

11. Nunnally JC. *Psychometric theory* (2nd edn). McGraw-Hill, New York, 1978.

12. Messick S. The once and future issues of validity: assessing the meaning and consequences of measurement. In: *Test validity* (ed. H. Wainer, H.I. Braun). Lawrence Erlbaum Associates, Hillside NJ, 1988.

13. Nunnally JC. *Psychometric theory* (2nd edn). McGraw-Hill, New York, 1978.

14. Patrick DL, Deyo RA. Generic and disease-specific measures in assessing health status and quality of life. *Med Care* 1989, **27** (Suppl 3), S217–S232.

15. Schag CA, Ganz PA., Heinrich RL. Cancer Rehabilation Evaluation System-short form (CARES-SF). A cancer specific rehabilitation and quality of life instrument. *Cancer* 1991, **68**, 1406–13.

16. Schag CA, Heinrich RL. Development of a comprehensive quality of life measurement tool: CARES. *Oncology (Huntingt)* 1990, **4**, 135–8.

17. Cella DF, Tulsky DS, Gray G *et al.* The Functional Assessment of Cancer Therapy scale: development and validation of the general measure. *J Clin Oncol* 1993, **11**, 570–9.

18. Aaronson NK, Ahmedzai S, Bergman B *et al.* The European Organization for Research and Treatment of Cancer QLQ-C-30: a quality-of-life instrument for use in international clinical trials in oncology. *J Natl Cancer Inst* 1993, **85**, 365–76.

19. Curran D, Fossa S, Aaronson N *et al.* Baseline quality of life of patients with advanced prostate cancer. European Organization for Research and Treatment of Cancer (EORTC), Genito-Urinary Tract Cancer Cooperative Group (GUT-CCG). *Eur J Cancer* 1997, **33**, 1809–14.

20. Bjordal K, Kaasa S, Mastekaasa A. Quality of life in patients treated for head and neck cancer: a follow-up study 7 to 11 years after radiotherapy. *Int J Radiat Oncol Phys* 1994, **28**, 847–56.

21. Sprangers MA, Groenvold M, Arraras JI *et al.* The European Organization for Research and Treatment of Cancer breast cancer-specific quality-of-life questionnaire module: first results from a three-country field study. *J Clin Oncol* 1996, **14**, 2756–68.

22. Borghede G, Sullivan M. Measurement of quality of life in localized prostatic cancer patients treated with radiotherapy. Development of a prostate cancer-specific module supplementing the EORTC QLQ-C30. *Qual Life Res* 1996, **5**, 212–22.

23. Borghede G, Karlsson J, Sullivan M. Quality of life in patients with prostatic cancer: results from a Swedish population study. *J Urol* 1997, **158**, 1477–85.

24. Albertsen PC, Aaronson NK, Muller MJ *et al.* Health-related quality of life among patients with metastatic prostate cancer. *Urology* 1997, **49**, 207–16.

25. Ackermann R, Frohmüller HGW. Complications and morbidity following radical prostatectomy. *World J Urol* 1988, **1**, 62–7.

26. Eggleston JC, Walsh PC. Radical prostatectomy with preservation of sexual function: pathological findings in the first 100 cases. *J Urol* 1985, **134**, 1146–8.

27. Dewitt L, Ang KK, van der Schueren E. Acute side-effects and late complications after radiotherapy of localized carcinoma of the prostate. *Cancer Treat Rev* 1983, **10**, 79–89.

28. Pilepich MV, Krall J, George FW *et al.* Treatment-related morbidity in phase III, RTOG studies of extended-field irradiation for carcinoma of the prostate. *Int J Radiat Oncol Phys* 1984, **10**, 1861–7.

29. Telhaug R, Fossa SD, Ous S. Definitive radiotherapy of prostatic cancer: the Norwegian Radium Hospital's experience 1976–1982. *Prostate* 1987, **11**, 77–86.

30. Bergman B, Damber JE, Littbrand B *et al.* Sexual function in prostatic cancer patients treated with radiotherapy, orchiectomy or oestrogens. *Br J Urol* 1984, **56**, 64–9.

31. Denis L, Robinson M, Mahler C. (study co-ordinators). *Protocol for a randomized prospective study of the treatment of patients with metastatic prostatic cancer to compare the therapeutic effect of orchidectomy versus LHRH-analog depot (zoladex) preparation supplemented by an anti-androgen.* EORTC Genito-Urinary Cooperative Group Protocol 30853, Brussels, 1986.

32. Aaronson NK. (Study Coordinator). *EORTC Protocol 15861: Development of a core quality-of-life questionnaire for use in cancer clinical trials.* EORTC Data Center, 1987.

33. Tannock I, Gospodarowicz M, Meakin W *et al.* Treatment of metastatic prostatic cancer with low-dose prednisone: evaluation of pain and quality of life as pragmatic indices of response. *J Clin Oncol* 1989, **7**, 590–7.

34. Fossa SD, Aaronson NK, Newling D *et al.* Quality of life and treatment of hormone resistant metastatic prostatic cancer. The EORTC Genito-Urinary Group. *Eur J Cancer* 1990, **26**, 1133–6.

27 | Palliative care for prostate cancer patients

Kevin J. Harrington and Konstantinos N. Syrigos

Introduction

The term palliative care is often seen as being synonymous with the treatment of patients in the terminal phase of a disease process, usually cancer. However, this narrow definition fails to embrace adequately the wide variety of clinical scenarios that can justifiably be included under this heading. It is more useful to consider palliative care as the specific treatment given to patients with incurable disease with the aim of relieving disease-related symptoms and promoting physical, psychological, and spiritual well-being. In the arena of malignant disease, palliative care legitimately includes such active therapeutic maneuvers as surgery, chemotherapy, and radiotherapy, as well as the more widely recognized palliative therapies such as pain relief. Many patients present with disease that is too advanced to allow for the possibility of cure, and others may have concomitant medical conditions, which preclude the use of aggressive therapy that might, under different circumstances, have offered the chance of a cure. In these patients, the aim of treatment from the very outset is to achieve symptom palliation and, if possible, prolongation of their lives. Therefore, palliative care of patients with cancer is a challenging and diverse discipline in which palliative-care physicians, oncologists, and surgeons can play an important part. In addition, the involvement of a variety of healthcare professionals including nurses, social workers, counsellors, physiotherapists, and occupational therapists as part of a multi-disciplinary team allows important psychosocial issues to be addressed as part of the overall care package.

In patients with prostatic cancer, failure to achieve a cure results mainly from the occurrence of distant metastatic disease, although in a significant proportion of patients local pelvic disease remains uncontrolled or recurs. During the course of such patients' illnesses, a wide variety of manifestations of the disease may arise, both locally in the pelvis and at more distant sites. In this chapter, an attempt will be made to review the most frequently encountered clinical situations and to give guidelines as to their most appropriate management. Those problems common to patients with a number of different tumor types will be reviewed initially, followed by a detailed discussion of problems more commonly related to prostate cancer.

General symptoms of cancer

Pain

Pain is defined as an unpleasant sensory and emotional experience associated with actual or potential damage or described in terms of such damage (1). It is the most feared symptom of cancer and occurs at some time in the majority of patients. Many patients avoid telling their carers about new or increasing pain because they fear that it may signify recurrent or progressive disease. This can represent a considerable obstacle to the accurate diagnosis and treatment of cancer-related pain. However, with appropriate assessment and therapy, cancer-related pain can be successfully controlled in most patients (2).

Careful diagnosis of the cause of each individual pain and selection of the most appropriate class of analgesic medication lies at the heart of successfully controlling pain due to malignant disease. Evaluation of pain should begin with an complete pain history, including the site, speed of onset, quality, radiation, and modifying factors, including the effect of previous analgesic medication. In addition, the impact of the pain on the patient's activities of daily living should be assessed. Certain distinct types of pain can be recognized by their specific clinical features (e.g. burning or shooting pains due to nerve compression or infiltration) (Table 27.1). Once these details are known, it is

Table 27.1   Cancer-related pain: type of pain and associated symptoms

Type of pain	Associated symptoms
Nerve compression or invasion	Continuous ache Burning or stinging Episodic stabbing (lancinating) pain Hyperesthesia/anesthesia
Bone metastases	Continuous ache Worsened by movement Sudden increase with pathological fracture
Obstruction of hollow viscus	Intermittent Colicky/cramping
Capsular/fascial stretch	Continuous dull ache Associated tenderness over the organ

possible to make a decision regarding the most appropriate analgesic medication and adjuvant therapy that should be prescribed.

The WHO analgesic ladder

The WHO analgesic ladder is a well-established and validated approach to the treatment of cancer-related pain (Table 27.2). The recommendations that it makes are that analgesic medication is administered by mouth (if possible), regularly, and according to an escalating response to the pain ('by mouth, by the clock, by the ladder'). There are three rungs to the analgesic ladder and the appropriate response to failure to control pain with medication from one level is to move up the ladder to a higher level rather than to prescribe a different drug at the same analgesic level. In addition to the conventional analgesic drugs, a number of adjuvant drugs are available, which can be useful in controlling atypical pain. If these general guidelines are followed, pain can be adequately controlled in up to 90% of cases.(2)

Level 1
Drugs in this level are the non-opioids. The most commonly used drugs in this class are paracetamol, aspirin, and the non-steroidal anti-inflammatory drugs

Table 27.2   The World Health Organization analgesic ladder

First level	Non-opioid +/- adjuvant therapy
Second level	Weak opioid and non-opioid +/- adjuvant therapy
Third level	Strong opioid and non-opioid +/- adjuvant therapy

(NSAIDS), which, in addition to their analgesic properties, may benefit symptoms by modifying the inflammatory response. When prescribing NSAIDs to patients with prostate cancer, it is important to ask about symptoms of dyspepsia or a prior history of peptic ulcer disease, in which case a prophylactic H_2-receptor antagonist (e.g. cimetidine or ranitidine) should also be prescribed. Drugs at this level of the analgesic ladder are useful in controlling mild to moderate pain (especially related to bone metastases) but, in patients with advanced disease, their main role is in conjunction with weak or strong opioid medication.

Level 2
Drugs at this level are the weak opioid analgesics, such as codeine, dihydrocodeine, and dextropropoxyphene. These agents are effective against moderately severe pain, which is not controlled by simple analgesics and/or NSAIDS. They should be used at full doses and as regular medication before they can be considered to have failed.

Level 3
Drugs at this level are the strong opioids, of which morphine is the drug of choice (2). Oral morphine is available in a number of different preparations aimed at facilitating the use of this drug. In the initial phase of converting a patient from a weak opioid to a strong opioid, it is preferable to prescribe an instant release formulation that ensures rapid delivery of pain control. Such preparations include oramorph liquid and sevredol tablets. The usual starting dose of these agents is 10 mg every 4 h. It is extremely important to reinforce the fact that the medication should be taken regularly and that the selected dose is simply a starting

level and that there is scope for altering the dose to tailor the delivery of analgesia to the individual needs of the patient. Furthermore, at this stage the patient should be told that if the pain persists or returns before the 4-h interval, he can take extra doses of morphine (so-called breakthrough doses), which should be the same as the 4-h regular doses. If the starting dose of morphine has failed to control the pain after 24 h, the regular 4-h doses should be increased (e.g. doubled), as should the breakthrough doses. Using this approach, if the pain is opiate-responsive, it should be possible to arrive at a dose of morphine that controls the pain within a relatively short space of time. A stable dose of morphine can be defined as one that controls pain for two consecutive days with only two breakthrough doses needed in each 24-h period. Once pain control has been stabilized, it is possible to convert the morphine prescription to a sustained-release preparation, which can be given once or twice daily. This is achieved by assessing the 24-h requirement of the instant-relief morphine preparation and converting on a 1:1 basis to a sustained-release preparation, such as MST Continus®, MXL®, and Morcap® SR, and oramorph® SR. For example, a patient requiring 120 mg of instant-release oramorph could be treated with MST Continue 60 mg twice daily or MXL 120 mg once daily.

When prescribing morphine for the first time, it is important that the patient is made aware of the possible side-effects of the drug and given appropriate medication to ameliorate such reactions, otherwise, there is a serious risk that the patient will take insufficient amounts of the drug and will suffer unnecessary uncontrolled pain and anxiety. Constipation, which may be severe, is almost invariable with the doses of morphine employed in a palliative setting. Importantly, this effect of the drug is not subject to tolerance and, therefore, will persist for as long as morphine is prescribed. Therefore, patients should be prescribed prophylactic laxatives with the aim of increasing bowel motility (e.g. senna, bisacodyl) and softening the stool (e.g. docusate sodium). Bulk-forming (e.g. ispaghula husk) and osmotic (e.g. lactulose) laxatives should not be used routinely in the prophylaxis of opiate-induced constipation. In patients with intractable opiate-induced constipation, oral naloxone may occasionally be of benefit (3). Naloxone does not antagonize the analgesic effects of morphine but is able to attenuate its local action on gastro-intestinal motility. Nausea and vomiting, induced by stimulation of the chemoreceptor trigger zone, are relatively common in the first few days of morphine therapy, occurring in approximately 30% of patients (4). This unpleasant side-effect often abates

spontaneously within the first week of treatment, with or without short-term use of anti-emetic medication (e.g. metoclopramide 10 mg thrice daily, haloperidol 1–2 mg at night). Occasionally, opiate-sensitive patients may require more prolonged use of prophylactic anti-emetics. Rarely, a patient may be unable to tolerate morphine despite the above measures, in which case a trial of an alternative opiate is indicated. Many patients experience sedation as an early side-effect of morphine medication, an effect that can be exacerbated by alcohol consumption. Therefore, patients should be warned of the risks of driving or operating heavy machinery in this situation. The sedative effect of morphine usually tends to wear off after the first week of treatment. Other adverse effects of morphine include xerostomia in approximately 40% of patients (5), urinary retention in approximately 5% (6) and myoclonic jerks in patients receiving high doses of the drug.

In addition to morphine, there are a number of alternative opiate drugs. These agents are generally used when the patient is unable to tolerate oral morphine or when administration by a different route (subcutaneous, transdermal, rectal) may improve efficacy and compliance. The most commonly used of these drugs is diamorphine. This drug is often used by the subcutaneous route (usually as a continuous infusion via a syringe driver) when patients are unable to receive morphine by mouth because of nausea and vomiting, dysphagia, general debility, or unconsciousness. This situation is a typical feature of the final days or hours of a patient's life. Diamorphine is a very convenient agent to use because of its high solubility and compatibility with other agents, which can be administered concomitantly in the same syringe driver. When converting a patient from oral morphine to subcutaneous diamorphine, a conversion factor of 3:1 applies, i.e. 3 mg of morphine is equivalent to 1 mg of diamorphine. Other alternative opiates include fentanyl, which can be delivered by transdermal patch, phenazocine, which can be useful in patients who are morphine intolerant, and dextromoramide, which can be useful as a short-acting analgesic when patients are undergoing unpleasant procedures such as regular dressing changes.

Nausea and vomiting

This distressing symptom occurs in up to 50% of patients with advanced cancer. The etiology of nausea and vomiting in this group of patients is often complex and may include factors relating to progression of the primary disease and its metastatic spread or the consequences of therapeutic manuevers aimed at treating the disease or disease-related symptoms (Table 27.3).

Table 27.3 Causes of nausea and vomiting in patients with advanced cancer

1. Metabolic derangement
   Hypercalcemia
   Uremia
   Hepatic failure
2. Drug-induced
   Cytotoxic chemotherapy
   Opiates (strong > weak)
3. Radiotherapy
   Abdomino-pelvic radiotherapy
   Cranial radiotherapy
4. Gastro-intestinal disturbance
   Bowel obstruction
   Constipation
   Gastric stasis
5. Central nervous system metastases
   Intracranial metastases
   Carcinomatous meningitis
6. Pain
7. Anxiety and fear

Vomiting may be induced by a number of stimuli acting at different receptor sites, both in the brain and the periphery. The chemoreceptor trigger zone, which lies in the region of the area postrema, lies outside the blood–brain barrier and is, therefore, exposed to circulating toxic agents. The vomiting centre lies within the blood–brain barrier and may be stimulated directly (e.g. cranial irradiation) or through signals from higher cortical centres or from vagal afferents from the gastro-intestinal and genito-urinary tracts. Direct stimulation of peripheral receptors, including those in the gastric antrum, can lead to stimulation of vagal afferents and release of mediators of vomiting directly into the bloodstream. The complexity of the whole system is increased further by the wide range of interconnections of neural pathways within the brain. One such connection to the so-called higher centers has a significant effect on the response of individuals to emetogenic stimuli. As yet, the detailed mechanisms underlying the causation of nausea and vomiting remain unclear, despite considerable improvements in knowledge in recent times.

The management of nausea and vomiting should be based initially on an attempt to define a reversible cause, such as metabolic disturbance, intestinal obstruction, or cerebral metastases. Specific treatment aimed at the individual cause may alleviate the symptoms without recourse to anti-emetic therapy. For example, patients with malignant hypercalcemia usually respond well to rehydration and treatment with intravenous bisphosphonates. Similarly, the use of high-dose steroids and whole-brain irradiation (see below) can often relieve nausea and vomiting due to cerebral metastases and raised intracranial pressure.

If a specific cause can not be pinpointed, as is often the case, treatment with anti-emetic medication should be commenced immediately. A large number of drugs from different pharmacological classes (anti-dopaminergic, anti-cholinergic, anti-histaminergic, anti-serotoninergic, and cannabinoids) will prevent nausea and vomiting. Some examples are provided in Table 27.4,

Table 27.4 Commonly prescribed anti-emetic medication

Class of Drug	Examples	Dose and route of administration	Specific uses
Anti-dopaminergic	• Metoclopramide	10 mg t.i.d.; p.o., s.c., i.v. 30 mg over 24 h via s.c. syringe driver	Gastric stasis
	• Domperidone	10–20 mg t.i.d.; p.o. 30–60 mg t.i.d.; p.r.	Gastric stasis
	• Haloperidol	1.5–3.0 mg o.d.; p.o., s.c., i.v. 3–10 mg over 24 h via s.c. syringe driver	Opiate-induced nausea Bowel obstruction
	• Prochlorperazine	5–10 mg t.i.d.; p.o., p.r. 3–6 mg b.i.d.; buccal.	Vertigo
	• Methotrimeprazine	6.25–12.5 mg o.d./b.i.d.; p.o., s.c. 12.5–150 mg over 24 h via s.c. syringe driver	Sedative Bowel obstruction
Anti-histaminergic	• Cyclizine	50 mg t.i.d.; p.o., s.c., i.v. 150 mg over 24 h via s.c. syringe driver	Vertigo Bowel obstruction
Anti-5HT$_3$	• Ondansetron	4–8 mg b.i.d.; p.o., i.v.	Drug-induced nausea
	• Granisetron	1 mg b.i.d.; p.o. 3 mg o.d.; i.v.	Bowel obstruction
Anticholinergic	• Hyoscine	400 μg t.i.d.; s.c. 500 μg q 3 days; transdermal 600–1200 μg over 24 h via s.c. syringe driver	Bowel obstruction
Steroid	• Dexamethasone	2–8 mg b.i.d.; p.o., i.v., s.c. 4–16 mg over 24 h via s.c. syringe driver	Brain metastases Hepatic capsular stretch
Cannabinoid	• Nabilone	1–2 mg b.i.d.; p.o.	Drug-induced nausea

along with general guidelines to appropriate dose and frequency of administration.

As in the case of analgesic medication, the preferred route of administration should be by mouth. However, uncontrolled vomiting can prevent effective dosing and many of the agents are available in a range of alternative formulations for delivery by other routes, including subcutaneous, intravenous, rectal, and buccal administration. Subcutaneous infusions of anti-emetics via a syringe driver are especially useful in the setting of the final days and hours of a patient's illness when oral medication may not be tolerated or accepted.

Anorexia and weight loss

Cancer cachexia is a familiar feature of advanced-stage disease. Patients are often pitifully thin and literally waste away as the disease progresses. Most patients do not have a clearly identifiable cause for their anorexia, they simply have a markedly decreased appetite and eat only small quantities despite encouragement. In some patients, direct local tumor progression, leading to bowel obstruction or reduced gastric capacity, may be responsible. In others, ill-defined changes in the sense of taste and smell can lead to an aversion to food and drink. Iatrogenic causes include opioid medication, palliative chemotherapy, and radiotherapy. In the absence of an identifiable cause, the syndrome is usually ascribed to circulating products from the tumor or altered levels of endogenous cytokines.

As yet, no specific treatment has been described to address this problem. Therapy involves provision of appetizing food and drink whenever the patient feels capable of eating it, even if this involves unconventional menus and mealtimes. Dietetic support with high-calorie supplements may be accepted and certainly has the benefit of seeming to provide a specific solution. Appetite stimulation with progestogens (e.g. medroxyprogesterone acetate or megesterol acetate) or corticosteroids (dexamethasone) can occasionally be of benefit but the adverse effects are often excessive. Despite these measures, most patients with the cancer cachexia syndrome will continue to lose weight and gradually become bed-bound. Under these circumstances, death usually occurs due to intercurrent infection. Enteral (e.g. nasogastric or gastrostomy) or parenteral nutrition is entirely inappropriate in such patients.

Constipation

Constipation occurs in as many as 50% of patients with advanced cancer (7) and can cause severe discomfort. Mis-diagnosis of symptoms such as abdominal fullness, loss of appetite, nausea and vomiting, pain, diarrhoea, and confusional states can result in subjecting the patient to unnecessary investigations, therapy, and physical and mental stress. The unfortunate, but not uncommon, situation of a patient with morphine-induced constipation being given ever-increasing doses of morphine to combat the pain of constipation is one that should be avoidable.

Constipation in patients with disseminated malignant disease can have a number of different causes, including dietary changes (e.g. low-residue diet and reduced-fluid intake), metabolic derangement (e.g. hypercalcemia), drug-induced reduction in bowel contractility, tumor-induced partial mechanical obstruction, and neurogenic constipation in patients with spinal cord lesions. In general, the commonest and most predictable cause of constipation in patients with terminal cancer is the use of medication. The opioid analgesics are a frequent cause of constipation, which can become severe if adequate doses of appropriate laxatives are not prescribed prophylactically (see above). Other drugs that can cause constipation include drugs with an anticholinergic action, such as the tricyclic anti-depressants, hyoscine hydrobromide, methotrimeprazine, and cyclizine. In patients receiving constipating drugs, prophylactic laxatives should be used regularly rather than waiting for constipation to occur and then instituting treatment. In most cases, one or two co-danthrusate (danthron 50 mg, docusate sodium 60 mg) capsules *nocte* will suffice, although the precise dose required will depend on the dose of the constipating agents and may vary widely between different patients.

For patients with metabolic derangement, such as hypercalcemia, effective treatment with rehydration with intravenous fluids (typically 4–6 l over the first 24-h) and intravenous bisphosphonates, if the calcium level is greater than 3.0 mM, can lead to clinical improvement in bowel function. However, many of these patients will be profoundly constipated and may need short-term treatment with laxatives that will soften the stool (e.g. docusate sodium) and increase bowel motility (e.g. senna). Patients with neurogenic constipation due to spinal cord lesions will need regular laxatives, but even with these measures they may remain severely constipated. Such patients can often be managed successfully by intermittent manual evacuation of feces. The management of constipation due to bowel obstruction is discussed in the next section.

Bowel obstruction

Malignant bowel obstruction in patients with prostate cancer can occur due to local spread of disease in the pelvis, nodal metastatic disease in the pelvis, or abdomen or large liver metastases. This clinical scenario is most common in patients with ovarian and colorectal cancers, but does occur in patients with locally advanced prostate cancer. The typical symptoms will depend on the level of the obstruction but usually include nausea and vomiting, constipation, colicky abdominal pain, and abdominal bloating. The obstruction usually evolves slowly and the patient may describe previous episodes that resolved spontaneously. Alternatively, the condition may present as acute bowel obstruction with no preceding symptoms. The diagnosis rests with the history, physical examination, and the aid of plain abdominal radiographs. Contrast studies may be useful in defining the level of obstruction and are of particular importance if a palliative surgical procedure is contemplated. It must be remembered that not all cases of bowel obstruction in patients with advanced cancer will be due to the malignant process. Patients who have undergone prior abdominal surgery, or who have received radical radiotherapy, may develop adhesions or benign strictures.

In most cases of bowel obstruction in the palliative setting, surgical intervention is not appropriate. However, patients with a single site of obstruction and the option of further palliative anti-cancer therapy may benefit from either a defunctioning procedure (e.g. defunctioning colostomy or ileostomy) or from excision of the obstructed segment and re-anastomosis. Similarly, patients with intractable symptoms that can not be controlled by medical means may be palliated effectively by a limited surgical approach. However, this group of patients has a poor prognosis and surgical procedures are often complicated by infection, anastomotic leak, the development of fistulae, and wound complications. Therefore, surgery should only be contemplated after careful consideration of each individual case.

Table 27.5 Causes of dyspnea in patients with advanced cancer

1. Pulmonary metastases
   Gross metastatic deposits
   Lymphangitis carcinomatosa
2. Pulmonary emboli
3. Anemia
   Secondary to hematuria
   Secondary to palliative chemotherapy
   Secondary to bone marrow infiltration
4. Serous effusion
   Pleural
   Pericardial
5. Respiratory infection
6. Superior vena caval obstruction
7. Anxiety

Most patients will be managed successfully by conservative means. The standard approach should be to make the patient 'nil by mouth' and provide intravenous hydration. The use of a nasogastric tube (drip and suck) may be useful in patients with upper gastrointestinal obstruction and high-output vomiting. Nausea and vomiting is relieved by regular antiemetics, which are best given by the parenteral route, usually as a continuous subcutaneous infusion by syringe driver. Cyclizine, haloperidol, and hyoscine are suitable agents (Table 27.5). The visceral pain of obstruction, which is usually a dull ache, along with episodes of severe spasm, can generally be controlled by the use of a level 3 analgesic with or without the aid of an anti-spasmodic drug, such as hyoscine. It is common to use a continuous subcutaneous infusion of diamorphine, titrating the dose upwards to control symptoms. All of the drugs that are used to treat this condition can be given via a single syringe driver, which improves compliance and ease of administration for the patient and staff. Where peri-tumor edema is thought to be a contributing factor to the obstructive process, the addition of high-dose dexamethasone may yield a therapeutic benefit, although the evidence in support of this therapy is somewhat anecdotal. Constipation may also exacerbate (or even cause) bowel obstruction and should be managed with suppositories and enemas. Using this approach, an episode of subacute or acute bowel obstruction will often settle but recurrence is frequent within a short period of time.

If the above measures fail, and surgery is not a palliative option, the prognosis is usually extremely bleak.

Attempts to control the symptoms with escalating doses of analgesia and more powerful anti-emetics (e.g. methotrimeprazine) can be successful, often at the expense of heavy sedation. If vomiting is a persistent and distressing symptom, symptomatic relief can be gained from placement of a naso-gastric tube or, if this is poorly tolerated, insertion of a percutaneous gastrostomy tube may allow venting of the stomach contents at intervals (8–10). This latter approach has the added advantage of allowing patients to eat and drink a little, which can be a major addition to the quality of life. The use of octreotide, a long-acting analog of the hypothalamic release-inhibiting hormone somatostatin, to reduce gastro-intestinal secretions has been reported as an effective means of palliating unresponsive obstructive symptoms in a number of cases (10–12). The usual starting dose is 300 μg as a subcutaneous infusion over 24 h and this can be increased up to 600 μg if indicated.

Edema

Leg, perineal, and abdominal edema are a frequent complication of locally advanced prostate cancer. The cause can be complex, with contributions due to general malnutrition and hypoalbuminemia, pelvic venous obstruction, and thrombosis (see below), and obstruction of the pelvic lymphatics. Efforts should be made to identify the cause of the oedema correctly since this has a direct bearing on the choice of therapy.

The treatment of cancer-related thrombosis is discussed in detail below. Peripheral edema due to a low albumin state in patients with advanced disease can be managed effectively by low pressure support stockings, which should be designed to provide an even but graduated pressure. Lymphedema should be managed actively by means of massage, skin care, support, and movement (13). Skin discomfort and pain should be treated with effective analgesia. Low-dose oral diuretics (e.g. frusemide 40 mg, amiloride 5 mg) may relieve the perception of skin tightness but are unlikely to affect the degree of swelling. High-dose steroids are sometimes of use if the lymphedema is secondary to lymphatic obstruction due to tumor infiltration and swelling. However, they should be prescribed only in the form of a short-trial course and should be withdrawn promptly if they prove to be ineffective. It should be remembered that steroid-induced fluid retention and procoagulant activity have the potential to exacerbate rather than relieve symptoms. Massage, even at sites distant from the edema, may have a beneficial effect on lymphatic return and can be useful.

Skin care is of enormous importance. Regular moisturisers (e.g. E45 cream) should be used and infection should be treated vigorously with appropriate antibiotics (e.g. amoxycillin and flucloxacillin). Recurrent episodes of cellulitis in a lymphedematous limb are an indication for prophylactic antibiotic use. Low-pressure compression hosiery may be of benefit but may succeed only in moving fluid from one place to another without promoting its resorption. If the patient is able to keep the limb moving, this is likely to promote lymphatic flow. If not, passive movement may be of benefit.

Cancer-related thrombo-embolic disease

Thrombo-embolic disorders have been reported in 1–11% of patients with malignant disease, and a further 10% of patients suffer hemorrhagic episodes, although only one in ten of these is directly related to disordered clotting function (14, 15). Disseminated intravascular coagulation (DIC), with its attendant risks of thrombosis and/or hemorrhage, occurs in 9–15% of patients to a degree sufficient to require intervention. These figures underlie the status of thrombo-embolic disease and hemorrhage as the second commonest cause of mortality in patients with cancer (14).

Venous obstruction and thrombosis should be sought actively. This complication of malignant disease is very common and can give rise to considerable morbidity and mortality. In a recent study (16), the incidence and resource implications of cancer-related thrombo-embolic disease was assessed over a 2-year period in a single, large cancer center. This study highlighted a number of important issues:

(1) cancer-related thrombo-embolic disease occurred frequently and accounted for approximately 6% of inpatient bed occupancy;

(2) most patients with this condition had advanced or relapsed/incurable disease;

(3) nearly half of the patients suffered additional thromboses, despite maintenance warfarin anticoagulation;

(4) a significant number of patients experienced anti-coagulation-induced hemorrhage.

Similar results were reported by Chan and Woodruff (1992) (17) who detailed major bleeding in 35% and further thrombo-embolism despite therapeutic levels of anticoagulation in 13% of patients. Specific data relating to patients cared for in a hospice setting are not available, but it is likely that cancer-related thrombo-embolic disease is at least as common as in a cancer center.

It is difficult to make general statements regarding the most appropriate management of patients with cancer-related thrombo-embolic disease in the context of terminal cancer. If the patient's life expectancy is very short, active management is likely to be inappropriate and compression hosiery and analgesia may be all that is required. However, if the patient's life expectancy is measured in weeks or months, anticoagulant treatment may provide significant symptomatic palliation. Where possible, patients should be investigated with Doppler ultrasound, since this is less traumatic than contrast venography. V/Q scanning is justified if there is a suspicion of recurrent symptomatic pulmonary emboli but, if a venous thrombosis has been confirmed and anticoagulant therapy is to be instituted, it can be omitted. Patients with confirmed thrombosis should be managed with intravenous heparin and oral warfarinization, aiming to achieve an International Normalized Ratio of 2.5–3.5. However, as mentioned above, oral anticoagulation can be particularly difficult to manage in this group of patients. A delicate balance must be struck between the risks of further thrombo-embolism in inadequately anticoagulated patients and the hemorrhagic complications of excessive therapy. Disease progression in the form of bone marrow, hepatic or vascular invasion may increase the chance of bleeding, whilst immobilization, due to general debility, pathological fractures, or paralysis, may accentuate the prothrombotic state. The situation is rendered even more complex by the observation that some patients with cancer-related thrombo-embolic disease appear to be relatively refractory to conventional heparin and warfarin-based anticoagulation regimens, which can lead to a situation in which either recurrent cancer-related thrombo-embolic disease or hemorrhagic sequelae of high-dose anticoagulation may occur. The use of low molecular-weight heparins (LMWH), given as a single daily subcutaneous injection, may offer improved efficacy with fewer complications and reduced morbidity. Further studies are required to elucidate the role of these agents in the prevention and treatment of cancer-related thrombo-embolic disease (18).

Dyspnea

Shortness of breath is an extremely frequent and distressing symptom of end-stage malignant disease (7).

There are a variety of possible causes for this symptom (Table 27.5). It should be remembered that patients may often have more than one of these conditions contributing to the sensation of breathlessness. Careful assessment is important, since specific measures may be available against each of the individual problems. A chest radiograph will reveal the presence of gross metastatic deposits, lymphangitis carcinomatosa, pleural fluid, pulmonary infections, and pulmonary emboli. Measurement of the arterial oxygen tension by sampling of arterial blood or pulse oximetry may give a useful index of the degree of hypoxia and can also guide the provision of safe levels of oxygen therapy. Dyspnea is a frightening symptom and in many cases the patient may gain considerable symptomatic benefit from the regular prescription of drugs aimed at reducing the stress of this sensation. Useful agents include diazepam at a dose of 2 mg twice or thrice daily and morphine elixir at a dose of 5 mg every 4 h.

Gross pulmonary metastatic disease or lymphangitis carcinomatosa are rarely suitable for specific anti-tumor therapy in the palliative setting. Instead, management should focus on relieving the symptoms of breathlessness by provision of oxygen with or without the addition of a trial of intermediate dose dexamethasone 4 mg twice daily. Respiratory infections are often the immediate cause of death in patients with end-stage cancer and the issue of whether or not to treat them is often a difficult one. In general, if a patient has reached the phase of his illness heralding a terminal decline, active treatment of a chest infection with antibiotics is inappropriate, unless such treatment may potentially relieve unpleasant symptoms such as fever and pleuritic chest pain. In fact, these symptoms may be palliated far better by the use of physical means of cooling and antipyretic drugs to control fever and analgesia to control pain. Similarly, the treatment of symptomatic pulmonary emboli is a matter for careful clinical judgement. Anticoagulation does not guarantee effective prevention of further emboli and carries the risk of severe side-effects (16). The placement of vena caval filters is associated with a number of potential complications and requires the use of maintenance anticoagulation. Most patients are unlikely to gain a net benefit from this procedure.

The management of malignant pleural effusions depends on the degree of symptoms caused by the fluid and the availability of systemic therapeutic manoeuvres. The option of treating malignant effusions with specific anti-cancer therapies is seldom available in the palliative care of patients with advanced cancer. In general, pleural effusions of a sufficient size to cause dyspnea should be managed by drainage. This can be achieved as a simple palliative procedure with a 22 G intravenous cannula inserted under local anesthesia through the intercostal space allowing drainage of the fluid by direct suction via a 50-ml Luer lock syringe. A 3-way tap arrangement allows preservation of an air-tight seal with the fluid being voided into a measuring cylinder. It is usually possible to drain up to 1000 ml of pleural fluid safely over 10–20 min using this set-up. Attempts to drain more than this by direct suction over a short space of time can be accompanied by coughing, a feeling of chest tightness, and paradoxical worsening of the shortness of breath. These symptoms are thought to be due to the development of pulmonary edema secondary to the rapid re-expansion of collapsed lung tissue and accompanying mediastinal shift. Contrary to popular belief, this procedure can provide a significant improvement in symptoms without rapid reaccumulation of the pleural fluid. In patients with a limited life expectancy, this may be all that is required to control symptoms before death occurs by other disease-related processes. In the presence of recurrent or very large pleural effusions, it may be necessary to insert a chest drain. This should be done using a medium bore tube (16–18 F) under local anesthesia. After placement of the tube, 500–1000 ml can be drained immediately via a system with an under water seal. Thereafter, the tube should be clamped for 60 min and then 500 ml can be drained each hour until the rate of flow decrease to less than 500 ml/h, after which time the tube can be left on free-drainage. Once the chest has been drained to dryness, it is common to attempt to achieve a chemical pleurodesis using a range of agents including tetracycline (1 g mixed with bupivicaine) and bleomycin (60 mg) (19, 20). In patients in whom this procedure fails, it may be worthwhile to attempt a talc pleurodesis at mini-thoracotomy, or insertion of a pleuroperitoneal shunt (21), although, in the palliative setting, this should be considered carefully before it is undertaken.

Bone metastases

Pain due to bone metastases is a common feature in patients with advanced cancer. The pattern of metastasis of prostatic cancer is typically to the bones and this event represents a significant problem in patients with this disease. Bone pain generally arises due to erosive metastases and can present as a gradually worsening pain over a number of weeks or as a sudden pain arising from the occurrence of a pathological fracture.

Mild to moderate pain may be controlled by simple analgesia from levels 1 and 2 of the analgesic ladder, such as an NSAID. However, if this medication fails to give symptomatic relief within 1 week it should be discontinued because of the risk of adverse effects, such as gastric irritation. For more severe pain, a combination of morphine and an NSAID can be effective. Evaluation of the cause of the bone pain is very important. Radiographs of the affected area should be performed and patients with osteolytic deposits at risk of fracture should be considered for a prophylactic surgical approach if their underlying illness suggests that they have a reasonable life-expectancy. In the presence of demonstrable bony metastatic disease, palliative radiotherapy is extremely effective and gives pain relief in approximately 80–90% of cases (22). The optimal dose and schedule of palliative radiotherapy in this situation have not been defined clearly. The available data from randomized studies suggest that a short course or single-fraction radiotherapy is well-tolerated and as effective as more protracted irradiation schedules (23–27). Therefore, most patients will be palliated by a dose of 8 Gy as a single fraction or 20 Gy in five fractions. However, there is an apparent reluctance on the part of many physicians to use single-fraction or short-course radiotherapy, especially in sites of disease where there is a perceived risk of pathological fracture or in patients with a good performance status and a life-expectancy measured in months rather than weeks (28, 29). In such patients, a schedule of 30 Gy in ten fractions is frequently employed. In patients with recurrent bone pain in a site that has previously been irradiated with good effect, there is a very high response rate to repeated irradiation (22).

The pattern of bone metastases in prostate cancer is very often one of very diffuse disease involving almost the entire skeleton. Patients afflicted by such disease often have multiple areas of pain in different bony sites. In such cases, the provision of localized palliative radiotherapy may necessitate the treatment of multiple areas at the same time. This can be unsatisfactory both to the patient and the clinician, because of the difficulties of adequately matching irradiation fields. Therefore, under such circumstances, hemibody irradiation is frequently used. For example, if the painful sites are mainly restricted to the lower limbs, pelvis, and lumbo-sacral spine, delivery of a single fraction of radiation to the lower hemibody (usually to a field extending from the iliac crests to the lower femur) to a dose of 8 Gy as at the mid-plane can be very helpful. When treating the upper hemibody (usually to a field extending from the clavicles to the iliac crests), the dose prescription is reduced to 6 or 7 Gy. Patients receiving this form of treatment should receive pre-medication with intravenous 5-HT3 receptor antagonists and dexamethasone in addition to intravenous fluids.

An alternative to this form of wide-field irradiation is the use of systemically administered radioisotope treatment. Strontium-89, samarium-153, rhenium-186, and yttrium-90 have all been investigated as possible therapeutic isotopes (30–36). As yet, however, most studies have focused on the use of strontium-89 and its comparison to external-beam radiotherapy. A phase III randomized placebo control trial performed by Porter *et al.* (1993) (31) evaluated the effectiveness of strontium-89 as an adjunct to local-field radiotherapy in 126 patients. Although no significant differences in survival or in relief of pain at the index site were noted, there was a significant reduction in the need for analgesic medication in the isotope-treated arm. In addition, there was a significant difference in the progression of pain as measured by new pain sites or the need for further radiotherapy. These results were achieved at the expense of increased hematological toxicity in the patients treated with strontium-89. Qulity *et al.* (1994) (32) treated 284 patients with prostatic cancer and painful bone metastases in a randomized phase III trial comparing local or hemibody radiotherapy with strontium-89 radioisotope therapy. All treatments provided effective pain relief, with no difference between any of the study groups at 3 months. However, fewer patients reported new pain sites after strontium-89 than after local or hemibody radiotherapy. Once again, mild hematological toxicity occurred in the isotope-treated patients without significant clinical sequele. In view of these findings, it is unlikely that strontium-89 therapy will find a place in the routine palliative therapy of prostatic cancer metastatic to bone, although it may have a role in patients with very widespread disease which relapses rapidly after local radiotherapy.

Cerebral metastases

Brain metastases from prostate cancer are uncommon. In a large single institution study, Castaldo *et al.* (1983) (37) reported eight patients with brain metastases among a cohort of 189 patients. Otherwise, reports of prostate cancer metastatic to the brain have been restricted to single-case reports. Therefore, there are no data to suggest that the management of patients with brain metastases from prostate cancer should be any different from that of patients with other malignant diagnoses.

The diagnosis of brain metastases should be considered in patients presenting with new neurological symptoms and should be confirmed by CT scanning if further treatment is contemplated. During the period of investigation, it is usual to commence treatment with high-dose dexamethasone 8 mg twice daily and this treatment, in itself, may lead to a considerable improvement in symptoms by virtue of its effect on peri-tumor vasogenic edema (38). In the unlikely clinical situation of a patient with prostate cancer presenting with a single brain metastasis as the sole site of relapse, a surgical approach would be appropriate. However, it is far more likely that cerebral metastases will arise in the setting of widespread metastatic disease, in which case the treatment approach is entirely palliative. Patients with confirmed brain metastases should be considered as candidates for palliative radiotherapy. Palliative treatment of brain metastases accounts for approximately 5% of the workload of UK radiotherapy departments (39). This form of treatment can be very effective at relieving the symptoms of raised intracranial pressure and may restore motor and sensory function in certain circumstances. The optimal radiotherapy schedule remains to be defined. In the 1970s the Radiation Therapy Oncology Group (RTOG) conducted a number of studies in which patients received doses of radiotherapy ranging from 20 Gy in 1 week to 50 Gy in 4 weeks. The studies showed no difference between the different fractionation regimens in terms of neurological improvement (approximately 80%), time to disease progression (median 2–3 months), or overall survival (median 3.5–5 months) (40–42). Thereafter, the emphasis switched towards assessment of abbreviated courses of radiation in an attempt to provide effective palliation without the need for prolonged and intensive treatment. The RTOG conducted a pilot study in which patients were treated with either 10 Gy as a single fraction or 12 Gy in two fractions (42). The results of this study demonstrated no significant difference between the rate of onset of improvement, the median survival and the morbidity for the two abbreviated fractionation regimens and the more prolonged treatments delivering 30–40 Gy, which had been used in the earlier studies. There was a difference in the duration of symptom relief in favor of the higher radiation dose, but this effect was considerably attenuated by the use of further single-fraction brain irradiation in patients with recurrent symptoms. In a recent prospective randomized trial, 544 patients with symptomatic cerebral metastases were treated with whole-brain radiotherapy to a dose of either 12 Gy in two fractions on consecutive days or 30 Gy in ten fractions over 2 weeks (43). The median survival was 11 weeks for the two-fraction treatment and 12 weeks for the ten-fraction treatment. The short duration of survival hampered an adequate assessment of the response rates, but overall responses were seen in 39% and 44% of those treated with two and ten fractions, respectively.

Specific urological symptoms

Neuropathic pain syndromes in pelvic malignancy

Neuropathic pain arises as a result of damage to nerves of the peripheral or central nervous system. Such pains may present in a number of different ways, including shooting or stabbing, burning or dull aching pains. Certain recognizable syndromes exist in which patients present with reproducible symptoms and signs. Recognition of these types of pelvic pain allows the physician to commence appropriate therapy immediately. This is of considerable importance since these conditions are rarely responsive to opiates alone and usual require the addition of one or more adjuvant drugs (Table 27.6).

Uncontrolled local pelvic disease frequently presents with a constant, dull, aching or dragging pain, which radiates to the lower back. This pain may occur in conjunction with the pain of lumbosacral plexus involvement that causes pain in the lower back, which may radiate to the buttock and down the leg. It may also be associated with weakness and numbness in the distribution of the affected nerve roots. Similarly, disease involving the perineal nerve roots can cause a very unpleasant perineal sensation of stabbing or burning perineal pain. This pain can be exacerbated by sitting and patients with this problem often appear to be unable to keep still as they constantly shift their position in an attempt to gain respite from their discomfort. Such pelvic, lumbosacral, and perineal pains can be extremely difficult to control completely but most patients will gain some benefit from opiate analgesia, an anti-neuropathic agent such as amitryptiline or sodium valproate, and an NSAID. In patients who have not already received full-dose radiotherapy, palliative irradiation of bulk disease may lead to a degree of tumor shrinkage and relief of pressure on the affected nerves.

Tenesmus describes a feeling of fullness of the rectum that is associated with the desire to evacuate, which often exacerbates the discomfort rather than relieving it. Tenesmus can result from direct tumor infiltration of the rectum or involvement of sacral nerve roots. Opiate analgesia often gives some relief, although additional adjuvant agents, such as amitryptiline, sodium valproate, and calcium channel antagonists, are frequently needed.

Hematuria

Whilst hematuria can be a presenting symptom of prostate cancer, its reappearance later in the course of the disease process generally signals the presence of locally recurrent disease invading the urethra or

Table 27.6 Drugs commonly used as adjuvants to conventional analgesics

Nature of pain	Class of drug	Typical examples, dose, and schedule
Neuropathic	• Tricyclic anti-depressants	• Amitryptiline 25–150 mg at night
	• Anticonvulsant	• Valproate 100–400 mg b.d., carbamazepine 100–200 mg t.i.d.
	• Local anesthetic (oral)	• Flecainide 100–200 mg b.d., mexilitine 150 mg b.d.
	• Corticosteroid	• Dexamethasone up to 8 mg b.d.
	• Calcium channel blocker	• Nifedipine—start 5 mg t.i.d., maximum 20 mg t.i.d.
	• Others	• Baclofen—start 5 mg t.i.d. maximum 100 mg per day
Bone	• Bisphosphonates	• Clodronate 800 mg b.d./q.i.d., pamidronate 60–90 mg i.v. q3–4 wk
	• Corticosteroid	• Dexamethasone 2–4 mg b.d.
Muscle spasm		
Skeletal muscle	• Benzodiazepine	• Diazepam 2–5 mg b.d.
	• GABA antagonist	• Baclofen—start 5 mg t.i.d., maximum 100 mg per day
Smooth muscle	• Anticholinergic	• Hyoscine butylbromide up to 20 mg q.i.d.
	• Calcium channel blocker	• Nifedipine—start 5 mg t.i.d. maximum 20 mg t.i.d.

bladder base. In the absence of previously documented recurrence or metastatic disease, this should be confirmed in all cases by repeat cystoscopy and biopsy. Patients with repeated hemorrhage may suffer recurrent episodes of clot retention and symptomatic anemia requiring multiple blood transfusions. The principle aim of palliative treatment should be to secure hemostasis, if possible. The presence of infection, which can exacerbate hematuria, should be sought actively and treated appropriately. In patients who have already been treated with radical radiotherapy to the prostate at their initial presentation, palliation of this distressing symptom can be very difficult to achieve because doses up to tolerance will already have been used. However, if there is scope within the limits of normal tissue tolerance, further doses of radiotherapy (e.g. 8 Gy single fraction or 30 Gy in ten fractions) can be very effective. There have been no direct studies on the palliation of hematuria due to prostate cancer, although the ability of two different radiotherapy fractionation regimens to palliate the symptoms of bladder cancer has been evaluated in a prospective study (44). Patients were treated in a non-randomized fashion with either 17 Gy in two fractions over 3 days or 45 Gy in 12 fractions over 26 days. Patient selection was based on the clinician's assessment of their general condition and performance status. The two-fraction treatment was more effective at palliating pain and hematuria than the more protracted conventional fractionation, although the survival was shorter in this group of patients. Therefore, by analogy, it would seem to be appropriate to deliver treatment with one of these abbreviated fractionation regimens to patients with hematuria due to prostate cancer.

Patients who have already received maximal doses of radiotherapy can be treated in other ways. Ethamsylate is a non-hormonal agent, which decreases capillary exudation and blood loss. Its putative mechanism of action is by increasing capillary vascular resistance and platelet adhesiveness in the presence of vascular lesions. It has no direct action on the normal coagulation mechanism. It can be used at a dose of 500 mg q.i.d in patients with intractable hematuria (7). The antifibrinolytic agent, tranexamic acid, should be avoided in this situation since the formation of very hard clots can cause clot retention and even ureteric obstruction (7). Bladder irrigation with a 1% alum solution can also be of benefit (45). Similarly, intravesical instillation of a 4% solution of formalin has been reported with good results (46). Physical measures such as balloon distention, diathermy and embolisation should be used with great caution (7, 47).

Recurrent urinary tract infections

Patients with locally recurrent prostate cancer are prone to repeated episodes of urinary tract infection. This tendency may be increased by the need for catheterization in patients with bladder outflow obstruction, incontinence, fistulae, or clot retention due to hematuria. Patients with an in-dwelling urinary catheter will almost always have evidence of bacteriuria, which does not require specific therapy in the absence of local or systemic symptoms of infection. Patients presenting with dysuria, frequency, suprapublic discomfort, loin pain, or fever should have a specimen of urine taken for microbiological analysis. If the symptoms are mild to moderate it may be possible to wait for the result of this test before commencing therapy. If the symptoms are more severe, or if there is constitutional upset, it is reasonable to treat patients with a single dose of 400 mg of trimethoprim by mouth. This treatment is especially effective in the case of urinary tract infections in females. Patients with in-dwelling urinary catheters should receive a more prolonged course of antibiotics for 5–7 days according to the drug sensitivities demonstrated by the microbiological culture. In the case of repeated infections, it may be necessary to give a 2-week course of antibiotics and repeat the culture of the urine to ensure eradication of the responsible pathogen.

Fistulae

The development of urinary fistulae can be extremely distressing and frightening to patients. Locally advanced pelvic cancers can infiltrate the bowel leading to persistent leakage of urine. Less commonly, skin involvement and subsequent breakdown can also lead to leakage of urine through the skin. Uncontrolled fistulae may have a dramatic impact on a patient's quality of life and may result in an otherwise relatively well patient remaining virtually housebound. Active palliative therapy of a malignant fistula can lead to considerable improvements in quality of life and should be pursued vigorously.

The optimal management of a malignant fistula is dictated by the clinical situation. The standard surgical approach of excision of the fistula (48) and repair is often impossible in these patients. Therefore, the aim of treatment is more usually directed towards limiting the extent of leakage, minimizing the deleterious effects of constant perineal irritation due to leakage of urine and/or feces over the skin of the perineum and attempting to maintain the quality of life of the patient. Leakage can be reduced by inserting an in-dwelling urinary catheter. If appropriate, in patients with good performance status and a reasonable life-expectancy, urinary diversion with percutaneous nephrostomy tubes or formation of an ileal conduit offers an alternative. Skin care is of considerable importance since, unless it is protected by barrier creams and/or protective dressings, it can become severely excoriated and infected. Malodorous lesions can be effectively treated by the use of topical metronidazole gel (49).

Urinary incontinence

Urinary incontinence is a particularly distressing symptom that can have a devastating impact on the patient's quality of life. It is often caused by locally advanced disease within the pelvis resulting in disruption of the intrinsic sphincter. However, reversible causes such as urinary tract infection and overflow incontinence due to bladder outflow obstruction should be sought and treated appropriately. If possible, local hypofractionated radiotherapy at a dose of 30 Gy in 10 fractions may lead to a reduction in tumor bulk, which may restore the functional anatomy of the urinary sphincter. Where no reversible cause can be isolated, urinary catheterization is effective. An in-dwelling catheter is frequently employed, but the technique of intermittent self-catheterization may also be very useful, especially in patients who are unable to tolerate a urinary catheter on a permanent basis due to local symptoms, such as bladder or trigone irritation, or for patients with a hypotonic bladder. A catheter is inserted under clean conditions (strict asepsis is not necessary) at least four times a day and the bladder is emptied. The same catheter can be used repeatedly so long as it is sterilized between insertions.

Obstructive nephropathy

Locally uncontrolled prostate cancer, by virtue of is anatomical site, frequently causes life-threatening urinary obstruction. This condition can be treated relatively easily by insertion of percutaneous nephrostomy tubes followed by internalization of urinary drainage with J-J ureteric stents. However, in recent years there has been considerable controversy surrounding the ethics of such treatment. Some authors have proposed that urinary diversion is not in the patient's best interest, since a peaceful death from uremia may be prevented, with only a short-term extension of life-span of

poor quality ending in death from another, potentially more symptomatic, complication of the malignant disease (50). The contrary view has also been advanced, based on the observation of improvement in quality and quantity of life following percutaneous nephrostomy and insertion of J-J stents (51,52).

The importance of clinical criteria that can assist in selection of patients for appropriate use of nephrostomies has been demonstrated in a number of studies. Fallon *et al.* (1980)(51) summarized the features predicting for a beneficial outcome of urinary diversion as being undiagnosed malignant disease, prostatic and cervical primary tumors, patients for whom there is an available treatment modality with a reasonable chance of a response, and patients who request urinary diversion as a means of prolonging life for legal or financial reasons. Feuer *et al.* (1991) (52) concluded that the following criteria contra-indicated the insertion of drainage tubes: progression of disease while on therapy, potentially life-threatening coincidental medical problems, poor performance status, no available effective salvage therapy, non-compliance with treatment, and uncontrolled pain.

The role of urinary diversion has been investigated in a prospective study in 42 patients who presented with renal failure secondary to malignant obstructive nephropathy (53). Eight of the patients had locally advanced and/or metastatic prostate cancer. The obstructive nephropathy was relieved in 33 of the 42 patients by insertion of percutaneous nephrostomies. The median survival of the entire group was 133 days (range 7–712 days). Survival of 6 months or more was seen in 17 patients, three of whom had prostate cancer. However, five patients died within 30 days of undergoing urinary diversion, one of whom had prostate cancer. This point exemplifies the importance of careful selection of patients for treatment. Analysis of patients by the number of therapeutic modalities that they had received prior to urinary diversion revealed that patients who had been heavily pretreated with combinations of surgery, radiotherapy, hormonal therapy, and chemotherapy had a short median survival following urinary diversion, whereas the availability of an effective therapeutic option was associated with a greater probability of prolonged survival.

There have been a number of studies specifically addressing the issue of urinary diversion in prostate cancer. Fallon *et al.* (1980) (51) treated 100 patients with a variety of malignant diseases by surgical urinary diversion. They reported a median survival of 7 months for 37 patients with prostate cancer, with 18 patients surviving more than 6 months. Again, prolonged survival was shown to be associated with the availability of a further therapeutic options. In a similar study in 51 patients, Sanhu *et al.* (1992) (54) reported a 2-year survival rate of 57%, although the majority of these patients were suitable for palliative local surgery (84%) and hormonal manipulation (71%). A different experience was reported by Dowling *et al.* (1991) (55) who treated 22 patients with hormone refractory prostate cancer with percutaneous urinary diversion after the onset of ureteric obstruction. The median survival of the entire group was only 4 months, with patients spending almost half of their remaining lifetime in hospital. Therefore, these authors concluded that in such patients the use of urinary diversion was not justified in the absence of available salvage hormonal therapy. In patients in whom the use of urinary diversion is felt to be inappropriate, high-dose dexamethasone may represent a reasonable alternative (56), at least as a short-term measure.

Management of the dying patient

Optimum management of patients in the last few days of their lives presents a number of specific problems. When a stage at which a terminal decline has been reached, it is extremely important that the medical staff recognize this fact and communicate it clearly and sensitively to the family. Unnecessary treatment should be withdrawn and investigations, including blood tests and radiographs, should be discontinued. Strenuous efforts must be made to ensure that the patient has adequate provision of analgesics and anti-emetics. At this stage, all medication is usually delivered by subcutaneous syringe driver. Assessment of the presence of pain may be difficult and it is important to heed the advice of family members and nursing staff who have greater contact with the patient at this time. If there is doubt, it is wise to err on the side of caution in providing increased doses of analgesia, rather than leaving a patient with suboptimal pain control. Terminal agitation is often a part of the natural process, but it is important to exclude and treat reversible causes such as pain, urinary retention, or bowel obstruction. In the absence of these causes, sedation with a benzodiazepine (e.g. midazolam 10–30 mg over 24 h) or methotrimeprazine (25–100 mg over 24 h) can be very effective. Retained secretions can cause noisy breathing, the so-called 'death rattle', which can be distressing to family members and other patients. This can be relieved effectively by fluid restriction and subcutaneous hyoscine. Wherever possible, provision of a quiet side-room to allow the patient and family members a measure of privacy is an important consideration.

References

1. International Association for the Study of Pain (IASP). Subcommittee on the taxonomy classification of chronic pain. *Pain* 1986, **42**, 216–21.
2. World Health Organisation (WHO). *Cancer pain relief*. WHO, Geneva, (1986).
3. Sykes NP. Oral naloxone in opioid-associated constipation. *Lancet* 1991, **337**, 1475.
4. Campora E, Merlini L, Pace M. The incidence of narcotic-induced emesis. *Journal of Pain and Symptom Management* 1991, **6**, 428–30.
5. White ID, Hoskin PJ, Hanks GW *et al.* Morphine and dryness of the mouth. *British Medical Journal* 1989, **298**, 1222–13.
6. Schug SA, Zech D, Grond S. A long term survey of morphine in cancer pain patients. *Journal of Pain and Symptom Management* 1992, 7, 259–66.
7. Regnard CFB, Tempest S. *A guide to symptom relief in advanced cancer* (3rd edn). Haigh and Hochland Ltd, Manchester, UK, 1991.
8. Baines M, Oliver DJ, Carter RL. Medical management of intestinal obstruction in patients with advanced malignant disease. A clinical and pathological study. *Lancet* 1985, ii, 990–3.
9. Ashby MA, Game PA, Devitt P. Percutaneous gastrostomy as a venting procedure in palliative care. *Palliative Medicine* 1991, 5, 147–50.
10. Campagnutta E, Cannizzaro R, Gallo A *et al.* Palliative treatment of upper intestinal obstruction by gynecological malignancy: the usefulness of percutaneous endoscopic gastrostomy. *Gynecologic Oncology* 1996, **62**, 103–5.
11. Khoo D, Hall E, Motson R *et al.* Palliation of malignant intestinal obstruction using octreotide. *European Journal of Cancer* 1994, **30**, 28–30.
12. Mangili G, Franchi M, Mariani *et al.* Octreotide in the management of bowel obstruction in terminal ovarian cancer. *Gynecologic Oncology* 1996, **61**, 345–8.
13. Badger C, Twycross RG. Management of lymphoedema – guidelines. Sobell Study Centre, Oxford, UK, 1988.
14. Ambrus JL, Ambrus CM, Mink IB, *et al.* Causes of death in cancer patients. *Journal of Medicine* 1975, 6, 61–71.
15. Belt RJ, Leite C, Haas CD *et al.* Incidence of haemorrhagic complications in patients with cancer. *Journal of the American Medical Association* 1978, **239**, 2571–4.
16. Harrington KJ, Bateman AR, Syrigos KN *et al.* Cancer-related thromboembolic disease in patients with solid tumors: a retrospective analysis. *Annals of Oncology* 1997, **8**, 1–5.
17. Chan A, Woodruff RK. Complications and failure of anticoagulation therapy in the treatment of venous

thromboembolism in patients with disseminated malignancy. *Australian and New Zealand Journal of Medicine* 1992, **22**, 119–22.

18. Kakkar VV. Prevention and management of venous thrombosis. *British Medical Bulletin* 1994, **50**, 871–903.

19. Tattersall MHN, Boyer MJ. Management of malignant pleural effusions. *Thorax* 1990, **45**, 81–2.

20. Ruckdeschel JC. Management of malignant pleural effusions. *Seminars in Oncology* 1995, **22** (Suppl 3), 58–63.

21. Petrou M, Kaplan D, Goldstraw P. Management of recurrent malignant pleural effusions: The complementary role of talc pleurodesis and pleuroperitoneal shunting. *Cancer* 1987, **75**, 801–5.

22. Mithal NP, Needham PR, Hoskin PJ. Retreatment with radiotherapy for painful bone metastases. *International Journal of Radiation Oncology Biology Physics* 1994, **29**, 1011–4.

23. Price P, Hoskin PJ, Easton D. Prospective randomised trial of single and multi-fractional radiotherapy schedules in the treatment of painful bony metastases. *Radiotherapy Oncology* 1986, **6**, 247–55.

24. Price P, Hoskin PJ, Easton D *et al*. Low dose single fraction radiotherapy in the treatment of metastatic bone pain: A pilot study. *Radiotherapy Oncology* 1988, **12**, 297–300.

25. Hoskin PJ, Price P, Easton D *et al*. A prospective randomised trial of 4 Gy or 8 Gy single doses in the treatment of metastatic bone pain. *Radiotherapy Oncology* 1992, **23**, 74–8.

26. Cole DJ. A randomised trial of a single treatment versus conventional fractionation in the palliative radiotherapy of painful bone metastases. *Clinical Oncology* 1989, **1**, 59–62.

27. Niewald M, Tkocz H-J, Abel U *et al*. Rapid course radiation therapy vs more standard treatment: a randomised trial for bone metastases. *International Journal of Radiation Oncology Biology Physics* 1996, **36**, 1085–9.

28. Bates T. A review of local radiotherapy in the treatment of bone metastases and cord compression. *International Journal of Radiation Oncology Biology Physics* 1992, **23**, 217–21.

29. Booth M, Summers J, Williams MV. Audit reduces the reluctance to use single fractions for painful bone metastases. *Clinical Oncology* 1993, **5**, 15–8.

30. Crawford ED, Kozlowski JM, Debruyne FM *et al. et al*. The use of strontium 89 for palliation of pain from bone metastases associated with hormone-refractory prostate cancer. *Urology* 1994, **44**, 481–5.

31. Porter AT, McEwan AJ, Powe JE *et al*. Results of a randomized phase-III trial to evaluate the efficacy of strontium-89 adjuvant to local field external beam irradiation in the management of endocrine resistant metastatic prostate cancer. *International Journal of Radiation Oncology Biology Physics* 1993, **25**, 805–13.

32. Quilty PM, Kirk D, Bolger JJ *et al*. A comparison of the palliative effects of strontium-89 and external beam radiotherapy in metastatic prostate cancer. *Radiotherapy Oncology* 1994, **31**, 33–40.

33. Dearnaley DP, Bayly RJ, A'Hern RP *et al*. Palliation of bone metastases in prostate cancer. Hemibody irradiation or strontium-89? *Clinical Oncology* 1992, **4**, 101–7.

34. Collins C, Eary JF, Donaldson G *et al*. Samarium-153-EDTMP in bone metastases of hormone refractory prostate carcinoma: a phase I/II trial. *Journal of Nuclear Medicine* 1993, **34**, 1839–44.

35. Graham MC, Scher HI, Liu GB *et al*. Rhenium-186-labeled hydroxyethylidene diphosphonate dosimetry and dosing guidelines for the palliation of skeletal metastases from androgen-independent prostate cancer. *Clinical Cancer Research* 1999, **5**, 1307–18.

36. Rosch F, Herzog H, Plag C *et al*. Radiation doses of yttrium-90 citrate and yttrium-90 EDTMP as determined via analogous yttrium-86 complexes and positron emission tomography. *European Journal of Nuclear Medicine* 1996, **23**, 958–66.

37. Castaldo JE, Bernat JL, Meier FA *et al*. Intracranial metastases due to prostatic carcinoma. *Cancer* 1983, **52**, 1739–47.

38. Kirkham SR. The palliation of cerebral tumors with high dose dexamethasone: a review. *Palliative Medicine* 1989, **2**, 27–33.

39. Maher EJ, Dische S, Grosch E. Who gets radiotherapy? *Health Trends* 1990, **22**, 78–83.

40. Borgelt B, Gelber R, Kramer S *et al*. The palliation of brain metastases: Final results of the first two studies by the Radiation Therapy Oncology Group. *International Journal of Radiation Oncology Biology Physics* 1980, **6**, 1–9.

41. Kurtz JM, Gelber R, Brady LW *et al*. The palliation of brain metastases in a favourable patient population: a randomised clinical trial by the Radiation Therapy Oncology Group. *International Journal of Radiation Oncology Biology Physics* 1981, **7**, 891–5.

42. Borgelt B, Gelber R, Larson M *et al*. Ultra-rapid high dose irradiation schedules for the palliation of brain metastases: the final results of the first two studies by the Radiation Therapy Oncology Group. *International Journal of Radiation Oncology Biology Physics* 1981, **7**, 1633–8.

43. Priestman TJ, Dunn J, Brada M *et al*. Final results of the Royal College of Radiologists' Trial comparing two different radiotherapy schedules in the treatment of cerebral metastases. *Clinical Oncology* 1996, **8**, 308–15.

44. Srinivasan V, Brown CH, Turner AG. A comparison of two radiotherapy regimens for the treatment of symptoms from advanced bladder cancer. *Clinical Oncology* 1994, **6**, 11–3.

45. Bullock N, Whittaker RH. Massive bladder haemorrhage. *British Medical Journal* 1985, **291**, 1522–3.

46. Vicente J, Rios G, Caffaratti J. Intravesical formalin for the treatment of massive haemorrhagic cystitis: retrospective review of 25 cases. *European Urology* 1990, **18**, 204–6.

47. Muefti GR, Virdi JS, Singh M. Reappraisal of hydrostatic pressure treatment for intractable postradiotherapy vesical haemorrhage. *Urology* 1990, **35**, 9–11.

48. Holmes SAV, Christmas TJ, Kirby RS *et al*. Management of colovesical fistulae associated with pelvic malignancy. *British Journal of Surgery* 1992, **79**, 432–4.

49. Newman V, Allwood M, Oakes RA. The use of metronidazole gel to control the smell of malodorous lesions. *Palliative Medicine* 1989, **3**, 303–5.

50. Kerby IJ. Strive to keep alive? *Clinical Oncology* 1993, 5, 192.

51. Fallon B, Olney L, Culp DA. Nephrostomy in cancer patients: to do or not to do? *British Journal of Urology* 1980, 52, 237–42.

52. Feuer GA, Fruchter R, Seruri E. Selection for percutaneous nephrostomy in gynecologic cancer patients. *Gynecologic Oncology* 1991, 42, 60–3.

53. Harrington KJ, Pandha HS, Kelly SA *et al*. Palliation of obstructive nephropathy due to malignancy. *British Journal of Urology* 1995, 76, 101–7.

54. Sanhu DPS, Mayor PE, Sambrook PA *et al*. Outcome and prognostic factors in patients with advanced prostate cancer and obstructive uropathy. *British Journal of Urology* 1992, 70, 412–6.

55. Dowling RA, Carrasco CH, Babaian RJ. Percutaneous urinary diversion in patients with hormone-refractory prostate cancer. *Urology* 1991, 37, 89–91.

56. Hamdy FC, Williams JL. Use of dexamethasone for ureteric obstruction in advanced prostate cancer: percutaneous nephrostomies can be avoided. *British Journal of Urology* 1995, 75, 782–5.

28 | *Pain and symptom management in prostate cancer patients*

Jessie A. Leak and D. Edward Supkis

Introduction

Prostate cancer is the most common malignancy diagnosed in men in the United States (excluding skin cancer) (1, 2) and it is the second most common cause of male cancer mortality (3). Although it rarely occurs before the age of 50 (1), estimates are that one in ten men will develop the disease over their lifetimes (2). Incidence is now estimated to exceed that of breast cancer (3). Statistically, each year prostate cancer represents 36–41% of all newly diagnosed cancers in men and 14% of all cancer deaths (3, 4). While the incidence of prostate cancer is increasing by about 2.8% per year (1), there is some age-adjusted data to suggest that from 1990 to 1995 there was a decrease in mortality from the disease for white men under 70 years of age at diagnosis (5). Overall, however, mortality is estimated to increase by 37% by the year 2000, from data published in 1993.

Incidence of prostate cancer varies considerably by race and geographic location. US black males have the highest incidence and mortality rates in the world: as high as 90 per 100 000 (6, 7). The incidence for US white males (40–60 per 100 000) is similar to those in northern Europe. In contrast, in Asian countries, rates are as low as 2 per 100 000 (7–9). Asians, Hispanics, and Native Americans in the United States are noted to have significantly lower incidence and mortality than blacks and whites in the US (8, 10).

Typically, at the time of diagnosis, patients have non-metastatic disease (11) and are asymptomatic. Initial detection of incidental, non-palpable tumors (T1) is generally by elevations in prostate-specific antigen (PSA) or as a result of incidental pathologic findings after surgery for presumed benign prostatic hypertrophy. Clinically confined, palpable tumors (T2 and T3) are frequently found by digital rectal examina-

tion. Confirmation in these instances, is by transrectal ultrasound (TRUS)-guided transrectal needle biopsy (TRNB) utilizing a biopsy gun (12). Those with advanced disease, signified by tumors penetrating the capsule, and other metastatic disease may present with symptoms consistent either with encroachment on the urethra or the further sequelae of urethral blockage, decreased compliance of the detrusor muscle. Presentation may include hesitancy, decreased force of urinary stream, frequency, nocturia, urgency, or urgency incontinence. Impotence may result from compression of the neurovascular bundles (12). Accompanying symptoms may include fatigue or weight loss. Not infrequently, with advanced disease, pain associated with bony metastasis, particularly in the axial and appendicular skeleton (13) is present at the time of diagnosis.

Once the suspicion of prostate cancer is present, the patient will likely be referred to an appropriate oncology specialist or team who will confirm the diagnosis, stage the disease, and recommend treatment options. During the course of diagnosis, staging, and/or treatment, an anesthesiologist and/or a pain and palliative-care specialist may become involved as a consultant for a number of indications. They may take an active role in managing both intra-operative and post-operative surgical pain. In this continuum, these consultants may also play a critical role in managing pain and symptoms associated, not only with disease progression, but those that arise from other treatments including chemotherapy and radiation modalities. During all stages of the disease, but in particular with advanced disease, this may include but is not limited to, symptom assessment and management (e.g. nausea, pain, constipation, or depression). Their services may also include help in coping with such issues as impotency and sexual loss, spiritual care, chaplaincy, social services, and most other aspects of palliative and end-of-life care.

Etiology of acute pain in prostate cancer

It is important to remember that pain in prostate cancer can present as an acute syndrome at any time during the course of the disease or that a more chronic pain situation may develop and persist even in the face of a new, more acute pain. The following sections will outline possible etiologies for both acute and chronic pain syndromes that may develop either as a result of the cancer itself and/or its treatment.

Acute pain associated with interventional procedures

During the staging process, transrectal ultrasound-guided biopsy (TRUS) of the prostate may cause pain, which is generally transient and mild in nature. In preparation for this procedure, the surgical oncology team will occasionally consult with the anesthesiology team to provide sedation for patients who either have extreme anxiety or significant co-morbid medical conditions that would mandate special monitoring and/or sedation.

Post-operative pain associated with diagnostic (TRUS) or more limited procedures, such as transurethral prostatic resection (TURP) or orchiectomy, is generally quite manageable. Those patients with pre-existing, unrelated pain syndromes and those with extensive and/or metastatic disease will have a greater propensity to have pain that is much more difficult to manage post-operatively. Patients undergoing retroperitoneal lymph node dissection may benefit from epidural analgesia post-operatively; however to date, there are no definitive studies showing better outcomes with epidural analgesia versus patient controlled analgesia (PCA).

It is absolutely critical for the pain and symptom control team to work closely with the anesthesiologist to provide adequate analgesia for both the more chronic background pain, as well as the more acute post-operative pain. Probably the most important caveat is pre-operative identification of these patients, so that an appropriate peri-operative care plan can be outlined prior to surgical intervention.

Acute pain associated with cancer treatment and symptom management

Spinal opioid hyperalgesia syndrome

This is an uncommon complication of intrathecal or epidural injection of high-dose opioids used for the treatment of generally refractory pain. Symptoms may include pain or hyperalgesia associated with possible myoclonus, piloerection, and priapism. These symptoms generally abate after discontinuation of the drug(s) (14–16).

Opioid headache

Patients receiving opioids rarely report the onset of a generalized headache. This may be secondary to the fact that opioids may increase cerebral blood-flow. This effect may be due to histamine release.

Post-dural puncture headache

These headaches are characterized by a dull, occipital discomfort that may radiate to the frontal region (17–22). The headache is position-dependent and is most severe with upright posture. The headache occurs hours to days after the dura has been punctured. The larger the needle that is used to puncture the dura, the higher the frequency of headache (18, 19). If a standard bevel needle is turned parallel to the dural fibers or if a non-traumatic needle is utilized (i.e. 'B' bevel), there is a lower incidence of a post-dural puncture headache. Conservative treatment is generally recommended including bed rest, hydration, and analgesics. If the headache persists, an epidural blood patch may be performed (22–25), which will generally relieve the symptoms of the headache fairly expeditiously.

Intravenous infusion pain

Pain at the site of an intravenous (IV) infusion is multifactorial. Common etiologies are: infiltration, extravasation, chemical phlebitis, venous spasm, and infection. Where there is pain at an IV site, without inflammation or phlebitis, it is generally caused by vascular spasm. This spasm can be relieved with the application of warm compresses and/or by reducing the rate of intravascular infusion (26). When there is pain and erythema, especially along the line of the vein, chemical phlebitis is usually present; it is generally the result of potassium chloride, hyperosmolar solution, or infusion of cytotoxic medications (27, 28). Extravasation usually is characterized by intense pain followed by ulceration at the IV site. It is important to make an early diagnosis between chemical phlebitis and extravasation.

Acute pain associated with chemotherapy toxicity

Steroid-induced perineal discomfort

Rapid infusion of high-dose (20–40 mg) dexamethasone may cause a brief burning pain or sensation in the perineum (29, 30). Slow infusion may mitigate this problem (31).

Steroid-induced pseudorheumatism

Abrupt cessation or slow tapering of steroids taken for any length of time may, in some individuals, cause a non-specific pain constellation of myalgias, arthralgias, and painful muscles and joints. The only known treatment is to restart the steroids at a higher dose and taper more slowly (31–33).

Acute pain associated with other chemotherapeutic agents

Many single agent and combination chemotherapy protocols have been used in the treatment of Stage C and D prostate cancer (34). Several of these agents may induce acutely painful syndromes. Cisplatin, a metal-containing agent, is known to frequently cause a dose-related peripheral neuropathy (35, 36). Patients with pre-existing coronary artery disease who receive continuous 5-fluorouacil (5-FU) infusions are known to be at an increased risk for anginal chest pain associated with ischemic changes on continuous EKG (37–39). Carboplatin, a metal-containing agent, may cause peripheral neuropathy in a small percentage of patients (40). Vinblastine, a vinca alkaloid and an antimitotic agent, may be associated with headache, jaw pain, paresthesias, or peripheral neuropathy (41). On rare occasions, headaches are also associated with hydroxyurea (42). Etoposide is also known to cause peripheral neuropathies or paresthesias (43). Tumor flare, characterized by increasing bone pain, may be seen in 5–25% of patients receiving leuprolide acetate, particularly during the first 2 weeks of therapy (44–46). These effects may be at least partially mitigated with concomitant administration of the antiandrogens flutamide or bicalutamide (47).

Post-chemotherapy induced painful gynecomastia

Painful gynecomastia may occur in up to 50% of patients who use estramustine phosphate secondary to its estrogenic effects (48). Nipple pain and gynecomastia have also been reported with the anti-androgenic agent, flutamide (49, 50).

Acute pain associated with infection

Acute herpetic neuralgia

Cancer patients, particularly those who have received immunosuppressive therapies, may experience up to a 2- to 3-fold increased risk of herpes zoster neuralgia with its attendant lancinating-type pain. Generally, the pain resolves within 2 months, however if pain persists, the patient may require further management for post-herpetic neuralgia. The infection is characterized by pain or itching, which may precede the typical skin rash by many days. It is not unusual for the dermatomal distribution of the eruption to coincide with the tumor location; prostate cancer patients may be predisposed to zoster infections in the lumbosacral segments (51–53).

Chronic pain syndromes associated with prostate cancer

Some practitioners define chronic pain as that which lasts for more than 3 months and which persists beyond a recognizable nociceptive stimulus or usual healing process. In many cases, cancer pain could be termed as chronic. However, in those cases presenting with a persistent painful stimulus, cancer pain might technically be difficult to classify as chronic, despite its longevity. Clearly, though, the impact on the cancer patient's functional ability, lifestyle, finances, and general sense of well-being must be carefully considered in the circumstance of pain with duration of less than 3 months.

Chronic pain associated with tumor

Bony metastasis pain

Bone pain in prostate cancer is not uncommon. Up to 70–80% of prostate cancer patients eventually develop skeletal metastasis to the pelvis, proximal long bones, or spine (54). There is a low incidence of pathologic fractures (unless the patient has been on corticosteroids), however, the high morbidity is generally related to the long clinical course of the disease process itself.

Malignant epidural spinal cord compression

Approximately 7% of patients with prostate cancer will develop malignant epidural spinal cord compressions. Of this subset, 12.2% will have poorly differentiated tumors and 2.9% will have well-differentiated tumors. Pain is the presenting complaint in approximately 30% of prostate cancer patients with malignant epidural spinal cord compressions (55–57). The lower thoracic, lumbar, and sacral levels are most often affected (56). During evaluation, its important to ask about bowel and bladder dysfunction, as over one-half of patients presenting with spinal cord or cauda equina compression show evidence of these abnormalities. Urinary retention and incontinence is generally preceded by constipation (58).

Neuropathic and somatic pain may occur as a result of epidural tumor. Neuropathic pain and dysfunction may arise secondary to nerve root injury or axonal injury arising from either demyelination, ischemia, compression or inflammatory process. Mechanical disruption or distortion of bone and soft tissue elements (i.e. ligamentous structures, periosteum, dura mater, or blood vessels), along with inflammatory mediators induced during the process, may activate afferent nociceptive neurons and cause somatic pain. Mechanical pain, generally worsened with weight bearing and shifting, may be due to vertebral collapse and the resultant intrinsic instability.

Musculoskeletal pain

Non-specific musculoskeletal pain in prostate cancer is frequently related to deconditioning, prolonged bed rest, muscle wasting or atrophy, or general debility. It is imperative to rule out metastatic disease with any new complain of pain. A rehabilitation program can be critical in some circumstances to provide the patient with maximization of quality of life. In general, opioids may not be that effective in treating this type of pain.

Colic

Pain secondary to colic is most commonly related to constipation. Bowel and other malignant obstructions are unusual in prostate cancer. Symptomatic treatment with laxatives and propulsive agents are generally recommended (59).

Pain secondary to capsular stretching

This type of pain is generally from liver metastasis. Opioids may be only moderately helpful in symptomatic management. Adjunctive treatments might include steroids or NSAIDs.

Pain secondary to tumor mass

Tumor encroachment on adjacent viscera as well as other structures such as soft tissue and nerve plexi, may cause extreme pain. This pain is partially opioid sensitive. However, depending on the pathology, surgery, radiation, chemotherapy, or embolization may be helpful.

Chronic pain associated with treatment

Post-chemotherapy neuropathies

Please see Acute pain syndromes associated with other post-chemotherapies.

Avascular necrosis of femoral or humoral head

While avascular necrosis of the femoral or humoral head may be a complication of intermittent or continuous corticosteroid therapy, this condition may also occur spontaneously (60–62). Predisposing factors may also include a history of alcohol abuse (63). Osteocyte toxicity results in an inflammatory exudative process and vascular insufficiency, which leads to irreversible osteonecrosis apparent radiologically only months after the process is underway (64, 65).

Osteonecrosis may be unilateral or bilateral and occurs most frequently in the femoral head, presenting with pain in the hip, thigh, or knee. Humoral head involvement generally is typified by shoulder, upper arm or elbow pain. In general, pain associated with this syndrome is incident-type pain worsened with movement (66). Diagnosis is best made with a bone scan and a MRI. Treatment is generally supportive in the early stages. In some circumstances, consideration might be given to core decompression (to theoretically reduce medullary hypertension and to improve ischemia) at this point (67), although in a cancer population this would need consideration on a case by case basis. Osteotomy or arthroplasty might be necessary with advanced stage bone destruction (60, 67).

Chronic pain associated with surgical approach to metastatic disease

Prostate cancer skeletal metastasis is most common to the spine, pelvis, and proximal long bones (54). Persistent, chronic, postsurgical pain after vertebrectomy, open reduction/internal fixation, or joint replacement is not unusual. Even in a palliative care setting, patient participation in a good multidisciplinary rehabilitation program is critical to maximize functionality and to decrease pain.

Gynecomastia associated with hormonal treatment

Pain associated with chemotherapy-induced gynecomastia can be persistent into a chronic phase. It is important to distinguish gynecomastia in this circum-stance from a primary breast cancer or a secondary cancer in the breast (68, 69). Please see section under Acute pain: post-chemotherapy induced gynecomastia.

Chronic post-surgical abdominal pain, non-specific

Patients may develop chronic, persistent, non-specific abdominal pain after surgery. Differential diagnosis might include ventral hernia, granuloma formation, neuroma, myofascial pain related to deconditioning, non-specific cutaneous neuritis, or a neuropathic pain syndrome related to surgery.

Pain associated with lymphedema

Patients with prostate cancer are at risk for development of pain secondary to lymphedema if they have undergone surgery or whole-pelvis radiation (70). Other risk factors for lymphedema development are: diabetes, renal failure, cardiac disease, as well as poor nutritional status and obesity, both of which lead to poor wound healing and an increased risk of lymphedema (71, 72). Treatment is best managed utilizing a multi-disciplinary approach, which includes education, massage, skin care, containment hosiery, and exercise (73).

Conclusion

Table 28.1 summarizes types of chronic pain associated with prostate cancer as well as each group's relative sensitivity to opioids.

Table 28.1 Opioids sensitivity to various pain syndromes.

Pain syndrome		Opioid sensitivity
CHRONIC TREATMENT ASSOCIATED PAINS IN PROSTATE CANCER	Post chemotherapy neuropathies	Insensitive
	Avascular necrosis	Partially sensitive
	Associated with surgical Approach to metastatic Disease	Partially Sensitive
	Painful gynecomastia	Partially sensitive
	Non-specific postsurgical, Abdominal	Insensitive
	Lymphedema	Partially sensitive
CHRONIC CANCER RELATED PAIN IN PROSTATE CANCER	Bony metastasis	Partially sensitive
	Metastatic epidural spinal cord Compression	artially sensitive
	Musculoskeletal pain	Insensitive
	Colic	Insensitive (may be due to opioid)
	Capsular Stretching	Partially sensitive
	Tumor Mass	Partially sensitive

Assessment and treatment of pain and other symptoms

In order to facilitate evaluation and the subsequent management of cancer pain, it is critical to observe the following five elements:

1. It is important to determine whether the pain is somatic, visceral, neuropathic, or idiopathic, or a combination of two or more of these inferred pain mechanisms. Qualitative descriptors, location, and distribution are useful in this assessment.
2. Of equal import, is whether the pain is associated with the cancer itself versus various treatment modalities or both. Portions of this chapter outline possible mechanisms for both acute and chronic pain syndromes associated with both prostate cancer alone as well as its treatment. Temporal relationships are important to determine. Chronic pain is defined as any pain lasting greater than 3 months beyond the acute phase of an injury or illness. Cancer pain may be insidious and much more difficult to define because of the myriad of factors playing into its course.
3. Determination of pain intensity is one of many elements in symptom management. Unfortunately, many practitioners may rely too heavily on variants of visual analog scales to determine pain intensity and treatment response to pain. Failure to accurately assess other symptomatology, mental status, psychosocial issues, and past history of chemical coping may lead to ultimate failure of pain treatment modalities. For this reason, it is important to assess the full picture when treating a presenting complaint of pain.
4. The impact of pain on activities of daily living (ADLs), as well as any role that it may play in the patient who is suffering, is an important part of realistically managing pain. Loss of independence (ADLs) and the management of suffering will be discussed further.
5. Always believe the patient's complaints of pain and other symptoms. Always investigate new complaints, no matter how vague.

Pain and symptom assessment

While pain is now being regarded as the 'fifth vital sign', it must be assessed in the context of the patient's entire symptom presentation, psychosocial milieu, level of cognitive function, and whether or not the patient has a history of chemical-coping strategies. There are a number of validated assessment tools in use that objectively quantify and qualify symptomatology, including pain. These provide some rational and consistent basis for treatment algorithms (74–79). The Symptom Assessment System used at MD Anderson Cancer Center (Fig. 28.1) utilizes many features of these inventories in a concise trendable fashion to maximize symptom recognition and treatment effectiveness (80). The Mini-Mental State Examination (MMSE) (Fig. 28.2), and The Cage Questionnaire (Fig. 28.3) help to quantify cognitive function and a history of chemical-coping, respectively (80–83). These three tools along with a functional assessment tool (i.e. the Edmonton Functional Assessment Tool (EFAT) or the Karnofsky Performance Status scale (KPS)) (84, 85), as well as a psychosocial assessment, are the basis of a comprehensive symptom control and/or palliative care intake. These tools are useful in both acute and chronic pain settings and provide meaningful data for a multidisci-

THE UNIVERSITY OF TEXAS
MD ANDERSON
CANCER CENTER

Patient Name: ______________
MDACC #: ______________
Date: ______________

SYMPTOM CONTROL & PALLIATIVE CARE
SYMPTOM ASSESSMENT

No Pain	0 1 2 3 4 5 6 7 8 9 10	Worst Pain Imaginable
No Fatigue	0 1 2 3 4 5 6 7 8 9 10	Worst Fatigue Imaginable
No Nausea	0 1 2 3 4 5 6 7 8 9 10	Worst Nausea Imaginable
No Depression	0 1 2 3 4 5 6 7 8 9 10	Worst Depression Imaginable
No Anxiety	0 1 2 3 4 5 6 7 8 9 10	Worst Anxiety Imaginable
No Drowsiness	0 1 2 3 4 5 6 7 8 9 10	Worst Drowsiness Imaginable
No Shortness Of Breath	0 1 2 3 4 5 6 7 8 9 10	Worst Shortness of Breath Imaginable
Best Appetite	0 1 2 3 4 5 6 7 8 9 10	Worst Appetite Imaginable
Best Sleep	0 1 2 3 4 5 6 7 8 9 10	Worst Sleep Imaginable
Best Feeling Of Wellbeing	0 1 2 3 4 5 6 7 8 9 10	Worst Feeling of Wellbeing Imaginable

Assessed by: ______________

Fig. 28.1 The Symptom Assessment System used at MD Anderson Cancer Center, aiming to maximize symptom recognition and treatment effectiveness.

plinary approach to the treatment of cancer-related symptoms and cancer treatment sequelae.

The Symptom Assessment System used at MD Anderson Cancer Center (Fig. 28.1) (80) is a tool used to assist the patient at each visit to qualify his or her symptoms. These symptoms include pain, fatigue, nausea, depression, anxiety, drowsiness, shortness of breath, appetite, sleep, and well-being. Patient opinion (not caregiver or healthcare professional) is the 'gold standard' for symptom assessment. Ideally, the patients should complete their own assessment. It is important to be aware of language barriers with any assessment tool and make appropriate arrangements for translation. For patients who are illiterate, a tool with faces may need to be made available. This tool is an excellent way to track symptoms over time, as each 'snapshot' may change with tumor progression as well as with treatment of the symptoms and the disease.

The Mini-Mental State Examination (Fig. 28.2) is a widely used, well-validated tool for cognitive impairment screening (82, 83). It measures orientation to time and place, immediate recall, short-term memory, calculation, language, and construct. This tool is excellent for detecting cognitive impairment, which may be masked or mistaken for symptoms of depression.

The Cage Questionnaire (Fig. 28.3) (81) should be completed at the time of the initial evaluation to avoid putting the patient on the defensive. The questions should apply to lifetime experience, even if the patient is not currently using alcohol. The questions should be asked prior to any questions regarding amount of alcohol ingested. A positive Cage (2/4 answered 'yes') indicates that the patient has had a history of chemical-coping and maladaptive behavior in stressful situations. Physicians frequently miss a history of alcoholism as part of their initial evaluation.

Pathophysiology of pain

Pain is thought to result from activation of peripheral nociceptors or mechanoreceptors via stimulation of mechanical (compression/infiltration) or chemical (i.e. prostaglandin, bradykinin) mediators. The resultant neuropathophysiology gives rise to four types of pain (Table 28.2).

THE UNIVERSITY OF TEXAS
MD ANDERSON CANCER CENTER

Patient Name: _____
MDACC #: _____
Date: _____

Mini-Mental State Assessment

MAXIMUM SCORE	SCORE	
5		What is the (day), (month), (date), (year), (season)?
5		Where are we: (city) (state) (country) (hospital) (floor)?
3		State 3 objects and ask patient to remember them: Glass Blanket Pencil
5		Spell WORLD backwards.
3		Ask for the 3 objects named above. If unable to name, give patient cues but score only for objects named without cues.
2		Ask patient to name these objects: Pen (or 2 other objects in the room) Watch
1		Ask the patient to repeat the following: "No ifs, ands or buts."
3		Have patient follow three stage command: "Take this sheet of paper in your right hand, fold it in half, and give it to me."
1		Read and obey the following: CLOSE YOUR EYES
1		Write a sentence (give the patient a topic).
1		Copy a design.
30		TOTAL SCORE

** Please make a note of any delay/hesitancy to respond or omissions. If score = 0, specify reason.

Years of Schooling:		Age					
		< 40	40-49	50-59	60-69	70-79	> 79
0 - 4 years		20	20	20	19	18	16
5 - 8 years		24	24	25	24	23	22
9 – 12 years		28	28	27	27	26	23
College or higher		29	29	28	28	27	26

Fig. 28.2 The Mini-Mental State Examination (MMSE) used at MD Anderson Cancer Center, aiming to quantify cognitive function.

THE UNIVERSITY OF TEXAS
MD ANDERSON CANCER CENTER

Patient Name: _____
MDACC #: _____
Date: _____

SYMPTOM CONTROL & PALLIATIVE CARE THE CAGE QUESTIONNAIRE

1. Have you ever felt that you should cut down on your drinking? Yes ☐ No ☐
   * do not continue if patient has NEVER had a drink*

2. Have you been annoyed by people criticizing your drinking? Yes ☐ No ☐

3. Have you ever felt bad or guilty about your drinking? Yes ☐ No ☐

4. Have you ever had a drink first thing in the morning or a drink to get rid of a hangover (eye-opener)? Yes ☐ No ☐

Assessed by: _____

Fig. 28.3 The Cage Questionnaire used at MD Anderson Cancer Center provides a history of chemical coping.

Table 28.2   Types of pain.

Type of pain	Descriptions	Examples	Opioid respond
SOMATIC	Dull, throbbing, aching, sharp Localized	Bone metastasis Muscle/soft tissue Tumor infiltration	Good to Excellent
VISCERAL	Deep, squeezing, cramping May be poorly localized	Liver or intra-abd Metastasis	Good
NEUROPATHIC	Burning, dysesthetic Lancinating "electric shock" like Generally at or near site of sensory loss or change	Trigeminal neuralgia Post herpetic Neuralgia	Poor
IDIOPATHIC	Variable	Variable	Variable to Poor

Somatic pain

Somatic pain, also known as nociceptive pain, implies pain associated with activation of primary afferent neurons stimulated by an ongoing noxious stimulus. This pain is generally well-localized in cutaneous or deep tissues and may be described as throbbing, sharp, aching, or dull. Examples might include post-surgical pain, metastatic bone pain, or myofascial/musculoskeletal pain, such as that resulting from prolonged bedrest (86). This type of pain may be quite opioid-responsive (87, 88).

Visceral pain

Visceral pain (actually a subset of somatic pain syndromes), in contradistinction to somatic pain, is frequently characterized as poorly localized. Pain descriptors may include deep, squeezing, pressure-like, or cramping when hollow viscus obstruction has occurred. With capsular involvement, such as with the liver, the patient may represent pain more as sharp or throbbing. Nociceptive activation occurs in these circumstances with infiltration, compression, extension, or stretching of thoracic, abdominal, or pelvic viscera (86). Autonomic dysfunction, such as nausea or diaphoresis, may accompany progression of this type of pain. When assessing pain, it is important to differentiate between referred visceral pain to a distant cutaneous site versus somatic pain. Clearly, this could profoundly influence indications for palliative pain therapies. An example might be a patient presenting with shoulder pain. The practitioner is faced with distinguishing a possible bony versus diaphragmatic irritation secondary to carcinomatosis.

Neuropathic pain

Neuropathic pain generally presents as a severe pain at or near the site of sensory loss characterized by burning, dysesthetic pain. Allodynia, perception of pain with a non-noxious stimulus (89), frequently is an accompanying feature. Central sensitization may be responsible for the paroxysmal, electric-shock type sensations commonly experienced with neuropathic pain. The pathophysiology of this type of pain is felt to be related to injury to peripheral or central neural structures. The resultant defects may include abnormal somatosensory processing at the site peripherally or in centrally mediated sympathetic pain as well as deafferentation syndromes. Autonomic dysregulation may be present with sympathetically mediated pain (i.e. swelling or vasomotor abnormalities). Examples might include lumbar plexopathies, peripheral neuropathies related to chemotherapeutic agents, paraneoplastic peripheral neuropathies or phantom limb pain. This type of pain may not be particularly responsive to opioids (87–91), the use of adjunctive agents (92–94), or interventional techniques may become critical in effective management of neuropathic pain.

Idiopathic pain

Idiopathic pain is sometimes perceived to be 'pain out of proportion with physical findings'. While rare in a cancer population, patients who tended toward somatization or who present with a functional somatic syndrome (95) prior to their cancer diagnosis will possibly have a greater propensity to manifest these tendencies after diagnosis, particularly with non-cancer related pain. The patient who has tended to cope chemically and somatically in the past will not likely change their coping strategies. It is important to identify these patients as such; however, punitive withholding of treatment based on this type of history is inappropriate. It is important to remember that no matter what the etiology, dealing effectively with pain in a cancer patient will require the practitioner to employ a variety of techniques to empower the patient to maximize their quality of life.

Conclusion

It is important to keep in mind that most cancer patients have more than one type of pain (96, 97). Neuropathic pain represents approximately 15–20% of all cancer-pain syndromes. This may be in combination with both visceral and somatic complaints. It is crucial to make these distinctions in order to maximize medication regimens (opioids and adjuvants), to discern those patients with undetected recurrence and to identify those that may benefit from other interventional and palliative therapies. When a patient presents with a new complaint of pain, it is critical to rule out further progression of the disease, particularly if further therapeutic or palliative treatments might be helpful.

The treatment of the symptom of pain

The treatment of pain focuses on the tiered, 3-step analgesic ladder advocated by the World Health Organization (WHO) (98). While opioids are the mainstay of cancer pain management, certain pain may be more or less sensitive to opioids. It is important to understand the pathophysiology of different types of pain so that a reasonable treatment plan can be implemented. In many circumstances, it may be essential to include non-narcotic adjuncts to either potentiate or to add to the opioid effect.

Narcotic analgesics in cancer-pain management

Pure opioid agonists in single-agent form are generally preferred for cancer pain treatment. These include fentanyl, hydromorphone, methadone, morphine, and oxycodone. Hydrocodone and codeine, also pure agonists, are manufactured as mixed agents with acetaminophen, although codeine is available singly. It is

important to remember that there is no 'ceiling effect' with opioids. Dosages can be extremely variable from patient to patient and should be increased until the desired analgesic effect is achieved or until problematic side-effects arise. Using combinations of pure agonists can produce additive effects.

The use of opioid partial agonists, such as buprenorphine, or mixed agonist–antagonists, such as butorphanol, nalbuphine, or pentazocine, should be avoided in the treatment of cancer pain. These medications have a dose-related ceiling effect and may cause problems with withdrawal.

Routes of administration

The oral route of administration is always preferred, but may be limited by dysphagia, delirium, bowel obstruction, or severe cognitive disturbance. Alternate administration routes include rectal, transdermal, transmucosal, parenteral, or neuraxial. Rectal administration can be safe and inexpensive but may be contraindicated for those patients with anorectal lesions or severe thrombocytopenia. Most opioids can be compounded for rectal use, but absorption may be variable. The transdermal route, most frequently used for fentanyl, may take several days to titrate and may therefore be more efficacious for stable pain syndromes. Transmucosal (i.e. oral transmucosal fentanyl) application may be extremely effective but expensive. Parenteral narcotics (equally efficacious intravenous or subcutaneous) may be given intermittently or by continuous infusion. The neuraxial route, either epidural or intrathecal, may be indicated in select situations.

Beginning and maintaining opioid therapy

The practitioner should start with conservative 'around-the-clock' (ATC) dosing and provide appropriate rescue medication for breakthrough pain. Once the medication has been titrated effectively over 3–4 days, a maintenance regimen can be established. Frequent intermittent assessments will be necessary to monitor for signs of toxicity or intolerant side effects, to assess the need for upward titration of medication as the disease progresses, and to verify satisfactory opioid effect.

Opioid toxicity

Toxic opioid metabolites may accumulate in patients who develop renal insufficiency, in those patients requiring high doses and/or those who have taken opioids for a prolonged period. Signs of toxicity may include intractable nausea, somnolence, pruritus, or evidence of neurotoxicity including delirium, myoclonus, or hyperalgesia. Treatment of toxicity includes symptomatic use of haloperidol for delirium, assessment and treatment of any underlying metabolic disorder, hydration and rotation of opioids. In the event of renal insufficiency, patients should have their opioid doses reduced empirically to avoid toxic accumulation of metabolites.

Rotation of opioids

Rotation of opioids may be needed when the following occur: pain is uncontrolled despite relatively high opioid doses, when administration of the current regimen becomes unwieldy due to large numbers of pills, etc., or when tolerance or toxicity occurs.

The procedure for rotation should be:

(1) calculate the current opioid dose in each 24-h period;

(2) determine a new opioid and find its equianalgesic dose conversion (Table 28.3);

(3) automatically reduce the new total opioid dose by at least 30–50% (per 24-h period) to compensate for incomplete cross-tolerance between narcotics and determine the new daily (24-h) dose of opioid;

(4) provide adequate opioids (short-acting) for break-through pain;

(5) assess frequently.

Cautions about methadone use

Methadone is a synthetic opioid agonist and N-methyl-D-aspartate (NMDA) antagonist. Advantages of this potent narcotic are excellent absorption, high lipid solubility, low cost, and high potency. The down side of methadone use is that the drug has an unpredictable half-life, decreased opioid cross-tolerance, and a lack of known metabolites.

Extreme caution is warranted when converting patients from other narcotics to methadone. Lawlor *et al.* observed that dosing ratios may be significantly underestimated for methadone. This same group noted dosing ratios of up to 11.36:1 when converting morphine to methadone (99). Other groups recommend ratios ranging from 1:1 up to 4:1 (oral route) (100–102). Methadone should not be administered as a subcutaneous infusion.

Table 28.3 Conversion from one opioid to another, in equianalgesic doses.

Conversion from another onioid to morphine (use table below):
a. Total amount of opioid that effectively controls pain in 24 hours.
b. Multiply by conversion factor in table below. Give 30% less of the new opioid to avoid partial cross-tolerance.
c. Divide by the number of doses/day.

Opioid	From parenteral opioid to parenteral morphine	From same parenteral opioid to oral opioid	From oral opioid to oral morphine	From oral morphine to oral opioid
Morphine	1	2.5	1	1
Hydromorphone (Dilaudid®)	5	2	5	0.2
Meperidine (Demerol®)	0.13	4	0.1	10
Levorphanol	5	2	5	0.2
Codeine	—	—	0.15	7
Oxycodone	—	—	1.5	0.7
Hydrocodone	—	—	0.15	7

The emerging view of opioid rotation, particularly when converting *to* methadone from other narcotics is that conversion ratios are not always the same both ways. In other words, converting *from* methadone *to* other narcotics may require different conversion factors. It is also notable that there is extreme interpersonal variability. Perhaps most importantly, it is now recognized that excitatory amino acids may play a significant role in the development of opioid tolerance and in the opioid-resistant pain associated with neuropathic pain. NMDA receptor antagonists, such as methadone, may actually work to reverse this tolerance (103, 104). It is therefore, extremely critical to be aware that previously published conversion factors may lead the practitioner into a false sense of security about using high doses of methadone in a drug-tolerant patient.

Adjuvant analgesics in cancer-pain management

While opioids are the mainstay of cancer-pain management, other medications may be used with narcotics to potentiate the opiate effect or to treat pain that is not sensitive to opiates. Not infrequently, treatment adjuncts may also be administered to treat opioid side-effects and thus allow the narcotic to work more effectively in treating the primary complaint of pain. Table 28.4 details treatment adjuncts that may be useful for different types of pain.

Table 28.4 Adjuvant analgesics in cancer pain management.

Adjuvant class	Examples of drug	Drug indication	Potential side effects
Antidepressants	Tricyclic antidepressant Amitriptyline	Non-specific cancer pain Postherpetic neuralgia Headache General cancer pain with depression	Cardiotoxicity (rare) Orthostatic hypotension Sedation Anticholinergic effects
	Doxepin	Headache	Same
	Clomipramine	Neuropathic pain Idiopathic pain	Same
	Nortriptyline	Mixed neuropathic pains Diabetic neuropathy	Neuroleptic malignant syndrome (rare) Cardiotoxicity (rare) Less likely to cause orthostatic hypotension Sedation Anticholinergic effects
	Non-tricyclic antidepressants Paroxetine	Non-specific pain adjuvant	Anxiety, 'activation', insomnia
	Trazodone		Cardiotoxicity, Sedation Orthostatic hypotension
Corticosteroids	Dexamethasone or Prednisone or Methylprednisolone	Neuropathic pain (RSD) Bone pain Pain secondary to obstruction of hollow viscus	Short term Delirium Mood changes Hyperglycemia Fluid retention Dyspepsia, ulcers Long term Cushingoid/body habitus changes Weight gain Severe osteoporosis Myopathy Increased infection risk Late neuropsychic effects
Neuroleptics	Methotrimeprazine	Non-specific cancer pain	Sedation Tardive dyskinestheia (late effect only) Neuroleptic malignant s.

Table 28.4 Adjuvant analgesics in cancer pain management *(continued)*

Adjuvant class	Examples of drug	Drug indication	Potential side effects
Oral or parenteral local anesthetics	Mexiletine (p.o.)	Neuropathic pain, dysesthetic-lancinating	Nausea and/or vomiting Tremor, dizziness Paresthesias
	Lidocaine (i.v.)	Neuropathic pain, dysesthetic-lancinating (conflicting views on efficacy in cancer patients)	Cardiac conduction Disturbances Dose-related dizziness, perioral numbness, paresthesias, progressing to encephalopathy and seizures
Anticonoulsants	Gabapentin	Neuropathic pain, lancinating	Drowsiness, fatigue
	Carbamazepine	Neuropathic pain, lancinating	Drowsiness, dizziness, nausea Leukopenia and/or thrombocytopenia (2%)
	Phenytoin	Neuropathic pain, Lancinating diabetic Neuropathy Post-herpetic Neuralgia	Dose dependent sedation, dizziness, unsteadiness Rare hepatotoxicity Cutaneous abnormalities
Alpha-2 adrenergic Agonists	Clonidine	Neuropathic, lancinating and dysesthetic, cancer pain (intraspinal route in clinical trials)	Sedation Hypotension (usually orthostatic) Dry mouth
N-methyl-D-aspartate Receptor antagonists	Ketamine	Experimental, may be helpful in certain neuropathic pain syndromes	Dissociative anesthetic agent
Osteoclast inhibitors	Biphosphonates Pamidronate	Metastatic bone pain	Rare hypocalcemia Nausea Flu-like syndrome related to release of cytokines (20%)
Radiopharmaceuticals	Strontium chloride-89	Metastatic bone pain (efficacious in endocrine-resistant)	Transitory pain flare Transient bone marrow suppression
Non-steroidal anti-inflammatory drugs (NSAIDs)	Non-selectiv Salicylates Acetates Propionates Fenamates Oxicams Preferential COX-2	Mild to moderate somatic pain (as recommended by WHO)	Dose-dependent GI: Nausea, vomiting, hemorrhage, perforation inhibition of platelet aggregation, nephrotoxicity, bronchospasm
	Inhibition Selective COX-2 Inhibition		Gastrointestinal side effccts May provide advantage of having no effect on platelet function

Constipation

Constipation affects up to 95% of palliative care patients taking chronic opioids (105) and has a prevalence of approximately 50–65% in terminal cancer patients as a group as a whole (106–109). It is impor- tant to remember that constipation in such a patient is not always solely due to opiate intake. The causes of constipation in this patient population can be multi-factorial and may include poor fluid intake or de-hydration, malnutrition with resultant autonomic neuropathy related to the anorexia/asthenia/cachexia of advanced cancer, decreased mobility, hypokalemia or hypercalcemia, or other drugs including iron, diuretics, anti-depressants, antacids, anti-hypertensive drugs, anticholinergics, anticonvulsants, or vinca alkaloids. Co-existing primary or secondary disease states including diabetes, pheochromocytoma, Parkinson's disease, or hypothyroidism may be contributing factors (109–111).

A presenting picture of any one or more of the following symptoms should raise the index of suspicion for constipation: irregular bowel movements, diarrhea, nausea and vomiting, abdominal discomfort or distension, or bowel obstruction should alert the practitioner to this problem (111, 112).

To fully assess the picture, a digital rectal examination should be performed to rule out impaction and to determine whether or not the vault has stool present (111). A plain abdominal radiograph may also be extremely helpful in documentation and assessment of this distressing symptom (111, 112).

It is also important to remember that just because a patient is not eating, there is still daily production of intestinal debris. Approximately one-eighth of a pound of accumulated matter must be eliminated each day no matter how much oral intake occurs. Therefore, under ideal circumstances, bowel movements should continue even without oral intake.

Treatment focuses on prophylaxis and therapeutic management. Aggressive attention to maintenance and prevention of these symptoms includes the prophylactic use of laxatives whenever constipating drugs, particularly opiates, are prescribed. In addition, sufficient oral fluid intake and ingestion of fiber-containing food will help to minimize the likelihood of constipation. Fiber alone, however, is not known to be a critical factor (113). Managing stress and maintaining daily activity levels will also help in prophylaxis (111, 114).

Laxative agents for prophylactic and therapeutic use may be by the oral and/or rectal route. Oral laxatives are generally of the softening/osmotic variety or peristaltic stimulants. Softening agents may include liquid paraffin preparations, surfactant laxatives such as docusate sodium, bulk-forming agents such as methyl cellulose, or osmotic laxatives such as lactulose or saline solutions of magnesium hydroxide or sulphate. Peristaltic stimulants might include senna-containing compounds or bisacodyl, a polyphenolic. In general, latency of action for oral agents varies from hours to days, thus making rectal laxatives a more desirable alternative in some cases. While distasteful for patient and staff alike, rectal laxatives generally have a faster

onset of action. These may include lubricant (e.g. olive oil), osmotic (glycerine or sorbitol), surfactant (e.g. sodium docusate), saline (e.g. sodium phosphate), or polyphenolic (bisacodyl) rectal laxatives (91).

Nausea and vomiting

Chronic and prolonged nausea, generally defined as that extending beyond 4 weeks (109, 115), is extremely prevalent in patients with advanced cancer. Estimates range from 21% to 68% in this patient population (115). The most common causes of nausea are noted below in Table 28.5 (109). In general, nausea is related to direct central effects, delayed gastric emptying, constipation, or vestibular dysfunction (115).

Treatment of nausea in these scenarios is two-pronged: elimination or amelioration of the underlying cause and careful and aggressive use of anti-emetic drugs. It is important to determine whether or not the patient has a bowel obstruction. In this scenario, metoclopramide is to be avoided. Otherwise, this drug may be quite effective as a first-line drug, particularly the slow-release form (109, 115, 116). Dexamethasone or other corticosteroids may potentiate the beneficial effects of metoclopramide (115, 116). In bowel-obstructed patients, the use of agents that minimize gastro-intestinal secretions and motility may be helpful.

Cognitive impairment and delirium

Cognitive impairment/failure and attendant delirium are extremely prevalent in patients with advanced cancer, particularly as they approach the active state of dying (117). Prevalence in this patient population ranges from 25% to 85% (118–125). This symptom is particularly distressing to the family and staff (124, 126). Delirium is defined as 'a transient organic brain

Table 28.5   The most common causes of nausea in prostate cancer patients

Major causes of chronic nausea in cancer patients
Constipation
Opioid therapy
Autonomic failure
Bowel obstruction
Metabolic abnormalities
Radiation therapy
Peptic/Gastric ulcer disease
Increased intracranial pressure
Other drugs

syndrome characterized by the acute onset of disordered attention and cognition, accompanied by disturbances of psychomotor behavior and perception' (127). Delirium is not infrequently misdiagnosed as depression; early delirium may easily be overlooked (119, 128).

Presenting signs and symptoms may include one or more of the following: cognitive failure, fluctuating levels of consciousness, changes in the sleep–wake cycle, psychomotor agitation, hallucinations, delusions, and other perception abnormalities (109). Frequent causes may include opioid toxicity, infection, dehydration, metabolic abnormalities particularly hypercalcemia or hyponatremia, as well as the masking effects of other drugs (e.g. benzodiazepines or other centrally-acting agents).

Adequate assessment using the MMSE or other tool is essential. Once it is determined that the patient is indeed experiencing delirium, it is sub-classified as hyperactive or hypo-active. In the case of hyperactive delirium, the symptoms should be managed with appropriate medication. Haloperidol is useful as a temporizing measure until reversible causes are systematically ruled out (197–130). Methotrimeprazine may be an attractive pharmacologic alternative in terminal delirium, although its limitations include hypotension and excessive sedation (131). If the delirium does not abate after judicious use of neuroleptics (generally will see improvement within 3–5 days), consideration should be given to using a short-acting benzodiazepine such as midazolam (109, 132).

Sedation

While sedation is a well-known consequence of medication effect, polypharmacy may amplify this problem. Sedating agents in this patient population may include opioid analgesics, ant-emetics, anxiolytics, neuroleptics, or tricyclic anti-depressants (133). It is important to titrate all medications carefully and to eliminate all non-essential drugs.

A certain number of patients, varying from 6% to 30%, are conscious until at least 15 min before death. Conversely, 8–34% of patients are unconscious for more than 24 h prior to death (134–136). Sedation, in this scenario, may therefore be related to the terminal nature of the illness.

The use of psychostimulants to enhance analgesic efficacy and to reduce opioid-induced somnolence and cognitive impairment is widely accepted (137, 138). Bruera *et al.* found that methylphenidate is generally well-tolerated with a minimal incidence of early toxicity (hallucinations in one patient and paranoid reaction in one patient) and no late toxicity in a survey of 50 patients (139). Dextroamphetamine and pemoline are also used for this indication. Pemoline is associated with at least three fatal cases of hepatoxicity (140), however, it may have lesser sympathomimetic effects. Treatment generally starts with a dose of 2.5–5 mg of methylphenidate or dextroamphetamine in the morning and may be repeated at noon (141).

Other neuropsychiatric disturbances

Cancer patients who report significant pain have a 39% chance of a concomitant psychiatric diagnosis, while only 19% of cancer patients without a psychiatric diagnosis reported significant pain (142). The most common psychiatric diagnoses in cancer patients with pain are adjustment disorder with depressed or anxious mood (69%) and major depression (15%) (143–145). The incidence of depression increases with advanced cancer; 25% of all cancer patients experience symptoms of depression and the prevalence increases up to 77% with advanced disease (146). There is a suggested association between depression and increased morbidity in this patient population (147–148).

Diagnosis of depression in cancer patients (149), particularly in those with advanced disease, presents an interesting dilemma because it is frequently difficult to differentiate signs and symptoms of depression versus those related to the cancer or cancer treatment (150, 151). When making a diagnosis of depression, it is important to rule out an organic mental disorder, cognitive impairment or delirium. A family history of depression and/or a history of depressive episodes in the past, may increase the index of suspicion for this diagnosis. Organic etiologies for depression related to cancer treatment include corticosteroids (152), use of chemotherapy drugs such as vinblastine (153), whole-brain radiation (154), or paraneoplastic syndromes (155–156). A number of methods, including diagnostic classification systems, structured diagnostic interviews, or self-report screening instruments, are used in assessment (149, 151, 157–160).

Optimal management of depression in a cancer patient, particularly in the terminal stages, involves supportive psychotherapy, cognitive behavioral therapies, and anti-depressant medications (161). Supportive counseling should include not only crisis management, but should leave an opportunity for patients to discuss some of the more existential issues that arise during the

Table 28.6 Anti-depressant medications used in the treatment of depression in cancer

Anti-depressant medications useful in the treatment of depression in terminal cancer
Tricyclic anti-depressants
Second-generation anti-depressants
i.e. Bupropion
Trazodone
SSRIs
Monoamine oxidase inhibitors
Psychostimulants
Benzodiazepines
Lithium carbonate

dying process. It may also be helpful for the patient to participate in a group process (162, 163). Behavioral therapies may include relaxation or distraction techniques, or guided imagery. These modalities may prove beneficial in mild to moderate depression (164). Pharmacologic intervention, however, is the most efficacious form of treatment for depression in this population (161). Unfortunately, in many cases the medications are prescribed too late in the disease process for maximum efficacy (165). It is essential to identify these patients early and to aggressively start appropriate medication management.

A number of different anti-depressant classes may be helpful in the treatment of depression in cancer (Table 28.6) (161). It is important to individualize these medications or combinations.

Asthenia

Asthenia is defined as an 'absence or loss of strength' (166). Three different symptom complexes are described by Neuenschwander and Bruera: fatigue or lassitude defined as easy tiring and decreasing ability to maintain performance; generalized weakness characterized by the expectation that a particular activity will not be able to be completed; and mental fatigue frequently accompanied by impaired ability to concentrate, memory loss, and emotional lability (166, 167). It is important to distinguish asthenia from localized or regional weakness secondary to neurologic deficit or muscular abnormality.

While it is recognized that asthenia may occur as an independent symptom, it frequently co-exists with cachexia, which is defined as 'progressive weight loss and catabolism of host body compartments such as muscle and adipose tissue' (166). Asthenia or fatigue is one of the most prevalent symptoms reported by cancer patients. It is a major impediment to reasonable quality of life and may be multi-factorial in nature. Prevalence is difficult to assess; however estimates range from 80% to 96% in patients undergoing chemotherapy and radiotherapy (168, 169).

Etiologies of cancer-related asthenia generally are either physiologic or psychosocial. Physiologic causes may include cancer-treatment, other unrelated disease processes, systemic disorders including, but not limited to anemia, infection, malnutrition, fluid and/or electrolyte abnormalities, or pulmonary, hepatic, cardiac or renal failure. Other causes of physiologic aberration may be due to sleep disorders, chronic pain, drug effect(s), or immobility and deconditioning (168). Psychosocial issues may involve anxiety disorders or mood disorders related to the environment (168).

Treatment of asthenia remains symptomatic and generally consists of patient education, individualized exercise regimens, activity modification, stress management, and attention to adequate nutrition and hydration. It is important to note that asthenia related to cachexia may not be related to malnutrition primarily, but in fact, may be an indication of major metabolic abnormalities (166, 170–172).

Myoclonus

Myoclonus in a terminal cancer patient is generally the result of high-dose opiate therapy. In the terminal phase, however it may be secondary to encephalopathy induced by multiple organ failure, particularly in those patients with renal and/or hepatic failure, or with hyponatremia (173). It is important to rule out any neurologic process that may cause myoclonus, i.e. tumor in the epidural space. Treatment should consist of elimination of any agents whose clearance is impaired by end-organ damage, empirical treatment with a low dose benzodiazepine, i.e. clonazepam (174), reduction in the current opioid dose, or rotation to an alternative opioid (175).

Interventional pain-management techniques

Neuraxial anesthesia

Some practitioners may choose to deliver narcotics via either the epidural or intrathecal (spinal) routes. Controversy still exists regarding the efficacy of this route of delivery. Narcotics most frequently used via the intraspinal route (either epidural or spinal) are fentanyl, morphine, hydromorphone, and methadone (176). Advantages of this mode of delivery may include an increase in potency and maintenance of more prolonged opiate CSF concentrations. Disadvantages may include a higher incidence of nausea, confusion, pruritus, urinary retention, and edema (177). Cost may be much greater (depending on life-expectancy) than oral administration or parenteral or subcutaneous infusions. Intraspinal delivery systems include either 'port' systems or internalized pump systems. Internalized pumps are the most expensive types of systems.

Miscellaneous blocks

Trigger-point injections may be useful for patients with concomitant myofacial pain syndromes. Subjective complaints may include stiffness and specific-point tenderness. Objectively, trigger points are noted to be firm palpable bands in the muscle that may restrict range of motion. Weakness without atrophy or neurologic deficit (178) may be present. Trigger points may be injected with a local anesthetic, with or without a steroid. Procaine, lidocaine, etidocaine, bupivacaine, and mepivacaine are local anesthetic options. Acupuncture or other dry-needling techniques may also be used (179–182). Garvey, *et al.* conducted a randomized double-blind study of all methods of treating trigger points and concluded that all treatment methods were equally effective (183).

Patients with bony-rib pain may experience significant pain relief with the judicious use of intercostal nerve blocks. These blocks are generally performed with local anesthetic and/or a neurolytic agent. Care should be exercised in performing these blocks as a systemic toxicity may occur with accidental injection of the local anesthetic into the vascular portion of the neurovascular bundle. Other complications may include pneumothorax or subarachnoid block.

A word about anticoagulation

In May of 1993, low molecular weight heparin (LMWH) was released in the United States for general use. The significant pharmacologic differences between LMWH and standard heparin were underestimated and in the following 5-year period, greater than 40 spinal hematomas were reported through the FDA's MedWatch system. The American Society of Regional Anesthesia (ASRA) complied with the FDA's 1997 request to develop practice guidelines on the management of patients undergoing neuraxial anesthesia (spinal or epidural anesthesia) in conjunction with the peri-operative use of LMWH (184).

The recommendations from ASRA (released in November, 1998) concerning neuraxial block and peri-operative LMWH, are as follows (185):

1. Monitoring of anti-Xa levels are not predictive of bleeding risk.

2. Concurrent use of anti-platelet drugs, standard heparin, or dextran, all increase the risk of spinal hematoma.

3. Delay LMWH therapy for 24 h with a traumatic or bloody needle or catheter placement.

4. Use a single-shot (no catheter placement) technique for patients already on LMWH therapy. The interval between the last dose of LMWH and the single-shot technique should be a minimum of 10–12 h. If higher doses of LMWH are used (e.g. Lovenox 1 mg/kg), wait a minimum of 24 h. Do not perform a neuraxial block on a patient who has received LMWH 2-h pre-operatively.

5. If a single-shot or a continuous catheter technique is used, wait 24 h post-operatively to start LMWH. If there is a catheter already in place, leave it in overnight and remove it the next day. Give the first dose of LMWH 2 h after the catheter has been discontinued.

6. If LMWH is started with a catheter in place, use extreme vigilance. Use opioid and/or dilute local anesthetic solutions and monitor neurological status frequently. LMWH therapy may be delayed if epidural analgesia is anticipated to last more than 24 h.

7. Timing of catheter removal with LMWH: delay removal for at least 10–12 h after last dose. Optimal: ideally removal at least 24 h after the last dose, which ideally allows for normalization of coagulation status. Further dosing should not occur for at least 2 h after removal.

Addiction vs. tolerance

Psychological dependence on, or addiction to, opioid analgesics is rare in a cancer-patient population. The few cancer patients who become addicted to opioids almost always have a history of substance abuse prior to their cancer diagnosis (186, 187).

It is important to differentiate between addiction or psychological dependence, tolerance, and physical dependence. Tolerance is the phenomenon of requiring a larger analgesic dose to maintain the original analgesic effect. Physical dependence generally accompanies tolerance and is used to describe a set of signs and symptoms characteristic of withdrawal if the opioid is stopped or chemically antagonized. Psychological dependence or addiction is characterized by a craving for the substance, drug-seeking behavior, and an overwhelming involvement in obtaining it for use other than for pain relief (188). Under-medication with opioids occurs frequently in cancer patients because of patient and physician fears regarding addiction (187, 189).

Suffering ... the forgotten symptom

As busy, evidenced-based practitioners, we often forget that no matter how well we manage pain and symptoms, some of our patients will do poorly. The dehumanization of medicine and our attempts to fit all treatments into algorithms both contribute to this phenomenon. Cassell (190) perhaps summed it up best when he stated that:

Suffering must inevitably involve the person; bodies do not suffer, persons suffer. The separation of the disease that underlies the suffering from both the person and the suffering itself, as though the scientific entity of disease is more real and more important than the person and the suffering, is one of the strange intellectual paradoxes of our times.

'Suffering is a symptom unique to each individual at any given time and given meaning by that individual's past, present and in most cases, real or perceived future' (191). It occurs 'not merely in the presence of great pain but also when the intactness of the person is threatened or sundered, and remains until the threat is gone or the intactness can be restored' (190). This is a critical distinction because one cannot make the assumption that pain always begets suffering. If we simply treat pain, then, we may still fail to treat the patient who is suffering the loss of wholeness. As we continue to treat pain and symptoms, we are just beginning to explore the role that suffering plays in patient satisfaction and quality of life (191).

References

1. Feig B, Berger D, Fuhrman G. Genitourinary cancer: prostate cancer—epidemiology and etiology. In: *The M.D. Anderson surgical oncology handbook* (2nd edn) (ed. M Delworth, C Dinney). Lippincott Williams & Wilkins, Philadelphia, PA, 1999, 360.
2. Ernstoff M, Heaney J, Peschel R. (1998). Epidemiology of prostate cancer. In: *Prostate cancer* (ed. F Keeley, L Gomella). Ch 1, p. 2.
3. Parker SL, Tong T, Bolden S *et al*. Cancer statistics. *CA* 1996, **46**, 5.
4. Wingo PA, Tong T, Bolden S. Cancer statistics, 1995. *CA* 1995, **45**, 8.
5. Shalala DE. *Cancer death rate declined for the first time ever in the 1990s* (press release). National Cancer Institute: Bethesda, MD, 14 November 1996.
6. Coffey DS. Prostate cancer: an overview of an increasing dilemma. *Cancer* 1993, **71** (Suppl), 880.
7. Muir CS, Nectoux J, Staszewski J. The epidemiology of prostatic cancer: geographical distribution and time trends. *Acta Oncol* 1991, **30**, 133.
8. Catalona WJ. *Prostate cancer*. Orlando, FL: Grune & Stratton, 1984.
9. Yu H, Harris RE, Gao YT *et al*. Comparative epidemiology of cancers of the colon, rectum, prostate and breast in Shanghai, China versus the United States. *Int J Epidemiol* 1991, **20**, 76.
10. Morra MN, Das S. Prostate cancer: epidemiology and etiology. In: *Cancer of the prostate* (ed. S Das, ED Crawford). New York, Marcel Dekker, 1993, 1–12.
11. Kaisary A, Murphy G, Denis L *et al*. The natural history of prostate cancer. In: *Textbook of prostate cancer: pathology, diagnosis and treatment* (ed. P Ekman, J Adolfsson, H Gronberg). Martin Dunitz Ltd, London. 1999, 2.
12. Stamey TA, Freiha FS, McNeal JE *et al*. Localized prostate cancer. *Cancer* 1993, **71**, 933.
13. Devita VT Jr, Hellman S, Rosenberg SA. Cancer of the prostate: history and physical examination. In: *Cancer principles & practice of oncology* (5th edn) (ed. J Oesterling, Z Fuks, C Lee, H Scher). 1997, p. 1335.
14. De Conno F, Caracenti A, Martini C *et al*. Hyperalgesia and myoclonus with intrathecal infusion of high-dose morphine. *Pain* 1991, **47**, 337–9.
15. Stillman MJ, Moulin DE, Foley KM. Paradoxical pain following high-dose spinal morphine. *Pain* 1987, **82**, 389.
16. De Castro MD, Meynadier MD, Zenz MD. Regional opioid analgesia. *Dev Crit Care Med Anesthesiology* 1991, **20**, 81–85.
17. Morewood GH. A rational approach to the cause, prevention and treatment of postdural puncture headache. *Can Med Assoc J* 1993, **149** (8), 1087–93.
18. Bonica JJ. Headache and other visceral disorders of the head and neck. In: *The management of pain*. Philadelphia, Lea & Febiger, 1953, 1263–309.
19. Tarkkila P, Huhtala J, Salminen U. Difficulties in spinal needle use. Insertion characteristics and failure rates associated with 25-, 27- and 29-gauge Quincke-type spinal needles. *Anaesthesia* 1994, **49** (8), 723–5.

20. Fink BR, Walker S. Orientation of fibers in human dorsal lumbar dura mater in relation to lumbar puncture. *Anesth Analg* 1989, **69** (6), 768–72.

21. Leibold RA, Yealy DM, Coppola M *et al*. Post-dural-puncture headache: characteristics, management, and prevention. *Ann Emerg Med* 1993, **22** (12), 1863–70.

22. Raskin NH. Lumbar puncture headache: a review. *Headache*. 1990, **30** (4), 197–200.

23. Martin R, Jourdain S, Clairoux M *et al*. Duration of decubitus position after epidural blood patch. *Can J. Anaesth* 1994, **41** (1), 23–25.

24. Olsen KS. Epidural blood patch in the treatment of post-lumbar puncture headache. *Pain* 1987, **30** (3), 293–301.

25. Heide W, Diener HC. Epidural blood patch reduces the incidence of post lumbar puncture headache. *Headache* 1990, **30** (5), 280–1.

26. Malloy HS, Seipp CA, Duffey P. Administration of cancer treatments: practical guide for physicians and oncology nurses. In: *Cancer: principals and practice of oncology* (3rd edn) (ed. De Vita VT, S Hellman SA Rosenberg). JB Lippincott, Philadelphia, 1989, 2369–402.

27. Mrozek-Orlowski M, Christi J, Flamme C *et al*. Pain associated with peripheral infusion of carmustine. *Oncol Nurses Forum* 1991, **18** (5), 942.

28. Hundrieser J. A non-invasive approach to minimizing vessel pain with DTIC or BCNU. *Oncol Nurses Forum* 1988, **15** (2), 199.

29. Zaglama NE, Rosenblum SL, Sartiano GP *et al*. Single, high-dose intravenous dexamethasone as an antiemetic in cancer chemotherapy. *Oncology* 1986, **43**, 27–32.

30. Cherny NI, Portenoy RK. Cancer pain: principles of assessment and syndromes. In: *Textbook of pain* (3rd edn) Edinburg, (ed. PD Wall, R Melzack). Churchill Livingston, 1994, 787.

31. Berger AM, Portenoy RK, Weissman DE. Corticosteroid-induced perineal discomfort. In: *Principles and practice of supportive oncology*. (ed. NI Cherny). Lippincott-Raven Publishers, Philadelphia, 1998, 13.

32. Twycross R. The risks and benefits of corticosteroids in advanced cancer. *Drug Safety* 1994, **11** (3), 163–78.

33. Rotstein J, Good RA. Steroid pseudorheumatism. *Arch Intern Med* 1957, **99**, 545–55.

34. Ernstoff MS, Heaney JA, Peschel RE. Chemotherapy for Prostate cancer. In *Prostate cancer* (ed. H Upadhyaya, NJ Vogelzang). Blackwell Science, Inc, 1998, 185.

35. Ignoffo RJ, Viele CS, Damon LE *et al*. Cisplatin. In: *Cancer chemotherapy pocket guide*. Lippincott-Raven, Philadelphia, 1998, 41.

36. Gregg RW, Molepo JM, Monpetit VJ *et al*. Cisplatin neurotoxicity: the relationship between dosage, time, and platinum concentration in neurologic tissues, and morphologic evidence of toxicity. *J Clin Oncol* 1992, **10**, 795–803.

37. Freeman NJ, Costanza ME. 5-fluorouracil-associated cardiotoxicity. *Cancer* 1988, **61**, 36–45.

38. Eskilsson J, Albertsson M. Failure of preventing 5-fluorouracil cardiotoxicity by prophylactic treatment with verapamil. *Acta Oncol* 1990, **29**, 1001–3.

39. Rezkalla S, Kloner RA, Ensley J *et al*. Continuous ambulatory ECG monitoring during fluorouracil therapy: a prospective study. *J Clin Oncol* 1989, **7**, 509–14.

40. Ignoffo RJ, Viele CS, Damonl LE *et al*. Carboplatin. In: *Cancer chemotherapy pocket guide*. Lippincott-Raven, Philadelphia, 1998, 31.

41. Ignoffo RJ, Viele CS, Damonl LE *et al*. Vinblastine sulfate. In: *Cancer chemotherapy pocket guide*. Lippincott-Raven, Philadelphia, 1998, 213.

42. Ignoffo RJ, Viele CS, Damonl LE *et al*. Hydroxyurea. In: *Cancer chemotherapy pocket guide*. Lippincott-Raven, Philadelphia, 1998, 118.

43. Ignoffo RJ, Viele CS, Damonl LE *et al*. Etoposide. In: *Cancer chemotherapy pocket guide*. Lippincott-Raven, Philadelphia, 1998, 87.

44. Ignoffo RJ, Viele CS, Damonl LE *et al*. Leuprolide Acetate. In: *Cancer chemotherapy pocket guide*. Lippincott-Raven, Philadelphia, 1998, 134–5.

45. Chrisp P, Sorkin EM. Leuprorelin. A review of its pharmacology and therapeutic use in prostatic disorders. *Drugs Aging* 1991, **1**, 487–509.

46. Thompson IM, Zeidman EJ, Rodriguez FR. Sudden death due to disease flare with luteinizing hormone-releasing hormone agonist therapy for carcinoma of the prostate. *J Urol* 1990, **144**, 1479–80.

47. Schellhammer P, Sharifi R, Block N *et al*. A controlled trial of bicalutamide versus flutamide, each in combination with luteinizing hormone-relapsing hormone analogue therapy, in patients with advanced prostate cancer. *Urology* 1995, **45**, 745.

48. Ignoffo RJ, Viele CS, Damonl LE *et al*. Estramustine phosphate. In: *Cancer chemotherapy pocket guide*. Lippincott-Raven, Philadelphia, 1998, 83.

49. Ignoffo RJ, Viele CS, Damonl LE *et al*. Flutamide. In: *Cancer chemotherapy pocket guide*. Lippincott-Raven, Philadelphia, 1998, 106.

50. Labrie F. Mechanism of action and pure anti androgenic properties of flutamide. *Cancer* 1993, **72**, 3816–27.

51. Rusthoven JJ, Ahlgren P, Elhakim T *et al*. Varicella-zoster infection in adult cancer patients: a population study. *Arch Intern Med* 1988, **148**, 1561–6.

52. Portenoy RK, Duma C, Foley KM. Acute herpetic and postherpetic neuralgia: clinical review and current management. *Ann Neurol* 1986, **20**, 651–64.

53. Rusthoven JJ, Ahlgren P, Elhakim T *et al*. Risk factors for varicella zoster disseminated infection among adult cancer patients with localized zoster. *Cancer* 1988, **62**, 1641–6.

54. Kaisary AV, Murphy GP, Denis L. Palliative care: In: *Prostate cancer: pathology, diagnosis, and treatment* pain (ed. A Tookman, A Kurowska). Martin Dunitz, London, 1999, 33.

55. Kuban DA, El-Mahdi AM, Sigfred SV *et al*. Characteristics of spinal cord compression in adenocarcinoma of the prostate. *Urology* 1986, **28**, 364.

56. Flynn DF, Shipley WU. Management of spinal cord compression secondary to metastatic prostatic carcinoma. *Urol Clin North Am* 1991, **18**, 145.

57. Berger AM, Portenoy RK, Weissman DE. Management of spinal neoplasm and its complications, Epidemiology In: *Principles and practice of supportive oncology* (ed. SM Weinstein). Lippincott-Raven Publishers, Philadelphia, 1998, 449.

58. Posner JB. Neurologic complications of cancer. *Contemporary Neurology Series* 1995, **45**, 119.

59. Kaisary AV, Murphy GP, Denis L *et al*. Palliative care In: *Prostate cancer: pathology, diagnosis, and treatment* (ed. A Tookman, A Kurowska). Martin Dunitz, London, 1999, 336.

60. Berger AM, Portenoy RK, Weissman DE. Cancer pain: principals of assessment and syndromes, postchemotherapy pain syndromes. In: *Principles and practice of supportive oncology* (ed. NI Cherny). Lippincott-Raven Publishers, Philadelphia 1998, 31.

61. Vreden SG, Hermus AR, van Liessum PA *et al*. Aseptic bone necrosis in patients on glucocorticoid replacement therapy. *Netherlands J Med* 1991, **39**, 153–7.

62. Watanabe S, Bruera E. Corticosteroids as adjuvant analgesics. *J Pain Sympt Manag* 1994, **9** (7), 442–5.

63. Matsuo K, Horohata T, Sugioka Y *et al*. Influence of alcohol intake, cigarette smoking and occupational status on idiopathic osteonecrosis of the femoral head. *Clin Orthop* 1988, **234**, 115–23.

64. Warner JJP, Philip JH, Brodsky GL *et al*. Studies of nontraumatic osteonecrosis; manometric and histologic studies of the femoral head after chronic steroid treatment: an experimental study in rabbits. *Clin Orthop* 1987, **225**, 128–40.

65. Cruess RL. Osteonecrosis of bone. Current concepts as to etiology and pathogenesis. *Clin Orthop* 1986, **208**, 31–9.

66. Foley KM. Pain syndromes in patients with cancer. *Med Clin North Am* 1987, **71**, 169–84.

67. Ombregt L, Bisschop P, ter Veer HJ *et al*. Disorders of the inert structures, the capsular patten. In: *A system of orthopaedic medicine*. WB Saunders, London, 1995, 740.

68. Ramamurthy L, Cooper RA. Metastatic carcinoma to the male breast. *Br J Radiol* 1991, **64**, 277–8.

69. Olsson H, Alm P, Kristoffersson U *et al*. Hypophyseal tumor and gynecomastia preceding bilateral breast cancer development in a man. *Cancer* 1984, **53**, 1974–7.

70. *PDQ supportive care/screening information-lymphedema*. Cancer Fax from the National Cancer Institute 208/00442. Current as of 09/01/93: 1.

71. Berger AM, Portenoy RK, Weissman DE. Lymphedema: patients at risk In: *Principles and practice of supportive oncology* (ed. ML Farncombe). Lippincott-Raven Publishers, Philadelphia, 1988, 276.

72. Foldi E, Foldi M, Weissleder H. Conservative treatment of lymphoedema of the limbs. *Angiology* 1985; Mar 85, 175.

73. Farncombe ML, Daniels G, Cross L. Lymphedema: the seemingly forgotten complication. *J Pain Sympt Manag* 1994, 9, 269.

74. Nishman B, Pasternak S, Wallenstein SL *et al*. The memorial pain assessment card: a valid instrument for the evaluation of cancer pain. *Cancer* 1987, **60**, 1151–8.

75. Daut RL, Cleeland CS, Flanery RC. Development of the Wisconsin brief pain questionnaire to assess pain in cancer and other diseases. *Pain* 1983, **17** (2), 197–210.

76. Bruera E, MacDonald S. Audit methods: the Edmonton symptom assessment system. In: *Clinical audit in palliative care* (ed. I Higginson). Oxford, Radcliff Medical Press, 1993, **8**, 61–77.

77. Cohen SR *et al*. Validity of the McGill Quality of Life Questionnaire in the palliative care setting: a multi-centre Canadian study demonstrating the importance of the existential domain. *Palliative Medicine* 1997, **11**, 3–20.

78. Cohen SR, Mount BM, Strobel MG *et al*. The McGill Quality of Life Questionnaire: a measure of life appropriate for people with advanced disease. A preliminary study of validity and acceptability. *Palliative Medicine* 1995, **9**, 207–19.

79. Price DD, McGrath PA, Rafii A *et al*. The validation of visual analogue scales as ratio scale measures for chronic and experimental pain. *Pain* 1983, **17** (1), 45–56.

80. Driver LC, Bruera E. *The M.D. Anderson Palliative Care Handbook* (1st edn). Department of Symptom Control and Palliative Care, The University of Texas M.D. Anderson Cancer Center, Houston, 2000.

81. Ewing JA. Detecting alcoholism. The CAGE questionnaire. *JAMA* 1984, **252** (14), 1905–7.

82. Folstein MF, Folstein SE, McHugh PR. 'Mini-Mental state'. A practical method for grading the cognitive state of patients for the clinician. *J Psychiatric Res* 1975, **12** (3), 189–98.

83. Folstein MF, Folstein SE, McHugh PR. Mini-Mental state. A practical method for grading the cognitive state of patients for the clinician. *J Psychiatric Res* 1975, **12** (3), 189–98.

84. Kasai T. *et al*. The Edmonton Functional Assessment Tool: preliminary development and evaluation for use in palliative care. *J Pain Sympt Manag* 1997, **13** (1), 10–9.

85. Yates JW, Cheloma B, McKinney PF. Karnofsky performance status. *Cancer* 1980, **45**, 2220–4.

86. Devita VT Jr, Hellman S, Rosenberg SA. Cancer of the prostate: supportive care and quality of Life—management of cancer pain—types of pain (5th edn) (ed. K Foley). 1997, 2810.

87. Arner S, Meyerson BA. Lack of analgesic effect of opioids on neuropathic and idiopathic forms of pain. *Pain* 1988, **33** (1), 11–23.

88. Cherny NI, Thaler HT, Friedlander-Klar H *et al*. Opioid responsiveness of cancer pain syndromes caused by neuropathic or nociceptive mechanisms; a combined analysis of controlled single dose studies. *Neurology* 1994, **44**, 857–61.

89. Kanner R. Overview: definitions. In: *Pain management secrets* Hanley & Belfus, Inc, Medical Publishers, 1997, 2.

90. Portenoy RK, Foley KM, Inturrisi CE. The nature of opioid responsiveness and its implications for neuropathic pain: new hypotheses derived from studies of opioid infusions. *Pain* 1990, **43** (3), 273–86.

91. Dubner R. A call for more science, not more rhetoric, regarding opioids and neuropathic pain. *Pain* 1991, **47** (1), 1–2.

92. Portenoy RK. Adjuvant analgesics in pain management. In: *Oxford textbook of palliative medicine* (ed. D Doyle, GW Hanks, N MacDonald). Oxford University Press, Oxford, 1993, 187–203.

93. McCleane GJ. Intravenous infusion of phentoin relieves neuropathic pain: a randomized, double-blinded, placebo-controlled, crossover study. *Anesth Analg* 1999, **89**, 985–8.

94. McQuay H, Carroll D, Alejandro AR *et al.* Anticonvulsant drugs for management of pain: a systematic review. *BMJ* 1995, **311** (7012), 1047–52.

95. Wessely S, Nimnuan C, Sharpe M. Functional somatic syndromes: one or many? *Lancet* 1999, **354** (9182), 936–9.

96. Coyle N, Adelhardt J, Foley KM *et al.* Character of terminal illness in the advanced cancer patient: pain and other symptoms during the last 4 weeks of life. *J Pain Sympt Manag* 1990, **5**, 83.

97. Portenoy RK. Cancer pain: pathophysiology and syndromes. *Lancet* 1992, **339**, 102.

98. World Health Organization. *Cancer pain relief* (2nd edn). WHO, Geneva. 1996.

99. Lawlor PG, Turner KS, Hanson J *et al.* Dose ratio between morphine and methadone in patients with cancer pain. *Cancer* 1998, **82** (6), 1167–73.

100. *Management of cancer pain. Clinical practice guidelines.* US Department of Health & Human Services, Rockville, MD, 1994, AHCPR Pub No. 94-0592.

101. *Cancer pain: a monograph on the management of cancer pain.* Health & Welfare Canada: Minister of Supply and Services, Canada, Ottawa, H42-2/5, 1984.

102. Twycross R, Lack S. Pain relief. In *Therapeutics in terminal cancer* (2nd edn) (ed. R Twycross, S Lack) Churchill Livingston, Edinburgh. 1990, 11–39.

103. Levy M. Pain management in advanced cancer. *Semin Oncol* 1985, **12**, 394–410.

104. Bruera E, Neumann CM. Role of methadone in the management of pain in cancer patients. *Oncology* 1999, 1275–1282.

105. Slykes N. Constipation and diarrhea. In: Oxford textbook palliative medicine (ed. D Doyle, G Hanks, N MacDonald). Oxford Medical Publications, Oxford, 1993, 293–310.

106. Doyle D, Hanks GWC, MacDonald N. Research into symptoms other than pain. In: Oxford textbook of palliative medicine (ed. E Bruera). Oxford University Press, New York, 1998, 179–85.

107. Coyle N *et al.* Character of terminal illness in the advanced cancer patient pain and other symptoms during the last 4 weeks of life. *J Pain Sympt Manag* 1990, **5**, 83–93.

108. Doyle D. Symptom relief in terminal illness. *Med Practice* 1983, **1**, 694–8.

109. Bruera E, Neumann CM. Management of specific symptom complexes in patients receiving palliative care. *Can Med Assoc J* 1998, **158**, 1717–26.

110. Berger AM, Portenoy RK, Weissman DE. Diarrhea, malabsorption, and constipation: pathophysiology In: *Principles and practice of supportive oncology.* Lippincott-Raven Publishers, Philadelphia, 1988, 201.

111. NP Sykes. Constipation and diarrhoea. In: *Oxford textbook of palliative medicine* (ed. Doyle D, Hanks GWC, MacDonald N). 1998, 513.

112. Bruera E, Suarez-Almazor M, Velasco A. *et al.* The assessment of constipation in terminal cancer patients admitted to a palliative care unit: a retrospective review. *J Pain Sympt Manag* 1994, **9** (8), 515–9.

113. Muller-Lissner SA. Effect of wheat bran on weight of stool and gastrointestinal transit time: a meta-analysis. *BMJ* 1988, **296**, 615–7.

114. Holdstock DJ, Misiewicz JJ, Smith T *et al.* Propulsion (mass movements) in the human colon and its relationship to meals and somatic activity. *Gut* 1970, **11**, 91–9.

115. Pereira J, Bruera E. Chronic nausea. In: *Cachexia-anorexia in cancer patients.* (ed. E Bruera, I Higginson). Oxford Medical Publications, Oxford University Press, Oxford, 1996, 23–37.

116. Bruera ED, MacEachern T, Spachynski KA *et al.* Comparison of the efficacy, safety, and pharmacokinetics of controlled release and immediate release metoclopramide for the management of chronic nausea in patients with advanced cancer. *Cancer* 1994, **74** (12), 3204–11.

117. Breibart W *et al.* Neuropsychiatric syndromes and psychological symptoms in patients with advanced cancer. *J Pain Sympt Manag* 1995, **10** (2), 131–41.

118. Massie MJ, Holland J, Glass E. Delirium in terminally ill cancer patients. *Am J Psychiatry* 1983, **140**, 1048–50.

119. Levine PM, Silberfarb P, Lipowski ZJ. Mental disorders in cancer patients. *Cancer* 1978, **42**, 1385–91.

120. Bruera E, Miller L, MacCallion J *et al.* Cognitive failure in patients with terminal cancer: a prospective longitudinal study. *Psychosocial Aspects Cancer* 1990, **9** (Abstract), 308.

121. Fainsinger R, Young C. Cognitive failure in a terminally ill patient. *J Pain Sympt Manag* 1991, **6**, 192–494.

122. Peipzig R, Goodman H, Gray G *et al.* Reversible narcotic associated mental status impairment in patients with metastatic cancer. *Pharmacology* 1987, **35**, 47–54.

123. Bruera E, Miller MJ, McCallion K *et al.* Cognitive failure in patients with terminal cancer: a prospective study. *J Pain Sympt Manag* 1992, **7**, 192–5.

124. Litchter I, Hunt E. The last 24 hr of life. *J Palliat Care* 1990, **6**, 7–15.

125. Bruera E. Case report: severe organic brain syndrome. *J Palliat Care* 1991, **7**, 36–8.

126. Stiefel F, Holland J. Delirium in cancer patients. *Int Psychogeriatr* 1991, **3**, 333–6.

127. Lipowski ZJ. Delirium (acute confusional states). *JAMA* 1987, **258**, 1789–92.

128. Lipowski ZJ. Transient cognitive disorders (delirium, acute confusional states) in the elderly. *Am J Psychiatry* 1983, **140**, 1426–36.

129. Lipowski ZJ. Update on delirium. *Psychiatr Clin North Am* 1992, **15**, 335–46.

130. Adams F, Fernandez F, Andersson BS. Emergency pharmacotherapy of delirium in the critically ill cancer patient. *Psychosomatics* 1986, **27**, 33–7.

131. Olive DJ. The use of methotrimeprazine in terminal care. *Br J Clin Practice* 1985, **39**, 339–40.

132. Bruera E, Pereira J. Neuropsychiatric toxicity of opioids. In: *Proceedings of the 8th World Congress on Pain, Progress in Pain Research and Management*, Vol. 8. (ed. TS Jensen, JA Turner, Z Wiesenfeld-Hallen. International Association for the Study of Pain Press, Seattle, 1997, 717–38.

133. Doyle D, Hanks GWC, MacDonald N. Psychiatric aspects of palliative care. In: *Oxford textbook of palliative medicine* (2nd edn) (ed. W Breibart, HM Chochinov, S Passkik). 1998, 939.

134. Doyle D, Hanks GWC, MacDonald N. The terminal phase. In: Oxford textbook of palliative medicine (2nd edn) (ed. R Twycross, I Lichter). 1998, 982.

135. Saunders C. Pain and impending death. In: *Textbook of pain* (ed. PD Wall, R Melzack) Churchill Livingstone, London, 1989, 624–31.

136. Lichter I, Hunt E. The last 48 hours of life. *J Palliative Care* 1990, **6** (4), 7–15.

137. Bruera E, Chadwich S, Brenneis C *et al.* Methylphenidate associated with narcotics for the treatment of cancer pain. *Cancer Treatment Report* 1987, **71**, 67–70.

138. Bruera E, Miller MJ, Macmillan K *et al.* Neuropsychological effects of methylphenidate in patients receiving a continuous infusion of narcotics for cancer pain. *Pain* 1992, **48**, 163–6.

139. Bruera E, Brenneis C, Paterson AH *et al.* Use of methylphenidate as an adjuvant to narcotic analgesics in patients with advanced cancer. *J Pain Sympt Manag* 1989, **4**, 3–6.

140. Berkovitch M, Pope E, Phillips J *et al.* Pemoline-associated fulminant liver failure: testing the evidence for causation. *Clin Pharmacol Therapeutics* 1995, **57**, 696–8.

141. RK Portenoy. Adjuvant analgesics in pain management. In: Oxford textbook of palliative medicine (2nd edn) (ed. Doyle D, Hanks GWC, MacDonald N). 1998, 380.

142. Derogatis LR, Morrow GR, Fetting J *et al.* The prevalence of psychiatric disorders among cancer patients. *J Am Medi Assoc* 1983, **249**, 751–7.

143. W Breibart, S Passik, D Payne. Psychological and psychiatric interventions in pain control. In: *Oxford textbook of palliative medicine* (2nd edn) (ed. Doyle D, Hanks GWC, MacDonald N). 1998, 439.

144. Ahles TA, Blanchard EB, Ruckdeschel JC. The multidimensional nature of cancer related pain. *Pain* 1983, **17**, 277–88.

145. Woodforde JM, Fielding JR. Pain and cancer. *J Psychosom Res* 1970, **14**, 365–70.

146. W Breibart, S Passik, D Payne. Psychological and psychiatric interventions in pain control. In: Oxford textbook of palliative medicine (2nd edn) (ed. Doyle D, Hanks GWC, MacDonald N). 1998, 440.

147. Kathol RG, Mutgi A, Williams J *et al.* Diagnosis of major depression in cancer patients according to four sets of criteria. *Am J Psychiatry* 1990, **147**, 1021–4.

148. Derogatis LR, Morrow GR, Schmale A *et al.* The prevalence of psychiatric disorders among cancer patients. *JAMA* 1983, **249**, 751–7.

149. American Psychiatric Association (APA). *Diagnostic and statistical manual of mental disorders* (3rd edn). DSM-III-R. APA, Washington, DC, 1987.

150. McDaniel JS, Nemeroff CB. Depression in the cancer patient diagnostic biological and treatment aspects. In: *Current and emerging issues in cancer pain: researcher and practice* (ed. CR Chapman, KM Foley). Raven, New York, 1993, 1–19.

151. Endicott J. Measurement of depression in patients with cancer. *Cancer* 1984, **53**, 2243–9.

152. Stiefel FC, Breibart W, Holland JC. Corticosteroids in cancer: neuropsychiatric complications. *Cancer Invest* 1989, 7, 479–91.

153. Weddington WW. Delirium and depression associated with amphotericin B. *Psychosomatics* 1982, **23**, 1076–8.

154. DeAngelis LM, Delattre J, Posner JB. Radiation-induced dementia in patients cured of brain metastases. *Neurology* 1989, **39**, 789–96.

155. Posner JB. Nonmetastatic effects of cancer on the nervous system. In: Cecil's textbook of medicine (ed. JB Wyngaarden, LH Smith). WB Saunders, Philadelphia, 1988, 1104–7.

156. Patchell RA, Posner JB. Cancer and the nervous system. In: The handbook of psychooncology: the psychological care of the cancer patient (ed. J Holland, J Rowland). Oxford University Press, New York, 1989, 327–41.

157. Spitzer RL, Endicott J, Robins E. Research diagnostic criteria, rationale and reliability. *Arch Gen Psychiatry* 1978, **35**, 773–82.

158. Spitzer R, Williams J. *Structured clinical interview for DSM-III-R*. Biometrics Research Department, New York State Psychiatric Institute, New York, 1988.

159. Zgmond AS, Sniath RP. The hospital anxiety and depression scale. *Acta Psychiatr Scand* 1983, **67**, 361–70.

160. Bech AT, Steer RA, Gerbin MG. Psychometric properties of the Beck Depression Inventory: twenty five years of evaluation. *Clin Psychol Rev* 1988, **8**, 77–100.

161. Massie MJ, Holland JC. Depression and the cancer patient. *J Clin Psychiatry* 1990, **51**, 12–17.

162. Massie MJ, Holland JC, Straker N. Psychotherapeutic interventions. In: *Handbook of psychooncology: psychological care of the patient with cancer* (ed. JC Holland, JH Rowland). Oxford University Press, New York, 1989, 455–69.

163. Spiegel D, Bloom JR, Yalom ID. Group support for patients with metastatic cancer: a randomized prospective outcome study. *Arch Gen Psychiatry* 1981, **38**, 527–33.

164. Pholland JC, Morrow G, Schmale A *et al.* Reduction of anxiety and depression in cancer patients by alprazolam or by a behavioral technique (abstract). *Proc Am Soc Clin Oncol* 1988, **6**, 258.

165. Williams ML, Friedman T, Rudd N. A survey of antidepressant prescribing in the terminally ill. *Palliative Medicine* 1999, **13**, 243–8.

166. Neuenschwander H, Bruera E. Asthenia-Cachexia. In: *Cachexia-anorexia in cancer patients* (ed. E Bruera, I Higginson). Oxford University Press, Oxford, 1996, 57–75.

167. Bruera E, MacDonald RN. Asthenia in patients with advanced cancer. *J Pain Sympt Manag* 1988, **3** (1), 9–14.

168. Portenoy RK, Itri LM. Cancer-related fatigue: guidelines for evaluation and management. *Oncologist* 1999, **4**, 1–10.

169. Irvine DM, Vincent L, Bubela N *et al.* A critical appraisal of the research literature investigating fatigue in the individual with cancer. *Cancer Nursing* 1991, **14** (4), 199–9.

170. Cella D, Peterman A, Passik S *et al.* Progress toward guidelines for the management of fatigue. *Oncology* 1998, **12**, 1–9.

171. Portenoy RK, Miaskowski C. Assessment and management of cancer-related fatigue. In: *Principles and practice of supportive oncology* (ed. A Berger, RK Portenoy, DE Weissman). Lippincott-Raven, Philadelphia, 1998, 109–118.

172. Neuenschwander H, Bruera E. Pathophysiology of cancer asthenia. In: *Topics in palliative care*, Vol. 2 (ed. R Portenoy, E Bruera). Oxford University Press, New York, 1998, 171–181.

173. R Twycross, I Lichter. The terminal phase. In: *Oxford textbook of palliative medicine* (2nd edn) (ed. Doyle D, Hanks GWC, MacDonald N) 1998, 988.

174. Eisele JH *et al.* Clonazepam treatment of myoclonic contractions associated with high dose opioids: a case report. *Pain* 1992, 49, 231–2.

175. Cherny Ni *et al.* Opioid pharmacotherapy in the management of cancer pain: a survey of strategies used by pain physicians for the selection of analgesic drugs and routes of administration. *Cancer* 1995, 76, 1283–93.

176. Mahaney GD, Peeters-Asdourian C. Cancer pain management. In: *Atlas of anesthesia: pain management*, Vol. VI (ed. RD Miller, SE Abram). Churchill Livingston, Philadelphia, 1998, 91–9.

177. Coombs DW, Maurer LH *et al.* Outcomes and complications of continuous intraspinal narcotic analgesia for cancer pain control. *J Clin Oncol* 1984, 2, 1414–20.

178. Travell J. Identification of myofascial trigger syndromes: a case of atypical facial neuralgia. *Arch Phys Med Rehabil* 1981, 62, 100–6.

179. Rubin D. Myofascial trigger point syndromes: an approach to management. *Arch Phys Med Rehabil* 1981, 62, 107–10.

180. Travel J. Myofascial trigger points: clinical view. In: *Advances in pain research and therapy* (ed. JJ Bonica, D AlbeFessard). Raven Press, New York, 1976.

181. Hameroff SR *et al.* Comparison of bupivacaine, etidocaine, and saline for trigger-point therapy. *Anesth Analg* 1981, 60, 752–5.

182. Frost FA, Jesen B, Siggaard-Anderson J. A controlled, double-blind comparison of mepivacaine injection versus saline injection for myofascial pain. *Lancet* 1980, 1, 499–501.

183. Garvey TA, Marks MR, Wiesel SW. A prospective, randomized double-blind evaluation of trigger point injection therapy for low back pain. *Spine* 1989, 14, 962–4.

184. Horlocker TT, Wedel DJ. Anticoagulation and neuraxial block: historical perspective, anesthetic implications, and risk management. *Reg Anesth Pain Med* 1998, 23 (6) (Suppl 2), 129–34.

185. Horlocker TT, Wedel DJ. Neuraxial block and low-molecular-weight heparin: balancing perioperative analgesia and thromboprophylaxis. *Reg Anesth Pain Med* 1998, 23 (6) (Suppl 2), 164–77.

186. Kanner RM, Foley KM. Patterns of narcotic use in a cancer pain clinic. *Ann New York Acad Sci* 1981, 362, 161–72.

187. Passik SD, Portenoy RK, Ricketts PL. Substance abuse issues in cancer patients, Part 1: prevalence and diagnosis. *Oncology* 1998, 12 (4), 517–21.

188. W Breibart, S Passik, D Payne. Psychological and Psychiatric interventions in pain control. In: *Oxford textbook of palliative medicine* (2nd edn) (ed. Doyle D, Hanks GWC, MacDonald N). 1998, 441.

189. Macaluso C, Weinberg D, Foley KM. Opioid abuse and misuse in a cancer pain population. (Abstract) *Second International Congress on Cancer Pain*, July 14–17, Rye, New York, 1988.

190. Cassell EJ. *The nature of suffering and the goals of medicine.* Oxford University Press, New York, 1991.

191. Leak JA. Suffering . . . the forgotten symptom. *Am Soc Anesthes Newsletter* 1999, 63 (10), 5–6.

Prostate cancer patients: psychological and sexual problems

Loukas Athanasiadis

Introduction

Prostate cancer is one of the commonest male cancers. The disease and its treatment can have a profound effect on the lives of both the patient and his family members (1). This chapter looks at the psychological, relationship, social, sexual, and other issues, associated with prostate cancer.

Psychological problems

Life-threatening acute illnesses and recurrent progressive conditions are particularly likely to provoke serious psychiatric problems. In chronic illness, psychiatric problems are more common in cases of distressing symptoms (e.g. severe pain), unpleasant treatment, demanding self-care, and disability. Psychological vulnerability, social circumstances, other life stresses, and the reactions of others (family, employers, doctors) are also important determinants of psychiatric morbidity (2).

The psychological consequences of prostate cancer are similar to those of cancer in general (3), or any other serious physical illness. Symptoms may be present even during the investigation period and before the diagnosis is made. Oncologists have noted in some patients the so-called 'PSA anxiety' that surrounds each PSA test and the anticipation before getting the results (3). Knowledge of the diagnosis of cancer in general, may cause shock, anger, disbelief, anxiety, and depression (2); the most common associated disorder appears to be adjustment disorder (4). The psychological reactions depend on psychiatric history, significant life changes, loss of friends or family to cancer (in particu-

lar prostate cancer), retirement issues and available support (3).

Important issues in patients with genito-urinary cancers include changes in sexuality, bladder and bowel function, relationships, body image, and lifestyle (3). Couples' issues include fear of the partner to be left alone (in case of death), role changes, attempts of the partner to 'put on a good face', sexual issues, and fear of transmission of cancer (e.g. through sexual activity) (5).

Physical issues, as a result of cancer, may cause irritability and psychological distress. Prostate cancer patients with pain are more anxious or depressed when compared with patients without pain (3) and they take more prescribed analgesics (6).

Distress about treatment options can also have a profound effect on irritability, anxiety, and mood (3). Surgery for cancer causes psychological problems that are similar to those for surgery in general, with the added meaning of cancer and the threat to life. It appears that psychological preparation for surgery facilitates post-operative adjustment and recovery. Extremely high anxiety or panic may be present in a few patients pre-operatively, especially if they had a pre-existing anxiety disorder. Major depression most often follows surgery when the results are ominous (e.g. surgery known to cause sexual dysfunction) (7).

Interventions for psychological problems include education, psychotherapy (individual, group, and couple's therapy), cognitive-behavioral interventions, and pharmacotherapy (3). Bindemann (8) proposes a supportive (reduction of anxiety related to illness and personal problems) and a directive strategy of management (recovery of confidence, hope for the future) for cancer patients. Pharmacotherapy may include the use of psychostimulants (e.g. pemoline, ritalin), anti-depressants (e.g. fluoxetine), and other drugs, as required (3).

Quality of life

Litwin (9) reports that older men without prostate cancer often present a degree of urinary, bowel function, and sexual function problems. Therefore, researchers assessing changes in the quality of life of prostate cancer patients need to have knowledge of pre-morbid functioning. Studies of older men with prostate cancer must be either longitudinal, or—if not feasible—a properly selected control group must be used.

In a quality-of-life study, Da Silva *et al.* (10) reported that pain, psychological distress, fatigue, and social and family life—confirmed in relation to objective parameters—were the most important parameters representing the patients' view of their conditions. It was found that there was a discrepancy between the doctors' evaluation and the patients' opinions about sexual status and pain. It also appeared that clinicians were reluctant to do quality-of-life research due to feasibility problems and doubts about the value of this effort.

Prostate cancer patients appear to present more problems in the sexual, urinary, and bowel function than men of similar age without prostate cancer, but not in general health related quality-of-life measures (11). According to preliminary findings (7) the overall quality of life of prostate cancer patients does not also appear to differ among patients undergoing different forms of treatment (prostatectomy, radiotherapy, cryotherapy, 'watchful-waiting'). However, specific quality-of-life domains may be influenced by treatment-specific complications.

Pain issues

A study assessed pain and quality of life following radical retropubic prostatectomy. The authors found that mild pain, associated with reduced quality of life (particularly social functioning) was common. Approximately one in two patients had some pain related to surgery at 3 months; the pain was associated with higher levels of pre-operative anxiety. Long-term

effects of intra-operative technique (epidural and/or general anesthesia) were not apparent (12). Daut and Cleeland (13) looked at the prevalence and severity of pain in selected groups of cancer patients (including prostate cancer). They reported that patients with metastatic cancer were more likely to report pain than patients with non-metastatic cancers. Patients reported a surprisingly high frequency of pain as a symptom when they were first diagnosed.

Form of treatment

Gaffo *et al.* (14) developed a self-administered questionnaire to assess the quality of life of patients with localized prostate cancer after treatment by radical radiotherapy. In a retrospective study of 70 patients, the main side-effects of treatment were sexual impairment and urinary symptoms. Physical, psychological, and relational issues did not suffer considerably. The degree of information about the disease and the therapy appeared to play an important role in adjustment after treatment.

McCammon *et al.* (15) compared quality-of-life evaluations from patients who received external-beam radiation therapy or radical prostatectomy for the treatment of localized prostate cancer. Gastro-intestinal problems were more frequent in the first group of patients and problems with urinary incontinence in the second. They concluded that patient satisfaction with treatment and choice of the same treatment varied according to function and current disease status. Incontinence, bowel dysfunction, and evidence of recurrent disease would make patients less likely to choose the same treatment again.

Shrader-Bogen *et al.* (16) attempted to identify and compare patients' self-reported quality of life and treatment side-effects 1–5 years after radical prostatectomy or radiotherapy. They used a mailed self-administered survey that included a demographic survey, the Functional Assessment of Cancer Therapy—General (to measure the overall quality of life) and the Prostate Cancer Treatment Outcome Questionnaire (to assess the patients' perceptions of the incidence and severity of specific changes in urinary, sexual, and bowel functions). The authors concluded that the prostatectomy group reported more sexual dysfunction and urinary problems whereas the radiotherapy group reported more bowel dysfunction. However, although complaints about problems in sexual and urinary function are common, global quality of life does not appear to be compromised following radical prostatectomy (17).

Goluboff *et al.* (18) looked at the incidence of urinary incontinence after radical prostatectomy and concluded that the operation was well-tolerated and presented excellent patient satisfaction. Early stage prostate cancer patients who were treated by radical prostatectomy also showed a steadily improved quality of life during the year after the surgery (19).

Recently there has been apparently some renewed interest in cryosurgery. In a study by Robinson *et al.* (20), men treated with cryosurgery for localized prostate carcinoma reported that their well-being had returned to pretreatment levels by 12 months, with the exception of sexual function.

Survivors

High prevalence of anxiety and depressive symptoms and decline in leisure activities from prior to the cancer diagnosis have been reported in survivors of prostate cancer (21). However, the actual prevalence of psychiatric problems in cancer survivors remains to be established (22). Post-traumatic stress disorder, fear of recurrence, body image, employment, relationship, and other issues may be present in cancer survivors. Sometimes cancer may even induce profound and radical personality changes and modify the survivor's values and philosophical approach to life (21). Family and social support, personality issues, and the disruption caused by the kind of treatment may play important role in adaptation. People who are positive about their lives in general and are willing to take on, can be expected to adapt relatively well (23).

Relatives

Relatives of cancer patients (including partner) can play a major supportive role. They are usually highly motivated in the direction of trying to assist, their relationship with the patient is often characterized by mutual fidelity and trust, and they are most likely to be available (8). The family of the cancer patient may be asked to contribute by offering support, sharing responsibility for decision-making, offering concrete care (e.g. home care), meeting financial and social costs, maintaining stability, and adapting to changes. However, there is a short- and long-term human cost to the family members and the family may not be able to adjust to the new circumstances. Immediate inter-

ventions or the creation of an extended system of support that deals with education of the family, communication skills, provision of services, mobilizing of social supports, and other issues, may be required (24).

Instruments

There are still considerable methodological problems regarding the development of optimal quality-of-life instruments (25). The use of a rapid screening for psychological distress in prostate carcinoma patients (who may be then referred for treatment), can be a very helpful tool in the hands of the oncologist. A screening method used in a pilot study by Roth *et al.* (26) has given encouraging results.

Rehabilitation

Rehabilitation plans must be discussed with the patient pre-operatively and put in action as soon as possible after surgery (7).

Sexual problems

Sexual problems are common in prostate cancer patients. Contributing factors include the disease itself and forms of treatment (radiation, surgery, hormonal therapy), aging, and psychological-relationship factors. However, concerns about fertility do not tend to be prominent, because of the patients'—usually advanced—age (27).

Assessment

The assessment of chronically ill, and other, patients with sexual difficulties may include questions about relationship strengths: the ability to show caring (e.g. 'has expression of caring changed since the illness began?'), ability to share feelings, role flexibility, ability to negotiate about disagreements, and similar needs for intimacy (e.g. 'how has the illness affected each of your needs for togetherness?'). The assessment of sexual skills may also include questions about flexibility in initiating sex, clear sexual communication, comfort with non-coital orgasms, focus on pleasure versus performance, agreement on sexual variety, and feeling sexual attractive despite physical changes (28). Questions about past medical history, the medical aspects of the disease, and treatment issues are also included.

Symptomatology

Early diagnosis of prostate cancer is often incidental and asymptomatic. Prostate cancer patients often have sexual dysfunction before the cancer diagnosis is made. Medical problems, that may or may not be related to the undiagnosed prostate carcinoma, may compromise pre-morbid sexual functioning (5). Each subsequent treatment following the cancer diagnosis increases the prevalence of sexual problems (29). Also, men with a pre-morbid history of sexual trauma or sexual problems are often more upset when cancer and its treatment interfere with sex (30).

Generally, the most frequent sexual side-effect of cancer and its treatment, is sexual avoidance, driven by anxiety about performance and partner reaction (31). However, in prostate cancer, medical factors appear to play a prominent role in the etiology of sexual dysfunction, in addition to the psychological-relationship ones.

Prostate cancer surgery causes erectile dysfunction in a large number of patients but the risk depends on the type of operation performed (32). Radical prostatectomy is associated with significant erectile problems and some decline in urinary function (33). However, Walsh *et al.* (34) reported that patient-reported rates of potency and continence after radical prostatectomy, performed by an experienced surgeon, were high. Kim *et al.* (35) reported a return of spontaneous partial erections in patients who were offered a new technique using sural nerve grafts to restore continuity of the cavernous nerves, which were resected during radical prostatectomy. It appears that nerve-sparing surgery presents a lower incidence of erectile dysfunction (36) than older surgery techniques. However, some of the reported benefits on sexual function may be the result of patient selection (men with more advanced cancers and pre-operative impotence receive nerve-sparing surgery less often) and not the technique *per se* (37). Schover (29) reports that even men who underwent nerve-sparing surgery and are defined as 'potent' may still present problems. They might then need additional sexual rehabilitation, with the inclusion of the partner.

In men whose semen-producing glands have been surgically removed, 'dry' orgasms (no ejaculation, but normal rhythmic orgasmic contractions in the rectal and pelvic area) occur. Most men complain that the orgasmic sensation is minimal (38). Retrograde ejaculation (result of bladder-neck dysfunction due to surgery) (27), may also incur adverse psychological reactions in some patients, particularly if they do not understand its significance (39).

Prostate cancer patients who had radiotherapy treatment, reported higher levels of sexual dysfunction than age-matched controls; however patients over 74 years of age did not perceive decreased sexual function as a significant problem (40). In another study (41), the same authors reported no changes in pelvic irradiation-induced urinary and intestinal late side-effects, and in sexual function, between 4 and 8 years after radiotherapy. The controls reported no changes in urinary or sexual problems but there was a decrease in intestinal problems. In a study by McCammon *et al.* (15), sexual dysfunction was similar in an external-beam radiation and a radical-prostatectomy group of patients. Preservation of sexual function in a nerve-sparing group was disappointingly low, although the patients in this group had fewer difficulties in achieving an erection than those in a non-nerve-sparing group.

A large proportion of men who undergo hormone-ablation treatment present sexual dysfunction. However, some patients maintain some level of sexual activity (5). Luteinizing-releasing hormone agonist therapy has been reported to strongly suppress erectile function and sexual activity (42). Estrogen treatment—often combined with radiation—reduces sexual drive and can be the key factor in this treatment regime that causes impotence (43).

In a study by Bergman *et al.* (44) men subjected to orchiectomy or treated by estrogens (12 patients from each group) were seldom capable of having intercourse or of experiencing orgasm. The latter group continued sexual activity with a partner more often than the first one, and scored higher for mental depression than the orchiectomy and a radiotherapy group. Nine of twelve patients who received radiotherapy preserved their erectile potency, however seven of them presented a reduced frequency of sexual activity.

Recovery of erectile functioning may be slow and may exceed 6 months in some patients (31). Recovery is more likely in younger men and men who did not present with bulky disease (5). Sexual dysfunction as a known result of therapy may be an important determinant of choice of treatment: Herr *et al.* (45) reported that newly diagnosed asymptomatic metastatic prostate cancer patients who chose to defer immediate intervention had better physical and sexual functioning than those who elected to receive hormonal therapy. The two groups were comparable except that the first group included more sexually active young men than the second group. Concerns over interference with sexual function was an important factor in the patients' decision to defer immediate treatment.

Therapy

Prevention and intervention programs for sexual difficulties with chronically ill (and other) patients (38) may include educational components, 'permission giving', cognitive restructuring techniques, graduated sexual tasks assignments (e.g. sensate focus exercises), techniques to increase sexual arousal and enhancement of general marital skills methods. A number of medical treatments are also available, and a combined (psychotherapy/medical) approach might be advisable for prostate cancer patients with sexual problems.

Prostate cancer patients who experience problems in their sexual function may have the following five options:

- decide to do nothing;
- have psychological treatment in order to try to adapt to the new circumstances in their lives (including sexual function);
- use vacuum pumps;
- try penile injections;
- use a penile prosthesis (46).

Recently, sildenafil (Viagra) can be a new treatment for erectile problems in this group of patients. Other new drugs for impotence, expected to be launched in the near future, may also offer further therapeutic options.

The results of recent studies that looked at prostate cancer patients who received sildenafil treatment for erectile dysfunction, are generally encouraging. Sildenafil was found to be effective (improved erections, ability to have intercourse) in more than half of 84 men who were included in a study by Lowentritt *et al.* (47). Age, pathological state, the degree of nerve-sparing surgery, and baseline post-operative erectile dysfunction had a significant impact on the outcome. In another study, Zippe *et al.* (48) concluded that successful treatment of erectile dysfunction in patients after prostatectomy with Viagra, may depend on the presence of bilateral neurovascular bundles (nerve-sparing approach). Kedia *et al.* (49) looked at a group of prostate cancer patients who presented erectile dysfunction after radiation therapy. They concluded that sildenafil citrate (Viagra) improved the ability to achieve and maintain an erection in most cases. Zelefsky *et al.* (50) observed improved erectile function in more than two-thirds of patients who were presenting post-radiotherapy impotence and were treated with sildenafil. In another study, sildenafil was also well-tolerated and could reverse erectile dysfunction after radiotherapy in a substantial proportion of prostate cancer patients (51). Early non-respondents to sildenafil may respond later. In a study by Hong *et al.* (52), the response to Viagra appears to be dependent upon the interval between nerve-sparing radical prostatectomy and the start of treatment with sildenafil, with a 60% peak between 18 and 24 months.

Intracavernosal injection of a papaverine/phentolamine mixture was shown to be effective in a group of patients who were treated by classical radical prostatectomy (53). Bahnson and Catalona (54) used intracavernous injections of papaverine to investigate the etiology of impotence following nerve-sparing radical retropubic prostatectomy in a group of patients and concluded that the predominant reason was vasculogenic in origin. Transurethral alprostadil (MUSE) was a well-tolerated and effective treatment for patients with erectile dysfunction following radical prostatectomy (55). The effectiveness of yohimbine in the treatment of erectile problems in general, remains a rather controversial issue. Several studies (56) conclude that this treatment is ineffective.

Erectile aids may be used in therapy. Perez *et al.* (17) looked at groups of patients who had nerve-sparing surgery, standard prostatectomy, prostatectomy/use of erectile aids, and a group awaiting radical prostatectomy. Self-reports showed that patients in the first group scored better in most areas of sexuality than patients in the second group. However, patients who were using erectile aids reported the best outcomes in sexuality, similar to patients awaiting surgery. The three surgery subgroups did not present differences in frequency of urinary leakage.

Initial results in 50 patients who underwent a combination procedure of non-nerve sparing radical retropubic prostatectomy and placement of a penile prosthesis showed an early return to sexual function. There was not an apparent increase in morbidity in this group when compared with patients who were submitted to radical prostatectomy alone (57).

Prostate cancer patients who undergo hormonal treatment present sexual-desire problems. In this group, testosterone replacement is not applicable and the only recourse is to attempt to enhance sexual fantasy and physical stimulation with erotic materials, prolonged and varied lovemaking, and vibrator stimulation (29).

Several psychological reactions to serious illness and surgery may also interfere with sexual function. Hawton (58) summarizes the main factors to consider:

- the reactions of the patient (anticipation of failure/harm/pain, impairment of self-concept, depression);

- the reactions of the partner (anxiety, guild);
- the nature of the relationship (discord, poor previous sexual adjustment);
- the response of the medical profession (avoidance of discussion, cursory discussion, inadequate information).

The trauma of having surgery in the area of the genitals may add a psychogenic component in the functional impairment (31). Also, men with retrograde ejaculation following transurethral resection of the prostate (not a direct cause of sexual dysfunction) may develop inhibited sexual desire and other sexual problems (5).

A wide range of cognitive factors may also play an important role in the sexual life of people whose sexual difficulties are related to a physical disorder (59). Common maladaptive thoughts and beliefs include:

- fears concerning the loss of masculinity/femininity;
- negative thoughts about sexual performance;
- taking the sick/disabled role;
- self and partner concerns about physical attractiveness;
- anticipation of pain;
- irrational beliefs about creation of further injury and other issues.

General psychological status (particularly depression and anxiety symptoms), fatigue, and a wide range of fears and concerns may also influence sexual functioning. The disease creates numerous stressors that may have a marked effect upon the couple's relationship. Change of roles, issues of dependence, financial problems, and other issues may make difficult for couples to adapt. Lack of adaptation, especially in cases of pre-existing relationship and sexual problems, may have a devastating effect on the relationship.

There is an important need for pre-operative counseling and opportunity to discuss sexual function in the post-operative period (39).

It appears that men who are clearly told pre-operatively what to expect after surgery, have fewer sexual problems than men who receive no sexual information (60).

Conclusion

The course and treatment of prostate cancer, can cause or aggravate a wide range of health, personal, relationship, sexual, social, employment, and other problems that the patient and partner/family are asked to deal with. A properly co-ordinated interdisciplinary approach is expected to provide optimal care to prostate cancer patients and their families.

References

1. Korda M. *Man to man, surviving prostate cancer*. Little, Brown & Company, London, 1996.
2. Gelder M, Gath D, Mayou R *et al. Oxford textbook of psychiatry* (3rd edn). Oxford University Press, Oxford, 1996, 358–62, 391–3.
3. Roth A, Scher H. Genitourinary malignancies. In: *Psychooncology* (ed. J Holland, W Breitbart, PB Jacobsen *et al.*) Oxford University Press, New York, 1998, 349–58.
4. Derogatis LR. Prevalence of psychiatric disorders among cancer patients. *J Am Med Assoc* 1985, **249**, 751–7.
5. Ofman U. Sexual quality of life in men with prostate cancer. *Cancer* 1995, **75** (7) (Suppl), 1949–53.
6. Heim HM, Oei TP. Comparison of prostate cancer patients with and without pain. *Pain* 1993, **53** (2), 159–62.
7. Jacobsen PB, Roth A, Holland J. Surgery. In: *Psychooncology* (ed. J Holland, W Breitbart, PB Jacobsen *et al*). Oxford University Press, New York, 1998, 257–68.
8. Bindemann S. Psychological impact of cancer its assessment, treatment, and ensuing effects on quality of life. In: *The quality of life of cancer patients* (ed. NK Aaronson, J Beckman). Raven Press, New York, 1987, 227–38.
9. Litwin MS. Health related quality of life in older men without prostate carcinoma. *J Urol* 1999, **161** (4), 1180–4.
10. Da Silva F, Reis E, Costa T *et al*. Quality of life in patients with prostatic cancer. *Cancer* 1993, **71** (3) (Suppl), 1138–42.
11. Litwin MS, Hays RD, Fimk A *et al*. Quality-of-life outcomes in men treated for localized prostate cancer. *JAMA* 1995, **273** (2), 129–35.
12. Haythornthwaite JA, Raja SN, Fisher B *et al*. Pain and quality of life following radical retropubic prostatectomy. *J Urol* 1988, **160** (5), 1761–4.
13. Daut R, Cleeland C. The prevalence and severity of pain in cancer. *Cancer* 1982, **50**, 1913–8.
14. Gaffo O, Fellin G, Graffer U *et al*. Assessment of quality of life after radical radiotherapy for prostate cancer. *Br J Urol* 1996, **78**, 557–63.
15. McCammon KA, Kolm P, Main B *et al*. Comparative quality-of-life analysis after radical prostatectomy or external beam radiation for localized prostate cancer. *Urology* 1999, **54** (3), 509–16.
16. Shrader-Bogen C, Kjellberg J, McPherson C. Quality of life and treatment outcomes. *Cancer* 1997, **79** (10), 1977–86.
17. Perez MA, Meyerowitz BE, Lieskovsky G *et al*. Quality of life and sexuality following radical prostatectomy in patients with prostate cancer who use or not use erectile aids. *Urology* 1997, **50** (5), 740–6.

18. Goluboff ET, Saidi JA, Mazer S *et al.* Urinary continence after radical prostatectomy: the Columbia experience. *J Urol* 1998, **159** (4), 1276–80.

19. Litwin MS, McGuigan KA, Shpall AI *et al.* Recovery of health related quality of life in the year after radical prostatectomy: early experience. *J Urol* 1999, **161** (2), 515–9.

20. Robinson JW, Saliken JC, Donnelly BJ *et al.* Quality-of-life outcomes for men treated with cryosurgery for localized prostate carcinoma. *Cancer* 1999, **86** (9), 1793–801.

21. Schag CA, Ganz PA, Wing DS *et al.* Quality of life in adult survivors of lung, colon and prostate cancer. *Quality of Life Research* 1994, 3, 127–41.

22. Kornblith AB. Psychosocial adaptation of cancer survivors. In: *Psychooncology* (ed. J Holland, W Breitbart, PB Jacobsen *et al*). Oxford University Press, New York, 1998, 223–40.

23. Spencer S, Carver C, Price A. Psychological and social factors in adaptation. In: *Psychooncology* (ed. J Holland, W Breitbart, PB Jacobsen *et al*). Oxford University Press, New York, 1998, 211–22.

24. Lederberg M. The family of the cancer patient. In: *Psychooncology* (ed. J Holland, W. Breitbart PB Jacobsen *et al*). Oxford University Press, New York, 1998, 981–93.

25. Fossa SD. Quality of life in prostate cancer: what are the issues and how are they measured? *Eur Urology* 1996, **29** (2) (Suppl), 121–3.

26. Roth A, Kornblith A, Batel-Copel L *et al.* Rapid screening for psychological distress in men with prostate carcinoma, a pilot study. *Cancer* 1998, **82**, 1904–8.

27. Champion A. Male cancer and sexual function. *Sexual and Marital Therapy* 1996, **II** (3), 227–44.

28. Schover LR. Sexual problems in chronic illness. In: *Principles and practice of sex therapy, update for the 1990's* (ed. S Leiblum, R Rosen). The Guilford Press, New York, 1989, 319–51.

29. Schover LR. Sexual rehabilitation after treatment for prostate cancer. *Cancer* 1993, **71** (3) (Suppl), 1024–30.

30. Schover LR. Sexual dysfunction. In: *Psychooncology* (ed. J Holland, W Breitbart, PB Jacobsen *et al.* Oxford University Press, New York, 1998, 494–9.

31. Ofman U. Preservation of function in genitourinary cancers: psychosexual and psychosocial issues. *Cancer Investig* 1995, **13** (1), 125–31.

32. Masters W, Johnson V, Kolodny R. *Human sexuality* (5th edn). Harper Collins College Publishers, New York, 1995, 620–1.

33. Stanford JL, Feng Z, Hamilton AS *et al.* Urinary and sexual function after radical prostatectomy for clinically localized prostate cancer: the prostate cancer outcomes study. *JAMA* 2000, **283** (3), 354–60.

34. Walsh PC, Marschke P, Ricker D *et al.* Patient-reported urinary continence and sexual function after anatomic radical prostatectomy. *Urology* 2000, **55** (1), 58–61.

35. Kim ED, Scardino PT, Hampel O *et al.* Interposition of sural nerve restores function of cavernous nerves resected during radical prostatectomy. *J Urol* 1999, **161** (1), 188–92.

36. Quinlan DM, Eptein JI, Carter BS *et al.* Sexual function following radical prostatectomy: influence of preservation of neurovascular bundles. *J Urol* 1991, **145**, 998–1002.

37. Talcott JA, Rieker P, Propert KJ *et al.* Patient-reported impotence and incontinence after nerve-sparing radical prostatectomy. *J Nat Cancer Inst* 1997, **89** (15), 1117–23.

38. Schover LR, Jensen SB. *Sexuality and chronic illness: a comprehensive approach.* Guilford Press, New York, 1988.

39. Bancroft J. *Human sexuality and its problems* (2nd edn). Churchill Livingstone, 1989, 582–4.

40. Fransson P, Widmark A. Self-assessed sexual function after pelvic irradiation for prostate carcinoma, comparison with an age-matched control group. *Cancer* 1996, **78** (5), 1066–78.

41. Fransson P, Widmark A. Late side-effects unchanged 4–8 years after radiotherapy for prostate carcinoma: a comparison with age-matched controls. *Cancer* 1999, **85** (3), 678–88.

42. Marumo K, Baba S, Murai M. Erectile function and nocturnal penile tumescence in patients with prostate cancer undergoing luteinizing-releasing hormone agonist therapy. *Int J Urol* 1999, **6** (1), 19–23.

43. Masters W, Johnson V, Kolodny R. *Heterosexuality.* Thorsons, New York, 1994, 336–338.

44. Bergman B, Damber JE, Littbrand B *et al.* Sexual function in prostatic cancer patients treated with radiotherapy, orchiectomy or oestrogens. *Br J Urol* 1984, **56** (1), 64–9.

45. Herr H, Kornblith A, Ofman U. A comparison of the quality of life of patients with metastatic prostate cancer who received or did not receive hormonal therapy. *Cancer* 1993, **71**, 1143–50.

46. Sprouce DO. Sexual rehabilitation of the prostate cancer patient. *Cancer* 1995, **75**, 1954–6.

47. Lowentritt BH, Scardino PT, Miles BJ *et al.* Sildenafil citrate after radical retropubic prostatectomy. *J Urol* 1999, **162** (5), 1614–7.

48. Zippe CD, Kedia AW, Nelson DR *et al.* Treatment of erectile dysfunction after radical prostatectomy with sildenafil citrate (Viagra). *Urology* 1998, **52** (6), 963–6.

49. Kedia S, Zippe CD, Agarwal A *et al.* Treatment of erectile dysfunction with sildenafil citrate (Viagra) after radiation therapy for prostate cancer. *Urology* 1999, **54** (2), 308–12.

50. Zelefsky MJ, McKee AB, Lee H *et al.* Efficacy of oral sildenafil in patients with erectile dysfunction after radiotherapy for carcinoma of the prostate. *Urology* 1999, **53** (4), 775–8.

51. Weber DC, Bieri S, Kurtz JM *et al.* Prospective pilot study of sildenafil for treatment of postradiotherapy erectile dysfunction in patients with prostate cancer. *J Clin Oncology* 1999, **17** (11), 3444–9.

52. Hong EK, Lepor H, McCullough AR. Time dependent patient satisfaction with sildenafil foe erectile dysfunction (ED) after nerve-sparing radical retropubic prostatectomy (RRP). *Int J Impotence Res* 1999, 1 (11) (Suppl), S15–22.

53. Dennis RL, McDougal WS. Pharmacological treatment of erectile dysfunction after radical prostatectomy. *J Urol* 1988, **139** (4), 775–6.

54. Bahnson RR, Catalona WJ. Papaverine testing of impotent patients following nervesparing radical prostatectomy. *J Urol* 1988, **139** (4), 773–4.

55. Costabile RA, Speval M, Fishman IJ *et al.* Efficacy and safety of transurethral alprostadil in patients with erectile dysfunction following radical prostatectomy. *J Urol* 1998, **160** (40), 1325–8.

56. Teloken C, Rhoden EL, Sogari P *et al*. Therapeutic effects of yohimbine hydrochloride on organic erectile dysfunction. *J Urol* 1998, **159** (1), 122–4.

57. Khoudary KP, DeWolf WC, Bruning CO. 3rd *et al*. Immediate sexual rehabilitation by simultaneous placement of penile prosthesis in patients undergoing radical prostatectomy: initial results in 50 patients. *Urology* 1997, **50** (3), 395–9.

58. Hawton K. *Sex therapy, a practical guide*. Oxford University Press, New York, 1985, 76–9, 235–9.

59. Spence S. Psychosexual therapy, a cognitive-behavioural approach (ed. D Marcer). Chapman & Hall, London, 1991, 264–74.

60. Reinish J, Beasley R. *The Kinsey Institute New Report on Sex. What you must know to be sexually literate*. St. Martin's Press, New York, 1990, 437–42.

Section VII

30 | Prostate cancer prevention

Keith Griffiths and Louis J. Denis

Introduction

In a symposium on the Biology of the Prostate and Related Tissues, at the National Cancer Institute in Washington in 1962, Professor Charles Huggins, in his opening remarks (1), talked of the fable of the three blind men who, for the first time, had encountered an elephant. In examining the different parts of the great beast, one was impressed by the tusks, reminiscent of a walrus, and another thought the hide was tough like a turtle. A third was taken by the snake-like trunk. The magnificence of the complete entity was not easy to envisage. In like manner, Professor Huggins emphasized, 'the importance of assembling the bits and pieces of prostatic problems in a unitary concept'. He emphasized the value of interdisciplinary discussion, the importance of bringing advances in science to the bedside and highlighted certain problems recognized at that time (Fig. 30.1), one of which, was the geographical differences in prostatic cancer incidence. Such problems still exercise the minds of today's investigators, but certain bits and pieces are coming together and this text relates to possible reasons for the high prevalence of prostate cancer in the developed countries of the

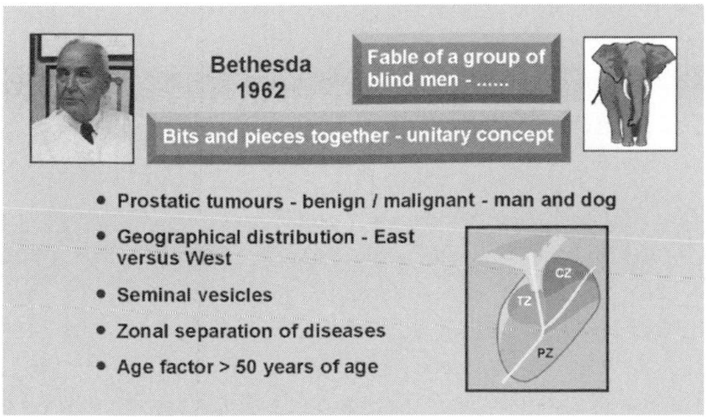

Fig. 30.1 Topics highlighted by Professor C Huggins in 1962 that he considered worthy of more investigation.

USA and Northern Europe, relative to that in the countries of Asia.

It would now be accepted that our knowledge and understanding of the endocrine, biochemical, and molecular processes implicated in the pathogenesis of prostatic disease is rapidly growing. Although long recognized that symptomatic clinical BPH, associated with bladder outlet obstruction is not a pre-malignant condition that leads to the development of prostatic cancer, current attitudes (2) are directed to the possibility that genetic instability associated with epithelial-cell hyperplasia of microscopic BPH may develop into transition zone cancer. Prostatic enlargement associated with bladder outlet obstruction is generally considered the consequence of dysfunctional growth regulatory processes (3, 4) within the gland, resulting from an androgen-estrogen imbalance at mid-life, the resultant estrogenic stimulus promoting the development of the benign stromal adenoma.

It is also clear from our understanding of the natural history of BPH (4–6) that similar risk factors are associated with the pathogenesis of both BPH and prostatic cancer. Particularly important is the age factor (7), both clinical conditions generally presenting in men beyond 50 years of age and also the fact that neither disease presents in men castrated early in life, suggesting that functional testes, but presumably androgens, are implicated in disease aetiology. Moreover, both conditions clinically respond to androgen-ablative therapy. Ethnicity and family history are other risk factors that are also recognized as exercising some influence on prostate cancer and the etiology of the disease. Also well accepted, is that early phases in the pathogenesis of cancer can be identified a number of years prior to the disease being clinically evident (Fig. 30.2). Certain pre-malignant lesions, prostatic intra-epithelial neoplasia (PIN), are recognized as an early stage in the multi-step process of carcinogenesis (8), although the evidence that atypical adenomatous

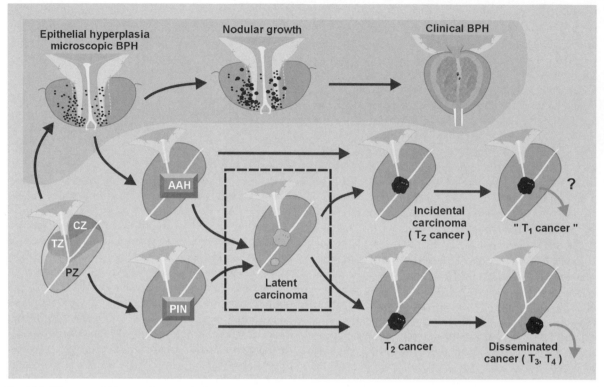

Fig. 30.2 The natural history of prostatic disease.

hyperplasia (AAH) is such a pre-malignant lesion remains equivocal (9). As with cancer of the breast, it may well be that some part of the commonality (10) of cancers of breast and prostate relates to initiation at the time of adolescence, or puberty, when younger people are 'inflicted' with marked hormonal changes that resulted in periods of rapid growth of the breasts and prostate. It is noteworthy, also, that certain 'bothersome' symptoms are now being recognized in men in their 40s (11, 12) and 'histological BPH', epithelial-cell hyperplasia and nodular hyperplasia, can be seen in the prostate glands of men in their early 20s (13, 14). Moreover, these classical studies of Coffey and his colleagues emphasized the increasing prevalence of these foci of epithelial hyperplasia with increasing age, in men from various parts of the world, both East and West.

The molecular biology associated with these early stages in the development of prostatic disease is of particular interest and was the essential basis of the discussions of a committee of the recent International Consultation on BPH (4). Its report highlighted the complexity of the processes concerned in the regulation

of prostate growth, but a consensus viewpoint was that on the basis of a better understanding of these processes, greater emphasis should now be directed to intervention initiatives, possibly related to dietary factors, that could lead to the prevention of prostatic cancer and BPH. Some of these dietary concepts are now considered in relation to molecular endocrinology implicated in the growth regulatory processes of the prostate gland.

Certain dietary factors and the risk of cancer of the prostate gland

The marked differences in the incidence of certain types of cancer between various countries or regions of the world, suggest that particular dietary factors can influence the biological processes related to carcinogenesis, either in a provocative or an inhibitory role. Estimates of the proportion of cancers attributable to dietary status habit vary from 10% to 70% (15–17), but data continues to accumulate supporting a role for such dietary factors (18, 19) and, although often contradictory, a pattern is recognizable, which directs attention to the potential benefits for healthcare of preventative studies related to the intake of these factors. This relationship between dietary status and cancer has recently been reviewed (20).

That geographical differences in cancer incidence are attributable to diet is supported by changes observed in the incidence rates in migrants who move from areas of low risk for particular cancers, to countries where the risk is higher (21–23). Such changes are illustrated by data from the migration of Japanese and Chinese men and women to Hawaii and to the mainland USA, whose risk of developing prostate or breast cancer, previously low, increases to match that of the indigenous population within a few generations.

Miller and his colleagues (19) considered that appropriate dietary changes could decrease the incidence of various cancers by reducing fat intake and increasing vegetable consumption in the case of breast and colorectal cancers, by reduction of obesity for endometrial cancer and diminishing intake of cured meats, salt-preserved foodstuffs and nitrite, whilst increasing fruit and vegetable consumption, in the case of stomach cancer. Such views are controversial (24, 25), particularly with regard to the relationship between dietary fat intake and cancer risk (24, 26).

'Cancers of the prostate and breast, cardiovascular disease, and osteoporosis feature prominently as 'Western Diseases'. The Western diet is characterized by high animal fat content and protein, and low fiber, which contrasts with the diet of the Asian communities, which is low in animal fat and rich in starches, legumes, fruit, and vegetables – all of which have a high-fiber content (Fig. 30.3). Predictably, therefore, animal fat is readily seen as a **causative factor**. More recently, however, has been the recognition (20, 27) that **certain constituents of the Asian diet and that of the Mediterranean region, protect against the development of these diseases**, and it is the lack of these constituents in the Western diet that is the important factor.

Geographical differences in the incidence of cancer of the prostate

Carcinoma of the prostate belongs to the group of hormone-dependent cancers, those of breast, ovary, and endometrium, the incidence and mortality rates of which, are high in the Western world, relative to those in Asia and in Mediterranean countries (Fig. 30.4).

Already, prostatic cancer is recognized as a serious healthcare problem, one of the most commonly diagnosed cancers in the West (28, 29), with the life-time risk in North American men being nearly 10%. A recent report (30) indicates that carcinoma of the prostate is now the second most common cancer after skin cancer in the male population of the USA, and the second most common cause of death from cancer, after that of the lung. The highest mortality rates occur in the black male population of the USA, twice that of the whites (31–33). The rate is 30 times less in Osaka, Japan, and 120 times less in Shanghai, China, than that of black males in North America (28, 34–36). The low prevalence prostate cancer in Japan is noteworthy, since their mean life-expectancy and socio-economic standards are as high as their counterparts in the West. The incidence in Japan is, however, rising and Japanese migrants to the United States manifest an increased risk to approximately half that of the indigenous Americans (28, 37).

Since prostate cancer, as well as benign prostatic hyperplasia (BPH), clinically present over the age of 50, the prevalence of both later in life in relation to the

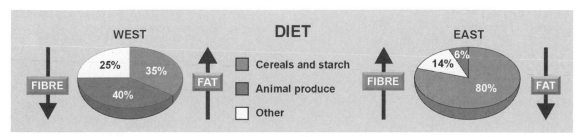

Fig. 30.3 General characteristics of Western and Eastern diets.

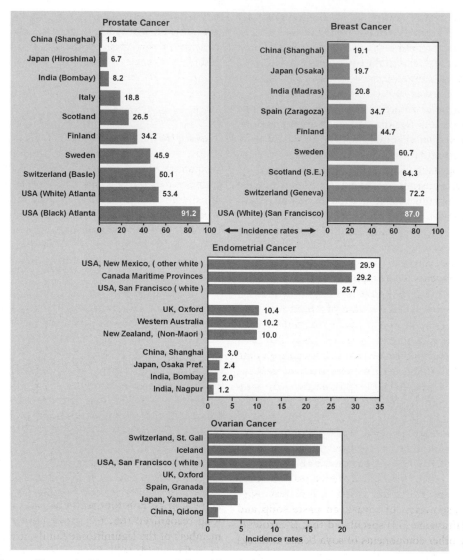

Fig. 30.4 Highest and lowest incidence rates recorded world-wide for prostate cancer, breast cancer, endometrial cancer and ovarian cancer.

increasing life-expectancy in developed countries, suggests that prostate disease will become an even more formidable health problem in the next millennium and emphasizes the importance of preventative measures.

Cancer etiology in relation to dietary habits

The Western diet is deficient in fiber and evidence supports the concept that high-fiber intake protects against colorectal cancer (38), possibly mammary cancer (39). Vegetables are a source of fiber, but their protective role (40, 41) may now additionally be attributable to other non-nutrient components of plant products (42–44).

The belief that prostate cancer risk was related to a high animal fat intake merely originated from international rates of prostate cancer mortality (45, 46) with the positive correlation between occurrence and mortality, and *per capita* fat consumption. The United States Health Professionals Follow-up Study of 47 855 men aged 40–75 (47) was one of the first studies to include an adjustment for total caloric intake. Total animal fat consumption was directly related to the risk of advanced cancer, although the linear trend fell just short of acceptable statistical significance. Other studies, however, (48–50) failed to find this association. Moreover, dietary fat did not influence the incidence of experimental prostate cancer (51), although total caloric intake rather than percentage fat, was associated with tumourigenesis, a concept supported by Albanes (52) in man.

Epidemiologists tend to support the hypothesis that prostate cancer risk is increased by high levels of dietary fat. Unfortunately, few studies have used a satisfactory dietary methodology and putative associations are thereby weakened. Most failed to adjust for total caloric intake and made little reference to fruits, vegetables, and cereals – rich sources of the non-nutrient components of the typical Asian diet (20, 27) and referred to as phyto-estrogens.

Some have, however, reported a protective effect of vegetables against the risk of cancer, in particular, a 17-year Japanese cohort study (53–55) of 265 118 adults, aged more than 40 years, which investigated the relationship between life-style and disease risk. Daily consumption of green-yellow vegetables was found to be an important protective factor against cancers of the stomach and prostate, as well as ischaemic heart disease, atherosclerosis, and liver cirrhosis. Green-yellow vegetables, defined as containing more than 600 μg of carotene/100 g, included pumpkin, carrots, spinach, green lettuce, and green asparagus. The mortality from cancer of the breast was lower with increased consumption of soya bean paste soup and soya milk. Hirayama (53) speculated that β-carotene, and possibly other components of soya beans and vegetables, were implicated in the reduction of mortality. In a case-control study on the effects of diet on breast cancer risk in Singapore (56), noteworthy was the finding that soya protein was recognized as a protective component of the diet.

Both investigations, therefore, suggested the potential influence of soya bean products on cancer risk and drew attention to components of certain vegetables, present in the traditional Asian diet, that may influence carcinogenesis. In a study of Japanese men in Hawaii, Stemmermann and colleagues (49) increased consumption of rice and soya were associated with a decreased risk of prostate cancer. Soya-based foods, such as tofu, are a rich source of the phyto-estrogens referred to as isoflavonoids (20, 27).

Several investigators have also demonstrated significant strong negative correlations between mortality from prostate cancer and dietary intake of cereals (57, 58). Cereals contain precursors of the lignans found in men and women, another group of phyto-estrogens (20, 59). Furthermore, a cohort study of diet, life-style, and prostate cancer in Seventh-Day Adventist men revealed that increasing consumption of beans, lentils, peas, tomatoes, raisins, dates, and other dried foods, were all associated with significantly decreased prostate cancer risk (60). The Mediterranean-style diet, considered protective against endocrine cancer as well as cardiovascular disease (61, 62), features a high intake of fresh fruit, vegetables, and pasta. Fresh fruit, citrus fruits, and raw vegetables were found to be protective against many cancers, including that of the prostate, in several Italian studies (63–65).

Dietary isoflavonoids and lignans: the phyto-estrogens

Many foods of plant origin contain constituents referred to as isoflavonoids, flavonoids, and lignans (Fig. 30.5) some of which possess weak estrogenic activity (Fig. 30.6) and therefore the potential for exerting an influence on hormone-dependent cancers, such as those of the breast and prostate (20). They can be equated with tamoxifen, the weakly estrogenic agent universally used in breast-cancer management. The presence of non-steroidal substances with estrogenic activity in certain foodstuffs of plant origin has been long recognized (66, 67). Soya bean and red clover, members of the leguminosae family, are major sources of isoflavonoids (67). Soya is consumed daily in large amounts in China and Japan and traditional diets of the Indian sub-continent, Africa, some Mediterranean countries, and South America, have a high-legume content including soya, lentils, and chick peas (67).

Soya beans contain the glycoside conjugates of the isoflavonoids, genistein, and daidzein and their methylated derivatives, biochanin A, and formononetin (Fig. 30.7). These can be metabolized by the enzymes of the normal microflora of the gut to the aglycones, genistein, and daidzein, which are then absorbed and appear in blood and ultimately in urine, primarily as glucuronide conjugates, and also sulphates (20).

The lignans also constitute a group of diphenolic compounds of plant origin (67, 68). The plant precursors, matairesinol and secoisolariciresinol, are metab-

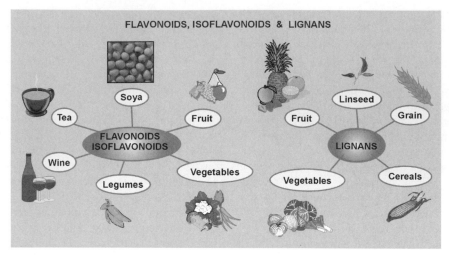

Fig. 30.5 Diagrammatic representation of certain sources of flavonoids, isoflavonoids and lignans.

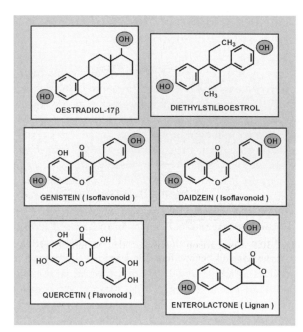

Fig. 30.6 Relationship between the chemical structures of estradiol-17β, the synthetic estrogen diethylstilboestrol, and weak dietary estrogens.

olized after ingestion by intestinal microflora to give rise to the weakly estrogenic enterolactone and enterodiol, respectively (Fig. 30.8). The lignans are absorbed from the gut to appear in blood and other body fluids. The precursors of the lignans are found in many cereals, grains, fruits, and vegetables but the richest source is linseed (flaxseed) (69).

The isoflavonoids and lignans are found in various body fluids (20), in urine, plasma, saliva, and in semen. Expressed prostatic fluid contains enterolactone and equol (70), suggesting that dietary estrogens can accumulate in the prostate and are components of prostatic secretion along with proteins such as prostate-specific antigen (PSA). The levels of isoflavonoids are high in the urine and plasma of the Japanese and Chinese men and women (Fig. 30.9). Lignans and isoflavonoids are also excreted in large amounts in the urine of vegetarians (71) who consume large quantities of whole-grain cereals, vegetables, and fruits, and who also have a lower incidence of prostate cancer than the general Western population.

Regulation of prostate growth: is there a role for phyto-estrogens?

The essential issue, therefore, relates to the growth regulatory mechanisms that is the manner. Essentially, in relation to these growth regulatory processes of the prostate gland and the potential role of the phyto-estrogens in influencing their activity. Most important, is the recognition that these phyto-estrogens have characteristics other than those directed to their well-established activity as weak estrogen agonists or indeed, estrogen antagonists (20). These will be considered in some depth, later, but are simply illustrated in Fig. 30.10.

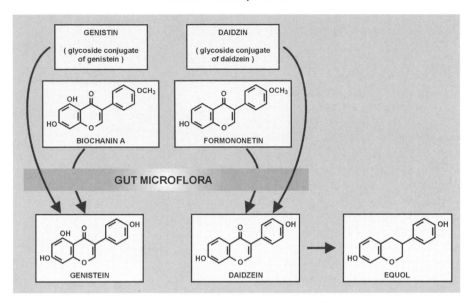

Fig. 30.7 Diagrammatic representation of metabolism by the normal gut microflora of dietary components into particular isoflavonoids and derivatives.

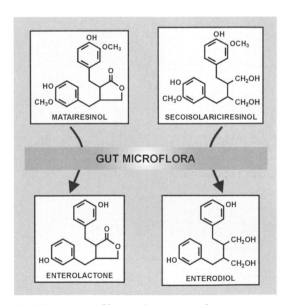

Fig. 30.8 Formation of lignans by gut microflora.

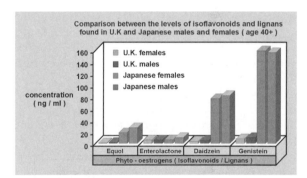

Fig. 30.9 Comparison between the serum levels of isoflavonoids and lignans found in UK and Japanese males and females (age 40+).

- 5α- reductase inhibition
- Tyrosine kinase inhibition
- Aromatase enzyme inhibition
- Angiogenesis inhibition
- DNA topoisomerase inhibition
- Tumourigenesis inhibition
- Antioxidant activity

Fig. 30.10 Biological properties of Isoflavonoids and lignans.

A brief discussion on some of the complexities of the growth regulatory mechanisms of the prostate gland is essential, however, in order to understand the probable means by which the phyto-estrogens could influence growth control.

Steroid hormones and growth-regulatory factors

The prostate is androgen-dependent and a source of testosterone is necessary for the growth and function of the gland (72), although it is 5α-dihydrotestosterone (DHT) that, as a DHT-androgen receptor (AR) complex, associates with specific hormone response elements (HREs) on the genome (73, 74) to modulate, in association with other transcription factors (TFs), the expression of androgen-responsive genes (Fig. 30.11). DHT is essential for prostate growth (75) and exercises an important role in the regulation of gene activity.

Androgens, however, as well as estrogens, glucocorticoids, and any other 'endocrine-related agents' that might, for example, be made available through the diet or even the environment, are often now referred to as extrinsic factors in the regulation of prostate growth (76, 77). Their biological effects on the gland are seen to be mediated by various peptide growth-regulatory factors. These intrinsic factors, which are produced by the gland, influence prostatic growth by promoting inter- and intra-cellular signalling between and within cell populations, through paracrine, autocrine, and intracrine effects (Fig. 30.12). It is the biological actions of these intrinsic factors, such as epidermal growth factor (EGF), keratinocyte growth factor (KGF), insulin-like growth factors (IGF-I &-II), and the fibroblast growth factors (FGFs), that promote the mitogenic effect and directly stimulate cell proliferation under the modulating influence of the steroid hormones. The inter-relationship, or crosstalk, between the signaling pathways influenced by DHT and those regulated by growth-stimulatory factors is pivotal to growth regulation in the prostate (Fig. 30.13).

Equally important in growth regulation is the intimate relationship between the stromal and epithelial compartments of the prostate, an interaction recognized many years ago by Franks (78), who reported that the stromal elements influence epithelial cell proliferation. The more recent studies of Cunha and his colleagues (79) have further emphasized the importance of this relationship. Essentially, DHT-mediated effects on the stromal compartment produce growth-stimulatory factors, which induce signal-transduction pathways within the epithelial cells that promote growth and differentiation (Fig. 30.14).

Interest at present, centers on KGF, one of the FGF family (FGF-7), and seen as a particularly important growth-promoting factor within the prostate (80–83).

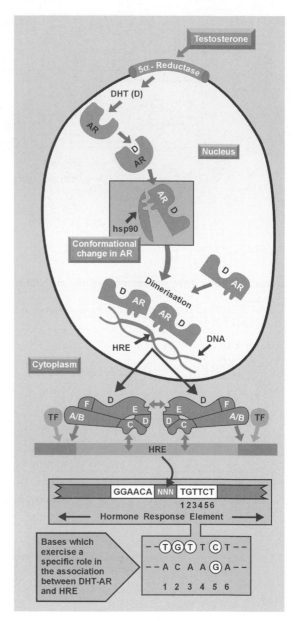

Fig. 30.11 Formation of the dihydrotestosterone–androgen receptor complex: DHT (D), dihydrotestosterone; AR, androgen receptor; HRE, hormone response element. TF, transcription factors.

KGF, produced by the fibroblasts within the stroma, elicits a paracrine mitogenic effect through an FGF-receptor (FGF-R) protein located on the epithelial-cell membrane. This receptor, FGF-R2-exonIIIb, a splice variant of the FGF-R2 (bek) gene, specifically recognizes KGF (84). Transforming growth factor (TGF)-β, originating in the smooth muscle-like cells of the

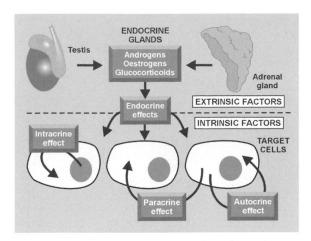

Fig. 30.12 Extrinsic and intrinsic growth regulatory factors.

stroma, inhibits this mitogenic action of KGF on epithelial-cell proliferation.

KGF has no effect on the stromal cells, whereas FGF-2 promotes an autocrine mitogenic action, mediated by the receptor FGF-R1, on the stromal elements (85), but it has no effect on epithelial cells. FGF-R1, encoded by the FGF-R1 (fig) gene, is normally localised only in stromal tissue.

The FGF family (FGF-1 to FGF-10) would appear to have a major role in the regulation of prostate growth. The FGFs, as well as other growth-stimulatory factors like EGF, associate with high-affinity receptors on the cell membrane, which have a tyrosine-specific protein kinase (TK) as part of the internal domain. The FGFRs are encoded by four distinct genes, but alternative

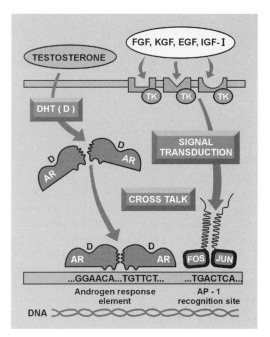

Fig. 30.13 Crosstalk between androgen- and growth factor-mediated signaling pathways.

splicing generates various isoforms, which consequently enhances the complexity of ligand–receptor interactions. FGF-8 mRNA was reported to be over-expressed in 71% of 31 human prostate cancers studied (86), has been identified in the androgen-independent Du-145 prostate cancer cells (87), and could well be concerned in cancer progression. A change in FGF-R2 expression, FGF-R2exonIIIb to FGF-

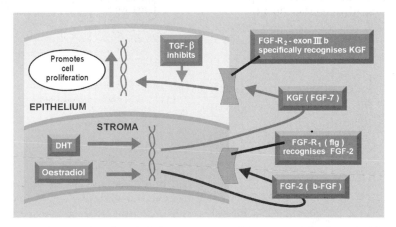

Fig. 30.14 Relationship between stromal and epithelial compartments of the prostate gland: DHT, dihydrotestosterone; TGF, transforming growth factor; FGF, fibroblast growth factors; KGF, keratinocyte growth factor.

R2exonIIIc, has been identified (88) in the Dunning prostate tumor of the rat, as it progresses to androgen independence. The different FGFs therefore associate with the FGF-Rs with varying affinities, although the precise part these interactions play in the growth-regulatory processes, both normal as well as dysfunctional, remains to be determined.

Estrogens and the prostate

Stromal hyperplasia is induced by estrogens and in relation to this, it has been seen to be relevant that the 'classical' estrogen receptor-α (ERα) is predominantly localized in the smooth muscle cells of the stroma of the human prostate (89). This would suggest that estradiol, as well as DHT, may be synergistically implicated in the production of FGF-2 by stromal cells (Fig. 30.14). Estrogens are clearly implicated in the growth-regulatory mechanisms of the prostate (4), although a precise role remains to be established. Nonetheless, exciting have been recent reports (90, 91) of a complementary DNA clone that encodes a new, distinct estrogen receptor, referred to as estrogen receptor β (ERβ). Especially of interest, is that the human and rat ERβ clones were identified within cDNA libraries from human testis and rat prostate. The ERβ also has a high affinity for estradiol. The ERα, however, predominates in the female reproductive system, whereas ERβ would appear to be the principal estrogen receptor component of the prostate, with cell-specific localization to the secretory epithelial cells of the gland (90) and research interest is now directed to the biological role of ERβ relative to that of ERα. Their roles may be quite distinct, complementary, or antagonistic and in relation to this, it is reported (92) that certain other estrogenic compounds preferentially bind to the ERβ (Fig. 30.15).

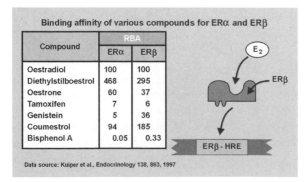

Binding affinity of various compounds for ERα and ERβ

Compound	RBA	
	ERα	ERβ
Oestradiol	100	100
Diethylstilboestrol	468	295
Oestrone	60	37
Tamoxifen	7	6
Genistein	5	36
Coumestrol	94	185
Bisphenol A	0.05	0.33

Data source: Kuiper et al., Endocrinology 138, 863, 1997

Fig. 30.15 The 'new' estrogen receptor, ERβ.

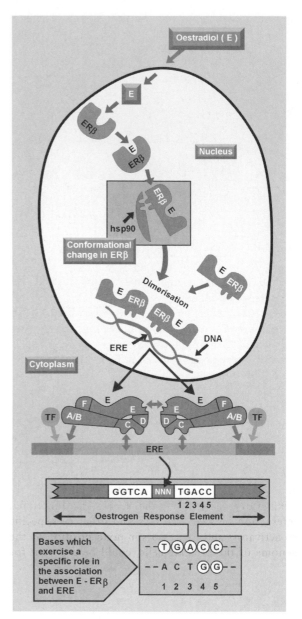

Fig. 30.16 Diagrammatic illustration of the intracellula processes relating to estrogen action.

Although similar amino acid sequences are recognized in both DNA and estrogen-binding domains of these receptor proteins, suggesting that they would associate with the same recognition sites on the genome, the estrogen-response elements (Fig. 30.16), the N-terminal A/B region, and related TAF-1 activa-

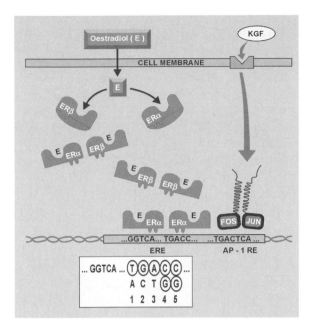

Fig. 30.17 Potential interrelationship between the estrogen-binding domain, of the receptor proteins and the genome: E, estradiol; ER, estrogen receptor; KGF keratinocyte-growth factor.

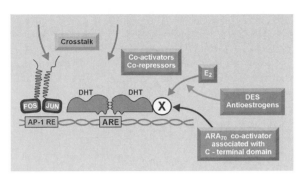

Fig. 30.18 Diagrammatic illustration of co-activator X, influenced by estradiol and part of the mechanism associated with androgen-receptor action.

The phyto-estrogens: biological effects with relevance to the prevention of prostatic disease

Estrogenic activity

Enterolactone, daidzein, genistein have weak estrogens activity (100), although anti-estrogenic properties have also been described. They compete with estradiol for binding to the nuclear estrogen receptor (101) and stimulate the synthesis of sex hormone binding globulin (SHBG) in the liver (102). Of the total testosterone in plasma, only 2% is free and this biologically active fraction enters the prostate. Any increase in SHBG levels would decrease free plasma-testosterone. Higher plasma SHBG and decreased free-testosterone have been reported for vegetarian men (103), Japanese and Chinese men (104).

Inhibition of steroid-metabolizing enzymes

Within the prostate, testosterone is metabolized to 5α-dihydrotestosterone (DHT) by the 5α-reductase (5α-R) enzyme (20). DHT associates with the androgen receptor (AR) and is the DHT–AR complex that influences gene transcription (105).

Recent studies (106) confirm that phyto-estrogens inhibit not only 5α-reductase, but also 17β-hydroxysteroid dehydrogenase, the latter regulating the reversible interconversion of testosterone and androstenedione, as well as estrone and estradiol.

There are substantial levels of plasma estrogens in the human male, approximately 30% of the plasma estrogen being synthesized and secreted by the testes and the remainder is derived from the peripheral aromatization of the adrenal C19-steroids, such as dehy-

tion functions are, however, different. Crosstalk (Fig. 30.17) between signaling pathways involving steroid-receptor function and those promoted by growth stimulatory factors (4), the synergistic functional interaction between the ERs and other cell-specific co-activators and -repressors in juxta-position on the genome of the prostate cells, could be different for the ERβ relative to ERα (93–97). The nucleotide recognition sequences could, for example, specifically interact with a ERα/ERβ heterodimer, and it is now necessary to further investigate these molecular events. Such work will revitalize interest in the precise biological role of estrogens within the human prostate gland, an interest that has already been particularly evoked by the recent studies of Rosner and his colleagues (98), with regard to the mitogenic effect of sex hormone binding globulin (SHBG) on the stromal tissue of the human prostate and of Chang and colleagues (99), which direct attention to the association of estradiol with the ALA70 co-activator, which, as part of a tripartite unit (Fig. 30.18), enhances the androgenic influence of DHT on gene transcription.

FGF family are recognized as potent angiogenic agents (115). Blocking angiogenesis could inhibit cancer progression. Genistein inhibited the FGF-2 induced invasion of collagen by bovine microvascular endothelial cells, with a reported IC50 of approximately 150 mM. Endothelial-cell proliferation *in vivo* was inhibited by lower concentrations of the isoflavonoid. Moreover, genistein significantly reduced the FGF-2 stimulated elevation of both the urokinase-type plasminogen activator (PA) and its physiological inhibitor (PAI-1) in vascular endothelial cells, factors associated with the proteolytic degradation of the extracellular matrix in angiogenesis. These effects may relate to the inhibition of the tyrosine kinase-associated FGF receptor (116).

There is therefore evidence for a protective role for genistein in restraining the progression and possible dissemination of foci of prostatic cancer by inhibiting neovascularization, the effects on angiogenesis, and tumor suppression opening up encouraging concepts for an innovative cancer preventative measures.

The complexity of the inter- and intracellular signaling pathways

The sophistication of the inter- and intracellular signaling pathways, between and within cells, and the intrinsic growth regulatory factors that influence these pathways, is becoming increasingly more apparent. The cell–cell interactions between glandular epithelial cells and the muscle cells and fibroblasts of the stromal compartment have been briefly described. The prostatic neuroendocrine cells, located within the epithelial compartment, are rarely mentioned. These cells are basally-orientated (Fig. 30.20) and morphologically, are either of the '**open type**', with apical processes extending to the lumen, or the '**closed type**', both having long dendritic processes extending under and weaving between adjacent epithelial cells (127). There is speculation regarding their role, but it generally would be considered to encompass the regulation of cell growth and differentiation, as well as neuroendocrine, endocrine, and exocrine secretion (128, 129). They are specialized, differentiated cells that contain and secrete:

- the biogenic amine, serotonin;
- bombesin/gastrin-releasing peptide;
- the chromogranin family of polypeptides;
- the calcitonin family of peptides;
- somatostatin;
- parathyroid hormone-related protein (PHTrP);
- thyroid-stimulating hormone (TSH)-like peptide;
- human chorionic gonadotrophin (HCG)-like peptide.

Although the high levels of calcitonin, bombesin, and somatostatin in semen suggest that these peptides are

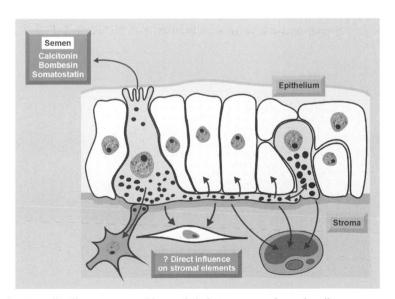

Fig. 30.20 Neuroendocrine cells, illustrating possible simple links to nerve and muscle cells.

directly secreted by the neuroendocrine cells, little is known about the inter-cellular autocrine and paracrine local regulatory mechanisms by which the neuroendocrine cells inter-relate with the neighboring cells. This may involve interaction between neuroendocrine cells, factors produced by the stromal compartment, extrinsic, blood-borne endocrine agents, or an input from the nervous system. Focal neuroendocrine cell differentiation is virtually ubiquitous in carcinoma of the prostate (127) and the extent of neuroendocrine cell proliferation correlates with poor prognosis.

A recent report from the Tenovus Cancer Research Centre (130) relating to the production of TGF-α and vascular endothelial growth factor (VEGF) by neuroendocrine cells of the human prostate is of particular interest. TGF-α expression, which mediates its biological action through the EGF receptor, is generally associated with the proliferation of human prostatic cancer cells and VEGF is now recognized as a powerful promoter of angiogenesis (Fig. 30.21). It is well-accepted that once a tumor attains a volume of approximately 2 mm, an improved new blood supply is required for continued growth (124–126, 131–133). The production of VEGF by the neuorendocrine cells of the tumor, and its activation of signaling pathways within the sprouting endothelial cells, may well be a factor associated with the promotion of angiogenesis and cancer progression (134, 135).

The inter-relationship between the intrinsic factors

The integrated response of the various populations of cells within the prostate to signaling language, reading sense from the many messages induced by the wide range of growth regulatory factors, as well as those initiated by the extrinsic endocrine factors that impact on the gland, is very clearly a finely-tuned and complex interactive system. As our understanding of these signaling pathways develops, the information that accumulates provides a greater insight into the potential consequences of their impairment and their relationship to the pathogenesis of prostate disease. Cells that respond to external stimuli, such as those induced by KGF or FGF-2, depend on the presence of cell membrane-localized receptor proteins (Fig. 30.22). The signaling pathways, sometimes referred to as the phosphorylation cascade, are complex and interest centers on the mechanisms by which these various kinases are controlled. As stated earlier, fundamental to the hormone responsiveness of the prostate gland is the inter-relationship between the signaling pathways that induce biological responses through steroid receptors and those activated through the binding of the peptide growth regulatory factors to the transmembrane cell receptors. It would now appear that the

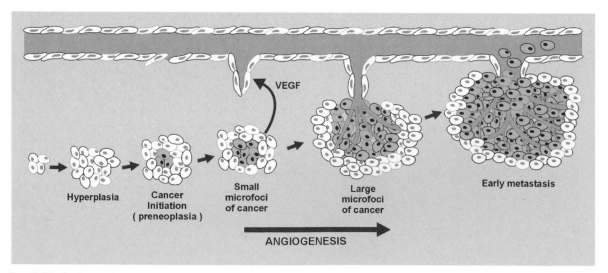

Fig. 30.21 Angiogenesis.

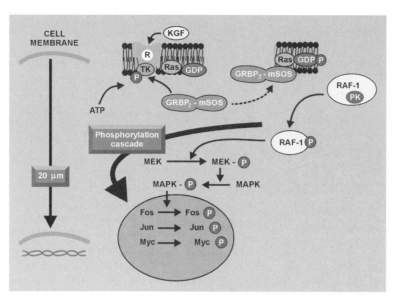

Fig. 30.22 Some complex aspects of signal transduction pathways.

mitogenic effect of DHT on prostate epithelial cells is mediated by peptide growth stimulatory factors, probably KGF (KGF-7), produced by the fibroblasts of the stromal compartment of the gland.

The association of the growth factor with the external domain of membrane receptor initiates the signaling processes related to mitogenesis. Through a tyrosine-specific protein kinase (TK) situated on the intracellular domain of the receptor, the binding of the peptide triggers a cascade of intracellular signaling events (Fig. 30.21) that ultimately lead to the activation of proto-oncogenes and gene transcription (136, 137). Such signals would activate the c-myc, c-fos, and c-jun proto-oncogenes, all encoding proteins that are involved in normal growth regulatory processes within the prostate gland and which are referred to as transcription factors (TFs). As well as encoding for transcription factors, proto-oncogenes would also encode growth regulatory factors and their corresponding membrane-receptor proteins, as well as for the many and various components of the signal transduction pathways (Fig. 30.22).

The fos and jun proteins, either as fos jun heterodimers, or as jun/jun homodimers, are components of the AP-1 transcription factor that specifically associates with the AP-1 recognition sequences on the genome (Fig. 30.13) characterized by the -TGACTCA-nucleotide sequence (138, 139). The interaction between the two proteins on the genome represents a specific interaction between the 'leucine zipper' structural domains of the proteins (140). The spatial disposition of the HREs, or androgen-response elements, alongside AP-1 recognition sites in juxtaposition along the promoter region of an androgen responsive gene (Fig. 30.13), would therefore lead to functional interaction or synergism (141, 142), the interaction referred to as crosstalk between signaling pathways. It would be considered (143, 144) that the association of the steroid receptor complex to the genome would change the spatial orientation of the DNA such that the DNA strands 'bend', thereby offering easier accessibility to the transcription factors for their recognition sites.

Little is known about the concentrations of DHT–AR necessary to support growth-factor signaling, nor of the sensitivity of these processes, which may be greater than hitherto believed. An even greater sensitivity may be conferred on cancer cells (145). AR expression is maintained in most androgen-resistant cancers of the prostate (146), and the presence of the AR itself may offer a growth advantage even in the presence of extremely low concentrations of androgen present in patients with prostate cancer on maximal androgenic blockade.

The complexity of these inter-relationships is further emphasized in Fig. 30.23, which illustrates how other receptor proteins can probably interact with the TFs, to influence gene transcription (147, 148). The illustration simply depicts the potential protein–protein interaction

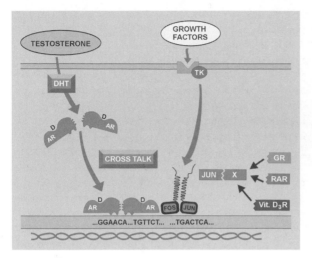

Fig. 30.23 Function interactions of crosstalk between signaling pathways: DHT; D, dihydrotestrosterone; AR, androgen receptor; TK, tyrosine kinase; GR, glucocortocoid receptor; RAR, retinoic acid receptor; Vit. D_3R, vitamin D_3 receptor.

of the retinoic acid receptor (RAR), the glucocorticoid receptor (GR), and the 1,25-dihydroxyvitamin D3 (1,25-diOHvitD3) receptor (VDR) with the fos/jun heterodimer complex that could thereby influence transcription activity (142).

Early stages in the natural history prostatic cancer

Impairment of the growth regulatory balance can lead to cellular hyperplasia with consequent genetic instability and subversion of the normal processes of growth restraint. Furthermore, proto-oncogenes that become dysfunctional through point mutations, deletions, amplification, or other changes that alter the structure or influence the expression of these growth regulatory genes, can induce carcinogenesis.

From a study of the ductal budding and branching patterns in the developing prostate, Timms and his colleagues (149) and Cunha *et al.* (150), re-emphasize the concept that the regional organization of the prostatic complex is determined by the regional heterogeneity of mesenchymal induction, with particular specific mesenchymal effects induced along a budding axis. The influence of stromal heterogeneity on prostatic growth and differentiation, effects that are 'imprinted' on the gland during fetal life by the action of the various steroid hormones *in utero*, including effects induced by

estrogens, is fundamentally important and relates to subsequent predisposition of various regions of the prostate to disease.

This concept of imprinting and predisposition to disease is particularly important with regard to the role of estrogens on the developing fetal prostate (151). Timms and colleagues (152) reported that a physiological, 50% increase in the estradiol concentration within the male mouse fetus, produced from a maternal silastic implant, subsequently resulted in the development of an enlarged adult prostate gland, with a 6-fold increase in AR levels relative to controls. A 5-fold increase in the total serum estradiol levels resulted in a smaller adult prostate gland.

The results suggest that estrogens can modulate the action of androgens by '*in utero*', enhancing the sensitivity of the prostate to androgen and, moreover, the effect is sustained throughout life, probably forming the basis of growth regulatory dysfunction and disease in later years. It is of interest, that the male mouse fetus, exposed to these physiological, small increases in estradiol levels, showed an immediate significant increase in the number of prostatic glands throughout the dorsal urogenital sinus, including the dorsocranial region, a region considered homologous to the areas of the human prostate in which BPH originates. It is certainly important to better understand the role of estradiol in the prostate gland.

Again, of particular interest, is that the biological action of estrogens on vasculature is associated with the production of nitric oxide, now seen as an important physiological regulator of endocrine systems, and implicated in the proliferation of smooth muscle cells. Moreover, in relation to intracellular signaling, the presence of a specific plasma membrane-located receptor for an estradiol–SHBG complex, which was found (153) in the stromal elements of the human prostate, provides another pathway by which estradiol may influence prostatic growth. The estradiol–SHBG complex can induce intracellular signaling by promoting an 8-fold elevation in cAMP levels, which in the absence of androgens, can induce PSA expression.

Furthermore, studies with the rat insulinoma RINm5F cell-line (154) suggest that the induction of nitric oxide (NO)-synthase and NO generation may influence apoptosis. The role of estrogens in relation to apoptosis in the prostate gland is, as yet, still to be precisely determined. It has also been suggested (153) that the reaction between NO and superoxide that gives rise to the toxic peroxynitrite, may be implicated in the process of apoptosis, by which phagocytes engulf and destroy foreign proteins, with 'apoptopic genes' encoding free radical scavengers.

Diet and prostate disease: the concept of prevention

The relationship of diet to prostate disease has been the subject of a recent major review (6) and interest now centers on certain isoflavonoids and lignans, products of vegetables, fruit, whole grains, and soya, that are metabolized by the gut microflora to give rise to compounds such as enterolactone, daidzein, and genistein, weak plant estrogens, referred to generally, as the phyto-estrogens.

The presence in plants of non-steroidal substances with estrogenic activity has been recognized for some time and may hundreds of plants manifest some degree of estrogenic activity. Soya bean and red clover are members of the leguminosae family, which is a major source of isoflavonoids, and soya is consumed daily in large amounts in a number of forms in China and Japan and in Asia generally. Many foods of plant origin contain varying amounts of isoflavonoids, flavonoids, and lignans and it is not unreasonable to assume that at least some of these polyphenolic phyto-estrogens could exercise a influence on estro-gen-sensitive growth regulatory processes of the prostate gland.

It is also necessary to consider the role of the dietary flavonoids in all discussions relating to the chemoprevention of cancer of the prostate. The thesis must be that they, together with the isoflavonoids and lignans (Fig. 30.24), may exercise a restraining role in preventing the development of the dormant, indolent latent carcinoma into the malignant aggressive cancer phenotype (156). The flavonoids are closely related in structure to the isoflavonoids (Fig. 24), the former having a 2-phenylchroman nucleus and the latter a 3-phenylchroman nucleus. Recently, several commonly occurring plant flavonoids have been shown to possess weak estrogenic activity (157). Unlike isoflavonoids, the flavonoids are ubiquitous in nature and are found in high concentration in many fruits, vegetables, and crop species. In particular, apigenin and kaempferol, both of which are estrogenic, are regarded as two of the major flavonoids because of their common occurrence among plants, and their significant concentrations when they are present. Apigenin, for example, is found in the leaves, seeds and fruits of flowering plants, with up to 7% of dry weight in leafy vegetables. Tea-leaves are an excellent source of apigenin.

The levels of isoflavonoids are high in the urine and plasma of the Japanese (Fig. 30.9) and Chinese whose traditional foodstuffs contain large amounts of soya in

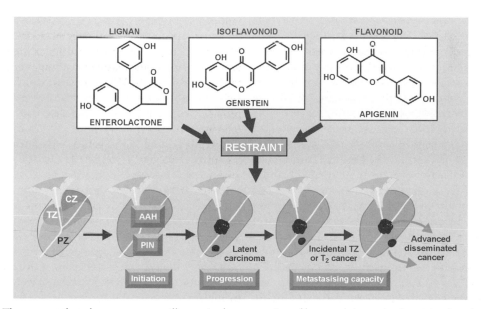

Fig. 30.24 The concept that phyto-estrogens will restrain the progression of latent carcinoma to the aggressive phenotype.

the form of bean curd (tofu), soya bean milk, miso, and tempeh. The concentration of lignans is high in the urine of vegetarians (158) whose diet contains whole-grain cereals, vegetables, and fruits. The concentrations of flavonoids in plasma and urine of different populations have yet to be determined and is an obvious program for future research. However, as tea, fruit, and vegetables are the principal sources of flavonoids, it is probable that Asians with their high consumption of tea, and vegetarians, have significant circulating levels of these compounds.

As already discussed earlier, it is not too difficult to envisage the growth restraining influence that such dietary factors could exercise on the development of prostatic disease (20, 159, 160).

The way forward

In proposing that dietary factors are responsible for the marked differences in the prostatic cancer incidence and mortality rates between East and West, there can rarely have been such convincing support than the identification of the large amounts relative to counterparts in the West, of isoflavonoids, flavonoids, and lignans in the body fluids of Asian people as a consequence of a their high dietary intake. Moreover, this and a greater understanding of particular specific effects of the phyto-estrogens on the biological processes associated with carcinogenesis thereby provide support for the belief that such compounds could restrain cancer development. Such information, which is currently accumulating at a most impressive rate, will be necessary to encourage those at the highest government level to strongly consider strategies for cancer, if not 'Western disease' prevention. The encouragement of individuals to recognize the probable healthcare benefits from such dietary changes, or an increase in the intake of such phyto-estrogens in food supplementation packages, throughout a lifetime, must also be seen as a major role for those now committed to such programm for prevention.

Associated with this new emphasis on prevention must be the realization that the ultimate proof of real benefit will reside in statistical evidence available some years into the new millennium. It must be seen that the strategy for prevention must firstly be health education directed specifically to the incidence, morbidity, and mortality associated with cancer, but particularly those of prostate and breast. The **'relative vulnerability' or degree of risk** to those people who enjoy a conven-

tional Western diet, high in animal protein and low in cereals legumes, fruit, and vegetables, compared with the lesser risk of those with a soya-based Asian or Mediterranean vegetarian style of diet, must be emphasized.

Dietary advice could follow. Already there is government encouragement for people to increase their consumption of vegetables, especially legumes, fruit, and cereals. More specifically, and with the intention of introducing soya and its isoflavonoid content into the diet, there would be mention of the availability of soya-based food supplements that taken daily, enhance the levels of the phyto-estrogens, genistein and daidzein, to those of the Chinese and Japanese people. Such soya preparations could be introduced into the regular diet such that there is minimal interference of the Western dietary style that most people would be loath to reject. The concept must be that the introduction of these dietary phyto-estrogens offers the possibility that their potential restraining influence on those biological processes implicated in carcinogenesis can provide at best significant health benefit, but at worst, can do little damage.

With the often stated reluctance, even hostility, to fundamental dietary change, the realization and acceptance that there is available an 'easy fix' that provides a specific, dietary supplementation of isoflavonoids and lignans to be taken along with the individual food preferences, must be seen as the way forward.

There have already been successful trials of a prototype supplement at the Tenovus Cancer Research Centre. Epidemiological studies have noted-lesser incidence of prostate cancer in Eastern Europe and Finland, and also in the immigrant communities of these peoples in Canada and Australia, where the original dietary customs tend to be preserved. Their traditional bread contains rye and buckwheat flour, which is significantly richer in lignans than wheat flour and loaves that often have whole flaxseeds added. The resultant multigrain loaf is therefore a rich source of dietary lignans and, as bread, is consumed daily in quantity. This may have some relevance to the reduced occurrence of prostate cancer in these communities.

A necessary strategy of health education must also be envisaged in Asian countries to ensure knowledge of the existing health benefits of their traditional soya-based dietary habit. This is particularly necessary when population groups in Asia acquire any degree of affluence, since there already has been recognized a willingness to encompass Western dietary habits that would be supported by the 'fast food' industry.

It remains to be determined whether the dietary constituents, the isoflavonoids, flavonoids, and lignans exercise their biological effect as antioxidants, weak estrogens, anti-estrogens or, indeed, as inhibitors of those signaling pathways driven by the ubiquitous growth regulatory factors. Tamoxifen, which is recognized as acting as a weak estrogen in its universal use in the clinical management of breast cancer as a weak estrogen, is being investigated as to its efficacy in the prevention of the disease in women considered 'at risk'. Already recognized, however, are the beneficial influence it elicits with regard to cardiovascular disease and osteoporosis in women.

Hormone replacement therapy (HRT), which is essentially low-dose estrogen therapy and controls menopausal problems, such as hot flushes, also provides longer term benefits in restraining cardiovascular disease and osteoporosis. It is noteworthy that menopausal Japanese women have a lower frequency of hot flushes than their Western counterparts (161) which presumably can be attributed to their soya-based diet and its associated weak estrogen content.

Although probably the benefits of dietary intervention can readily be promulgated, there might be concern amongst men that a greater intake of weak estrogens could produce certain undesirable side-effects, such as feminization. Although understandable, reassurance would come from the absence of such effects in the vast male population of Asia, consuming a life-long traditional soya diet. The traditional Asian male assumes all aspects of a healthy male life and is abundantly fertile, whilst at the same time enjoying a significantly reduced risk of prostatic malignancy.

Appropriate chemopreventive trials of phyto-estrogens may be difficult to establish and certainly may be seen as expensive. They must, however, be supported and although certain mild adverse side-effects may emerge from current lack of knowledge of biological processes, this must be seen from our current understanding of the Asian people as being of minimal risk. Certainly, if the aim of such studies is to evaluate the influence of enhancing the concentrations of particular isoflavonoids or lignans in the study groups merely to the pre-determined levels of the Asian people, it is reasonable to anticipate that any adverse effects would be negligible.

Acknowledgements

The authors are grateful to CompGraphics Services, Cardiff, for providing the illustrations for which they hold all copyrights.

References

1. Huggins CH. Introduction. In: *Biology of the prostate and related tissues*, National Cancer Inst. Monograph 12 (ed. EP Vollmer, G Kauffmann). NIH, Bethesda, 1963, xi–xii.
2. Bostwick DG. Origins of prostatic carcinoma. *Cancer* 1996, **78**, 230–6.
3. Griffiths K, Coffey D, Cockett ATK *et al.* The regulation of prostatic growth. In: *The 3rd International Consultation on Benign Prostatic Hyperplasia* (ed. ATK Cockett, S Khoury, Y Aso *et al.* S.C.I., Paris, 1996, 73–115.
4. Griffiths K, Cockett ATK, Coffey DS *et al.* Regulation of prostate growth. In: *4th International Consultation on BPH* (ed. L Denis S.C.I. Paris, 1998, 83–128.
5. Girman C, Panser L, Chute C *et al.* Natural history of prostatism: urinary flow rates in a community-based study. *J Urol* 1993, **150**, 887–92.
6. Guess HA. Epidemiology and natural history of benign prostatic hyperplasia. *Urol Clin North Am* 1995, **22**, 247–61.
7. Franks LM. Benign nodular hyperplasia of the prostate: a review. *Ann R Coll Surg England* 1954, **14**, 92–106.
8. Bostwick DG, Pacelli A, Lopez-Beltran A. Molecular biology of prostatic intraepithelial neoplasia. *Prostate*, 1989, **29**, 117–34.
9. Harper ME, Glynne-Jones E, Goddard L *et al.* Expression of androgen receptor and growth factors in premalignant lesions of the prostate. *J Path* 1998, **186**, 169–77.
10. Lopez-Otin C, Diamandis EP. Breast and prostate cancer: an analysis of common epidemiological, genetic and biochemical features. *Endocrine Rev* 1998, **19**, 365–96.
11. Barry MJ, Boyle P, Fourcroy J *et al.* Epidemiology and natural history of BPH. In: *The 3rd International Consultation on Benign Prostatic Hyperplasia* (ed. ATK Cockett, S Khoury, Y Aso *et al.*) S.C.I., Paris, 1996, 21–36.
12. Garraway WM, Collins GN, Lee RJ. High prevalence of benign prostatic hypertrophy in the community. *Lancet* 1991, **338**, 469–71.
13. Berry SJ, Coffey DS, Walsh PC *et al.* The development of human benign prostatic hyperplasia with age. *J Urol* 1984, **132**, 474–9.
14. Isaacs JT, Coffey DS. Etiology and disease process of benign prostatic hyperplasia. *Prostate* 1989, **29**, 33–50.
15. Wynder E, Gori G. Contribution of the environment to cancer incidence: an epidemiologic study. *J Natl Can Inst* 1977, **58**, 825–32.
16. Higginson J, Muir C. Environmental carcinogenesis: misconceptions and limitations to cancer control. *J Natl Can Inst* 1979, **63**, 1291–8.
17. Doll R, Peto R. The causes of cancer: quantitative estimates of avoidable risks of cancer in the United States today. *J Natl Can Inst* 1981, **66**, 1191–308.
18. Hill MJ. Dietary fat and human cancer (review). *Anticancer Res* 1987, **7**, 281–92.
19. Miller AB, Berrino F, Hill M *et al.* Diet in the aetiology of cancer: a review. *Eur J Cancer* 1994, **30A**, 207–20.
20. Griffiths K, Adlercreutz H, Boyle P *et al. Nutrition and cancer.* ISIS Medical Media, Oxford, 1996.

21. Haenzel W, Kurihara M. Studies of Japanese migrants. Mortality from cancer and other diseases among Japanese in the United States. *J Natl Cancer Inst* 1968, **40**, 43–68.

22. Buell P. Changing incidence of breast cancer in Japanese-American women. *J Natl Cancer Inst* 1973, **51**, 1479–83.

23. Shimizu H, Ropp RK, Bernstein L *et al.* Cancers of the breast and prostate among Japanese and white immigrants in Los Angeles County. *Br J Cancer* 1991, **63**, 963–6.

24. Skrabanek P. Invited viewpoints. *Eur J Cancer* 1994, **30A**, 220–1.

25. McMichael AJ. Invited viewpoints. *Eur J Cancer* 1994, **30A**, 221–3.

26. Anon. Diet and breast cancer. *Nature* 1992, **359**, 76.

27. Adlercreutz H. Western diet and Western diseases: some hormonal and biochemical mechanisms and associations. *Scand J Clin Lab Invest* 1990, **50**, (Suppl 201), 3–23.

28. Zaridze DG, Boyle P, Smans M. International trends in prostatic cancer. *Int J Cancer* 1984, **33**, 223–30.

29. Sondik E. Incidence, survival and mortality trends in prostate cancer in the United States. In: *A multidisciplinary analysis of controversies in the management of prostate cancer* (ed. DS Coffey, MI Resnick, FA Dorr *et al.*). Plenum Press, New York, 1981, 9–15.

30. World Health Organization. Trends in prostate cancer 1980–1988. *WHO Weekly Epidemiological Record* 1992, **67**, 281–8.

31. Dhom G. Epidemiology of hormone-dependent tumors. In: *Endocrine dependent tumors* (ed. KD Voigt, C Knabbe). Raven Press Ltd, New York, 1991, 1–42.

32. Muir CS, Waterhouse JAH, Mack T *et al.* (ed.) *Cancer incidence in five continents, Vol V.* IARC Scientific Publications, No. 88, IARC, Lyon, 1987.

33. Zaridze DG, Boyle P. Cancer of the prostate: epidemiology and aetiology. *Br J Urol* 1987, **59**, 493–503.

34. Skeet RG. Epidemiology of urological tumours. In: *Scientific Foundations of Urology*, Vol. II (ed. DI Williams, GD Chisholm). William Heineman Medical Books, London, 1976, 199–211.

35. Miller GJ. Diagnosis of stage A prostatic cancer in the People's Republic of China. In: *A multidisciplinary analysis of controversies in the management of prostate cancer* (ed. DS Coffey, MI Resnick, FA Dorr *et al.*) Plenum Press, New York, 1988, 17–24.

36. Parkin DM, Muir CS, Whelan S *et al. Cancer incidence in five continents*, Vol. V1. IARC Scientific Publication No. 120, IARC, Lyon, 1992.

37. Boyle P, Levi F, Lucchini F *et al.* Trends in diet-related cancers in Japan: a conundrum. *Lancet* 1993, **342**, 752.

38. Burkitt DP. Epidemiology of cancer of the colon and rectum. *Cancer* 1971, **28**, 3–13.

39. Rose DP. Dietary fibre, phytoestrogens, and breast cancer. *Nutrition* 1990, **8**, 47–51.

40. Trock B, Lanza E, Greenwald P. Dietary fibre, vegetables, and colon cancer: critical review and meta-analysis of the epidemiologic evidence. *J Natl Cancer Inst* 1990, **82**, 650–61.

41. Macquart-Moulin G, Riboli E, Cornee J *et al.* Case-control study on colorectal cancer and diet in Marseilles. *Int J Cancer* 1986, **38**, 183–91.

42. Steinmetz K, Potter J. Vegetables, fruit and cancer. I. Epidemiology. *Cancer Causes Control* 1991, **2**, 325–57.

43. Steinmetz K, Potter J. Vegetables, fruit and cancer. II. Mechanisms. *Cancer Causes Control* 1991, **2**, 427–42.

44. Ingram DM, Nottage E, Roberts T. The role of diet in the development of breast cancer: a case-control study of patients with breast cancer, benign epithelial hyperplasia and fibrocystic disease of the breast. *Br J Cancer* 1991, **64**, 187–91.

45. Wynder EL, Mabuchi K, Whitmore WF. Epidemiology of cancer of the prostate. *Cancer* 1971, **28**, 344–60.

46. Boyle P, Zaridze DG. Risk factors for prostate and testicular cancer. *Eur J Cancer* 1993, **29A**, 1048–55.

47. Giovannuucci E, Rimm EB, Colditz GA. *et al.* A prospective study of dietary fat and risk of prostate cancer. *J Natl Cancer Inst* 1993, **85**, 1571–9.

48. Severson RK, Nomura AM, Grove AS *et al.* A prospective study of demographics, diet and prostate cancer among men of Japanese ancestry in Hawaii. *Cancer Research* 1989, **49**, 1857–60.

49. Stemmerman GN, Nomura AM, Heilbrun LK. Cancer risk in relation to fat and energy intake among Hawaii Japanese: a prospective study. *International Symposium of the Princess Takamatsu Cancer Research Fund* 1985, **16**, 265–74.

50. Kolonel LN, Hankin JH, Nomura AM *et al.* Dietary fat intake and cancer incidence among five ethnic groups in Hawaii. *Cancer Research* 1981, **41**, 3727–8.

51. Simopoulos AP. Nutritional cancer risks derived from energy and fat. *Med Onco Tumor Pharm* 1987, **4**, 227–39.

52. Albanes D. Caloric intake, body weight and cancer: a review. *Nutr Cancer* 1987, **9**, 199–217.

53. Hirayama T. A large scale cohort study on cancer risks by diet – with special reference to the risk reducing effects of green-yellow vegetable consumption. In: *Diet nutrition And cancer*, (ed. Y Hayash) Tokyo/VNU Sci. Press, Utrecht: Japan Sci Soc Press, 1986, 41–53.

54. Hirayama T. Epidemiology of prostate cancer with special reference to the role of diet. *Natl Cancer Inst Monographs* 1979, **53**, 149–55.

55. Hirayama T. Life-style and cancer: from epidemiological evidence to public behaviour change to mortality reduction of target cancers. *Monographs Natl Cancer Inst* 1992, **12**, 65–74.

56. Lee HP, Gourley L, Duffy SW *et al.* Dietary effects on breast cancer risk in Singapore. *Lancet* 1991, **337**, 1197–200.

57. Kodama M, Kodama T. Interrelation between Western type cancers and non-Western type cancers as regards their risk variations in time and space. II Nutrition and cancer risk. *Anticancer Res* 1990, **10**, 1043–9.

58. Rose DP, Boyar AP, Wynder EL. International comparisons of mortality rates for cancer of the breast, ovary, prostate and colon and per capita food consumption. *Cancer* 1986, **58**, 2363–71.

59. Setchell KDR, Adlercreutz H. Mammalian lignans and phytooestrogens. Recent studies on their formation, metabolism and biological role in health and disease. In:

Role of gut flora in toxicity and cancer London (ed. Roland IR). Academic Press, 1988, 315–45.

60. Mills PK, Beeson WL, Phillips RL *et al.* Cohort study of diet, lifestyle and prostate cancer in Adventist men. *Cancer* 1989, **64**, 598–604.

61. Block G, Patterson B, Subar A. Fruit, vegetables and cancer prevention: A review of the epidemiological evidence. *Nutrition & Cancer* 1992, **18**, 1–29.

62. Negri E, La Vecchia C, Franceschi S. *et al.* The role of vegetables and fruit in cancer risk. In: *Epidemiology of diet and cancer* (ed. MJ Hill, A Giacosa, CPJ Caygill). Ellis Horwood, Chichester, 1994, 327–34.

63. Buiatti E, Palli D, De Carli A *et al.* A case-control study of gastric cancer and diet in Italy. *Int J Cancer* 1989, **44**, 611–6.

64. Buatti E, Palli D, De Carli A *et al.* A case-control study of gastric cancer and diet in Italy. II. Association with nutrients. *Int J Cancer* 1990, **45**, 896–901.

65. La Vecchia C, De Carli A, Negri E *et al.* Epidemiological aspects of diet and cancer: a summary review of case-control studies from Northern Italy. *Oncology* 1988, **45**, 364–70.

66. Bradbury RB, White DC. Oestrogens and related substances in plants. *Vitam Horm* 1954, **12**, 207–33.

67. Price KR, Fenwick GR. Naturally occurring oestrogens in food – a review. *Food Add Contam* 1985, **2**, 73–106.

68. Rao CBS. (ed.) *The chemistry of lignans*. Andra University Press, and Publications, Waltair, India, 1978, 1–377.

69. Thompson LU, Robb P, Serraino M, *et al.* Mammalian lignan production from various foods. *Nutr Cancer* 1991, **16**, 43–52.

70. Finlay EMH, Wilson DW, Adlercreutz H, *et al.* The identification and measurement of 'phyto-oestrogens' in human saliva, plasma, breast aspirate or cyst fluid, and prostatic fluid using gas chromatography-mass spectrometry. *J Endocrinol* 1991, **129**, (Suppl), 49.

71. Adlercreutz H, Fotsis T, Bannwart C *et al.* Determination of urinary lignans and phytooestrogen metabolites, potential antiestrogens and anticarcinogens, in urine of women on various habitual diets. *J Steroid Biochem* 1986, **25**, 791–7.

72. Bruchovsky N, Lesser B, VanDoorn E *et al.* Hormonal effects on cell proliferation in rat prostate. *Vit & Horm* 1975, **33**, 61–102.

73. Truss M, Beato M. Steroid hormone receptors: Interaction with deoxyribonucleic acid and transcription factors. *Endocr Revs* 1993, **14**, 459–79.

74. Gronemeyer H. Transcription activation by estrogen and progesterone receptors. *Ann Rev Genet* 1991, **25**, 89–123.

75. Imperato-McGinley J, Guerro L, Gautier T *et al.* Steroid 5I-reductase deficiency in man: An inherited form of male pseudohermaphroditism. *Science* 1974, **186**, 1213–5.

76. Griffiths K, Akaza H, Eaton CL *et al.* Regulation of prostate growth. In: *The 2nd International Consultation on Benign Prostatic Hyperplasia.* (ed. ATK Cockett, S Khoury, Y Aso *et al.*). S.C.I., Paris, 1993, 49–75.

77. Lee C, Kozlowski JM, Grayhack JT. Intrinsic and extrinsic factors controlling benign prostatic growth. *Prostate* 1997, **31**, 131–8.

78. Franks LM, Riddle PN, Carbonell AW *et al.* A comparative study of the ultrastructure and lack of growth capacity of adult human prostate epithelium mechanically separated from its stroma. *J Pathol* 1970, **100**, 113–9.

79. Cunha GR, Chung LWK, Shannon JM *et al.* Hormone-induced morphogenesis and growth: role of mesenchymal-epithelial interactions. *Rec Prog Hom Res* 1983, **39**, 559–5.

80. Yan G, Fukabori Y, Nikoloropolous S *et al.* Heparin-binding keratinocyte growth factor is a candidate stromal to epithelial cell andromedin. *Mol Endocrinol* 1992, **6**, 2123–8.

81. Peehl DM, Wong ST, Rubin JS. KGF and EGF differentially regulate the phenotype of prostatic epithelial cells. *Growth Regul* 1996, **6**, 22–31.

82. Sugimura Y, Foster BA, Hom YK *et al.* Keratinocyte growth factor (KGF) can replace tesosterone in the ductal branching morphogenesis of the rat ventral prostate. *Int J Develop Biol* 1996, **40**, 941–51.

83. Culig Z, Hobixch A, Cronauer MV *et al.* Androgen receptor activation in prostatic tumour cell lines by insulin-like growth factor I, keratinocyte growth factor and epidermal growth factor. *Cancer Res* 1994, **54**, 5474–8.

84. Miki T, Bottaro DP, Fleming TP Determination of ligand-binding specificity by alternate splicing: Two distinct growth factor receptors encoded by a single gene. *Proc Natl Acad Sci* 1992, **89**, 246–50.

85. Sherwood ER, Fong CJ, Lee C, Kozlowski JM. Basic fibroblast growth factor: A potential mediator of stromal growth in the human prostate. *Endocrinology* 1992, **130**, 2955–63.

86. Leung HY, Dickson C, Robson CN *et al.* Over-expression of fibroblast growth factor-8 in human prostate cancer. *Oncogene* 1996, **12**, 1833–5.

87. Schmitt JF, Hearn MT, Risbridger GP. Expression of fibroblast growth factor-8 in adult rat tissues and human prostate carcinoma cells. *J Steroid Biochem Mol Biol* 1996, **57**, 173–8.

88. Yan G, Fukabori Y, McBride G *et al.* Exon switching and activation of stromal and embryonic fibroblast growth factor (FGF)-FGF receptor genes in prostate epithelial cells accompany stromal independence and malignancy. *Mol Cell Biol* 1993, **13**, 4513–22.

89. Krieg M, Bartsch W, Thomsen M *et al.* Androgens and estrogens: their interaction with stroma and epithelium of human benign prostatic hyperplasia and normal prostate. *J Steroid Biochem* 1983, **19**, 155–61.

90. Kuiper GGJM, Enmark E, Pelto-Huikko M *et al.* Cloning of a novel estrogen receptor expressed in rat prostate and ovary. *Proc Natl Acad Sci* 1996, **93**, 5925–30.

91. Mosselman S, Polman J, Dijkema R. ERB: Identification and characterisation of a novel human estrogen receptor. *FEBS Letters* 1996, **392**, 49–53.

92. Kuiper GGJM, Carisson B, Grandien J *et al.* Comparison of the ligand binding specificity and transcript tissue distribution of estrogen receptors I and β. *Endocrinology* 1997, **138**, 863–70.

93. Berry M, Metzger D, Chambon P. Role of the two activating domains of oestrogen receptor in the cell-type

and promoter-context dependent agonistic activity of the anti-oestrogen 4-hydroxytamoxifen. *EMBO J* 1990, **9**, 2811–8.

94. Tzukerman MT, Esty A, Santiso-Mere D *et al.* Human estrogen receptor transactivational capacity is determined by both cellular and promoter-content and mediated by two functionally distinct intramolecular regions. *Mol Endocrinol* 1994, **8**, 21–30.

95. Kraus WL, McInerny EM, Katzenellenbogen BS. Ligand-dependent, transcriptionally productive association of the amino- and carboxy-terminal regions of a steroid hormone nuclear receptor. *Proc Natl Acad Sci* 1995, **92**, 12314–8.

96. Montano MM, Muller V, Trobaugh A, Katzenellenbogen BS. The carboxy-terminal F domain of the human estrogen receptor: role in the transcriptional activity of the receptor and the effectiveness of antiestrogens as estrogen antagonists. *Mol Endocrinol* 1995, **9**, 814–25.

97. Katzenellenbogen JA, O'Malley BW, Katzenellenbogen BS. Tripartite steroid hormone receptor pharmacology: interaction with multiple effector sites as a base for the cell- and promoter-specific action of these hormones. *Mol Endocrinol* 1996, **10**, 119–31.

98. Nakhla AM, Khan MS, Romas NP *et al.* Estradiol causes the rapid accumulation of cAMP in human prostate. *Proc Natl Acad Sci* 1994, **91**, 5402–5.

99. Yeh S, Miyamoto H, Shima H, Chang C. From estrogen to androgen receptor: A new pathway for sex hormones in prostate. *Proc Natl Acad Sci* 1998, **10**, 5527–32.

100. Pope GS, Wright HG. Oestrogenic isoflavones in red clover and subterranean clover. *Chem & Ind* 1954, 1019–1020.

101. Martin PM, Horwitz KB, Ryan DS *et al.* Phytooestrogen interaction with estrogen receptors in human breast cancer cells. *Endocrinology* 1978, **103**, 1860–7.

102. Adlercreutz H, Hockerstedt K, Bannwart C *et al.* Effect of dietary components, including lignans and phytoestrogens on enterohepatic circulation and liver metabolism of estrogens and on sex hormone binding globulin (SHBG). *J Steroid Biochem* 1987, **27**, 1135–44.

103. Belanger A, Locong A, Noel C *et al.* Influence of diet on plasma steroids and sex hormone-binding globulin levels in adult men. *J Steroid Biochem* 1989, **32**, 829–33.

104. Vermeulen A. Metabolic effects of obesity in men. *Verhandelingen-Koninklijke Academie Voor Geneeskunde Van Belgie* 1993, **55**, 393–7.

105. Griffiths K, Eaton CL, Harper ME *et al.* Somes Aspects of the Molecular Endocrinology of Prostatic Cancer (review). In: *Antiandrogens in prostate cancer* ed. L Denis Springer-Verlag, 1996.

106. Evans BAJ, Griffiths K, Morton M. Inhibition of 5a-reductase and 17b-hydroxysteroid dehydrogenase in genital skin fibroblasts by dietary lignans and isoflavonoids. *J Endocrinol* 1995, **147**, 295–302.

107. Vermeulen A. Testicular hormone secretion and aging in males. In: Benign prostatic hyperplasia (ed. JT Grayshack, JD Wilson, MJ Saherbenske DHEW Publ., No. (NIH) 76–1113, 1976, 177–182.

108. Griffiths K *et al.* The regulation of prostatic growth. In: *3rd International Consultation on BPH* (ed. ATK Cockett *et al*). S.C.I. Paris, 1995, 71–115.

109. Kellis JT, Vickery LE. Inhibition of human estrogen synthetase (aromatase) by flavones. *Science* 1984, **225**, 1032–4.

110. Kellis JT, Nesnow S, Vickery LE. Inhibition of aromatase cytochrome P-450 (estrogen synthetase) by derivatives of Â-naphthoflavone. *Biochem Pharmac* 1986, **35**, 2887–91.

111. Ibrahim AR, Abui-Hajj YJ. Aromatase inhibition by flavonoids. *J Steroid Biochem Molec Biol* 1990, **37**, 257–260.

112. Adlercreutz H, Bannwart C, Wahala K *et al.* Inhibition of human aromatase by mammalian lignans and isoflavonoid phytoestrogens. *J Steroid Biochem Molec Biol* 1993, **44**, 147–153.

113. Campbell DR, Kurzer MS. Flavonoid inhibition of arose enzyme activity in human preadipocytes. *J Steroid Biochem Molec Biol* 1993, **46**, 381–8.

114. Aaronson S. Growth factors and cancer. *Science* 1991, **254**, 1146–53.

115. Griffiths K *et al.* Regulation of prostatic growth. In: *4th International Consultation on BPH* (ed. LJ Denis *et al.*). S.C.I. Paris, 1997, 85–128.

116. Akiyama T, Ishida J, Nakagawa S *et al.* Genistein, a specific inhibitor of tyrosine-specific protein kinases. *J Biol Chem* 1987, **262**, 5592–5.

117. Kiguchi K, Glesne D, Chubb CH *et al.* Differential induction of apoptosis in human breast cells by okadaic acid and related inhibitors of protein phosphatases 1 and 2A. *Cell Growth Differ* 1994, **5**, 995–1004.

118. Scholar EM, Toews ML. Inhibition of invasion of murine mammary carcinoma cells by the tyrosine kinase inhibitor genistein. *Cancer Lett* 1994, **87**, 159–62.

119. Iisala S, Majuri ML, Carpen O *et al.* Genistein enhances the ICAM-mediated adhesion by inducing the expression of ICAM-1 and its counter receptors. *Biochem Biophys Res Comm* 1994, **203**, 443–9.

120. Spinozzi F, Pagliacci MC, Migliorati G *et al.* The natural tyrosine kinase inhibitor genistein produces cell cycle arrest and apoptosis in Jurkat T-leukemia cells. *Leuk Res* 1994, **18**, 431–9.

121. Matsukawa Y, Marui N, Sakai T *et al.* Genistein arrests cell cycle progression at G2-M. *Cancer Res* 1993, **53**, 1328–31.

122. McCabe MJ Jr., Orrenius S. Genistein induces apoptosis in immature human thymocytes by inhibiting topoisomerase-II. *Biochem Biophys Res Comm* 1993, **194**, 944–50.

123. Fotsis T, Pepper M, Adlercreutz H *et al.* Genistein, a dietary-derived inhibitor of in vitro angiogenesis. *Proc Natl Acad Sci* 1993, **90**, 2690–4.

124. Folkman J, Watson K, Ingber D *et al.* Induction of angiogenesis during the transition from hyperplasia to neoplasia. *Nature* 1989, **339**, 58–61.

125. Folkman J. Toward an understanding of angiogenesis: search and discovery. *Perspectives in Biol Med* 1985, **29**, 10–36.

126. Weidner M, Semple JP, Welch WR *et al.* Tumour angiogenesis and metaplasia-correlation in invasive breast cancer. *New Eng J Med* 1991, **324**, 1–8.

127. Di Sant Agnese P. Neuroendocrine differeniation in carcinoma of the prostate. Diagnostic, prognostic and therapeutic implications. *Cancer* 1992, **70**, 254–68.

128. Larsson LI. On the possible existence of multiple endocrine, paracrine and neuroendocrine messengers in secretory cell systems. Invest. *Cell Pathol* 1980, **3**, 73–85.

129. Bishop A, Polak J. Gut endocrine and neural peptides. *Endocrinol Pathol* 1990, 1–24.

130. Harper ME, Glynne-Jones E, Goddard L *et al.* Vascular endothelial growth factor (VEGF) expression in prostatic tumours and its relationship to neuroendocrine cells. *Br J Cancer* 1996, **74**, 910–16.

131. Folkman J. What is the evidence that tumors are angiogenesis dependent? *J Natl Cancer Inst* 1990, **82**, 4–6.

132. Folkman J, Klagsbrun M. Angiogenic factors. *Science* 1987, **235**, 442–7.

133. Weidner N, Carroll PR, Flax J *et al.* Tumor angiogenesis correlates with metastasis in invasive prostate carcinoma. *Am J Pathol* 1993, **143**, 401–9.

134. Cockett ATK, Di Sant Agnese PA, Gopinath P *et al.* Relationship of neuroendocrine cells of prostate and serotonin to benign prostatic hyperplasia. *Urology* 1993, **42**, 512–9.

135. Di Sant'Agnese PA, Cockett AT. Neuroendocrine differentiation in prostatic malignancy. *Cancer.* 1996, **78**, 357–61.

136. Aaronson S. Growth factors and cancer. *Science* 1991, **254**, 1146–3.

137. Weinberg RA. The action of oncogenes in the cytoplasm and nucleus. *Science* 1983, **230**, 770–6.

138. Curran T, Bravo R, Muller R. Transient induction of c-fos and c-myc is an intermediate consequence of growth factor stimulation. *Cancer Surv* 1985, **4**, 655–81.

139. Jones N. Transcriptional regulation by dimerisation: two sides to an incestuous relationship. *Cell* 1990, **61**, 9–11.

140. Landschultz, WH, Johnson PF, McKnight SL. The leucine zipper: a hypothetical structure common to a new class of DNA binding proteins. *Science* 1986, **240**, 1759–64.

141. Schule R, Muller M, Kaltschmidt C, *et al.* Many transcription factors interact synergistically with steroid receptors. *Science* 1988, **242**, 1418–20.

142. Shemshedini L, Knauthe R, Sassone-Corsi P *et al.* Cell specific inhibitory and stimulatory effects of fos and jun on transcription activation by nuclear receptors. *EMBO J* 1991, **10**, 3839–49. .

143. Sabbah M, Le Recousse S, Redeuilh G *et al.* Estrogen receptor-induced binding of the xenopus vitellogenin A2 gene hormone response element. *Biochem Biophys Res Commun* 1992, **185**, 944–52.

144. Nardulli AM, Shapiro DJ. Binding of the estrogen receptor DNA-binding domain to the estrogen response element induces DNA binding. *Mol Cell Biol* 1992, **12**, 2037–42.

145. Griffiths K, Morton MS, Nicholson RI. Androgens, androgen receptors, antiandrogens and the treatment of prostate cancer. *Eur Urol* 1997, **32** (Supll 3), 24–40.

146. Chodak GW, Krane DM, Puy LA *et al.* Nuclear localization of androgen receptor in heterogeneous samples of normal, hyperplastic and neoplastic human prostate. *J Urol* 1992, **147**, 798–803.

147. Beato M, Herrlich P, Schutz G. Steroid hormone receptors: many actors in search of a plot. *Cell* 1995, **83**, 851–7.

148. Mangelsdorf DJ, Evans RM. The RXR heterodimers and orphan receptors. *Cell* 1995, **83**, 841–50.

149. Timms BG, Mohs TJ, Didio LJA. Ductal budding and branching patterns in the developing prostate. *J Urol* 1994, **151**, 1427–32.

150. Sugimura Y, Norman JT, Cunha GR *et al.* Regional differences in the inductive activity of the mesenchyme of the embryonic mouse urogenital sinus. *Prostate* 1985, **7**, 253–60.

151. Santti R, Newbold RR, Makela S *et al.* Developmental estrogenization and prostatic neoplasia. *Prostate* 1994, **24**, 67–78.

152. Vom Saal FS, Timms BG, Montano MM. Prostate enlargement in mice due to fetal exposure to a low dose of estradiol or diethylstilbestrol, and opposite effects at high doses. *Proc Natl Acad Sci* 1997, **94**, 2056–61.

153. Ding VHD, Moller DE, Feeney WP *et al.* Sex hormone-binding globulin mediates prostate androgen receptor action via a novel signaling pathway. *Endocrinology* 1998, **139**, 213–8.

154. Suarez-Pinzon WL, Strynadka K, Schulz R *et al.* Mechanisms of cytokine-induced destruction of rat insulinoma cells: the role of nitric oxide. *Endocrinology* 1994, **134**, 1006–10.

155. Sarafian TA, Bredesen DE. Is apoptosis mediated by reactive oxygen species? *Free Radic Res* 1994, **20**, 1–6.

156. Mcguire MS, Fair WR. Prostate cancer and diet: Investigations, interventins and future considerations. *Mol Urol* 1997, **1**, 3–9.

157. Miksicek RJ. Commonly occurring plant flavonoids have estrogenic activity. *Mol Pharmacol* 1993, **44**, 37–43.

158. Adlercreutz H, Fotsis T, Bannwart C *et al.* Determination of urinary lignans and phytoestrogen metabolites, potential antiestrogens and anticarcinogens, in urine of women on various habitual diets. *J Steroid Biochem* 1986, **25**, 791–7.

159. Morton MS, Griffiths K, Blacklock N. The preventive role of diet in prostatic disease. *Br J Urol* 1996, **77**, 481–93.

160. Griffiths K, Denis L, Turkes A *et al.* Possible relationship between dietary factors and pathogenesis of prostate cancer. *Int J Urol* 1998, **5**, 195–213.

161. Adlercreutz H, Hamalainen E, Gorbach S. Dietary phyto-oestrogens and the menopause in Japan. *Lancet* 1992, **339**, 1233.

31 | *Genetic counseling for prostate cancer*

Sherry Campbell Grumet

Introduction

Into your practice walks a man with a family history of prostate cancer. There are several questions that may arise in your discussion, including: What is my risk to develop prostate cancer? How does my family history factor into this risk? Is genetic testing available? How can I reduce my risk or prevent prostate cancer? What screening is available and how well does it detect prostate cancer? Who else in my family is at risk? How do I get reliable and up-to-date information about prostate cancer issues? Genetic counseling is the process of answering some of these questions (1).

Recent advances in cancer genetics have resulted in the discovery of genes responsible for the inherited predisposition of certain types of cancer. As a result, protocols for cancer genetic counseling have been developed to accommodate the growing demand for genetic information. Cancer genetic counseling protocols were researched and developed in response to the discovery of the breast/ovarian cancer predisposition genes, BRCA1 and BRCA2, and the hereditary colon cancer predisposition genes for FAP and HNPCC. Cancer risk assessment and genetic testing has enabled some high-risk individuals to receive more accurate information about their risk status. Genetic information is already being applied to clinical practice, in which a genetic diagnosis may dictate screening frequency, prophylactic surgery, or chemoprevention strategies. Once prostate cancer predisposition genes are identified and characterized, the options for clinical management based on a genetic diagnosis may be possible. In this chapter, genetic counseling methods used for other hereditary cancer syndromes have been adapted and combined with our knowledge of prostate cancer into a prostate cancer genetic counseling protocol (Tables 31.1 and 31.2).

Table 31.1 Components of a prostate cancer genetic counseling session

Assessing patient's needs
Contracting
Education
Generate and expand family pedigree
Risk assessment/information
Screening/life-style recommendations
Genetic testing options/issues
Referrals

Patient assessment

The first and most important step in genetic counseling is to assess the patient's educational and psychosocial needs. The goal is to elicit, understand, and adapt the counseling to the knowledge, experience, assumptions, and beliefs that are unique to the patient (2). If not already familiar with the patient's background, asking him to describe the circumstances that led him to seek information and counseling gives the patient the opportunity to 'tell their story' and the healthcare professional the opportunity to build a rapport with the patient. The patient's personal narrative may include references to personal issues within their family, risk perceptions, specific concerns, and information that they may have already gathered (2). Concerns, questions, gaps in information, and misconceptions can now be addressed during the counseling process. Also, allowing the patient to 'tell their story' and state their concerns invites the patient to be more involved in structuring their genetic counseling session and gives the counselor direction as to what topics or concerns the patient is interested in discussing.

The next step is contracting. Contracting between the patient and healthcare professional is the process of discussing and agreeing on the specific goals of the

Table 31.2   Prostate cancer genetic counseling checklist

Prostate cancer education session
   Prostate anatomy and function
   Epidemiology of prostate cancer
   Risk factors for prostate cancer
   Chromosomes, genes and their function
   Role of genes in cancer initiation and progression
   Sporadic vs. hereditary cancer
   Inheritance pattern (autosomal dominant, recessive of
   X-linked)
   Review sporadic, familial and hereditary pedigrees
   Prostate cancer risk based on ethnicity or family history
   Signs and symptoms of prostate cancer
   Current prostate cancer screening or prevention methods
   Nutrition and exercise guidelines
   (When available) genetic testing options and the risks,
   limitations and benefits of genetic testing

Individualized components
   Document personal health, screening and exposure history
   Expand and discuss family history of cancer and
   non-cancerous conditions
   Discuss risk for cancer based on ethnicity or family history
   Discuss the influence of environment and/or a genetic
   predisposition on their risk
   Review screening guidelines for prostate cancer
   Explain current options for reducing the risk for prostate
   cancer
   When available and when appropriate, discuss their option
   for genetic testing
   Identify other family members that are at increased risk
   for prostate cancer
   Discuss screening guidelines for other types of cancer
   Explore psychosocial issues surrounding their personal
   risk for cancer and their family dynamics

session. Review the topics of information that will be discussed during the meeting and inquire as to the patient's specific concerns and questions. When possible, it is often helpful to address specific concerns or questions at the beginning of the session. Clarifying goals and involving the patient at the beginning of the session benefits both the counselor and the patient, and helps make the session more productive.

Education

Many people believe knowledge is power. For those individuals affected by or at risk for a genetic condition, having knowledge or access to knowledge about the diagnosis, etiology, and management implications imparts the power to respond to their particular life situation. A person who has unanswered questions, who is confused by the information they have received,

and who has extreme fear may have trouble seeking medical attention (2). The communication of information in a manner that is compatible with the patient's level of education, attitudes, and beliefs may empower that individual.

A person undergoing counseling and screening for a potentially hereditary disease must assimilate a great deal of complicated information about genetics and cancer. The basic principles of cancer genetics as it pertains to prostate cancer, patterns of inheritance, risk factors for prostate cancer, nutritional information, signs and symptoms of prostate cancer, and prostate cancer screening and diagnosis are generally reviewed with the patient (Tables 31.2 and 31.3, Fig. 31.1). Educating the patient at the beginning of the session allows the individual to use this information as it pertains to their situation as the counselor takes a family history and assesses risk. Information may give the patient a sense of power over their situation and their questions and discussion during the session will be more targeted and meaningful.

Taking a family history

Risk assessment and counseling is dependent on obtaining accurate and detailed information about the family's physical and psychological health, and the dynamics of the relationships between family members. The family history is the basis for determining the inheritance pattern of a disease, determining risk, and

Table 31.3   Prostate cancer genetic counseling history, containing a list of commonly asked questions during the pedigree expansion

Clinical history questions

- Full name
- Date of birth/date of death
- Risk factors for prostate cancer or other types of cancer
  (i.e. exposures, occupation, life-style)
- History of surgeries, medical procedures or chronic
  illnesses
- History of cancer biopsies
- History of cancer diagnosis;
  What was the primary site of the cancer?
  How was the cancer discovered?
  What was the specific diagnosis?
  What was the stage at diagnosis?
  What was the course of treatment?

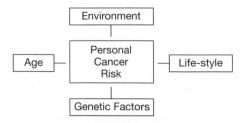

Fig. 31.1 A man's risk of developing prostate cancer is dependent on genetic and non-genetic factors.

assessing educational and psychosocial counseling needs for the patient.

A family pedigree is the diagram that records the family history information and provides an easy-to-follow picture of the family's cancer status. The person seeking information and risk assessment is considered the proband. A three-generation pedigree containing information on the patient, their first-degree relatives (children, siblings, parents), second-degree relatives (half-sibling, aunts, uncles, nieces, nephews, grandparents, and grandchildren), and third-degree relatives (first cousins) should be completed for each patient. It is also helpful in assessing cancer risk to ask about the patient's grandparent's siblings. Documenting the history of family members who did not develop cancer is just as important as documenting those who did develop cancer when assessing cancer risk. Information on affected family members should include the primary site of cancer, age of diagnosis, potential environmental factors or exposures, which may have contributed to the development of the cancer, and their ethnicity. In some cases, it may be necessary to request medical records to verify this information. Table 31.3 contains a list of commonly asked questions during the pedigree expansion. Please refer to Bennett *et al.* (3) for a detailed step-by-step explanation on constructing a pedigree.

Although the focus of the pedigree may be cancer, asking questions about other medical conditions is also necessary. For example, it may become apparent that the patient has a greater risk for developing heart disease than prostate cancer, or other genetic disorders may be identified in the family when reviewing the pedigree. In these cases, non-cancerous conditions should be discussed; however, it may be necessary to make referrals to other healthcare specialists. In addition, asking about other medical conditions may give the counselor an idea of what the patient's experience has been with disease and the healthcare system, which

may have an impact on the patient's willingness to follow through with screening and their ability to psychologically deal with the information presented to them during genetic counseling (1).

Risk assessment

All men are at risk of developing prostate cancer. A man's risk is dependent on genetic and non-genetic factors (Fig. 31.1). African-American ancestry, age, and family history of prostate are the most significant risk factors and can be used to determine risk for developing prostate cancer. In addition, there is data that suggests a family history of breast/ovarian cancer may also be a risk factor for prostate cancer. A diet high in fat and certain environmental exposures may also contribute to the initiation or progression of prostate cancer.

Diet and environmental factors

Risk assessment may include analyzing the patient's diet and making suggestions as to how to improve nutritional habits. More research is needed to determine the role diet plays in the initiation and progression of prostate cancer. Thus far, the strongest evidence indicates that some component of animal fat intake appears to be a promoter of prostate cancer. Although more research is needed, other dietary factors, such as vitamin C, vitamin D, vitamin E, beta-carotene, and lycopene may confer protection (4). Promoting a healthy diet and exercise may not only decrease the risk for prostate cancer, but for other cancers and medical conditions as well.

The link between certain environmental exposures and prostate cancer still remains allusive. Men with occupations involving heavy physical labor, rubber manufacturing, and newspaper printing may have a slightly higher incidence of prostate cancer. There has been some suggestion that long-term exposure to cadmium, a compound used in battery, paint, and cigarette manufacturing, may increase the risk for prostate cancer (5,6). Cigarette smoking, vasectomy, and sexually transmitted diseases have also been under investigation; however, conflicting data has yet to implicate these factors with an increased incidence of prostate cancer (7). At this time, not enough conclusive information is known about environmental exposures to incorporate them into the risk-assessment process.

African-American ancestry

African-American men have the highest incidence of prostate cancer in the world and are two to three times more likely to die from prostate cancer compared to American-Caucasian men. The clinical incidence of prostate cancer is 30–50% greater among African-Americans than Caucasian-American men (8); however, there appears to be no significant difference in the incidence of the latent form of prostate cancer between these two groups (9). It is speculated that African-Americans consume a diet higher in fat, which may account for the difference in the progression of latent prostate cancer in African-American men (10). In addition, there is some evidence that African-American men may be exposed to elevated levels of androgens throughout life and that there may be other genetic differences that may contribute to the variations in incidence and aggressiveness of prostate cancer between races (11).

The mortality rate from prostate cancer is two to three times greater in African-American men between the ages of 40–70 compared to age-matched Caucasian-American men (12). The difference in mortality rate could be due to a more virulent form and/or the delayed diagnosis of prostate cancer in the African-American population (13). The delay in diagnosis may be a result of certain barriers to healthcare, including the distrust of the healthcare system, fear of being diagnosed with prostate cancer, associating prostate cancer with death, concerns about treatment side-effects, and the lack of health insurance (14).

Age

The incidence of prostate cancer sharply increases with advancing age. In fact, prostate cancer risk increases faster with age compared to any other cancer. Approximately 77% of men diagnosed with prostate cancer are over the age of 65 and the average age of diagnosis is approximately 70 years.

Inherited genetic factors are particularly important if there is a history of early onset prostate cancer (< 65 years). First-degree relatives of men who developed prostate cancer before the age of 53 years had a cumulative lifetime risk of 40% for developing prostate cancer compared with the risk of 18% in men with a relative that was diagnosed over the age of 65 (15). However, research indicates that relying on age of diagnosis as a guideline to determine whether a case of prostate cancer is a result of heritable factors may not

always be useful. Hereditary prostate cancer cases may only occur 6–8 years younger than sporadically occurring cases (15). In addition, the counselor must keep in mind that the age a family member was diagnosed with prostate cancer may depend on how advanced medical care and prostate cancer screening was at the time and place the person was diagnosed. As our detection methods improve and more men seek medical attention annually, the age at which sporadically occurring prostate cancer is detected may decrease.

Family history and hereditary prostate cancer

The Mormon population in the state of Utah has served as an important epidemiological cohort for the study of hereditary cancers, due to their extensive genealogical records, which makes it possible to collect information on hundreds of individuals that are descendants from a common ancestor. Case control analysis of this population found that overall, cancer of the prostate appeared the most 'familial' of all cancer sites (16).

Approximately 25% of all men diagnosed with prostate cancer have a known family history (17). Family history of prostate cancer can be divided into three categories: sporadic, familial, and hereditary.

The majority of prostate cancer occurs sporadically, and the family history usually includes only one known case of late-onset prostate cancer (Fig. 31.2). First-degree relatives of a man diagnosed with prostate cancer have a 2- to 3-fold increased risk for developing prostate cancer compared to the general population (18). However, there may be an additional risk if this single case of prostate cancer occurred at a young age.

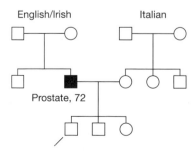

Fig. 31.2 A family pedigree is the diagram that records the family history information and provides an easy-to-follow picture of the family's cancer status.

Familial Family History

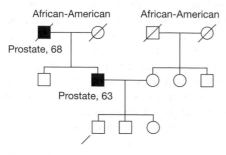

Fig. 31.3

Also, there is evidence that a diagnosis of prostate cancer in a brother results in a greater risk than a diagnosis in a father. One study found that, compared with men with no family history of prostate cancer, men with a history of prostate cancer in a father had a 2–3-fold increased risk, but men with a family history of prostate cancer in a brother had a 4–5-fold increased risk (19).

Familial prostate cancer appears as a clustering of prostate cancer in a family, which may include two brothers or a father and son (Fig. 31.3). The etiology of familial prostate cancer may involve the combination of several mechanisms, such as shared environmental factors, similar diets, and a genetic predisposition (20). In general, first-degree relatives of a man diagnosed with prostate cancer have a 2- to 3-fold increased risk, and this risk increases as the number of affected relatives increases, i.e. men with two first-degree relatives with prostate cancer may have a 5-fold increased risk, and men with three first-degree relatives may have an 11-fold increased risk (18, 21, 22). In addition, first-degree relatives of men with early onset prostate cancer have a greater risk compared to men whose relatives had a late onset cancer.

Hereditary prostate cancer

It has been estimated that approximately 9% of all prostate cancers occurring by age 85 and 43% of prostate cancers diagnosed under the age of 55 are a result of an inherited predisposition (15). Hereditary prostate cancer should be considered for families that present with multiple cases of prostate cancer and/or with early-onset prostate cancer (20). General guidelines for identifying hereditary prostate cancer include a clustering of three or more affected relatives within a nuclear family, such as a father and two sons, or two

relatives with early onset prostate cancer (< 55 years), or the occurrence of prostate cancer in each of three generations (Fig. 31.4) (17, 20). Since hereditary prostate cancer can be inherited from a individual's mother (Fig. 31.5), the maternal family history must also be considered.

Genetics of prostate cancer

Despite the fact that prostate cancer is the leading cancer in men and approximately 9% are believed to be hereditary, the genetics of hereditary prostate cancer have not been uncovered. Attempts to identify and characterize genes predisposing to prostate cancer (prostate cancer predisposition genes) have been hampered by:

(1)   locus heterogeneity (more than one prostate cancer gene);

Hereditary Family History

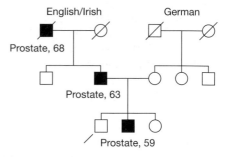

Fig. 31.4

Maternal Family History

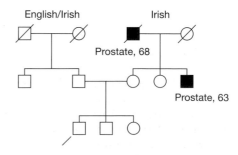

Fig. 31.5

(2) high phenocopy rate (a sporadic prostate cancer in a family with hereditary prostate cancer syndrome);

(3) late age of onset of the disease;

(4) absence of distinguishing clinical features;

(5) difficulty in finding extended pedigrees with large numbers of living affected members who are informative for linkage analysis (23).

Early research demonstrated the existence of one or several autosomal dominant prostate cancer predisposition genes with a penetrance (proportion of individuals who inherit a prostate cancer gene mutation who will develop prostate cancer) as high as 88% (15). Once prostate cancer predisposition genes are identified and characterized, more precise risk estimates for prostate cancer will be known.

Genome-wide screens of putative hereditary prostate cancer families have yielded four proposed loci (location of a gene on a chromosome) for prostate cancer. The first prostate cancer predisposition locus, 1q24–q25 (HPC1), was discovered by linkage analysis of 91 families from the USA and Sweden. Smith *et al.* (24) estimated that germline mutations in HPC1 accounted for approximately 34% of prostate cancer in the studied families and roughly estimates that 1 in 500 individuals in the United States may be a carrier of a mutated HPC1 gene. This study also found the average age of diagnosis was 65 years, with an age range of 39–85 years (24). Early onset cancer, higher grade tumors, and more advanced-stage disease at diagnosis may predict the families who carry a mutation in HPC1 (25). A linkage study using 47 French and German families with three or more prostate cancers diagnosed per family, resulted in linkage to a possible prostate cancer predisposition locus at 1q42.2–q43 (HPC2 or PCAP) (26). In addition to HPC1 and HPC2, there is evidence for a third prostate cancer predisposition locus at the chromosome 1p36 region. In fact, a significant portion of families with both a high risk for prostate cancer and a family member with brain cancer show linkage to the chromosome 1p36 region (27).

In the past, several population-based studies have reported a statistically significant excess risk of prostate cancer in men with affected brothers when compared to those with affected fathers. This is consistent with an X-linked or autosomal recessive mode of inheritance (23, 28). In fact, a study by Xu *et al.* discovered four independent family collections that provided evidence for linkage to the Xq27–28 locus (23).

There may be indirect genetic factors, called modifier genes, that play a minor role in prostate cancer initiation and progression. For example, there is the possible involvement of genes that affect the metabolism or circulating levels of androgens (29). Inheriting a certain combination of alleles (variations of a gene) could allow for an increased amount of circulating androgens, possibly increasing the risk for prostate cancer, while another combination of alleles may result in a better metabolism of androgens, resulting in a reduction of risk. The inheritance of modifier genes may be more complicated than a simple Mendelian pattern like autosomal dominant or X-linked inheritance, which are discussed later in this chapter.

Inheritance patterns of hereditary prostate cancer

Based on the previously described loci implicated as potential sites for prostate cancer predisposition genes, hereditary prostate cancer is believed to follow two inheritance patterns: autosomal dominant and X-linked.

In the Mendelian model, humans have two copies (alleles) of each gene, one paternal and one maternal, that determines a physical trait or disease. Autosomal dominant diseases are those in which only one mutated gene (heterozygous state) is required, compared to autosomal recessive diseases in which both alleles are required to be mutated (homozygous state) for the disease to be expressed. A person who is a carrier of a germline mutation (mutation in a gene that may be inherited from a parent and passed to offspring) in a prostate cancer predisposition gene will pass the mutant allele to his or her children 50% of the time (Fig. 31.4). A male child that inherits a germline mutation in a prostate cancer predisposition gene has the potential to develop prostate cancer. The percentage of risk is dictated by the penetrance of that particular prostate cancer predisposition gene. The siblings of the individuals who carry a germline mutation *each* have a 50% chance of inheriting the same mutation. Both men and women can pass an autosomal dominant prostate cancer predisposition gene mutation to their children.

Characteristics of an X-linked inheritance pattern are different from autosomal dominant inheritance. The X and Y chromosomes are the human sex-determining chromosomes and determine if a child will be female (XX) or male (XY). Therefore, a father who carries a

BRCA1 Family History

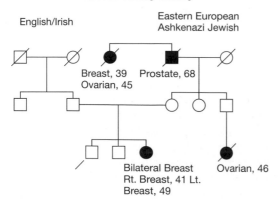

Fig. 31.6

X-Linked Pattern of Inheritance

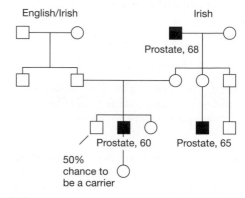

Fig. 31.7

germline X-linked prostate cancer predisposition gene mutation will not pass the mutation to his sons; however, all of his daughters will inherit the X-linked prostate cancer predisposition gene mutation (Fig. 31.6). Each child, sons and daughters, of a women who is a carrier of a germline X-linked prostate cancer predisposition gene has a 50% chance of inheriting the mutant allele. Again, the risk for men who inherit an X-linked prostate cancer predisposition gene mutation depends on the penetrance of that particular gene.

Family history of breast cancer

There are data to suggest that a family history of breast and/or ovarian cancer is a risk factor for prostate cancer. In addition, the combination of a family history of breast/ovarian and prostate cancer (on the same side of the family) may be an even stronger risk factor. A population-based cohort study of family history and risk of incident prostate cancer that adjusted for major confounding factors discovered that men with a family history of breast and/or ovarian cancer were at a 70% increased risk to develop prostate cancer. If there was a history of prostate and breast/ovarian cancer, the risk to develop prostate cancer was increased 480% (19).

Part of the increased risk for prostate cancer observed when there is a family history of breast/ovarian may be due to the inheritance of a mutation in the BRCA1 or BRCA2 gene. A woman who is found to be a carrier of a BRCA1 or BRCA2 germline mutation has a significantly increased risk of developing breast and/or ovarian cancer (Fig. 31.7). These cancers tend to be early onset, especially cancers associated with BRCA1, which tend to present prior to

menopause. Men who carry a germline mutation in BRCA1 or BRCA2 have a 2–4-fold increased risk for developing prostate cancer due to a BRCA1 or BRCA2 mutation segregating in their family (30, 31). BRCA1 and BRCA2 follow an autosomal dominant pattern of inheritance.

Genetic testing

In the future, genetic testing for a prostate cancer predisposition gene may help determine if the prostate cancer observed in a family is hereditary. Genetic testing is the process of determining if a person has inherited a germline mutation in a particular gene. But genetic testing is more than just a blood test, in fact there are substantial ethical, legal, and social implications associated with genetic testing.

Genetic information possesses unique characteristics when compared to other diagnostic tests, therefore, genetic testing requires a thorough informed consent process. For example, genetic test results affect an entire family. Once a family member is found to be a carrier of a genetic mutation that predisposes to cancer, other family members could potentially be at risk. Psychosocial issues may arise within the family, including guilt for passing a gene mutation to their children, or even conflict over having genetic testing and learning test results. Genetic information has symbolic meaning in our culture because our genetic material may determine our physical and psychological destiny (2). Genetic information may stigmatize a particular person or ethnic group. Also, genetic test results present a new category and challenge for medical professionals. A patient is suddenly reclassified from healthy to at-risk and the level of predicting whether that person will develop cancer may be uncertain. In addition, the genetic test process is sometimes complicated by uninformative or ambiguous test results, which can be confusing and frustrating to the patient and the physician.

The benefits, risks, and limitations of genetic testing must be reviewed with the patient before they can give informed consent for genetic testing. Potential benefits gained by genetic test results include:

(1) better estimation of personal cancer risk;

(2) better able to make informed decisions about screening and cancer-prevention methods;

(3) able to identify other family members at risk;

(4) reduced anxiety and screening for family members who are negative for a known family mutation;

(5) to know why prostate cancer is in their family.

Potential limitations of genetic testing include the fact that genetic information does not predict if, or when, the cancer will occur, and sometimes test results may be uninformative of ambiguous. Potential risks associated with genetic testing may include the potential for:

(1) employment or insurance discrimination;

(2) social stigmatization;

(3) negative emotional reaction;

(4) conflict within the family over learning and discussing genetic information and cancer risk.

Because of the potential risk and limitations of genetic testing, the decision to proceed with testing is a personal decision the patient and his family must make once they are fully informed about the implications of genetic testing. The genetic counselor plays a non-directive role, helps facilitate the decision-making process and promotes patient autonomy.

Screening guidelines

Prostate cancer screening, including annual digital rectal exam (DRE) and prostate-specific antigen (PSA) testing beginning at the age of 40, for men at increased risk for developing prostate cancer may help detect prostate at an early, curable stage. Individuals who could benefit from screening should be informed about potential benefits and limitations of prostate cancer

screening. Inform the patient of the sensitivity, specificity, and positive predictive value of the screening test. In addition, explaining the criteria for biopsy and the diagnostic process will prepare the patient in the event of an abnormal result. Based on family history, personal risk factors, or general population screening recommendations, it may also be beneficial to discuss screening guidelines for other cancers and medical conditions.

Psychosocial counseling

By communicating cancer risk information and genetic test results in medical practice, healthcare professionals have the potential to motivate high-risk individuals to adhere to cancer prevention and surveillance; however, there might be adverse psychologic and social consequences as well (32). Men seeking information about their risk of developing prostate cancer, or who receive genetic test results, must come to terms not only with their risk of developing cancer, but also the possibility that other members of their family, even their children, may be similarly at risk. Emotional reactions such as anger, guilt, fear, and grief may be experienced by learning cancer-risk information. In addition, supportive and grief counseling may be important for an unaffected family member dealing with the diagnosis of prostate in a relative and the potential loss of a loved one (33). For these reasons, it is important to set aside time during the genetic counseling session to inquire about the feelings the patient may have concerning his risk and family history of prostate cancer, and how the family has dealt with the diagnosis of cancer. Discuss with the patient support systems that have helped him cope with anxiety and or problems in the past. In addition, identify referrals for more information or counseling, when appropriate.

Support groups/educational resources

Support groups and educational resources are offered through two organizations based in the United States. These groups offer men education, support, and promote the awareness of prostate cancer and screening through newsletters, educational presentation, websites, and support groups. In addition, contact your social services department at your institution to find local recourses and support groups.

- Us TOO International, Inc. is based at PO Box 3083, Oak Brook, IL, 60522-9767, USA., 1-800-808-7866, www.ustoo.com.There are over 500 US TOO chapters located in the US, Canada, Australia and Europe.
- Man-to-Man group is offered through the American Cancer Society and can be contacted at 1-800-227-2345, www.cancer.org/m2m/m2mgoals.html.

Case examples

Case 1

A 46-year-old man reports that his father developed prostate cancer at the age of 73. He has two paternal uncles and a paternal grandfather who lived into their 70s and did not develop prostate cancer. His maternal and paternal family histories are negative for other types of cancer. Based on the fact that his father's prostate cancer was late-onset, and the fact that his paternal family history includes several men who lived into their 70s without cancer, the proband's risk to develop prostate cancer is increased 2–3-fold. The counselor should advise the patient on the guidelines, limitations, and benefits of prostate cancer screening. In addition, psychosocial issues regarding anxiety associated to his risk should be addressed in addition to other issues the patient may raise during the session.

Case 2

A 50-year-old man reports that his father, an only child, developed prostate cancer at the age of 51 and subsequently died from the cancer. His paternal grandfather died in a car accident at the age of 40. His maternal family history is negative for cancer. Risk assessment for this man is difficult since his paternal family size is small and his paternal grandfather died at a young age. The fact that his father was diagnosed at a young age with prostate cancer raises the possibility that there may be a hereditary predisposition in his family. First-degree relatives of men who developed prostate cancer before the age of 53 years may have a cumulative lifetime risk of 40% for developing prostate cancer (15). The counselor should advise the patient on the guidelines, limitations, and benefits of prostate cancer screening. The counselor should also identify

other at-risk family members and offer counseling or referrals for counseling. In addition, psychosocial issues regarding anxiety with regards to his risk should be addressed. This is especially important since the patient is nearing the age his father was diagnosed with prostate cancer. The counselor should try to help the patient understand that feeling anxious as he nears the age his father was diagnosed is a normal reaction. In addition, explore support systems and provide referrals for information and counseling, if needed.

Case 3

The patient is a 52-year-old man who reports that his brother was just diagnosed with prostate cancer at the age of 56. In addition, his father was also diagnosed at the age of 63 and his paternal grandfather at the age of 68. This family history fits an autosomal dominant hereditary pattern of inheritance. The patient may have a 50% chance of having inherited the prostate cancer predisposition gene mutation in his family. His risk for developing cancer if he did in fact inherit the mutated allele may be as high as 88% (15). The counselor should advise the patient on the guidelines, limitations, and benefits of prostate cancer screening. Also, the counselor should identify other at-risk family members and offer counseling or referrals for counseling for these individuals. In this case, searching for a hereditary prostate cancer research program may allow the patient and his family to gain more information about their risk and allow them to further research on hereditary prostate cancer. Genetic testing in the future would be an option for this family. In addition, psychosocial issues regarding anxiety with regards to his risk should be addressed. This is especially important since his brother was recently diagnosed. The counselor may also inquire about the family's beliefs with regard to what is causing cancer in the family and how well the family is coping with the diagnoses. Since there is the possibility that this is an inherited form of prostate cancer, the counselor may also want to explore feelings of anger and guilt due to the possibility of inheriting a predisposition to prostate cancer, and also the possibility that he may have passed this risk to his children. In addition, explore support systems and provide referrals for information and counseling, if needed.

Conclusion

Cancer genetic counseling is the communication process between healthcare professionals and their patients concerning the occurrence, or risk of occurrence, of cancer in his or her family (1). The counseling process combines education, risk assessment, and health promotion. Genetic counseling also includes facilitating decision-making surrounding genetic testing, addressing psychosocial concerns, assisting the patient with coping and reducing anxiety, and helping the patient identify support systems. Once prostate cancer predisposition genes are identified and characterized, more precise risk estimates for prostate cancer will be known, the option of genetic testing can be provided to men with a family history of prostate cancer, and the molecular mechanisms of prostate cancer will be better understood. Genetic information may be the key to answering many of the questions men have about their family history and their risk to develop prostate. The genetic counseling process is responsible for imparting this information to the patient and promoting patient autonomy.

References

1. Peters JA. Familial cancer risk part 1: impact on today's oncology practice. *J Oncology Management* 1994, **12**, 20–30.
2. Baker DL, Schuette JL, Uhlmann WR (ed.) *A guide to genetic counseling*. Wiley & Sons, Inc, New York, 1998.
3. Bennett RL, Steinhaus KA, Uhrich SB *et al*. Recommendations for standardized human pedigree nomenclature. *Am J Hum Genet* 1995, **56**, 745–52.
4. Giovannucci E, Rimm EB, Colditz GA *et al*. A prospective study of dietary fat and risk of prostate cancer. *J Natl Cancer Inst* 1993, **85**, 1571–9.
5. Le Marchand L, Wilkens LR, Kolonel LN *et al*. Lifetime occupational physical activity and prostate cancer risk. *Am J Epidemiol* 1991, **133**, 103–11.
6. van der Gulden JW. Prostate cancer and work environment. *J Occup Med* 1992, **34**, 402–9.
7. Haas GP, Sakr WA. Epidemiology of prostate cancer. *CA Cancer J Clin* 1997, **47**, 273–87.
8. Parker S, Tong T, Boldey S. *et al*. Cancer statistics, 1997. *CA Cancer J Clin* 1997, **47**, 5–27.
9. Sakr WA. Epidemiology of high grade prostatic intraepithelial neoplasia. *Patholo Res Practice* 1995, **191**, 838–41.
10. Gao X, Grignon DJ, Chbihi T *et al*. Elevated 12-lipoxygenase mRNA expression correlates with advanced stage and poor differentiation of human prostate cancer. *Urology* 1995, **46**, 227–37.
11. Eyre HJ, Feldman GE. Status report on prostate cancer in African Americans: a national blueprint for action. *CA Cancer J Clin* 1998, **48**, 315–8.
12. Ries LAG. *Cancer statistics review, 1973–1987*, NIH publication no. 90-2799. Bethesda, MD, United States Public Health Service, 1990.
13. Powell IJ. Prostate cancer and African-American men. *Oncology* 1997, **11**, 599–605.
14. Gelfand DE, Parzuchowski J, Cort M *et al*. Digital rectal examinations and prostate cancer screening: attitudes of African American men. *Oncol Nurs Forum* 1995, **22**, 1253–5.
15. Carter BS, Beaty TH, Steinberg G *et al*. Mendelian inheritance of familial prostate cancer. *Proc Nat Acad Sci USA* 1992, **89**, 3367–71.
16. Cannon L. Genetic epidemiology of prostate cancer in the Utah Mormon genealogy. *Cancer Surv* 1982, **1**, 47–68.
17. Carter BS, Bora GS, Beaty TH *et al*. Hereditary prostate cancer: epidemiologic and clinical features. *J Urol* 1993, **150**, 797–802.
18. Bratt O, Kristoffersson U, Lundgren R, *et al*. The risk of malignant tumors in first-degree relatives of men with early onset prostate cancer: a population-based cohort study. *Eur J Cancer* 1997, **33**, 2237–40.
19. Cerhan JR, Parker A, Putnary SD *et al*. Family history and prostate cancer risk in a population-based cohort of Iowa men. *Cancer Epidemiol, Briomarkers & Prevention* 1999, **8**, 53–60.
20. Walsh PC, Partin AW. Family history facilitates the early diagnosis of prostate carcinoma. *CA* 1997, **80**, 1871–4.
21. Spitz MR, Currier RD, Fueger JJ *et al*. Familial patterns of prostate cancer: a case-control analysis. *J Urol* 1991, **146**, 1305–7.
22. Steinberg GD, Carter BS, Beaty TH *et al*. Family history and the risk of prostate cancer. *Prostate* 1990, **17**, 337–47.
23. Xu J, Meyers D, Freije D *et al*. Evidence for a prostate cancer susceptibility locus on the X chromosome. *Nat Genet* 1998, **20**, 175–9.
24. Smith JR, Freije D, Carpten J *et al*. Major susceptibility locus for prostate cancer on chromosome 1 suggested by a genome-wide search. *Science* 1996, **274**, 1371–1374.
25. Gronberg H, Bergh A, Damber J *et al*. Characteristics of prostate cancer in families potentially linked to hereditary prostate cancer 1 (HPC1) locus. *JAMA* 1997, **278** (15), 1251–5.
26. Berthon P, Valeri A, Cohen A *et al*. Predisposing gene for early-onset prostate cancer, localized on chromosome 1q42.2–43. *Am J Hum Genet* 1998, **62**, 1416–24.
27. Gibbs M, Stanford JL, McIndoe RA *et al*. Evidence for a rare prostate cancer-susceptibility locus at chromosome 1p36. *Am J Hum Genet* 1999, **64** (3), 776–87.
28. Monroe KR, Yu MC, Kolonel LN *et al*. Evidence of an X-linked or recessive genetic component to prostate cancer risk. *Nat Med* 1995, **1**(8), 827–9.

29. Bankhead C. Clues to prostate cancer gene are few, but possibilities emerge. *J Natl Cancer Inst* 1996, **88** (1), 11–2.

30. Streuwing JP. The risk of cancer associated with specific mutations of *BRCA1* and *BRACA2* among Ashkenazi Jews. *N Engl J Med* 1997, **336**, 1401–8.

31. The Breast Cancer Linkage Consortium. Cancer Risks in BRCA2 mutation carriers. *J Natl Cancer Inst* 1999, **91** (15), 1310–16.

32. Lerman C, Rimer BK, Engstrom PF. Cancer risk notification: psychosocial and ethical implications. *J Clin Oncol* 1991, **9** (7), 1275–82.

33. Peters JA, Stopfer JE. Role of the genetic counselor in familial cancer. *Oncology* 1996 **10** (2), 159–75.

32 | Prostate cancer clinical trials meta-analyses

Nancy A. Dawson and Jon L. Hopkins

Introduction

Meta-analysis is a procedure to systematically research and collect published and (ideally) unpublished randomized clinical trials (RCTs) of treatments and quantitatively summarize their results, in order to obtain an objective assessment of efficacy. Randomized trials are effective, and usually unbiased, for showing the average results in a selected outcome variable for treatment. A versus treatment B, and meta-analyses will produce an average of these averages. The number of meta-analysis or overviews appearing in the literature is rapidly increasing and are now widely used to provide evidence to support clinical strategies (1). The objectives of a meta-analysis include increasing power to detect an overall treatment effect, estimation of the degree of benefit associated with a particular study treatment, assessment of the amount of variability between studies, or identification of study characteristics associated with particularly effective treatments (2). Assuming there were a large number of published RCTs with available, high-quality data, meta-analysis of clinical trials in prostate cancer could potentially demonstrate clinically meaningful treatment effects. This unfortunately is not yet the case.

In the United States, cancer of the prostate is the most common malignancy in men with an estimated 179 300 new cases diagnosed in 1999 (3). According to information collected by the National Cancer Institute's Surveillance, Epidemiology, and End Results (SEER) program, the incidence of this cancer peaked at greater than 300 000 new cases in 1993 and then decreased, suggesting an adjustment to the initial influence of mass screening (3, 4). The medical research communities have correspondingly increased their focus on the disease but major questions remain unresolved. Although current or planned clinical trials are addressing many of the important issues, the number of completed large randomized clinical trials suitable for meta-analysis is relatively small (5). One blatant exception is the greater than 25 randomized clinical trials comparing monohormonal therapy to combined androgen blockade in hormone-sensitive metastatic disease.

Addressing the earliest point of intervention, the prevention of prostate cancer emerges as a very attractive option when faced with the problems inherent in both early detection and treatment of metastatic disease (6). Some research has suggested that populations of patients with diets high in fiber or low in fat have a lower incidence of prostate cancer. In a randomized trial from Finland, originally designed to determine if vitamin E and/or A could prevent lung cancer, instead there was a significant reduction in the number of diagnosed prostate cancers in patients receiving vitamin E. Agents that block or suppress gene mutation such as selenium, vitamin C, and the isofllavenoids, have all been suggested as possible chemopreventive agents. Difluromethylorithine DFMO has been recognized as a potent inhibitor of ornithine decarboxylase (ODC), which catalyzes the synthesis of polyamines found in high concentrations in the prostate (7). Since high polyamine levels enhance cell proliferation, DFMO has been suggested as a potential preventive agent.

Current studies examining the effect of chemoprevention include a University of Wisconsin phase I/II trial designed to determine whether DFMO could modulate a number of markers for prostate carcinogenesis. A second much larger study of greater than 18 000 men, the Prostate Cancer Prevention Trial (PCPT), is testing the hypothesis that finasteride, which prevents the conversion of testosterone to the more potent dihydrotestosterone via inhibition of the enzyme $5\ \alpha$-reductase, can prevent the development of prostate cancer (3). A third trial, the Selenium and Vitamin E Chemoprevention Trial (SELECT) of over 32 000 men, is scheduled to begin in mid-2000. These trials will provide much information about potential methods to prevent prostate cancer, and may even identify strategies that can reduce the morbidity and mortality of this common disease.

Currently there are far more questions than there are answers in the diagnosis and treatment of prostate cancer. Beginning with screening, there are several potential confounding factors and problems to include:

- over diagnosis;
- unknown impact on mortality;
- potential morbidity of subsequent treatment;
- significant cost of screening and treatment (4, 6).

To date there is only one completed randomized screening trial. This trial reported a survival advantage for screened patients, but has been criticized for a number of selection biases and for not performing an intention-to-screen analysis. A second screening trial, the Prostate, Lung, Colorectal Ovarian cancer (PLCO) study will hopefully help to resolve the controversy over secondary prevention (i.e. early detection and treatment) of prostate cancer (7). The aim of this trial is to determine whether annual screening will reduce mortality from prostate cancer. Men enrolled in the study will receive screening with PSA and DRE of the prostate as well as chest X-ray and flexible sigmoidoscopy to screen for lung and colorectal cancer annually for 4 years. This cohort will be compared with whatever regular testing is provided in the community (5).

Another of the important fundamental questions is what treatment is best for localized disease. Studies have demonstrated that the majority of tumors detected by screening tests, including PSA and DRE, are clinically confined to the prostate (T1–T2 tumors) (6). Opinions have varied concerning the relative benefits of treating these clinically localized tumors. Many authors have advocated that observation or 'expectant management' will lead to acceptable outcomes during 5- and 10-year follow-ups. However, more recent analysis of the literature has suggested that with longer follow-up, mortality from the untreated disease increases dramatically. While several authors have demonstrated excellent survival among patients with clinically localized prostate cancer treated with radical prostatectomy, concerns have been raised about the high rates of positive surgical margins, PSA recurrence, and patient-reported morbidity.

There are several ongoing randomized trials for clinically localized prostate cancer. The Veterans Administration and National Cancer Institute are co-sponsoring the Prostate Cancer Intervention versus observation trial (PIVOT), which randomizes patients with clinically confined prostate carcinoma to either radical prostatectomy or observation (7). Powered to detect differences in survival, the results of this trial will not be available for many years but promises to provide some of the most important answers regarding the management of early localized disease. Since the PLCO chemoprevention trial does not mandate specific treatment for detected prostate cancers, this study fits quite well with PIVOT. The combination of the two trials may provide evidence of the relative efficacy of both screening and treatment.

Although there are numerous phase II trials currently assessing different treatment modalities in patients with clinically localized disease, the current and planned phase III trials providing a head to head comparisons to assess the relative worth of brachytherapy, cryotherapy, radical prostatectomy, external-beam radiotherapy, hormonal therapy, and watchful waiting are few (8). The initial course of many diagnosed prostate cancers is indolent. Thus it is difficult to reliably assess efficacy of any treatment from studies in which patients at relatively low risk of short-term progression are treated and in whom follow-up is less than 10 years. Current phase III trials include the NCIC trial of hormonal therapy versus hormonal therapy and radiation therapy, and PIVOT. The American College of Surgeons Oncology Group (ACSOG) will initiate a randomized trial of 1500 men comparing prostatectomy and brachytherapy in mid-2000.

Hormonal therapy has been the mainstay of therapy for advanced prostate cancer, since the work of Huggins and Hodges in the 1940s (7, 8). Unfortunately, there is little evidence that significant advances in the treatment of metastatic disease have been made since that time. In the early 1980s Labrie and colleagues introduced the concept of combined androgen blockade (CAB) utilizing an LHRH agonist or orchiectomy (to ablate testicular androgens) plus an anti-androgen (to block remaining adrenal androgens) (9). In 1989 the National Cancer Institute (NCI) and the Southwestern Oncology Group (SWOG) completed a trial comparing a LHRH-a plus an anti-androgen to an LHRH-a alone (10). The results of the trial suggested that combined androgen deprivation significantly improved median time to progression in patients with metastatic disease. However, a follow-up SWOG study comparing orchiectomy with or without flutamide in patients with metastatic disease, demonstrated no difference in progression free or overall survival (11). Numerous other comparative studies have led to one of the few areas in prostate cancer where there has been a major role for meta-analysis.

A number of therapies for metastatic prostate cancer are currently being investigated in clinical trails. One of the more intriguing potential approaches involves intermittent hormonal therapy. Intermittent therapy employing LHRH agonists has the potential advantage of:

- lower cost compared to continuous therapy;
- periods during which side-effects are reduced;
- lower risk of long-term complications, such as osteoporosis and anemia;
- the possibility that delaying the development of androgen-independent disease may enhance survival (7).

A current SWOG study randomizes patients who achieve an undetectable PSA following initial hormonal therapy to either continuous therapy or intermittent hormonal therapy. This trial will address one of the most important new potential treatment approaches for patients with metastatic disease.

Although PSA has not been validated as an early surrogate endpoint that may be used in clinical trials, there is no question that patients who exhibit biochemical failure are at higher risk of death from metastatic disease (4, 6). The optimal treatment for these patients is unknown. Radiotherapy to the prostatic fossa is commonly employed for patients who relapse following radical prostatectomy without evidence of distant disease. Although initial studies suggested that freedom from progression could be affected by this treatment, the long term, PSA-free recurrence rate has been disappointing. Clinical trials employing adjuvant radiotherapy, with or without hormonal therapy, are ongoing. The European Organization for Research and Treatment of Cancer (EROTC) (12) trial will assess the efficacy of early versus delayed hormonal therapy for PSA recurrence. An ideal study to assess potential treatments for relapse after definitive therapy would stratify patients according to their risk of recurrence and might include newer methods of ascertaining whether the biochemical recurrence was due to a local or systemic failure. Patients could then be randomized, so that the contribution of radiotherapy and hormonal therapy could be evaluated. Such a study has yet to be mounted.

At present there is no conclusive evidence that additional treatment improves survival of patients who relapse after initial hormonal therapy. Numerous chemotherapeutic regimens and other methods of treatment are being studied in this setting. Historically, relative chemotherapeutic insensitivity was evidenced by significant (> 50%) objective tumor regression in less than 10–15% of patients, by the rare attainment of complete remission (CR). However, recent phase II trials of estramustine combined with vinblastine, paclitaxel, etoposide, or doxetaxel have demonstrated objective tumor regression in 30–40% patients with measurable disease, pain improvement in up to 50%, and significant declines in PSA in 50% of patients with androgen-independent prostate cancer (13). Randomized phase III trials of mitoxantrone plus steroids versus steroids, estramustine plus vinblastine versus vinblastine, and suramin plus hydrocortisone versus hydrocortisone have shown significantly longer survival for patients with greater than 50% decline in PSA (14, 15, 16). In the setting of secondary hormonal manipulation, declines in PSA of this magnitude in men treated megestrol acetate was also correlated with improved survival (17).

The role of meta-analysis in assessment of clinical trials

Meta-analysis of clinical trials offers the opportunity to pool results from a number of randomized studies so increasing the statistical ability to detect the value of treatment (18). For a meta-analysis to give definitive information, it should at least meet the minimum standard that would be expected of a well-designed, adequately powered, and carefully conducted randomized, controlled trial (1, 5). These minimum standards include both quantitative standards – and assessment of whether the total sample is large enough to provide reliable results and the use of appropriate statistical monitoring guidelines to indicate when the results of the accumulating data of a meta-analysis are conclusive. The quality of meta-analysis depends essentially on the completeness of the collection of trials. Apart from this problem, the limits of a meta-analysis are the limits of the trials it includes; the addition of ill-designed and ill-conducted trials can only be a bad meta-analysis. Meta-analyses based on individual data provided by each trialist allows a better appreciation of the quality of a trial, increases the statistical power, and allows for some covariates to be taken into account (19, 20). The most reliable type of meta-analysis uses individual patient data and includes all cri-teria, published and unpublished (21, 22). If the inade-quacies of previous trials have led to a performance of a suitable new trial, the numbers emerging from meta-analyses of prior non-pertinent results should not stop it.

Factors needed to evaluate a meta-analyses are: description of the problem; definition of the outcome(s) (primary and secondary); methods for identifying the selecting trials for inclusion; statistical problems such as the detection of bias, the validity of the information provided by the meta-analysis, quality criteria for a meta-analysis, and how to locate published meta-analyses (19). Well-conducted meta-analyses or overviews are the best method of summarizing all available unbiased evidence on the relative effects of treatments. Recently meta-analysis has expanded to cover non-randomized studies, including evaluation of diagnostic tests and pooling of epidemiological studies (15, 18). There is growing concern for standards, and several methodological issues remain unresolved (21). Meta-analysis of randomized trials of adjuvant therapy in early breast cancer illustrates the value of such analy-ses. These have helped, not only routine clinical practice, but have thrown light upon biological mechanisms and directed future research (20). Due to the emergence of evidence-based medicine (EBM), the role of meta-analy-sis is expanding. EBM is taking advantage from the Cochrane Collaboration, an international network of experts performing, updating and disseminating meta-analyses of important treatments, according to common models and established procedures (19). Meta-analysis in prostate cancer clinical trials has been of limited use to date primarily due to a lack of RCTs.

Screening

The goal of cancer screening is the early detection of tumors in the hope that the added lead-time will permit curative intervention for some patients who would oth-erwise die of their disease (4, 6). This assumes localized disease is found at the time of detection. However, cure is not the only objective of cancer care. Prolongation of life and improvement in the quality of life in the absence of cure is also valuable. In the case of prostate cancer, improving the quality of life translates into delaying the appearance of metastases and local symp-toms, and avoiding iatrogenic morbidity.

A prostate cancer screening program needs two essential attributes to be successful: the screening test must be capable of advancing the time of diagnosis, and the earlier treatment interventions must have an impact on the eventual course of the disease (6). A bal-anced assessment of the evidence suggests that in appropriately selected men, screening will allow cura-tive treatment of presymptomatic cancers that other-wise would cause substantial morbidity and mortality.

The true value of screening requires randomized trials where the screened and unscreened populations are identical with regard to risk factors of prostate cancer. The sample size of such trials must be very large because an asymptomatic population will only contain a small proportion of patients with detectable cancer, and an even smaller size proportion of patients who will either die of the disease or be potentially impacted by the early treatment intervention permitted by early detection (4, 22). Endpoints such as cancer inci-dence, stage of diagnosis, and case survival, though inter-esting and informative about the natural history of the disease, are inappropriate for comparisons of screened and unscreened groups because they are affected by pro-found sampling biases, namely, length-based sampling and lead-time biases. Other important aspects of screen-ing that merit evaluation in a trial are the 'costs' of the screening program. This must be evaluated in relation to the 'benefits', i.e. reduced mortality (6).

The most striking aspect of the literature on screen-ing is the relatively small percentage of cancers that will be detected. Using the preferred method for first-line prostate cancer screening, the PSA and DRE, Catalona *et al.* (23) reported 8% of the patients screened had an elevated PSA and a corresponding figure for an abnormal DRE is 7% from the study by Metlin *et al.* (24) The real sensitivity of any screening strategy will necessarily be very low. However, the cancers that are missed will typically be very small tumors. The rational for screening is based on the sup-position that the great majority of the tumors that would become clinically significant during the patients' lifetimes will be detected by screening. In three studies involving a total of 19 880 men, a significant stage migration in tumors was detected through PSA-based screening (4). In two large multicenter studies involving 6630 and 2299 men, the combined percentage of pathologically organ-confined cancers detected through PSA screening was 98% (6). In the other study, the per-centage of pathologically organ-confined cancers detected by PSA-based screening was 66% in men who had undergone radical prostateectomy. This represents a 100% increase over the percentage of organ-confined cancers detected in historical series.

Under the direction of The National Cancer Institute, an ambitious and potentially informative large screening trial involving the three major cancers affecting men (prostate, lung, colorectal) is ongoing (3): 74 000 men from 64 to 74 to will be randomized to a screening battery including DRE and PSA or to a control arm of standard medical care. It is likely that many cancers will be detected in the screened group, and using a more aggressive screening strategy could increase the advancement of lead-time. Nine countries in Europe and North America are half-way to recruiting about 300 000 men to randomized trials to determine whether prostate cancer screening with prostate-specific antigen can save lives. Nine randomized controlled trials, collectively called the International Prostate Screening Trials Evaluation Group, hope to have all participants through the first round of screening in 1999 (8). Critics of screening trials claim that there is a risk for the over diagnosis of 'innocent cancers' and that none of the potentially curative treatment options available have demonstrated the capacity to reduce survival. One of the major threats to prostate cancer screening trials everywhere is the perceived acceptance of screening in the US. European investigators have shown restraint and slower acceptance of prostate cancer screening, while waiting for completion of prostate cancer screening clinical trials.

As these trials are ongoing and analysis of long-term impact will not follow for several years, meta-analysis of screening trials will not be feasible for 5–10 years. In fact, to date there is only one published randomized PSA era prostate cancer screening trial. Labrie *et al.* (25) randomized 46 193 men ages 45–80 on the Quebec City electoral roll between screening and no screening. However, only 8137 of the men in the screening arm were actually screened. There were 137 prostate cancer deaths in the 38 056 unscreened men compared to 5 deaths in the screened group (3.25 odds ratio favoring screening, $P < 0.01$). Although his study has been highly criticized because of the large number of men randomized to be screened but not screened, and the failure to analyze on an intent-to-screen basis, the results are nonetheless titillating.

Localized disease

Treatment of localized prostate cancer is among the most controversial areas in oncology today. Available options include: radical prostatectomy, external-beam radiation therapy, brachytherapy, watchful waiting, cryosurgery, hormonal therapy, and combinations of these modalities. These approaches appear to have

similar 5-year survival rates. However, these approaches may lead to different rates of disease-free survival and overall survival with clear differences in morbidity. Because the results of single-modality treatment have been disappointing, there has been a trend within the last decade toward multi-modality combination therapies, with a particular emphasis on combining hormonal therapy with surgery or radiation therapy (26). More recent clinical trials have added chemotherapy for patients with high-risk pathologic features. Large randomized trials comparing these different approaches have only been recently initiated and hence there are sparse meta-analyses of clinical trials in localized prostate cancer. Nonetheless, the areas that deserve comparative analysis and the current ongoing studies need to be addressed.

Radical prostatectomy has the potential for cure in T1 and T2 lesions of the prostate with PSA progression-free survival rates of 70–80% at 5 years and 50–70% at 10 years (26). Surgery has been shown to have limited ability to cure locally advanced (T3) prostate cancer. In two recent series of patients who underwent surgery for clinical T3 disease, only 9–22% of patients had pathologically organ-confined disease. Van den Ouden *et al.* (27) reported only 22% of patients free of clinical or biochemical progression at a mean follow-up time of 43.9 months.

From surgical series in patients with organ-confined disease, 85% remain free from biochemical failure at 10 years, but only 42% of those with extracapsular penetration or high-grade pathology and 43% with seminal vesicle involvement had a similar disease-free survival rate. Of patients with lymph node involvement, 15% remain free of biochemical progression at 5 years, and none had an undetectable PSA level at 10 years follow-up. Thus it appears that an aggressive surgical approach for patients with locally advanced cancer rarely results in long-term disease-free survival (28).

In a recent series of external-beam radiation therapy (EBRT) alone for clinical stage T3 prostate cancer, 10-year survival rates of 35–45% and 15-year survival rates from 17% to 31% were shown. Zietman *et al.* (29) recently reported a 10-year biochemical disease-free survival rate of only 18% in 540 clinical stage T3–4 patients who underwent ERBT. These disappointing results have led to the widespread use of the combination of hormonal therapy and radiation therapy. This concept dates back to 1967, when a randomized prospective study comparing androgen ablation with diethylstilbestrol (DES) plus radiation therapy, to radiation therapy alone, was initiated at the MD Anderson Cancer Center in men with clinical stage T3 prostate cancer (26). In 78 randomized patients, there was a statistically significant improvement in disease-free survival and freedom from metastasis for the patients who received early hormonal therapy, but there was no difference in overall survival, despite a median follow-up duration of 14.5 years. Three subsequent studies showed improved disease-free survival and improved local control with combined therapy. Most recently, Bolla *et al.* (30) demonstrated a survival benefit of combination therapy using goserelin acetate for 3 years compared to radiation alone in men with localized disease, the majority of whom where stage T3. The National Cancer Institute of Canada (NCIC) is currently assessing whether radiation adds therapeutic efficacy, both in terms of local control, progression free and overall survival in a clinical trial of hormone therapy versus hormone therapy plus radiation.

Most patients who have persistent disease after primary radiation therapy are given subsequent salvage hormonal therapy; the question becomes whether early versus late hormonal therapy makes a survival difference in patients who undergo ERBT. The randomized prospective study by Fellows *et al.* (31) included three treatment groups: an orchiectomy-only group, a radiation therapy-only group, and a combined orchiectomy plus radiation group. There was no statistical difference between the combined orchiectomy plus radiation therapy group, and the combined therapy treatment groups with regard to distant disease progression and overall survival.

The placement of radioactive seeds using an open retropubic or open perineal approach became popular in the 1970s. Results of brachytherapy in this era were particularly poor for patients with poorly differentiated or clinical stage C lesions; local recurrence rates approached 50% and 5- and 10-year disease-free survival rates were as low as 23% and 14%, respectively. In recent series limited to favorable cases with clinical stage T1–2, 76–98% of men have no biochemical progression at median follow-ups of 2–3 years (7, 30).

Most investigators feel that brachytherapy alone is insufficient for locally advanced lesions and have advocated combining the brachytherapy with ERBT. However, this has not been assessed in a randomized prospective fashion. The question of the superiority of radical prostatectomy versus brachytherapy will be assessed in a 1500-patient trial spearheaded by the American College of Surgeons Oncology Group (ACSOG) planned to activate in mid-2000. Eligible

men will have T1c or T2a low-grade prostate cancer (Gleason score < 7 and PSA < 10). Primary endpoints will be comparative overall survival, quality of life, and satisfaction with procedure received. Concern has been raised whether this trial can be completed, in light of the failure of the MRC PR06 trial to accrue patients.

Watchful waiting is the selected option by some men desiring to avoid the complications of surgery or radiation. This approach is supported by two studies from Europe showing comparable survival in population-based studies where treatment was only initiated when symptomatic compared to treated cohorts. The current ongoing prostate intervention versus observation trial (PIVOT) addresses this question (7, 27). Enrolled men are randomized to prostatectomy versus observation. Men progressing on observation may later choose surgery.

Cryotherapy has re-emerged as a potential local therapy in the management of prostate cancer in the early 1990s, when it was realized that transrectal ultrasound could be used to monitor the extent of prostatic freezing (26). Despite initial enthusiasm for this procedure, it has not been widely adopted. Furthermore, planned large trials of cryosurgery versus radiation have never actualized.

Another approach to improved resectability is the use of neoadjuvant hormonal therapy to eliminate the bulk of tumor cells that are sensitive to hormones in the hope that these cells may be the ones that are primarily responsible for the extra-prostatic extension. Then, if adequate tumor shrinkage has occurred, it may be possible to eliminate any residual, hormonally unresponsive cells by surgical extirpation. The results of recent randomized prospective studies comparing neoadjuvant hormonal therapy with surgery for clinical sage T1–T3 prostate cancer, show statistically significant reduction in the frequency of positive surgical margins but the incidences of seminal invasion and lymph node metastasis were not statistically different. In a meta-analysis of seven similarly designed RCT, despite differences in risk factors, neoadjuvant androgen deprivation was significantly associated with lower pathologic T stage and negative surgical margins (Bonney) (32). However, at present there remains no obvious long-term survival benefit within the context of randomized prospective trials.

Locally advanced prostate cancer remains a difficult problem and although the results of single-modality treatments have been disappointing, this problem represents a paradigm for multi-modality therapy. In a recently reported trial by the Eastern Cooperative

Oncology Group (ECOG), 98 men with positive lymph nodes post-prostatectomy, randomized to immediate initiation of androgen deprivation, had a significant improvement in progression-free and overall survival compared to those treated at time of progression (33). Post-operatively in patients with high-risk disease based on Gleason score > 7 or positive surgical margins, local lymph nodes or seminal vesicles are being assessed for added benefit of hormonal therapy, chemohormonal therapy, or radiation. RTOG 96–01 is a randomized trial evaluating the role of adjuvant bicalutamide in addition to radiation in men with pT3 prostate cancer (7). In a second US Intergroup trial, men with high-risk disease will be randomized after prostatectomy to hormone therapy with or without chemotherapy consisting of mitoxantrone and prednisone (34). Again an inadequate number of comparable trials have been completed to allow for meta-analysis.

Hormone-sensitive metastatic disease

For more than five decades, the preferred treatment for advanced prostate cancer has been suppression of testicular androgen production by medical or surgical castration. However, until recently there was little data to support initiating early androgen deprivation in the asymptomatic man. In 1998, the Medical Research Council reported their randomized trial of early versus delayed hormonal therapy in men with locally advanced (T2–4) or metastatic disease (35). They demonstrated improvements in all causes of mortality, disease-specific mortality, rate of local and metastatic progression, catastrophic complications (spinal cord compression urinary obstruction, and pathological fractures). However, the optimal form of this therapy with either monotherapy, in the form of bilateral orchiectomy, or a LHRH agonist, or combined androgen deprivation adding an anti-androgen, remains a source of controversy.

Researchers from Italy and Spain initially investigated the use of anti-androgens in metastatic disease in the late 1960s and 1970s. The first randomized controlled trials using an anti-androgen was the European Organization for Research and Treatment of Cancer (EROTC) Genitourinary (GU) Group protocol 30805 developed in 1979. This study compared cyproterone acetate (CPA) vs. DES vs. castration as a standard treatment. In the final analysis of 335 patients showed no differences in time to progression and overall survival among the three treatment arms (36). In 1983,

Labrie *et al.* (9) proposed the use of combined androgen blockade to obtain better results than those obtained with the most widely used techniques of surgical or hormonal castration alone. Since that time, many randomized comparative trials using various forms of CAB have been carried out to examine the question of whether CAB would significantly delay the progression to endocrine independence of prostate cancer and eventually prolongation of survival.

A review of the efficacy of the anti-androgen nilutamide plus orchiectomy compared to orchiectomy plus placebo in previously untreated patients with stage D prostate cancer was published by Bertagna *et al.* (36) in early 1992. The results of seven randomized double-blind trials with similar design and involving (1056) patients were analyzed. The short-term results reported by all of the studies were similar in that there were significant improvements in metastasis-related bone pain and levels of tumor markers with nilutamide. In addition, the combination of nilutamide and ochiectomy resulted in a marked improvement in response rate. Disease progression measured at 6 months was reduced by one-third by the administration of nilutamide. This review illustrated the advantage of meta-analysis in providing a means to detect moderate differences observed between different treatment regimens. Although this analysis only provides data on a single method of preventing the effects of androgens, the results provided were important in the evolving discussion on the endocrine treatment of metastatic prostate cancer (37).

The Prostate Cancer Trialists' Collaborative Group (PCTCG) conducted an important meta-analysis in 1995 of 25 trials that compared conventional castration (surgical or medical) versus maximum androgen blockade (castration plus prolonged use of an anti-androgen such as flutamide, cyproterone acetate, or nilutamide) (38). Previous trials had not provided consistent and convincing evidence of approved survival with CAB. These trials were small and did not provide randomized evidence on a large enough scale. Data from individual patients could be obtained from 22 of the 25 studies identified, involving 5710 patients with a median follow-up of 40 months. The results involved 3283 deaths among the 5710 patients, and included approximately 90% of the randomized evidence from studies that began before December 1989. Mortality rates were 58% for castration alone and 56% for CAB. Corresponding 5-year survival rates were 22.8% and 26.2%, which represented an insignificant improvement in survival of 3.5%. Logrank time-to-death analysis found no significant differences between trials or the effects of the different types of CAB, and there was no evidence of additional benefit in an overview of all CAB trial results. A few of the studies included in the analysis produced results that may indicate that CAB may be more effective in patients with minimal disease or with good prognosis. However, these results consisted of a small subgroup of a few hundred patients and must be interpreted with caution. At the time of its release, this meta-analysis provided the best randomized evidence on whether CAB had any effect on survival in advanced prostate cancer.

In 1997 Caubet and colleagues (39) recognized that the PCTCG meta-analysis included trials containing two different classes of anti-androgens: non-steroidal anti-androgens (NSAAs) and progestational steroids (with intrinsic androgenic activity and lower anti-androgenic activity than NSAAs flutamide and nilutamide). As a result, a meta-analysis of published randomized controlled trials was designed to assess the survival benefit in advanced prostate cancer of MAB using NSAAs versus castration alone. The results were compared to meta-analysis of data summaries provided in the PCTG report and showed a statistically significant prolongation of overall survival and progression-free survival in patients with advanced prostate cancer for CAB using NSAAs compared with castration alone. A 22% decrease in hazard rate for survival and a 26% decrease in hazard rate for time to progression were found with CAB using NSAAs. Study selection and a focus on NSAAs was the primary reason for the different results obtained in this meta-analysis as compared to the PCTCG analysis. Sensitivity analysis based on PCTG data showed that a favorable survival result for CAB was associated with NSAAs but not with steroidal anti-androgens and depended on randomization blinding and overall trial quality. A criticism of this meta-analysis is the small number of trials and relatively small number of patients included in the analysis. However, the results illustrated important concepts for the design of future trials in regards to study quality that may significantly affect trial results.

One of the more important and recent meta-analyses of CAB was conducted by Bennett *et al.* (40) as an attempt to address confusion presented by the conflicting results of randomized controlled trials conducted during a 10-year period (1989–98), which included treatment with flutamide as the non-steroidal anti-androgen agent in maximal androgen blockade. Their results compiled from nine studies and 4128

patients supported earlier findings of a 10% improvement in overall survival with flutamide in MAB therapy. The focus on flutamide has served to limit the applicability of data obtained from this meta-analysis but was appropriate in that the two largest individual studies of maximal androgen blockade based on phase III clinical trial results from the South West Oncology group (SWOG) involved this agent (41). Reports from ongoing meta-analysis by the PCTG, the agency for healthcare policy and research evidenced based literature review of hormonal therapies, and the American Society of Clinical Oncology Metastatic Prostate Cancer Guidelines Panel may provide data to permit clearer evaluation of the effect of CAB therapy.

One of the more interesting of several treatments currently being tested in clinical trials for metastatic prostate cancer involves intermittent hormonal therapy. The concept was initially investigated by Klotz and colleagues (42) in the early 1980s in patients on DES therapy. Patients were cycled on and off therapy up to three times with improved quality of life before disease progression was noted. Subsequent clinical trials have demonstrated the reversibility of the adverse effects of androgen deprivation and improvement in quality of life. Current phase III clinical trials, involving men with metastatic disease or recurrent disease after localized therapy, will provide additional quality-of-life data and examine the possibility of a delay in disease progression, along with the possibility of prolonged survival, which has been demonstrated in some models. Undoubtedly, meta-analytic review of these trials will be important and valuable as completed data becomes available.

Hormone-refractory disease

Despite initial responses to androgen deprivation, eventually resistant disease develops, manifested by rising levels of prostate-specific antigen (PSA), progressive disease on imaging studies, and, ultimately, worsening symptoms. Virtually all of the mortality and a significant portion of the morbidity of the disease are associated with the hormone-refractory state (43). Therapy for the disease in this stage is primarily palliative, consisting of second-line hormonal therapy and chemotherapy. Phase II and III clinical trials are ongoing and no meta-analysis yet exists to summarize results.

Secondary hormonal manipulation, after the failure of primary androgen deprivation, is one of the important new treatment strategies. This approach is based on the recognition that hormone-refractory prostate cancer is a heterogeneous disease, and some patients may respond to alternative hormonal interventions despite the presence of castrate levels of testosterone (44). Furthermore, some patients with disease progression will experience subjective and objective improvement upon removal of that agent. At present, over 200 patients have been evaluated in clinical trials for the anti-androgen-withdrawal syndrome. Withdrawal responses occur in 15–30% of patients, although prospective identification of patients most likely to respond has proven difficult. Clinical variables such as the castration method, the inclusion or exclusions of anti-androgen as part of combined androgen blockade or added after disease progression, age, performance status, and biochemical data, such as PSA level, have not been reliable independent predictors of response. The Cancer and Leukemia Group B (CALGB) is presently comparing the response rate and duration of response to anti-androgen withdrawal alone versus anti-androgen withdrawal combined with ketoconazole and hydrocortisone (43). In addition, a planned phase III study conducted through the Eastern Cooperative Oncology Group will compare second-line hormone therapy using ketoconazole and hydrocortisone, a chemotherapy regimen involving paclitaxel and estramustine and vitamin D analog as a biological agent.

Megestrol acetate, which suppresses the release of luteinizing hormone, blocks binding of DHT to the androgen receptor, and inhibits 5α-reductase has been modestly effective in hormone-refractory prostate cancer. Patel and colleagues treated 29 men with hormone-refractory disease with megestrol acetate and noted three objective responses and 20 patients with stable disease. Other small series have demonstrated the same small response rate. In CALGB 9181, 149 men were randomized to two doses of megestrol acetate with no dose response and a disappointing 11.3% PSA response (18). Thus, although megestrol acetate may produce responses in some patients, it is generally less effective than other secondary hormonal manipulations, and should only be offered to those patients unable to tolerate other therapies.

In the past 10 years, several chemotherapy agents have shown activity when used alone or in combination with other agents. Estramustine phosphate, a stable conjugate of nornitrogen mustard and estradiol, was synthesized to allow selective delivery of the alkylating agents into estrogen receptor-positive cancer cells (45). As a single agent it has reported response rates of up to 20%. The first clinical trials involving its use in a combination regimen occurred in the early 1990s when estramusine was combined with vindblastine. In three phase-II trials, the overall response rate of 24% in patients with measurable disease, with 54% of patients having a sustained decrease in serum prostate-specific antigen (15, 46). These promising results prompted a randomized trial comparing the two-drug combination with vindblastine alone (14). The two-drug combination showed an improvement in progression-free survival but no statistically significant overall survival. It was evident that estramustine seemed to protect against vindblastine-induced granulocytopenia. The results obtained from the estramustine/vindblastine trials spurred further development of combinations of estramustine with other anti-microtuble agents. Although initial clinical studies with paclitaxel alone showed little activity with prostate cancer, when combined with estramustine there was significant antimitotic activity in prostate cancer cell-lines. With paclitaxel given as a 96-h continuous infusion, the combination paclitaxel and estramustine produced a 50% decline in PSA reproduced in at least three phase I and II clinical trials (47). The combination of estramustine and docetaxel has produced similar high results in phase II trials. A median survival of 24 months reported with this latter combination, suggests a possible impact of chemotherapy on survival (48).

Another active chemotherapy agent in HRPC is mitoxantrone. The Cancer and Leukemia Group B have conducted a trial comparing mitoxantrone plus hydrocortisone to hydrocortisone alone with survival as its primary endpoint (16). No crossover was allowed and quality of life was a secondary endpoint. Although there was no difference in overall survival, there was an indication that quality of life, in particular pain control, was improved in the mitoxantrone-treated patients. Overall, the studies of mitoxantrone plus glucocorticoids have shown up to 40% of patients demonstrating improvement in pain and quality of life with this treatment; but without an apparent impact on overall survival (16). The toxicity profile is acceptable and this combination is a useful palliative treatment. The promising results of the mitoxantrone and taxane combinations have prompted a current phase-III intergroup trial comparing mitoxantrone and prednisone to estramustine and doxetaxel.

No recent meta-analysis exists on the currently used chemotherapy regimens in HRPC. Given the recent number of randomized phase III trials, a meta-analysis may soon be warranted with regard to the palliative effects of chemotherapy. The newer taxane regimens suggest potential impact on survival, however randomized phase III trials to address this issue have only recently been launched rendering meta-analysis for survival premature (7).

Suramin, a polysulfonated napthylurea that acts as a competitive inhibitor for a variety of cellular enzymes and growth factors, has shown *in vitro* activity against human prostate cancer cell-lines. In initial clinical trials, partial response rates of 35% were seen in patients with measurable disease, and a decrease in serum PSA by 75% was shown in 34% of the patients (49). There were also significant improvements in bone pain. Sequential studies at the University of Maryland to define optimal dosing schedules for suramin have shown a decrease in PSA by at least 50% in 48 of 61 patients but nearly half of the patients had treatment discontinued because of does-limiting toxicity (50). A large multicenter randomized double-blind trial comparing suramin plus hydrocortisone with placebo plus hydrocortisone has recently been completed. There was an improvement of bone pain and PSA response, but no overall improvement in survival (15). The future of suramin as a therapy for hormone-refractory prostate cancer remains unclear.

No meta-analysis exists to review results of clinical trials involving radiotherapy in hormone refractory disease. However, at least three randomized controlled trials have shown a clear benefit for external-beam radiotherapy for localized bony lesions or support the use of strontium-89 for multiple uncontrolled sites of pain on both sides of the diaphragm (51).

Conclusions

Many important questions about the prevention, early diagnosis, and treatment of patients with prostate cancer remain unanswered. However, a host of prospective, well-designed clinical trials are underway that should answer many of these questions. Meta-analysis has recently become a popular tool for synthesizing the information from available studies on a specific clinical problem. It has been successful at showing the efficacy of adjuvant therapy in breast cancer, for which many individual studies appeared to give conflicting results. Many of the large, randomized, breast cancer trials had large sample sizes and long follow-ups and so the meta-analysis was able to show convincingly a small but clinically meaningful treatment effect on long-term disease recurrence and sur-

vival. This is similar to the situation in localized prostate cancer in all respects except for the availability of randomized trials. Unfortunately there is no free lunch. This technique can only be applied if high-quality data are available. One must be similarly cautious in applying analytic techniques (and also cost-effectiveness analysis) to try to resolve clinical dilemmas. Although these techniques can be valuable in identifying the important components of clinical decisions, the results are often crucially dependent on critical input data, such as the comparative efficacy of alternative treatments. The methodology of meta-analysis is limited by the availability of high quality data from randomized trials.

The various cooperative groups have committed a vast amount of resources to the evaluation of a series of important questions regarding the optimal management of prostate cancer. These trials are extremely broad in scope, encompassing preventions, organ-confined disease, locally advanced disease, metastatic disease, and hormone-refractory disease. A variety of treatment modalities, such as chemopreventive agents, surgery, radiation, hormones, and chemotherapy, will all play an important role, reflecting the fact that the treatment of prostate cancer is becoming a true multi-disciplinary process. Given the broad array of problems associated with managing prostate cancer, this trend has been well received in the investigative community.

A quantitative syntheses of the data in similar randomized, controlled trials can potentially be more useful to the practicing physician than a traditional narrative review article, but such syntheses must be properly performed to warrant serious attention. In many cases, conducting an inter-group trial by partnering the major co-operative groups has and will facilitate accrual and timely completion and analysis. Such large trials are essential and will allow clinicians to make future decisions on data derived from controlled multi-institutional studies, rather than interpolation of information from less reliable sources. The complexity of the clinical research questions and the enormity of the public health problem will not only force the clinical trial world into global collaboration and megatrials, but also into surrounding endpoints where the financial savings and the emphasis on quality of life may prove to be as important as the sacred overall survival endpoint.

Despite a recent decrease in newly diagnosed patients, prostate cancer remains the most commonly diagnosed visceral malignancy in the United States today. Thus, information derived from these trials will influence therapeutic decisions affecting literally hundreds of thousands of patients in the years ahead. Many aspects of prostate cancer treatment will remain controversial until results of large, randomized trials with longer follow-up are available. Although meta-analysis will be critical if these multiple randomized studies yield conflicting results, sufficiently large-well conducted megatrials, may actually be adequate to answer the many current questions and controversies.

References

1. Sacks HS, Reitman DR, Pagano BA *et al*. Meta-analysis: an update. *The Mount Sinai J Med* 1996, **63**, 216–24.
2. Egger M, Smith GD, Phillips AN. Meta-analysis principles and procedures. *Br Med J* 1997, **315**, 1533–7.
3. Landis SH, Murray T, Bolden S *et al*. Cancer statistics 1999. *CA*, **49**, 8–31.
4. Austenfeld MS, Thompson JR, Middleton R. Meta-analysis of the literature: guideline development for prostate cancer treatment. *J Urol* 1994, **152**, 1866–9.
5. Pogue J, Yusef S. Overcoming the limitations of current meta-analysis of randomized controlled trials. *Lancet* 1998, **351**, 47–52.
6. Aziz DC, Barathur RB. Prostate-specific antigen and prostate volume: a meta-analysis of prostate cancer screening criteria. *J Clinic Labor Analysis* 1993, **7**, 283–92.
7. Thompson I, Seay T. Will current clinical trials answer the most important questions about prostate adenocarcinoma? *Oncology* 1997, **11**, 1109–21.
8. Huggins C, Hodges CV. Studies on prostate cancer I: the effect of castration, estrogen, and androgen injection on serum phosphatases in metastatic carcinoma of the prostate. *Cancer Res* 1941, **1**, 293–7.
9. Labrie F, Dupont A, Belanger A. New hormonal therapy in prostate carcinoma: Combined treatment with an LHRH agonist and an antiandrogen. *Clin Invest Med* 1982, **5**, 267.
10. Crawford ED, Eisenberger MA, McLeod DG *et al*. A controlled trial of leuprolide with and without flutamide in prostatic carcinoma. *N Engl J Med* 1989, **321**, 419–24.
11. Eisenberger MA, Blumenstein BA, Crawford ED *et al*. Bilateral orchiectomy with or without flutamide for metastatic prostate cancer. *N Engl J Med* 1998, **339**, 1036–42.
12. Denis L. European organization for research and treatment of cancer (EORTC) prostate cancer trials, 1976–1996. *Urology* 1998, **51** (Suppl 5A), 50–7.
13. Smith DC. Chemotherapy for hormone refractory prostate cancer. *Urol Clin N Am* 1999, **26**, 323–31.
14. Hudes GR, Greenberg R and Kriegel RL. Phase II study of estramustine and vindblastine, two microtubule inhibitors, in hormone refractory prostate cancer. *J Clin Oncol* 1992, **10**, 1754–61.
15. Small EJ, Marshall ME, Reyno L. Superiority of suramin + hydrocortisone (S+H) over placebo + hydro-

cortisone (P+H): results of a double-blind phase III study in patients with hormone refractory prostate cancer. *J Clin Oncol* 1992, **10**, 1754–61.
16. Kantoff PW, Halabi S, Conway M *et al*. Hydrocortisone with or without mitoxantrone in men with hormone-refractory prostate cancer: results of the cancer and leukemia group B 9182 study. *J Clin Oncol* 1999, **17**, 2506.
17. Dawson NA, Conaway M, Halabi S *et al*. A randomized study-comparing standard versus moderately high dose megestrol acetate in advanced prostate cancer: cancer and leukemia group b (CALGB) study 9181. *Cancer* 1999 (in press).
18. Sacks HS, Berrier J, Reitman D *et al*. Meta-analysis of randomized controlled trials. *New Engl J Med* 1997, **316**, 450–5.
19. Normand SL. Meta-analysis: formulating, evaluating, combining, and reporting. *Stat Med* 1999, **18**, 321–59.
20. Feinstein AR. Meta-analysis and meta-analytic monitoring of clinical trials. *Stat Med* 1996, **15**, 1273–80.
21. Begg CB. The role of meta-analysis in monitoring clinical trials. *Stat Med* 1996, **15**, 1299–306.
22. LeLorier J, Gregoire G, Benhaddad AJ *et al*. Discrepancies between meta-analyses and subsequent large randomized, controlled trials. *New Engl J Med* 1997, **337**, 536–42.
23. Catalona W, Smith D, Ratliff T. Measurement of prostate-specific antigen in serum as a screening test for prostate cancer. *New Engl J Medicine* 1991, **324**, 1156–61.
24. Mettlin C, Murphy G, Ray P. Results from multiple-examinations using transrectal ultrasound, digital rectal examination, and prostate specific antigen. *Cancer* 1993, **71**, 891–8.
25. Labrie F, Canadas B, Dupont A *et al*. Screening decreases prostate cancer death: First analysis of the 1988 Quebec prospective randomized controlled trial. *Prostate* 1999, **1**, 83–91.
26. Pisters LL. The challenge of locally advanced prostate cancer. *Semin Oncol* 1999, **26**, 202–6.
27. Van den Ouden D, Davidson P, Hop W. Radical prostatectomy as a monotherapy for locally advanced (stage T3) prostate cancer 1994. *J Urol* 1994, **151**, 646–51.
28. Oh W, Kantoff P. Treatment of locally advanced prostate cancer: is chemotherapy the next step? *J Clinic Oncol* 1999, **17**, 3664–75.
29. Zeitman AL, Shipley WU. Progress in the management of T3–4 adenocarcinoma of the prostate. *Eur J Cancer* 1997, **33**, 555–9.
30. Bolla M, Gonzalez D, Warde P. Improved survival in patients with locally advanced prostate cancer treated with radiotherapy and goserelin. *New Engl J Med* 1999, **337**, 295–300.
31. Fellows G, Clark P, Beynon L. Treatment of advanced localized prostatic cancer by orchiectomy, radiotherapy, or combined treatment: a Medical Research Council Study–Urological Cancer Working Party-Subgroup on Prostatic Cancer. *Br J Urol* 1992, **70**, 304–9.
32. Bonney WW, Schned AR, Timberlake DS. Neoadjuvant androgen ablation for localized prostatic cancer: pathology methods, surgical end points and meta-analysis of randomized trials. *J Urol* 1998, **160**, 1754–60.

33. Messing EM, Manola J, Sarosdy M *et al.* Immediate hormonal therapy compared with observation after radical prostatectomy and pelvic lymphadenectomy in men with node-positive prostate cancer. *N Engl J Med* 1999, **24**, 1781–8.

34. The Medical Research Council prostate Cancer Working party Investigators Group. Immediate versus deferred treatment for advanced prostatic cancer: initial results of the Medical Research Council Trial. *Prostate Cancer* 1997, **2**, 235–46.

35. Robinson MR, Smith PH, Richards B *et al.* The final analysis of the EORTC Genito-Urinary Tract Cancer Co-perative Group phase III clinical trial (protocol 30805) comparing orchidectomy, orchidectomy plus cyproterone acetate and low dose stilboestrol in the management of metastatic carcinoma of the prostate. *Eur Urol* 1995, **28**, 273–83.

36. Bertagna C, De Gery A, Hucher M *et al.* Efficacy of the combination of nilutamide plus orchidectomy in patients with metastatic prostatic cancer. A meta-analysis of seven randomized double-blind trials. (1056 patients). *Br Med J* 1992, **73**, 396–402.

37. Dawson N, Wilding G, Oliver S. New Developments in prostate cancer treatment. *CME News Letter for Health Care Professionals*, **4**, 30–5.

38. Prostate Cancer Trialist'Collaborative Group. Maximum androgen blockade in advanced prostate cancer: an overview of 22 randomized trials with 3283 deaths in 5710 patients. *Lancet* 1995, **346**, 265–9.

39. Caubet J, Tosteson TD, Dong EW *et al.* Maximum androgen blockade in advanced prostate cancer: a meta-analysis of published randomized controlled trials using nonsteroidal antiandrogens. *Urology* 1997, **49**, 71–8.

40. Bennett CL, Tosteson D, Schmitt B *et al.* Maximum androgen-blockade with medical or surgical castration in advanced prostate cancer: a meta-analysis of nine published randomized Controlled trials and 4128 patients using flutamide. *Prostate Cancer Prostat Dis* 1999, **2**, 4–8.

41. Crawford ED, DeAntoni EP, Hussain M *et al.* Prostate cancer clinical trials of the southwest oncology group. *Oncology* 1997, **11**, 1154–63.

42. Klotz L, Herr H, Morse M. Intermittant endocrine therapy for advanced prostate cancer. *Cancer* 1986, **58**, 2546–50.

43. Vogelzang NJ, Crawford ED, Zeitman A. Current clinical trial design issues in hormone-refractory prostate carcinoma. For the Consensus Panel. *Cancer* 1998, **82**, 2093–101.

44. Reese DM, Small EJ. Secondary hormonal manipulations in hormone refractory prostate cancer. *Urol Clin N Am* 1999, **26**, 311–21.

45. Janknegt RA. Estramustine phosphate and other cytotoxic drugs in the treatment of poor prognostic advanced prostate cancer. *Prostate* 1992, **4**, (Suppl) 105–10.

46. Waselenko JK, Dawson NA. Management of progressive metastatic prostate cancer. *New Engl J Med* 1997, **11**, 1551–67.

47. Hudes GR, Nathan FE, Khater C. Phase II trial of 96-hour paclitaxel plus oral estramustine phosphate in metastatic hormone-refractory prostate cancer. *J Clin Oncol* 1997, **15**, 3156–63.

48. Petrylak DP, Macarthur RB, O'Connor J *et al.* Phase I trial of doxcetaxel with estramustine in androgen-independent prostate cancer. *J Clin Oncol* 1999, **3**, 3160–66.

49. Myers C, Copper M, Stein C *et al.* Suramin: a novel growth factor antagonist with activity in hormone-refractory metastatic prostate cancer. *J Clin Oncol* 1992, **10**, 881–9.

50. Eisenberger MA, Sinibaldi VJ, Reyno LM *et al.* Phase I and clinical evaluation of a pharmacologically guided regimen of suramin in patients with hormone-refractory prostate cancer. *J Clin Oncol* 1995, **13**, 2174–86.

51. Kuyu H, Lee W, Bare R *et al.* Recent advances in the treatment of prostate cancer. *Ann of Oncol* 1999, **8**, 891–8.

33 | Social and economic implications of prostate cancer

Ronald M. Benoit and Michael J. Naslund

Introduction

The introduction of prostate-specific antigen (PSA) testing for use in the early detection of prostate cancer has led to controversy regarding the appropriateness of prostate cancer screening and any subsequent treatment. This controversy is in part due to the fact that the effect of early treatment of prostate cancer on mortality is not yet known. However, other cancer screening programs, such as breast and cervical cancer, were implemented without knowledge of the effect of such screening on mortality. In fact, proof of the efficacy of these other screening programs was based on their widespread use in the community and not on controlled, randomized trials. One critical difference between these other cancer screening programs and prostate cancer screening is that prostate cancer screening became available when cost control was a dominant concern in the health system. The rising cost of healthcare has made payers (employers, insurance companies, and federal and state governments) less willing to approve new benefits for their members.

The etiology of the current cost consciousness in healthcare is well known. American companies are now forced to compete globally. The relatively high cost of healthcare for American businesses has decreased productivity and hampered their ability to compete internationally. The rising cost of healthcare has also placed an increasing burden on federal and state governments and compelled them to better control their healthcare costs. The current debate regarding the solvency of Medicare illustrates this point.

Regardless of the present healthcare environment, the cost of care must always be considered. Very few interventions in medicine offer actual cost savings. Most add cost while hopefully providing a reasonable benefit to patients. Supplying endless 'cost-effective' interventions could conceivably bankrupt our government and businesses. Patients, whether they are young or old, curable or incurable, afflicted with cancer or benign disease, have always competed for healthcare resources. In today's healthcare environment they are competing for more limited resources as cost-control efforts intensify.

In the current healthcare marketplace, proof of efficacy and cost-effectiveness are central requirements for the implementation of new medical interventions. Practitioners must decide whether the dollars spent on a new intervention, such as prostate cancer screening, are worth the benefits (defined in terms of years of life saved, improved quality of life, or discomfort avoided), compared to alternative uses of the same dollars on more established interventions. The cost and benefits of prostate cancer screening and subsequent treatment can be definitively determined only by controlled, randomized trials with long-term follow-up. Until such studies become available, doctors and patients must make decisions regarding the appropriateness of prostate cancer screening based on the currently available evidence. This article will review the possible effect of widespread prostate cancer screening on total healthcare costs, followed by a review of several studies that have attempted to define the effectiveness and the cost-effectiveness of PSA screening and treatment.

Effect of PSA screening on costs of prostate cancer treatment

From a strict financial perspective, the most 'cost-effective' method of treating prostate cancer is probably not to treat it at all. Treatment of a disease usually costs more than no treatment.

The benefits of saving years of life, years of life with full activity, or years of discomfort avoided are difficult to quantify in a strict financial perspective. However, to let men die of prostate cancer, or even to let prostate cancer progress locally without intervention, would be morally unacceptable in most countries. While most countries are certainly willing to commit some portion of its healthcare resources to the treatment of prostate cancer, the level of such commitment is not known. The proportion of total healthcare resources to be spent on treating prostate cancer is not merely an economic decision, but a social and ethical decision as well. The controversy surrounding the costs of prostate cancer treatment is not due to the cost of treating prostate cancer detected by traditional methods (biopsy performed due to local symptoms, palpable nodule on digital rectal exam (DRE), or bone pain), but rather to the increased costs from the widespread use of PSA screening. Society must decide whether this additional cost, resulting from the use of PSA screening for prostate cancer, is a worthwhile expenditure of healthcare resources. This decision will be in part based on the magnitude of these additional costs and the benefits they produce for patients.

Any discussion of the increased costs of prostate cancer due to PSA screening must address the issue of clinically insignificant prostate cancer. The incidence of prostate cancer has increased markedly with the introduction of PSA. If this increased incidence is due to the detection of a large amount of clinically insignificant prostate cancer, the cost of prostate cancer treatment will rise with little benefit in terms of increased survival but with some increase in morbidity and mortality due to that treatment. This would not represent a wise use of healthcare resources.

Several studies indicate that concern regarding increased incidental prostate cancer detection from PSA screening is unfounded (1, 2). By the strict pathologic criteria currently available, prostate cancer screening with PSA does not diagnose a larger proportion of clinically insignificant cancers than were diagnosed by traditional methods of detection (biopsy performed due to local symptoms, abnormal DRE, or symptoms of metastatic disease). Much of the recent increase in prostate cancer detection is due to the detection of prevalence cancers (3). These are cancers that would have been detected in later years by the traditional methods mentioned previously, but are being detected earlier due to PSA screening. Once these prevalence cancers have been removed from the population by prostate cancer screening, the incidence of prostate cancer detection should return to approximate historical levels (3).

Widespread use of PSA screening will certainly increase healthcare costs. The cost of a serum PSA (with or without the cost of a DRE) will be incurred for all men screened. The use of PSA will lead to a portion of screened men undergoing (and incurring the charges for) a transrectal ultrasound (TRUS) and prostate biopsy. These costs must also be attributed to screening. However, even without PSA screening, a significant number of these men would still undergo PSA testing and subsequent TRUS and prostate biopsy due to local symptoms or abnormal DRE. Several investigators have developed models to calculate the additional costs to the healthcare system due to screening. Optenberg and Thompson estimated the cost resulting from the first year of screening men aged 50–70 would be 27.9 billion dollars (4). They compared this to the 255 million dollars currently spent for prostate cancer treatment for men in this age range. Kramer *et al.* estimated the total costs of the first year of prostate cancer screening with PSA for men aged 50–74 would be 11.9 billion dollars (5). These estimates include the costs of screening, diagnosis, treatment, and complications resulting from such treatment.

These types of analyses can potentially lead to a gross over-estimation of the costs of screening. First, not all men aged 50–70 will be eligible for screening due to various co-morbidities, which will decrease their life-expectancy to less than 10–15 years. Second, not all men will submit to the screening exam. Virtually every medical group recommends serial mammography for women over age 50 and this recommendation has received widespread publicity for many years. Yet, less than 50% of eligible women have a mammogram on a yearly basis (6). Furthermore, one-third of men who volunteered for PSA screening as part of a research protocol, and subsequently had a suspicious examination, refused further evaluation (1, 7). Given these facts, it seems likely that only a minority of eligible men would receive PSA screening and that only a portion of these men would receive further evaluation if indicated. Since the costs of screening and diagnosis represent only approximately 10% of the total costs resulting from prostate cancer screening (the remaining costs come from subsequent treatment of the prostate cancers detected) (8), it is unlikely that the increased costs due to prostate cancer screening and subsequent diagnosis will significantly increase overall healthcare costs.

Treatment resulting from prostate cancer screening with PSA will, however, increase overall healthcare costs. This increase will not be due to the detection of clinically insignificant prostate cancer. The majority of prostate cancers detected as a result of PSA screening are clinically significant and, therefore, would have eventually required treatment (provided screening is done in men with greater than 10 years of life-expectancy) (1, 7). PSA screening diagnoses cancers earlier than those same cancers would have been diagnosed by traditional methods of prostate cancer detection. This early detection increases healthcare costs by two factors: cost discounting and stage migration.

Since treatment of prostate cancers detected by PSA screening will be treated several years earlier than if PSA screening was not in effect, treatment costs will be paid in present dollars rather than future dollars. The present value cost of treatment today is more than the cost of that treatment at some point in the future, just as a dollar paid to someone today is worth more to that person than a dollar to be paid one year from today. The reason for the increased value today is that the recipient does not have to wait one year to obtain the money and therefore will have access to that dollar for investment, consumption, or spending. Carter *et al.* have estimated that PSA screening will detect a prostate cancer on average 2.6–11.2 years earlier than that same cancer would have been detected by traditional methods (9). Table 33.1 demonstrates the increased costs in present value dollars, which occurs when

radical prostatectomy is performed several years earlier than otherwise would have occurred. A cost of $14 000 is assumed for radical prostatectomy with discount rates of 6%, 8%, 10%, and 15%.

The concept of present value recognizes that money paid in the future is worth less than the same amount of money paid today. This difference in value occurs because the recipient of money in the future misses the advantages of a purchase or investment, which would have been possible if that money were paid today. This difference in value can be quantitated using the following relationship:

$$PV = C/(1 + r_t)^1, \qquad (33.1)$$

where *PV* is present value, *C* is the amount of money paid, *r* is the risk-adjusted discount rate and *t* is the time period when future money is to be paid.

The risk adjusted discount rate (*r*) represents the opportunity cost of money for the individual or company in question. Both objective and subjective factors are used to estimate *r*. The risk-adjusted discount rate will vary among different individuals and different companies based on the cost of obtaining capital through debt and/or equity financing, the investment/business portfolio of the individual or company, the risk profile of the individual's/company's business and the risk of non-payment of the money that has been promised at some point in the future. The estimation of *r* is complex for a large company and is

Table 33.1 Impact on charges for radical prostatectomy if surgery is performed earlier (i.e. due to detection by PSA) than would have otherwise been performed (due to detection by traditional methods). A charge of $14 000 is assumed for radical prostatectomy, and impact on charges by discount rates of 6%, 8%, 10%, and 15% are calculated. For example, if surgery is performed 3 years earlier due to PSA screening, and assuming a discount rate of 8%, the charge for radical prostatectomy will increase from $14 000 to $17 979.

Year	Discount rate 6%	8%	10%	15%
0	$14 000	$14 000	$14 000	$14 000
1	$14 894	$15 217	$15 556	$16 471
2	$15 844	$16 541	$17 284	$19 377
3	$16 856	$17 979	$19 204	$22 797
4	$17 932	$19 542	$21 338	$26 820
5	$19 076	$21 242	$23 709	$31 552
6	$20 294	$23 089	$26 343	$37 121
7	$21 589	$25 097	$29 271	$43 671
8	$22 967	$27 279	$32 523	$51 378
9	$24 433	$29 651	$36 136	$60 445
10	$25 993	$32 229	$40 152	$71 111
11	$27 652	$35 032	$44 613	$83 661
12	$29 417	$38 078	$49 570	$98 424

difficult to derive without detailed financial knowledge of that company. Because of the uncertainty regarding the appropriate risk-adjusted discount rate for a diverse group such as healthcare payers, a range of possible *r* values was used to generate Table 33.1. The rationale for this range of values was that health insurance is a predictable business using actuarial analysis. Because of this predictability, an *r* of 15% is a reasonable high-end estimate. For a healthcare payer with at least some degree of business risk to have an *r* as low as 6%, the yield on long-term (20–30 years) federal treasury bonds, which are perceived to be 'risk-free', would probably have to fall below 4%. Given the range of interest rates and inflation rates over the past 30 years, this scenario appears to be unlikely and thus 6% is a good low-end *r* value.

The second reason for the higher costs resulting from PSA screening is due to the stage-migration effect caused by PSA screening. Greater than 95% of prostate cancers detected by PSA screening will be clinically localized and therefore eligible for early treatment (1, 7), while prostate cancers detected by traditional methods are clinically localized in only approximately 63% of cases (10). Therefore, a larger proportion of men will be candidates for early treatment when PSA screening is practiced as opposed to traditional methods of detection. This stage migration due to prostate cancer screening will increase costs because treatment of clinically localized disease (such as radical prostatectomy and external-beam radiation) is more costly than treatment of metastatic disease (androgen ablation) (11).

Although PSA screening detects clinically localized disease in greater than 95% of cases, only 65–75% of these cases will have pathologically organ-confined disease (1, 7). The percentage of extra-prostatic cancers detected by screening is consistent with reports that 30% of men receive adjuvant therapy after radical prostatectomy. This adjuvant treatment will also add additional costs to the group of men detected by PSA screening. In contrast, while traditional methods of detection result in approximately 63% of cases being clinically localized, only half of these men have pathologically organ-confined disease (12). Therefore, an approximately equivalent number of men in both groups will be candidates for adjuvant therapy. The timing of therapy (and subsequent cost-discounting) will again be a factor as the PSA-detected group of men will be candidates for adjuvant therapy several years earlier than the men detected by traditional methods. Adjuvant treatment options for men who have under-

gone radical prostatectomy and are found to have residual cancer include radiation therapy or early or delayed androgen ablation. Both groups of men will likely be candidates for delayed hormonal therapy at similar times, negating the effect of discounting. No data exists to estimate the ratio of different adjuvant treatment modalities utilized in the PSA-detected and traditionally detected groups of men.

The costs of palliative treatment for local symptoms (medical therapy, TURP, androgen ablation) will be decreased by screening and subsequent early treatment, since radical prostatectomy and radiation therapy decrease the risk of local progression. This saving must be balanced by the increased spending needed to treat the complications of early treatment (incontinence, impotence, and bladder neck contracture). The net effect of these countering forces cannot be accurately calculated since no adequate control groups exist from which to estimate the need for and timing of palliative treatment for local symptoms in men who do not undergo PSA screening.

Some have suggested that curative treatment of prostate cancer at an early stage by radical prostatectomy or radiation therapy will result in lower costs because the patient will be spared (and the payers will be saved the cost of) a death from metastatic prostate cancer. These costs would include palliative treatment of local disease (TURP, androgen ablation), palliative treatment of distant disease (radiation for bone pain, ureteral bypass for obstruction, pain control), and chemotherapy for hormone-refractory disease. However, one issue on which everyone can agree is that all men, with or without prostate cancer, will die. No evidence exists that a death from metastatic prostate cancer is more or less costly than other causes of death. A patient with prostate cancer who is cured of his disease will eventually die from another cause, e.g. coronary artery disease. It is certainly possible that this type of death is more costly than the death from prostate cancer, which was avoided in this patient.

Estimates of the effectiveness of prostate cancer screening

Krahn *et al.* (11) and Fleming *et al.* (13) have published analyses of the effectiveness of the treatment of early stage prostate cancer and have found little or no clinical benefit from treatment of clinically localized prostate cancer. These studies received widespread attention in the popular media and medical literature, resulting in an increased emphasis on watchful waiting for early stage prostate cancer.

Both of these studies utilized decision-analysis (Markov) models. These models place patients in different disease states (e.g. no evidence of disease, local symptoms, metastatic disease, death), which may change over designated periods of time. Utility factors are assigned to patients who suffer complications of treatment (impotence, incontinence, bladder-neck contracture). The outcomes from decision-analysis models are heavily dependent on the assumptions used to construct the model. Given the publicity these studies have received, and the controversy they have generated, it is worthwhile to evaluate the validity of the assumptions on which these models are based.

Rate of progression

The most important assumption in models of the effectiveness of prostate cancer treatment is the rate of disease progression. Both analyses based their rate of progression for untreated patients on a Swedish cohort of men with clinically localized prostate cancer who were said not to have received treatment (14). Risk of progression was stratified by clinical stage in the Krahn study (11), and by grade in the Fleming study (13). The yearly rate of metastatic progression in the Fleming study was 2.7 per 1000 patients for men with well differentiated tumors, 13 per 1000 patients for men with moderately differentiated tumors, and 42 per 1000 patients for men with poorly differentiated tumors.

There are several reasons why this cohort of patients may not be a representative sample for men with clinically localized prostate cancer detected by screening. The average age of the men in the Swedish study was 72, which is older than the ages recommended for screening (men aged 50–70). Moderately or poorly differentiated disease was present in 34.2% of men with cancer in the Swedish study (14), while 77.6% and 78.2% of men diagnosed with cancer in large-scale United States screening trials had moderately or poorly differentiated disease (1, 7). In addition, a large proportion of these men were diagnosed by cytology, which leads one to question the diagnosis of cancer in at least some of these men (15). All of the men in this study were not untreated as the title of the article suggests, since almost half of the men underwent hormonal therapy at some point during follow-up. This

study occurred prior to the PSA era, so biochemical progression due to rising PSA could not be measured. In addition, serum acid phosphatase, although available, was not measured.

This cohort may also represent a group of men destined not to progress. Although the death rate from prostate cancer in Sweden is among the highest in the world, the men in this study demonstrate a very low rate of progression. The low rate of progression found in these men may represent a 'reverse length time bias'. Since these men were diagnosed by traditional methods of detection (resulting in late detection) and not by PSA (leading to earlier detection), by the time of diagnosis the men who were destined to progress may have selected themselves out of the cohort already. There is no question that some men with clinically localized prostate cancer will not progress. This group of men may simply represent a group with a large proportion of 'non-progressers', and not a true spectrum of clinically localized prostate cancers.

As previously mentioned, the outcomes of decision-analysis models are heavily influenced by the assumptions used to construct the model, most importantly the rate of progression. Although sensitivity analyses were performed in both studies using different treatment efficacies, no sensitivity analysis was performed using different estimates of the natural history of prostate cancer. A sophisticated computer model is not necessary to determine that men with a 0.0027 annual risk of progression do not need treatment!

Other studies can be used to represent the natural history of untreated localized prostate cancer. Beck *et al.* performed a sensitivity analysis using the Fleming Markov model but with more realistic progression rates (16). In this sensitivity analysis, Beck *et al.* used progression rates from a meta-analysis of recent watchful waiting series (14) and progression rates of men treated with brachytherapy at the Scott Department of Urology (17) (Table 33.2). Results were calculated with and without the quality-of-life adjustments used in the Fleming model and are shown in Table 33.3. By using these more realistic assumptions of the natural history of prostate cancer, the years of life saved by treatment of early stage prostate cancer increase by as much as 13-fold. Treatment of moderately differentiated disease results in 2.58–3.06 years of life saved, while treatment of poorly differentiated disease results in 2.34–2.78 years of life saved. The years of life saved, using these assumptions of the natural history of prostate cancer, compare very favorably to the years of life saved by other cancer screening programs (18).

Table 33.2 Comparison of the risk of progression over 10 years in the Fleming decision-analysis model, a meta-analysis of recent watchful waiting series, and the Scott Department of Urology brachytherapy series

Grade of disease	Fleming (13)	Meta-analyis (17)	Scott brachytherapy (16)
Well-differentiated	2.7%	19%	30%
Moderately differentiated	13%	42%	50%
Poorly differentiated	42%	64%	70%

Table 33.3 Beck *et al.*'s sensitivity analysis of the years of life saved (with and without quality-of- life adjustment) by prostate cancer screening using the various estimates of the natural history of prostate cancer which appear in Table 33.2

	Years of life saved					
	Without QOLA			With QOLA		
	Fleming	meta-analysis	Scott	Fleming	meta-analysis	Scott
Grade of disease						
Well-differentiated	0.16	1.35	2.06	(–)0.34	1.01	1.81
Moderately differentiate	0.75	2.58	3.06	(–)0.33	2.41	2.94
Poorly differentiated	1.30	2.78	2.47	1.0	2.68	2.34

QOLA = quality of life adjustment

Data From Ref. 16.

Quality-of-life adjustment

The decision-analysis models also adjust for changes in quality of life due to side-effects of treatment, such as impotence and incontinence. These complications are assigned utility values, which are incorporated into the health states (e.g. no evidence of disease, local progression, metastatic disease) in which the patient progresses throughout his life.

While not as important as the rate of progression, the quality-of-life adjustment is certainly of critical importance in these models. Given the low rate of progression of disease assumed in these models, most men will have many years of life after treatment, whether or not they are cured by treatment. Therefore, quality-of-life differences are multiplied by many years and will markedly affect the results. The quality-of-life adjustment assigned to complications of treatment, were not based on standardized, validated questionnaires. In the Krahn study, the effect of complications on quality of life were based on estimates from a small group (10 members) of urologists, radiologists, and oncologists. In the Fleming study, utility values were assigned to each health outcome state based on a consensus of clinicians involved in outcomes research and treatment of prostate cancer. Patients with prostate cancer were not surveyed in either study.

In both decision-analysis models, patients with no evidence of disease were assigned a utility value of 1.0. No quality-of-life benefit was assigned to men who were cured of disease. Many urologists, familiar with the satisfaction that a patient who undergoes radical prostatectomy expresses when told his prostate cancer is pathologically organ-confined and his post-operative PSA is undetectable, may disagree with this assignment. In addition, no decrease in quality of life was given for men who did not receive treatment and were left with the knowledge that they have cancer and have a risk of progression.

The studies by Krahn *et al.* and Fleming *et al.* assume the impotency rate for radical prostatectomy is 31–65%. However, the baseline impotency rate is not discussed. Men who were impotent pre-operatively should not have their quality of life adjusted downward due to pre-existing impotence. In addition, a potent 60-year-old man who becomes impotent post-operatively will have his quality of life adjusted downward for the remainder of his life using these models. The models do not account for the fact that a significant portion of men would become impotent later in life even if they were not treated for prostate cancer. Furthermore, in these models, the quality-of-life adjustment remains steady for a given complication for the remainder of a patient's life. It is unlikely the quality-of-life adjustment from impotence for a man at age 50 is the same as at age 70.

This method of assigning quality-of-life changes has questionable validity. But even if a large-scale standard was developed that had validity and reproducibility, its ability to measure quality-of-life changes for individual patients would remain suspect. It appears likely that each patient will process the stated risk of complications according to his own unique values, motivations, and priorities. Only that individual can weigh the importance in his life of continence, potency, the risk of local progression, the risk of distant disease, and the risk of death. If a patient is given full, informed consent, he will select his treatment option, including watchful waiting, based on his own preference and priorities. If he is willing to accept a risk of complications for the perceived benefit of aggressive treatment, his quality-of-life adjustment may be less than expected if a complication does occur because he will have accepted the risk of complications pre-operatively.

Discounting future years of life

The discounting of future years of life, similar to the way future costs are discounted, is a controversial issue. The decision to discount future life-years is especially important for screening or preventive programs in which the costs are immediate but the health benefits are realized at some time in the future. For screening programs, the cost-effectiveness relies heavily upon whether future benefits are discounted. This is particularly true for prostate cancer screening because of the lead-time associated with PSA and the generally slow growth of prostate cancer.

As discussed previously, present value analysis is a widely accepted technique of weighting future dollars by a discount factor to make them comparable to present dollars. Some authors argue that for consistency, the same discount factor should be applied to future health benefits as well. The reason for discounting future years of life saved is not that life-years can be invested to yield more life-years, in the same way that dollars can be invested to yield more dollars, but rather that future years of life are being valued relative to dollars. If a dollar in the future is discounted relative to a present dollar, a year of life in the future should be discounted relative to a year-life in the present. If a constant steady state relationship between dollars and

health benefits is assumed, then health benefits must be discounted as well as health costs. However, discounting future years of life assumes that life-years in the future are less valuable than life-years today, not only from a financial perspective, but in a utilitarian sense as well.

The rate used to discount the future years of life is also a matter of uncertainty. The discount rate depends on many factors, including the interest rate. Interest rates reflect differences between the productive potential of investment capital and individual preferences versus future consumption of goods and services. Although historical trends are available to predict future interest rates, a large degree of uncertainty exists with these predictions. Medical knowledge and technology may improve in the future, which would make saving lives in the future less expensive, further discounting future years of life saved. Societal attitudes concerning willingness to pay for years of life saved are subject to change, which could increase or decrease the 'value' of future years of life. The cost of healthcare may also change, becoming more or less expensive compared to the opportunity cost of money. In the computer models reviewed in this article, the discount rate applied is 5%. For this approach to achieve validity, extensive questioning of people of different ages over a multi-year time horizon to determine whether a year of life is worth more to a 60-year-old man than it is to a 70-year-old man, and if so, whether 5% is the appropriate discount rate. Until such data is available, the validity of discounting the future value of human life remains questionable.

Cost-effectiveness of prostate cancer screening and treatment

Benoit *et al.* have estimated the cost-effectiveness of prostate cancer screening in terms of cost per year of life saved (8). In this study, no attempt was made to estimate the rate of progression of untreated, clinically localized prostate cancer diagnosed by screening. Although no randomized, controlled study of the effectiveness of prostate cancer screening has been performed, several studies have demonstrated that men with pathologically organ-confined prostate cancer treated with radical prostatectomy have the same life-expectancy as age-matched men without prostate cancer (19–21). However, there is no available data that shows how many years of life would have been lost in this cohort of men if they were not treated for their prostate cancer. To estimate this important information, Benoit *et al.* used a cohort of men from Northern Sweden that was studied by Grönberg *et al.* which compared the survival rate of those men with prostate cancer to the survival rate of the men in the national standard population (22). These men with prostate cancer were treated by non-curative methods (watchful waiting, androgen ablation) and were not treated with radical prostatectomy. The difference in survival rates between the men with cancer and the overall population of men were the years of life lost due to prostate cancer. These results are similar to the years of life lost due to prostate cancer in American men as calculated by Albertsen (Table 33.4) (23).

Table 33.4 Years of life lost due to prostate cancer for men aged 65–74 as calculated by Gronberg *et al.* (22) and Albertsen *et al.* (23)

Grade of cancer	Gronberg years	Albertsen years
Well-differentiated	2.2	0
Moderately differentiated	4.9	4–5
Poorly differentiated	7.1	6–8

In the screening model created by Benoit *et al.* it was assumed that men with pathologically organ-confined cancer, detected by screening and treated by radical prostatectomy, benefit from screening. The benefit will be a regaining of the years of life that would have been lost from prostate cancer if the cancer had been detected at a later stage by traditional methods when it was no longer curable. It is important to note that this model did not assume that radical prostatectomy cures pathologically organ-confined prostate cancer. Rather, it is assumed that men with pathologically organ-confined prostate cancer treated by radical prostatectomy will have the same life-expectancy as age-matched men without cancer, which has been confirmed by several studies (19–21).

Costs were calculated by adding the costs of screening, diagnosis, treatment, and complications from treatment. By dividing the total costs by the years of life saved, the cost per year of life saved by prostate cancer screening was estimated (Table 33.5). These costs compare favorably to the costs per year of life saved for more established cancer screening programs such as breast, cervical, and colon cancer screening (Table 33.6).

Table 33.5 Cost per year of life saved by prostate cancer screening and treatment as calculated by Benoit *et al.* (8)

Age range (years)	PSA and DRE	PSA alone
50–59	$2339–$3005	
60–69	$3905–$5070	
50–69	$3574–$4627	$3574–$4956

PSA, prostate-specific antigen; DRE, digital rectal exam.

Table 33.6 Cost per year of life saved for various medical interventions

Intervention (ref. no.)	Cost per year of life saved
Smoking cessation counseling (24)	$5429–$15 833
Hypertension control (25)	$32 600
Coronary artery bypass (25)	$62 900
Renal dialysis (26)	$42 000–$80 300
Liver transplantation (25)	$225 000
Screening mammography (25)	$20 000–$50 000
Cervical cancer screening (27)	$33 572
Colon cancer screening (28)	$28 848–$113 348

Accuracy of cost-effectiveness analyses

Society's objective in the expenditure of healthcare resources is to maximize the health benefits for the dollars spent. To facilitate these allocation decisions, the best information available on both the efficacy of medical practices and their costs must be made available to decision-makers to allow valid comparisons among alternative uses of resources. For these comparisons to have any degree of precision, accurate information on the cost and efficacy of medical practices involved must be available. If these studies do not contain this data, society (or the decision-makers society has appointed) cannot make valid comparisons among alternative uses for the available resources.

The costs of prostate cancer screening, diagnosis, and treatment that would result if PSA screening was implemented nationally is unknown. This lack of information is due to several factors. The number of men who would undergo screening, subsequent diagnosis, and treatment is difficult to predict. National cost data for radical prostatectomy or external-beam radiotherapy is not available. Likewise, longitudinal cost data, which would demonstrate the short and long-term costs associated with routine follow-up care and complications resulting from treatment, have not been published.

Less data is available on the efficacy of prostate cancer treatment. The technique of several treatment options for clinically localized prostate cancer (radical prostatectomy, external-beam radiotherapy, cryosurgical ablation of the prostate, and interstitial radiotherapy) has been changing during the last several years. This fact, combined with the long follow-up needed to determine the efficacy of prostate cancer treatment, leaves little solid data on the long-term results of current treatments for clinically localized prostate cancer.

Given the paucity of data regarding the cost and efficacy of prostate cancer screening and treatment, a cost-effective analysis cannot accurately predict the benefit (or lack of benefit) of prostate cancer screening. A cost-effective analysis must limit uncertainties and intangibles to achieve accuracy. The lack of solid data regarding the cost and efficacy of prostate cancer results in these uncertainties dominating any analysis. Several studies have been published that have evaluated the effectiveness and cost-effectiveness of prostate cancer screening and treatment. Despite the inaccuracies inherent in such analyses, these studies have received widespread attention in the medical and lay literature, and have been used to justify the denial of prostate cancer screening.

The particular objective of the cost-effective analyst must also be considered. Patients, physicians, and payers all have an interest in the outcome of these studies. Patients in a third-party payer system are interested only in the benefits of screening and treatment, and are not concerned about the costs involved. Physicians are certainly not disinterested participants in this controversy. Urologic surgeons stand to benefit both financially and in terms of prestige. The perceived ability to cure a very common cancer will also serve to enhance urologists' self-worth. Other specialists also have a stake in this issue, since resources spent on prostate cancer screening and treatment will reduce the dollars available for treatment of other diseases.

The payers of healthcare have an obvious interest in the outcome of these analyses. Their objective is to limit expenditures while maintaining client satisfaction. PSA screening will increase the resources expended to treat prostate cancer because of the lead time and stage migration associated with the early detection of prostate cancer. Additionally, private insurers generally cover their clients until the age of 65, at which time Medicare coverage begins. The lead time associated with PSA screening will result in a substantial proportion of men being diagnosed with prostate cancer prior

to the age of 65 rather than after the age of 65, therefore transferring costs from Medicare to the private insurer. Studies that demonstrate the lack of effectiveness or cost-effectiveness of prostate cancer screening and treatment, allow the payers of healthcare to deny these benefits without resulting in client discontent.

Conclusions

Widespread PSA screening will increase overall healthcare costs. This increase will not result from the detection of clinically insignificant prostate cancer, but rather the stage migration caused by prostate cancer screening. This stage migration will result in a larger percentage of men with prostate cancer undergoing early treatment options, which are more expensive than treatment of late disease. More importantly, early detection of prostate cancer will lead to treatment several years earlier than would have occurred otherwise. Since treatment will then be paid for in current rather than future dollars, the opportunity costs of money will make treatment costs resulting from PSA screening greater than treatment costs resulting from traditional detection.

The critical question is what benefits will be obtained by the expenditure of these additional healthcare dollars. If early treatment of clinically localized cancer has little or no effect on cause-specific survival, the additional healthcare costs will have been spent only to limit eventual treatment of local symptoms in the screened men. If early treatment of prostate cancer can increase survival, the added expense would be more worthwhile. Since there is not adequate data available to address this issue, several approaches have been used to develop models to estimate cost-effectiveness.

Decision-analysis models have been used to evaluate the effectiveness of prostate cancer screening and treatment, and have found little or no benefit. The current review has demonstrated how assumptions used in the models can influence the results. Benoit *et al.* have also constructed a model of the effectiveness and cost-effectiveness of prostate cancer, but in this study only concrete parameters such as cost, published complication rates, and survival data were used. This quantitative analysis demonstrated that prostate cancer screening may well be an effective and cost-effective healthcare intervention, compared to currently accepted medical interventions.

Although men aged 50–70 will potentially benefit the most from PSA screening, this benefit will not be realized until these men are in their seventh and eighth decade of life. Society must decide if the years of life saved in these men warrants the use of its limited healthcare resources. This decision will be easier when randomized, controlled trials are available to quantify the costs and benefits of PSA screening.

References

1. Catalona WJ, Smith DS, Ratliff TL *et al*. Detection of organ confined prostate cancer is increased through prostate-specific antigen-based screening. *JAMA* 1993, **270**, 948–54.

2. Benoit RM, Naslund MJ. Detection of latent prostate cancer from routine screening: comparison with breast cancer screening. *Urology* 1995, **46**, 533–7.

3. Jacobsen SJ, Katusic SK, Bergstrath EJ *et al*. Incidence of prostate cancer diagnosis in the eras before and after serum prostate-specific antigen testing. *JAMA* 1995, **274**, 1445–9.

4. Optenberg SA, Thompson IM. Economics of screening for carcinoma of the prostate. *Urol Clin North Am* 1990, **17**, 719–37.

5. Kramer BS, Brown ML, Prorok PC *et al*. Prostate cancer screening: what we know and what we need to know. *Ann Intern Med* 1993, **119**, 914–23.

6. Mammography and clinical breast exams among women aged 50 years and older Behavioral Risk Factor Surveillance System, 1992. *MMWR* 1993, **42**, 737–46.

7. Richie JP, Catalona WJ, Ahmann F *et al*. Effect of patient age on early detection of prostate cancer with serum prostate-specific antigen and digital rectal examination. *Urology* 1993, **42**, 365–74.

8. Benoit RM, Gronberg H, Naslund MJ. A quantitative analysis of the costs and benefits of prostate cancer screening. *J Urol* 1996, **155**, 564A.

9. Carter HB, Pearson JD, Metter EJ *et al*. Longitudinal evaluation of prostate specific antigen levels in men with and without prostate disease. *JAMA* 1992, **267**, 2215–20.

10. Jones GW, Mettlin C, Murphy GP *et al*. Patterns of care for carcinoma of the prostate gland: results of a national survey of 1984 and 1990. *J Am Coll Surg* 1995, **180**, 545–54.

11. Krahn MD, Mahoney JE, Eckman MH *et al*. Screening for prostate cancer: a decision analytical view. *JAMA* 1994, **272**, 773–80.

12. Chodak GW, Keller P, Schoenberg HW. Assessment of screening for prostate cancer using the digital rectal examination. *J Urol* 1989, **141**, 1136–8.

13. Fleming C, Wasson JH, Albertsen PC *et al*. A decision analysis of alternative treatment strategies for clinically localized prostate cancer. Prostate Patient Outcomes Research Team. *JAMA* 1993, **269**, 2650–8.

14. Johansson JE, Adami HO, Andersson SO *et al*. High 10-year survival rate in patients with early, untreated prostatic cancer. *JAMA* 1992, **167**, 2191–6.

15. Chodak GW, Steinberg GD, Bibbo M *et al*. The role of transrectal aspiration biopsy in the diagnosis of prostatic cancer. *J Urol* 1986, **135**, 299–302.

16. Beck JR, Kattan MW, Miles BJ. A critique of the decision analysis for clinically localized prostate cancer. *J Urol* 1994, **152**, 1894–9.

17. Chodak GW, Thisted RA, Gerber GS *et al*. Results of conservative management of clinically localized prostate cancer. *New Engl J Med* 1994, **330**, 241–8.

18. Rosen MA. Impact of prostate-specific antigen screening on the natural history of prostate cancer. *Urology* 1995, **46**, 757–68.

19. Jewett HJ, Bridge RW, Gray GF *et al*. The palpable nodule of prostatic cancer: results 15 years after radical excision. *JAMA* 1968, **203**, 403–6.

20. Myers RP, Fleming TR. Course of localized adenocarcinoma of the prostate treated by radical prostatectomy. *Prostate* 1983, **4**, 461–72.

21. Paulson DF, Moul JW, Walther PJ. Radical prostatectomy for clinical stage T1-2N0M0: long term results. *J Urol* 1990, **144**, 1180–4.

22. Grönberg H, Damber J-E, Jonnson J *et al*. Patient age as a prognositic factor in prostate cancer. *J Urol* 1994, **152**, 892–5.

23. Albertsen PC, Fryback DG, Storer BE *et al*. Long-term survival among men with conservatively treated localized prostate cancer. *JAMA* 1995, **274**, 626–31.

24. Cummings SR, Rubin SM, Oster G. The cost effectiveness of counseling smokers to quit. *JAMA* 1989, **261**, 75–9.

25. Mushlin AI, Fintor L. Is screening for breast cancer cost-effective? *Cancer* 1992, **69**, 1957–62.

26. Garner TI, Dardis R. Cost-effectiveness analysis of end-stage renal disease treatments. *Med Care* 1987, **255**, 25–34.

27. Fabs MC, Mandelblatt J, Schechter C *et al*. Cost effectiveness of cervical cancer screening for the elderly. *Ann Intern Med* 1992, **117**, 520–7.

28. Byers T, Gorsky R. Estimates of costs and effects of screening for colorectal cancer in the United States. *Cancer* 1992, **70**, 1288–95.

Index

finasteride 23, 39–40
  and cell lines derived from tumors 87
  effect on PSA levels 155, 212
  Prostate Cancer Prevention Trial (PCPT) 441
  vs alpha-blockers 40–2
fine-needle aspiration biopsy (FNAB) 186
fine-needle aspiration (FNA) in PIN 106
fistulae
  recto-urethral 262
  urinary 369–70
flow rate *see* uroflow rate
fluoroquinolines 31, 32
flutamide 278, 280*n*, 285, 303–4, 315–16
  clinical trials 448
  and combined androgen blockade 309
  withdrawal syndrome 316–17
FNA *see* fine-needle aspiration (FNA)
follicle-stimulating hormone (FSH) 22, 24–5
food *see* diet
Food and Drug Administration (FDA) of the United States 39, 43
formalin 369
fractures in systemic disease 154
free fatty alcohols 39
fructose 15
fruit in diet 60
FSH *see* follicle-stimulating hormone (FSH)
Functional Assessment of Cancer Therapy (FACT) 354, 397

G-protein 18
gadopenetate dimeglumine (gadolinium-DTPA) 183–4
Gallup Organization of Princeton (NJ) 35
ganciclovir (GCV) 320
GDEPT *see* gene-directed enzyme prodrug therapy (GDEPT)
gender and cancer 72
gene therapy 94–6, 320–1, 324
  ablative 334–5, 399
  categories 324
  cell-adhesion molecules (CAM) 331–2
  corrective 94–5
    pre-clinical models 330–2
  cytoreductive 332–4, 337
  cytotoxic-reduction in pre-clinical models 95–6
  immunomodulatory 320, 335–7
  new therapies 204
  non-viral vectors 324–6
    cationic liposomes 325–6
    DNA-coated gold particles 325
    naked (plasmid) DNA 320, 325
    polymer–DNA complexes 316

p21 protein 331
p53 331
  retinoblastoma *Rb* 331
  strategies 330–32
  suicide genes 332
  tumor-suppressor genes (TSG) 332
  with vaccines 320–1
  vectors 324–30
  viral vectors 320, 326–30
    adeno-associated 329–30
    adenoviral 328–9
    retroviral 327–8
  see also genes; genetic counseling
gene-directed enzyme prodrug therapy (GDEPT) 332–3
general practitioner (GP) *see* primary care physician (PCP)
genes
  amplification 56
  genetic alterations 138–42
    apoptosis-related genes 139–40
    gain 139
    ploidy 139
  genetics of PCA 434–6
  metastasis-associated 127
  proto-oncogenes 55
  relationship between PIN and prostate cancer 138
  susceptibility 54
  tumor-suppressor (TSG) 55, 141–2, 203, 332
  see also gene therapy; genetic counseling;
genetic counseling 430
  case examples 438
  family history 431–2, 433–4, 436, 438
  genetic testing 436–7
  genetics of PCA 434–6
  patient assessment 430–2
  psychosocial counseling 437
  risk assessment 432–4
    African-American ancestry 433
    age 433
    diet and environmental factors 432
    hereditary PCA 433–4, 435–6
  screening guidelines 437
  support groups/educational resources 437–8
genetics of PCA 434–6
genistein 417
genital prolapse, female 4
genomic action of steroid hormones 12
geography and incidence 374, 407, 409, 418
  see also race
GH *see* growth hormone (GH)
GH receptor (GH-R) 23
Giemsa solution 9
Gleason's grade/score 5, 73, 77, 80, 112
  cell–substrate attachment 125
  and imaging 177
  in improving data reporting 292

loss of cell–cell adhesion 124
  and morphobiology of PCA 126
  prognostic value 128–9, 196
glucose transport 15
glutathione peroxidase 60
glycolysis 14, 15
glycoprotein expression 138
GO cells 16
gonadotropin levels 12
gonadotropin receptors 24
gonadotropinoma 25
goserelin 280*n*, 316
grading 196, 197, 345
  morphobiology of cancer progression 125–6
granulocytic sarcoma 194
granulocytopenia 318
growth factors 9, 11, 22, 57
  epidermal 136
  and gene therapy 320
  and growth factor receptors 140
  growth kinetics 135–7
  paracrine-mediated 87
  peaks 12
  polypeptide 136
  as prognostic/predictive markers 201
growth hormone (GH) 22
  deficiency 24
  receptors 23–4
growth kinetics in genesis and progression of PCA 135–7
guinea pig prostate 84, 85
gynecomastia 40, 376

haloperidol 360, 363, 383
halter monitor findings 39
headache, opioid/post-dural puncture 375
Health Care Financing Administration BESS Data (1998) 37
hematoma, peri-prostatic 164
hematospermia 40, 153, 164
hematuria 36, 153, 368–9
  after TRUS 164
  and carcinoma of bladder 35
  controlled by finasteride 40
heme oxygenase enzyme (HO-1) 16–17
hemorrhage
  during radical prostatectomy 5, 6
  repeated 369
  in thrombo-embolic disease 364
hemostasis 5, 369
  pelvic (in radical prostatectomy) 235
heparin 365, 389
heredity 54, 78, 139, 192
  and gene counseling 433–4
  inheritance patterns 435–6
  see also family history
herpes simplex virus thymidine kinase gene (HSV-tk) 320, 332–3
heterozygosity, loss of (LOH) 55, 138–9